I0044526

# Advances in Molecular Medicine

# Advances in Molecular Medicine

Edited by Jim Remington

hayle
medical

New York

Hayle Medical,
750 Third Avenue, 9th Floor,
New York, NY 10017, USA

Visit us on the World Wide Web at:
www.haylemedical.com

© Hayle Medical, 2020

This book contains information obtained from authentic and highly regarded sources. Copyright for all individual chapters remain with the respective authors as indicated. All chapters are published with permission under the Creative Commons Attribution License or equivalent. A wide variety of references are listed. Permission and sources are indicated; for detailed attributions, please refer to the permissions page and list of contributors. Reasonable efforts have been made to publish reliable data and information, but the authors, editors and publisher cannot assume any responsibility for the validity of all materials or the consequences of their use.

ISBN: 978-1-63241-856-2

**Trademark Notice:** Registered trademark of products or corporate names are used only for explanation and identification without intent to infringe.

**Cataloging-in-Publication Data**

Advances in molecular medicine / edited by Jim Remington.
    p. cm.
Includes bibliographical references and index.
ISBN 978-1-63241-856-2
1. Medical genetics. 2. Molecular biology. I. Remington, Jim.
RB155 .A28 2020
616.042--dc21

# Table of Contents

**Permissions**

**List of Contributors**

**Index**

# Preface

Molecular medicine is concerned with the study of molecular structures and mechanisms, identification of molecular and genetic errors of disease and the design of molecular interventions for correcting these. Such studies are aided by various physical, biological, bioinformatics, medical and chemical techniques. The molecular medicine perspective lays emphasis on cellular and molecular interventions for the management of disease. In molecular pathology, diseases are studied based on an examination of body fluids, tissues or organs. Various techniques, such as DNA microarray, quantitative polymerase chain reaction, multiplex PCR, in situ hybridization, DNA sequencing, in situ RNA sequencing, etc. are used in molecular pathology. Molecular diagnostics refers to a collection of techniques that analyze biomarkers in the genome and proteome, the genetic code of individuals and how cells express their genes as proteins. These allow the diagnosis and monitoring of diseases, detection of risks and formulation of individual-specific therapies. Molecular diagnostics are widely used in prenatal testing for chromosomal abnormalities, identification of infectious diseases, disease risk management, etc. This book discusses the fundamentals as well as modern approaches of molecular medicine. It consists of contributions made by international experts. The extensive content of this book provides the readers with a thorough understanding of the subject.

After months of intensive research and writing, this book is the end result of all who devoted their time and efforts in the initiation and progress of this book. It will surely be a source of reference in enhancing the required knowledge of the new developments in the area. During the course of developing this book, certain measures such as accuracy, authenticity and research focused analytical studies were given preference in order to produce a comprehensive book in the area of study.

This book would not have been possible without the efforts of the authors and the publisher. I extend my sincere thanks to them. Secondly, I express my gratitude to my family and well-wishers. And most importantly, I thank my students for constantly expressing their willingness and curiosity in enhancing their knowledge in the field, which encourages me to take up further research projects for the advancement of the area.

**Editor**

# IL-6 is associated to IGF-1Ec upregulation and Ec peptide secretion, from prostate tumors

A. Armakolas[1*], A. Dimakakos[1], C. Loukogiannaki[1], N. Armakolas[2], A. Antonopoulos[2], C. Florou[3], P. Tsioli[4], E. Papageorgiou[1], T. P. Alexandrou[4], M. Stathaki[1], D. Spinos[1], D. Pektasides[3], E. Patsouris[4] and M. Koutsilieris[1]

## Abstract

**Background:** Ec peptide (PEc), resulting from the proteolytic cleavage of the IGF-1Ec isoform, is involved in prostate cancer progression and metastasis, whereas in muscle tissue, it is associated with the mobilization of satellite cells prior to repair. Our aim is to determine the physiological conditions associated to the IGF-1Ec upregulation and PEc secretion in prostate tumors, as well as, the effect of tumor PEc on tumor repair.

**Methods:** IGF-1 (mature and isoforms) expression was examined by qRT-PCR, both in prostate cancer cells co-incubated with cells of the immune response (IR) and in tumors. PEc secretion was determined by Multiple Reaction Monitoring.

The effect of PEc, on mesenchymal stem cell (MSC) mobilization and repair, was examined using migration and invasion assays, FISH and immunohistochemistry (IHC). The JAK/STAT signaling pathway leading to the IGF1-Ec expression was examined by western blot analysis. Determination of the expression and localization of IL-6 and IGF-1Ec in prostate tumors was examined by qRT-PCR and by IHC.

**Results:** We documented that IL-6 secreted by IR cells activates the JAK2 and STAT3 pathway through IL-6 receptor in cancer cells, leading to the IGF-1Ec upregulation and PEc secretion, as well as to the IL-6 expression and secretion. The resulting PEc, apart from its oncogenic role, also mobilizes MSCs towards the tumor, thus promoting tumor repair.

**Conclusions:** IL-6 leads to the PEc secretion from prostate cancer cells. Apart from its oncogenic role, PEc is also involved in the mobilization of MSCs resulting in tumor repair.

**Keywords:** Immune response, IGF-1Ec, Il-6, Il-6R, JAK2/STAT3 pathway, MSCs mobilisation

## Background

The IGF-1 gene gives rise to three premature isoforms, all of which, after proteolytic cleavage, result in the mature IGF-1 (IGF-1) that consists of the peptide products of parts of exon 3 and 4. Under normal conditions, the major isoform produced is the IGF-1Ea (peptide products of exons 3, 4 and 6), whereas IGF-1Eb (peptide products of exons 3, 4 and 5) and IGF-1Ec (peptide products of exons 3, 4 and parts of exons 5 and 6) are expressed in almost negligible amounts. The Ec peptide (PEc or MGF) consists of the last 24 aa of the IGF-1Ec (Philippou et al., 2014). The results of the overexpression and silencing of PEc in prostate cancer cell lines in in vitro and in vivo models suggest that PEc is one of the key players in prostate cancer progression and metastasis by activating the ERK 1/2 pathway and therefore inducing cellular proliferation and Epithelial to Mesenchymal Transition (EMT), in prostate cancer cells. PEc seems to act in an autocrine and/or paracrine mode of action, through an unknown receptor. Other than the IGF-1R, Insulin Receptor, or any of the IGF-1/Insulin Receptor hybrids that are involved in the IGF-1 system (Armakolas et al., 2010; Armakolas et al., 2015). Consistent with our laboratory evidence, PEc expression in

* Correspondence: aarmakol@med.uoa.gr
[1]Physiology Laboratory, Medical School, National & Kapodistrian University of Athens, 115 27 Goudi-Athens, Greece
Full list of author information is available at the end of the article

human prostate cancer biopsies was significantly associated to tumor grade and stage (Armakolas et al., 2015; Savvani et al., 2013).

Despite the involvement of PEc in cancer and its lack of expression in normal tissue, the physiological role of PEc, up to now, is closely interwoven with skeletal and cardiac muscle as part of their repair and regeneration process. PEc has been proposed to mobilize the satellite cells (myogenic stem cells) as a response to stimuli such as injury or exercise in the former case and myocardial infarction in the later (Kandalla et al., 2011; Matheny Jr. et al., 2010; Philippou et al., 2009; Stavropoulou et al., 2009; Mavrommatis et al., 2013; Hill et al., 2003; Hill & Goldspink, 2003).

There is, therefore, the possibility that prostate tumor damage may lead to PEc secretion and PEc itself may be associated with the tumor repair process, by inducing human mesenchymal stem cell (HMSC) mobilization, similarly to its effects in skeletal and cardiac muscle. The expression level of the IGF-1Ec isoform in normal prostate is negligible (Dai et al., 2010), as is the case in advanced prostate cancer cell lines when growing in in vitro condition (Armakolas et al., 2010; Armakolas et al., 2015). This indicates that the IGF-1Ec isoform that leads to the production of PEc is expressed only when required.

A previous study where subcutaneous tumors had been generated in SCID mice using PC-3 prostate cancer cells (advanced prostate cancer), resulted in the interesting observation that, 1 week after palpable tumor detection, IGF-1 Ec was moderately expressed (Armakolas et al., 2015).

It is now widely accepted, that human tumors are immunogenic (Blankenstein et al., 2012; Hernandez et al., 2016), therefore the immune response (IR) has an adverse effect on tumor growth. SCID mice do not possess T or B lymphocytes, the cells that are responsible for the adaptive IR but retain their innate immune response mechanism (IIR) intact (Bastide et al., 2002).

Our aim was to determine the in vivo physiological mechanism that leads to the IGF-1Ec upregulation and PEc secretion in prostate tumors. In addition, since PEc is also associated with MSC mobilization and repair in healthy tissue, we also examined the effects of tumor secreted PEc on HMSC mobilization and tumor repair.

## Methods
### Subjects
Human bone marrow was collected from three male healthy donors 32, 37, 29 years old with open femur fractures. Lymphocytes were isolated from whole blood from two 26 and 37 year old healthy males. A written

informed consent (IC) was obtained by all subjects in any case. These IC as well as the entire study had been approved by the Institutional Ethics Committee. Animal studies have been approved by the Ministry of Rural Development and Food, General Directorate of Veterinary and all the experimental procedures conformed to the Declaration of Helsinki.

### Cell cultures
The PC-3 cells, an androgen resistant, p53-negative and Kirsten-Ras (K-Ras) mutated human prostate cancer cell line and the DU-145 human prostate cancer cell lines were obtained from American Type Cell Culture (ATCC, Manassas, VA, USA). Low passage (passage 10–15) PC-3 cells were maintained in Dulbecco's modified Eagle's medium (Cambrex, Walkersville, MD, USA) supplemented with 10% heat-inactivated foetal bovine serum (FBS) (Biochrom, Berlin, Germany) and 100 U/ml penicillin/streptomycin (Cambrex, Walkersville, MD, USA). Low passage DU-145 cells were maintained in Minimum essential media supplemented with FBS and 100 U/ml penicillin/streptomycin (all from GIBCO BRL, Invitrogen Corp, Carlsbad, CA, USA) at 37 °C in a humidified atmosphere of 5% CO2.

Subcutaneous injections in SCID mice.

Male SCID mice (7 weeks old) were obtained from Democretos Laboratory. Mouse handling and experimental procedures were approved by the Hellenic Ministry of Rural Development and Food, General Directorate of Veterinary. Animal handling and experimental procedures were obtained in the Experimental Surgery Laboratory of the Athens Medical School. Implantations were carried out as previously described (Armakolas et al., 2015). Briefly, a suspension of 1 X 107 cells in 200 µl in 1X PBS was injected subcutaneously in each mouse.

### Quantitative real-time PCR (qRT-PCR)
Total RNA was isolated using Trizol (Invitrogen, Carlsbad, CA, USA). Quantitative real-time PCR was performed in the Biorad IQ5 multicolor Real Time PCR detection system, as previously mentioned,). Each reaction was obtained in 25 ml using 12 ml SYBR green Supermix (Bio-Rad Laboratories Hercules, CA, USA), 0.5 mg/ml oligo dTs (Fermentas, Glen Burnie, MD, USA), 2 ml cDNA, and 0.3 mM primers. Each reaction was performed in triplicate and values were normalized to GAPDH. The primers used are summarized in Table 1. The PCR conditions were the same in all cases: 95 °C for 30 s 1 cycle, 94 °C 20 s, 60 °C 30 s 72 °C 30 s for 35 cycles and 72 °C for 5 min. The normalization of qRT-PCR experiments was carried out according to ΔΔct method using as a

**Table 1** Primers used in this study

| Gene | Forward | Reverse |
|---|---|---|
| IGF-1Ec (PEc) | 5'-TATCAGCCCCCATCTACCA-3' | 5'-CTTGCGTTCTTCAAATGTACTTCCT-3' |
| IGF-1Ea | 5'-GTATTGCGCACCCCTCAAG-3' | 5'-CAAATGTACTTCCTTCTGGGTC-3' |
| IGF-1Eb | 5'-GTATTGCGCACCCCTCAAG-3' | 5'-CTACTTCCAATCTCCCTCCTCTG-3' |
| E- cadherin | 5'-TGGAGGAATTCTTGCTTTGC-3' | 5'-CGTACATGTCAGCCAGCTTC-3' |
| Vimentin | 5'-GACAATGCGTCTCTGGCACGTCTT-3' | 5'-TCCTCCGCCTCCTGCAGGTTCTT-3' |
| Mouse MIG-1 | 5'-TGAAGTCCGCTGTTCTTTCC-3' | 5'-GGGTTCCTCGAACTCCACACT-3' |
| Mouse IFNγ | 5'-CTGCGGCCTAGCTCTGAGA-3' | 5'-CAGCCAGAAACAGCCATGAG-3' |
| Human IFNγ | 5'-CTAATTATTCGGTAACTGACTTGA-3' | 5'-ACAGTTCAGCCATCACTTGGA-3' |
| Human NCAM | 5'CATGGAATTAGAGGAGCAGGTCAC-3' | 5'-CAGTGTACTGGATGCTCTTCAGG-3' |
| Mouse NCR1 | 5'-TGGCTCTTACAACGACTATGC-3' | 5'-AGAAGAAGTAGGGTCGGTAGGTG-3' |

reference gene GAPDH and is the unscaled analysis from the software Biorad IQ-5 vs 2.0.

## Lymphocyte isolation

Ficoll-Paque Plus (GE-Healthcare Bio-Sciences, Pittsburgh, PA 15264–3065 USA) was used according to manufacturers instructions. Briefly, one volume of blood in EDTA was mixed with one volume of PBS and was then gently poured on top of the Ficoll-Paque plus and centrifuged at 400 X g for 30 min at 20 °C. The middle lymphocyte layer was then transferred into a clean tube. The obtained cells were incubated in DMEM 10% FBS media. Each sample was analyzed for the presence of lymphocytes with flow cytometry on a FACS Calibur CyFlow ML Partecflow cytometer, using a mouse anti-human APC conjugated CD-45 antibody and a mouse anti-human FITC conjugated CD-3 antibody for T lymphocytes and CD-45 and a mouse anti-human FITC conjugated CD-20 antibody for B lymphocytes detection all from (Abcam, Cambridge, UK). The results obtained were analyzed using the ModFit software (Flowmax3.0 Software (1997–2007) Version 3.0 (b4)) (Additional file 1: Figure S1).

## Lymphocyte sensitization

PC-3 and DU-145 prostate cancer cells were treated for 30 min at 37 °C with 20 μg/ml Mitomycin C (Sigma Aldrich, St. Louis, MO, USA. These cells provided the monolayer upon which the Lymphocytes were to be sensitized. Approximately $2 \times 10^7$ lymphocytes were added in 3 ml of DMEM medium to each sensitizing culture flask (Kall et al., 1976).

## Human polymorphonuclear cell isolation

human polymorphonuclear cells were obtained from the blood of healthy donors after the depletion of lymphocytes using a combination gradient composed of equal volumes of Ficoll HistoPaque 1077 and Ficoll Histopaque 1119 (both from Sigma Aldrich, St. Louis, MO,

USA). One volume of blood in EDTA was mixed with one volume of PBS and was then gently poured on top of the Ficoll-Paque plus and centrifuged at 400 X g for 30 min at 20 °C. The polomorphonuclear layer was then transferred into a clean tube. The obtained cells were incubated in DMEM 10% FBS media. Characterisation and counting of the cells was carried out by using a blood analyser (Sysmex XE 5000, Sysmex Sverige, Marios Gata 13, S-434 37 Kungsbacka, Japan) where it was determined that our cells were > 95% polymorphonuclears.

## Co-incubation protocol

Approximately 150–200,000 prostate cancer cells were co-incubated with $0.5 \times 10^6$ cells of the IIR or human lymphocytes for 24 and 48 h standard in vitro killing assay conditions (Hicks et al., 2006).

## Trypan blue exclusion assay

PC-3 and DU-145 cells were plated at a cell density of $12 \times 10^3$ cell/well in 24-well plates and grown with DMEM containing 10% FBS. These cells were co-incubated with cells of the IR. After 24 h and 48 h of seeding cells, the cells of the IR (lymphocytes or polymorphonuclears) were washed away and the cell number of the adhering prostate cancer cells was counted as previously described (Armakolas et al., 2010).

## Western blot analysis

Cell extracts were obtained, by lysis in RIPA buffer (50 mmol/L Tris-HCl, 150 mmol/L NaCl, (Sigma Aldrich, St. Louis, MO, USA) containing 0.55 Nonidet P-40, protease 1 mmol/L phenylmethylsulfonyl fluoride (PMSF) (Sigma Aldrich, St. Louis, MO, USA), 10 μg/mL aprotinin, 10 μg/mL leupeptin; (Sigma Aldrich, St. Louis, MO, USA) and phosphatase inhibitors (1 mmol/L sodium ortovanadate, 1 mmol/L NaF) (Sigma Aldrich, St. Louis, MO, USA) as previously described. Protein concentrations were determined by Bio-Rad Protein Assay (Bio-Rad Laboratories, Hercules, CA, USA). Equal amount of cell lysates (20 µg) were heated at 95 °C for 5 min, electrophoresed on 12% SDS–PAGE under denaturing conditions and transferred onto nitrocellulose membrane (Bio-Rad Laboratories, Hercules, CA, USA). The blots were blocked with TBS-T (20 mmol/L Tris–HCl [pH 7.6], 137 mmol/L NaCl and 0.1% Tween 20) containing 5% nonfat dried milk or 3% Bovine Serum Albumin (BSA) in the case of phospho antibodies, at room temperature for 1 h. The membranes were probed overnight with primary antibodies at 4 °C.

The primary antibodies used were: mouse monoclonal anti-human phospho STAT1–6 antibodies and rabbit polyclonal anti-human antibodies for total STAT1–6 (all at 1/1000 dilution, all from (Santa Cruz Biotecnology, CA, USA), and mouse monoclonal anti–human total JAK1–3 antibodies and rabbit monoclonal anti-human pJAK1–3 antibodies (all were used at 1/1000 dilution, (Abcam, Cambridge, UK) as an internal control we used the GAPDH. Detection was carried out by using an HRP goat anti-rabbit IgG or a goat anti-mouse IgG (both used at 1/2000 dilution, (Santa Cruz Biotecnology, CA, USA) and the Supersignal West Pico Chemiluminescent substrate kit (Thermo Scientific, Waltham, MA, USA).

Multiple reaction monitoring (MRM).

This analysis was performed as a fee for service in the centre de Recherche Protéomique, CHUL, G1V 4G2, Quebec, (Quebec) Canada. Briefly media from prostate cancer cells before and after the co-incubation with cells of the IR were collected and treated with dithiothreitol (DTT) and iodoacetamide and they were then digested overnight with trypsin. The samples were applied on a stage tip before mass spectrometry analysis.

Samples have been solubilised into 50 µL of 0.1% formic acid containing 5 fmol/µL of a standard peptide (ASSILAT). For each sample, 2 µL were injected into a 5500 Qtrap (AbSciex, Framingham, MA, USA). Peptides were eluted over an 18 min acetonitrile gradient and three peptides were monitored: YQPPSTNK and GSTFEER (PEc fragments) and ASSILAT (normalization). For each peptide, at least five transitions were monitored to improve the signal specificity.

## Human mesenchymal stem cell (HMSC) isolation
The whole procedure was carried out as previously described (Soleimani & Nadri, 2009; Armakolas et al., 2016). Briefly the obtained bone marrow was filtered through a 70-mm filtered mesh and the obtained cells were cultured at a density of 25 X 106 cells in DMEM, 20% FBS. The cells were incubated in a standard tissue culture incubator (37 °C and 5% CO2) the media was changed initially at 3 h and then every 8 h for the rest 72 h. The adherent cells were then trypsinised for 2 min

at 25 °C and the obtained cells were examined for E-cadherin (epithelial marker) and Vimentin (mesenchymal marker) expression by immunofluorescence (Additional file 2: Figure S2).

## Immunofluorescence staining
Cultured cells on chamber slides were stained by an indirect immunofluorescence method. Cells were rinsed in PBS and fixed with ice cold 80% methanol for 10 min at room temperature. They were permeabilized with PBS plus 0.5% Triton X-100 (Sigma Aldrich, St. Louis, MO, USA) for 10 min. They were then incubated with primary antibodies overnight at 4 °C: rabbit anti-E-cadherin (1:100) (Abcam, Cambridge, UK) or mouse anti-Vimentin (1:100) (Abcam, Cambridge, UK) in PBS. After 3 washes with PBS, 5 min at room temperature, cells were incubated for 30 min with goat anti-rabbit IgG conjugated to the fluorescent Alexa 488 dye (1:2000) (Abcam, Cambridge, UK) or with goat anti-mouse IgG conjugated to the fluorescent Alexa 555 dye (1:2000) (Abcam, Cambridge, UK) in PBS. After 3 washes, samples were stained with DAPI (1 µg/ml) for viewing with microscope (Olympus BX40, Tokyo, Japan) (Armakolas et al., 2015).

## Migration/invasion assay
The effect of the secreted Ec peptide on HMSC migration and invasion was analyzed using Cultrex cell invasion assay (Trevigen, Gaithersburg, MD, USA) according to the manufacturer's instructions. Briefly, for the invasion assay, the membrane in the upper chamber of 96-well plate was coated with 0.5 × basement membrane matrix/Matrigel. For the migration assay, the membrane was left uncoated. Human Mesenchymal Stem Cells were starved in the serum-free medium for 8 h prior to the assay, then seeded at the upper chamber at a density 5 × 104/well. Media from PC3, DU-145 and PC-3 PEcKD cells under the effect of the IR (48 h) was introduced at the bottom chamber. After 16 h, the cells on the lower surface were dissociated and counted using an inverted microscope prior to quantify the relative cell migration/invasion.

Fluorescence IN SITU Hybridisation (FISH) in Paraffin-Embedded Tissues Sections.

FISH was carried out according to the manufacturers instructions (Cambio Ltd., The Irwin Centre, Scotland Road, Dry Drayton, Cambridge, UK). Briefly slides were deparafinized in xylem and dehydrated in a sequential series of ethanol baths (100%, 96%, 80%, 70%). They were incubated in Pepsin solution (ZytoVision GmbH Fischkai 1D-27572 Bremerhaven, Germany) Quench the pepsin in Glycine solution. Post-fix in paraformaldehyde solution for 2 min. and apply 10 µl paint mix to the centre of the slide (Cambio Starfish Pan Centromeric

Chromosome Paint 1697-MF-01, Scotland Road, Dry Drayton, Cambridge, UK). The slides were then denatured at 60 °C for 10 min and hybridised at 37 °C overnight. After washing in formamide and detergent wash solution the slides were incubated with DAPI (Life Technologies, Carlsbad, CA, 92008, USA) for 5 min at room temperature and they were then covered with Fluorescence Mounting Media (DAKO, 2966 Industrial Row Troy, Michigan 48084, USA). Visualization took place using a microscope (Olympus BX40, Tokyo, Japan) and the software used was the Case Data Manager 5.5 (Applied Spectral Imaging, Inc. 5315 Avenida Encinas, Suite 150 Carlsbad, CA 92008, USA).

### IL-6 blocking
IL-6 was blocked with a mouse anti-human IL-6 antibody (1/100), (Thermo Fisher Scientific, Waltham, MA, USA) and IL-6R was blocked with 100 nM Tocilizumab (Acterman, Roche Ltd. 2015 F. Hoffmann-La, Basel, Switcherland) an anti-IL-6 receptor antibody, in two different occasions. Briefly each antibody was added in cell culture just after the incubation of prostate cancer cells with human cells of the innate or adaptive IR or 1 h before the administration of IL-6. Cells were then collected and analyzed for the IGF-1Ec expression, for IL-6 expression and for JAK2 and STAT-3 activation.

### Immunohistochemistry
Formaldehyde-fixed tumors were paraffin wax embedded. Microtome sections of 3 μm were allowed to adhere to glass slides, dried at 37oC overnight, de-waxed in xylene and rehydrated in serial dilutions of ethanol. Antigen retrieval was obtained by heating the slides in a steamer in Envision Flex Retrieval Solution pH 9 (DAKO 50X in ddH2O), (DAKO, Glostrup, Denmark) covered with aluminum foil for 30 min. Serial sections of the tumors were then incubated with either anti-human IL-6 (1/20 in PBS) (Santa Cruz Biotecnology, CA, USA) or the polyclonal rabbit anti-PEc antibodies (1/5000 in PBS) or the rat anti-mouse CD-45 (1/20) (Thermo Fisher Scientific, Waltham, MA, USA) overnight at 4oC. The samples were then incubated with Biotinylated Link Universal (LSAB+ Kit, DAKO) (DAKO, Glostrup, Denmark) at RT in a humidified chamber for 30 min. Tissue sections were then visualized under light microscopy (Nikon Eclipse 80i; Nikon, Tokyo, Japan), while negative and positive control staining procedures were also included in all immunohistochemical analyses. Samples were photographed using a digital camera (Nikon DS-2 MW; Nikon, Tokyo, Japan). Image analysis was performed in six random fields from each slide using the Image Pro Plus 5.1 software (Media Cybernetics, Bethesda, MD, USA). IGF-1Ec (brown staining) average

intensity levels, measured using arbitrary units on a linear scale from 0 (black) to 255 (white), and the average percentage of the extent of brown staining are combined in the following equation: PEc or IL-6 expression = 255 − average intensity levels of brown staining × average percentage of extent of brown staining. The mean intensity and extent of levels of brown staining for the six representative optical fields was estimated in each case and compared.

### Statistical analysis
Comparisons of IGF-1 isoform expression and mature IGF-1 expression between groups, was obtained and one-way Anova test Samples remained significant after Bonfferoni correction was applied whenever ANOVA test used and each pair of variables was also compared using the 2-tailed equal variance Student's t test whereas the normal distribution was tested with the Kolmogorov-Smirnov (K-S) test (SPSS v. 11 statistical package, SPSS Inc. Headquarters, Chicago, USA). Statistical significance was set at $p$ values less than 0.05, error bars refers to standard deviations (s.d), n = the number of experimental repeats.

### Results
PC-3 and DU-145 cells as well as their tumors respectively, were quantitatively examined for the expression of the IGF-1Ec isoform. It was determined that the tumors arising from both cell lines presented a statistically significant IGF-1Ec elevation compared to the levels of their corresponding cell lines ($p < 0.0001$ in both cases, students t test, $n = 3$) (Fig. 1a). The IGF-1Ec expression levels in the subcutaneous tumors were also examined at different time intervals at 1, 2 and 4 weeks after palpable detection (n = 3 tumors per different time interval). IGF-1Ec expression was significantly increased as tumors progressed for both PC-3 and DU145 tumors (week 2 vs week 4 $p = 0.005$ and $p = 0.0046$ respectively, week 1 vs week 4 $p = 0,00038$ and $p = 0,00033$ respectively one-way Anova test, $n = 3$) (Fig. 1b). The activation of the IIR generated by the prostate cancer establishment in vivo was examined by assessing the expression of mouse MIG-1, an angiostatic cytokine induced by IFNγ, that can be secreted by the natural killer cells of SCID mice and plays physiologically important roles in promoting innate and adaptive IR (Haabeth et al., 2011). MIG-1 was elevated in white blood cells isolated from blood extracted from SCID mice after the establishment of subcutaneous tumors (Additional file 3: Figure S3 A) indicating a tumor associated activation of the IR. The attack of the SCID mice IR on prostate tumors was determined by IHC. An increased amount of mouse CD-45 (pan-leucocyte marker) positive cells, was observed to co-localize to the tumors (periphery

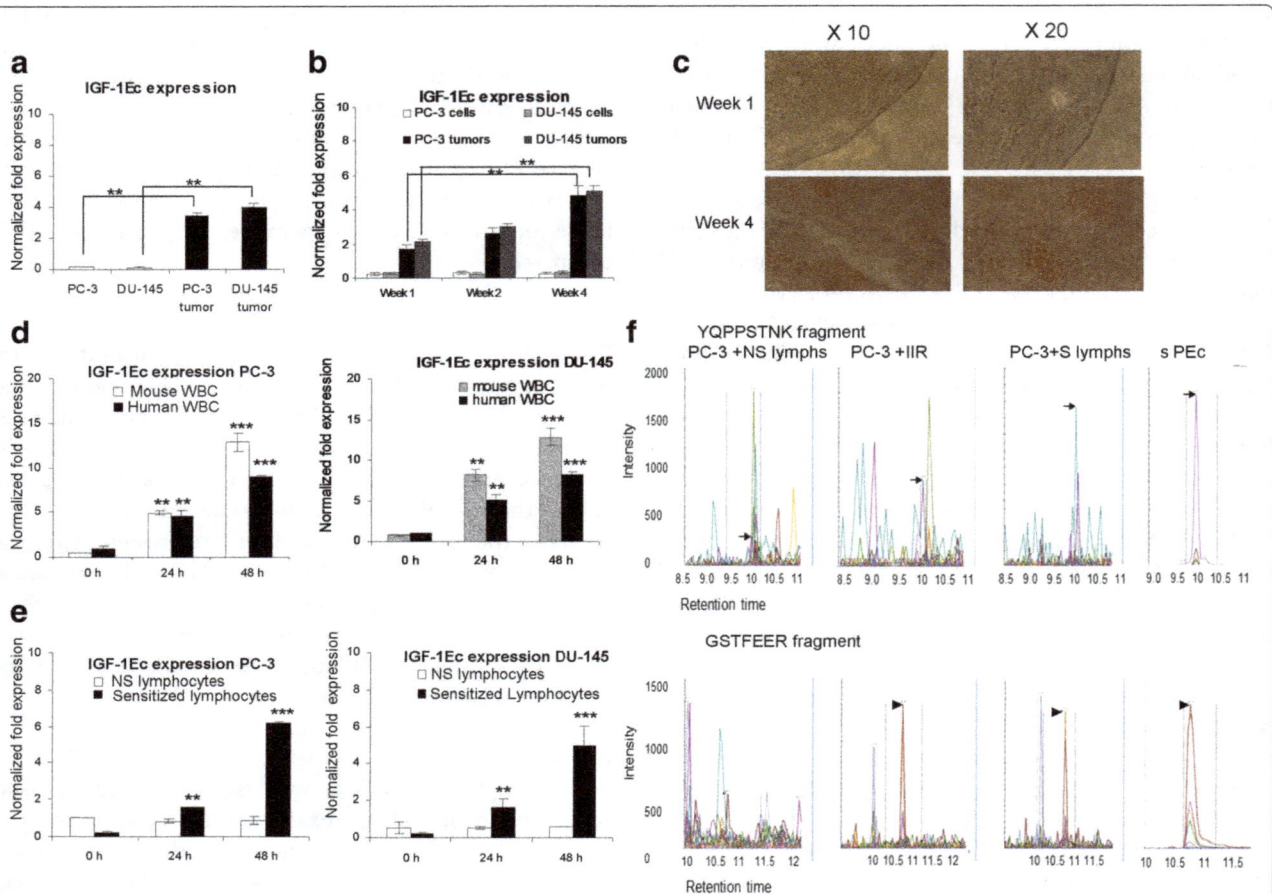

**Fig. 1** PEc expression is induced in prostate cancer cells as a response to the immune system attack. **a**: Analysis of IGF-Ec expression in PC-3 and DU-145 cell lines and their corresponding tumors in SCID mice, by qRT-PCR. The PC-3 and the DU-145 tumors produced significantly higher IGF-1Ec expression when compared to their corresponding cell lines. **b**: Analysis of IGF-1Ec expression in PC-3 and DU-145 tumors (qRT-PCR) at different time intervals. In both cases IGF-1Ec expression is increased as tumor progresses. **c**: Detection of mouse CD-45 positive cells in human tumors extracted from SCID mice (IHC). A significant increase of CD-45 cells was observed as tumor progresses. **d**: Effect of the mouse and human cells of the IIR in the IGF-1Ec expression levels in PC-3 and DU-145 cells. In both cases human and mouse IR seems to be associated with significant IGF-1Ec upregulation in prostate cancer cells at 24 and 48 h. **e**: Co-incubation of PC-3and DU-145 cells with human sensitized lymphocytes indicated a significant increase of the IGF-1Ec expression at 48 h compared to the prostate cancer cells treated with non-sensitized lymphocytes. **f**: Multiple Reaction Monitoring (MRM) analysis of protein in the media obtained from co-cultures of PC-3 cells with human lymphocytes or with cells of the IIR. Both PEc specific digest products (**YQPPSTNK** and **GSTFEER**), were detected into the media of PC-3 cells after co incubation with either the human cells of the IIR (sample 2) or with sensitized lymphocytes (sample 3) (**: $p < 0.005$, ***:$p < 0.0005$)

and inside), that increased as the tumors progressed (Fig. 1c).

### In vitro innate immune response (IIR) activation by prostate cancer cells

Blood was extracted from SCID mice and after red cell lysis the rest of the cells (neutrophils, eosinophils, basophils and macrophages), were incubated with PC-3 or DU-145 cells for 0, 6 and 12 h. Mouse MIG-1 levels were significantly induced after 6 and 12 h coincubation with prostate cancer cells and SCID mouse blood cells (Additional file 3: Figure S3 B).

### In vitro effect of the immune response (IR) in prostate cancer cells

Cells of the IIR or sensitized lymphocytes were coincubated with either PC-3 or DU-145 cells and cellular viability of the prostate cancer cells was measured at 24 h. It was found that prostate cancer cell numbers were statistically significant decreased ($p < 0.009$ for every case, students t test, $n = 3$, Additional file 3: Figure S3 C), indicating the in vitro activation of the innate and adaptive IR.

### Effect of IIR on IGF-1Ec expression

The effect of the mouse and human IIR was also examined on IGF-1Ec expression. SCID mouse blood cells were incubated with PC-3 and DU145 cells for 0, 12, 24 h. A statistically significant increase in the IGF-1Ec expression was determined at 24 h (Fig. 1d, e). Similar results were obtained after co-culturing freshly isolated human white blood cells with PC-3 and DU-145 cells ($p = 0.0048$ and $p = 0,0034$ respectively, students t test, $n = 3$).

### Adaptive IR

Prior to determining the effect of the human adaptive immune response to cancer produced PEc, freshly isolated human lymphocytes, were sensitised to PC-3 and DU-145 cells and were then co-cultured with PC-3 and DU-145 respectively. The intracellular expression of the IGF-1Ec isoform presented a 6 fold increase after 48 h incubation of PC-3 cells with human sensitized lymphocytes (SL), compared to the PC-3 cells treated with non-sensitized lymphocytes ($p < 0.001$, students t test $n = 3$, triplicate) Similar were the results for DU-145 cells ($p < 0.001$ students t test, $n = 3$, triplicate), (Fig. 1d, e). Determination of the secreted PEc in PC-3 cells was obtained with MRM by examining the extracellular content of the PC-3 cells after incubation with SL for the presence of PEc. It was confirmed that PC-3 cells secreted PEc as a response of the immune system attack (Fig. 1f).

### Effect of the human IR on IGF-1 isoforms

The IGF-1 isoforms expression ratio under the effect of either the human IIR was also examined. It was found that in both prostate cancer cell lines, the expression of the IGF-1Ea isoform was not significantly affected by the innate or adaptive IR (results not shown). Similarly to the IGF-1Ec, IGF-1Eb isoform presented a significant increase at 24 and 48 h compared to the untreated cell lines (in PC-3 cells $p = 0.0001$ and in DU-145 $p = 0,00009$), students t test, $n = 3$) (Additional file 4: Figure S4 A-D). This increase of the two isoforms was not reflected on the mature IGF-1 levels, where no statistically significant increase was observed (results not shown).

### Effect of PEc on the HMSC mobilization

Serum free media obtained from the co-culturing of PC-3 or DU-145 cells with the SL or with cells of the IIR stimulated the migration and invasion of HMSC in an identical fashion to the effect generated by the synthetic PEc peptide alone. This effect was significantly higher compared to the effect obtained by the media from all the controls ($p < 0.0001$ for every case, $n = 5$, triplicate). This effect was reversed when the media was incubated for 1 h at room temperature with a polyclonal anti-PEc antibody ($p < 0.0001$, $n = 5$, triplicate) (Fig. 2 a, b). Similarly media from prostate cancer cells that had silenced the expression of PEc (PC-3 or DU-145 IGF-1Ec KD cells), collected 48 h after exposure to SL or cells of the human IIR, presented a significantly lower effect on

HMSC migration and invasion when compared to the effect caused by the media of PC-3 cells under the same conditions (Student's t test, $p = 0.001$, $p = 0.002$ respectively, $n = 5$. Error bars refers to s.d) (Fig. 2c, d). This evidence suggests that PEc secretion, induced by the effect of activated lymphocytes or by the innate immunity on prostate cancer cell lines, seems to induce HMSC mobilization. In in vivo conditions tumors from SCID mice were collected at different time intervals and examined simultaneously for the presence of mouse CD-45 and for the existence of mouse centromeric sequences. Mouse mesenchymal cells do not express CD-45.

A number of cells localized in the human tumors collected from SCID mice were observed to express mouse CD-45 and present positive signal for the mouse centromeric sequences. In some of those cells DAPI and FITC (representing the mouse centromeric probe) were exactly aligned, probably representing recruited MSC whereas in other cases FITC was only partially aligned with DAPI suggesting fusion of the mouse MSC with the cells of the human tumor (Fig. 2e).

### Defining the pathway that leads to the IGF-1Ec upregulation

The IGF-1 gene possesses multiple binding sites for STAT proteins (Varco-Merth & Rotwein, 2014). STAT proteins are activated (phosphorylated) as a response to interleukin receptor (ILR) activation. Interleukins (ILs) are molecules that are involved in the process of the IR and they are secreted by leucocytes. The activation status of all the STAT and JAK proteins was examined by WB analysis. It was found that STAT3 and JAK2 were phosphorylated in both prostate cancer cell lines as a response to immune attack (Fig. 3a).

The JAK2/STAT3 pathway is most commonly activated by the IL-6 receptor. Recent evidence suggests that both prostate cancer cell lines used in this study also possess IL-6 receptor. Treatment of the cancer cells (PC-3 and DU-145) with IL-6 led to significant IGF-1Ec isoform upregulation in both prostate cancer cell lines ($p = 0.0096$ and $p = 0,001$ respectively, students t test, $n = 5$). Blocking of IL-6 using an anti-human IL-6 monoclonal antibody in prostate cancer cell lines treated with IL-6, inhibited the IGF-1Ec production. Similar were the results when an anti-IL-6 receptor antibody used ($p = 0.001$ and $p = 0,00087$ respectively, students t test, $n = 5$) (Fig. 3b).

The treatment of the PC-3 and DU-145 cells under the influence of IL-6 with either anti-IL-6 or anti-IL-6R led to inhibition of IGF-1Ec expression. Prior to determine if this effect is associated with the JAK2/STAT3, protein extracts from prostate cancer cells under the influence of IL-6 with and without the treatment of anti-IL-6R antibody were examined for the phosphorylation of JAK2 and STAT3. It was found that treatment of the

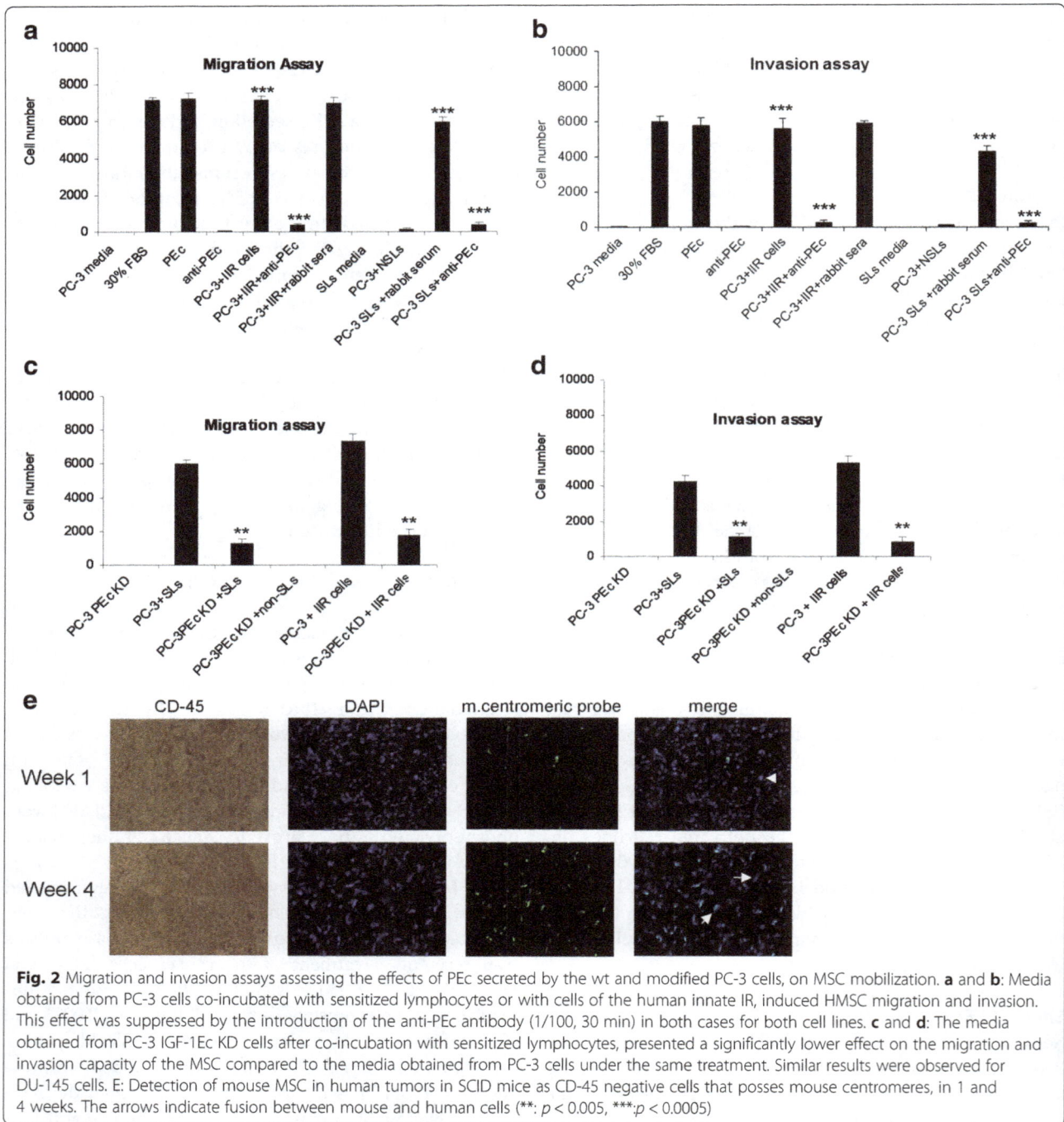

**Fig. 2** Migration and invasion assays assessing the effects of PEc secreted by the wt and modified PC-3 cells, on MSC mobilization. **a** and **b**: Media obtained from PC-3 cells co-incubated with sensitized lymphocytes or with cells of the human innate IR, induced HMSC migration and invasion. This effect was suppressed by the introduction of the anti-PEc antibody (1/100, 30 min) in both cases for both cell lines. **c** and **d**: The media obtained from PC-3 IGF-1Ec KD cells after co-incubation with sensitized lymphocytes, presented a significantly lower effect on the migration and invasion capacity of the MSC compared to the media obtained from PC-3 cells under the same treatment. Similar results were observed for DU-145 cells. E: Detection of mouse MSC in human tumors in SCID mice as CD-45 negative cells that posses mouse centromeres, in 1 and 4 weeks. The arrows indicate fusion between mouse and human cells (**: $p < 0.005$, ***:$p < 0.0005$)

prostate cancer cell lines with the IL-6 lead to the activation of the JAK2/STAT3 pathway and this activation was abolished when these cells were treated with each of the aforementioned antibody (Fig. 3c).

Prostate cancer cell lines under the influence of the IR (innate or adaptive) presented a significant increase of IGF-1Ec upregulation (similar to the one observed after IL-6 treatment) ($p < 0.001$, students t test, $n = 3$) which was abolished when these cells were treated with anti-

IL-6R antibody (Fig. 3d). Furthermore the co-cultures of prostate cancer cell lines with either the cells of the innate or adaptive IR was associated with JAK2/STA3 pathway activation. This effect was abolished when these cells were treated with the anti-IL-6R antibody (Fig. 3e).

Evidence obtained from prostate cancer biopsies suggests that human prostate tumors express IL-6 in many instances (Kall et al., 1976). Due to the fact that mouse IL-6, secreted by mouse macrophages and natural killer

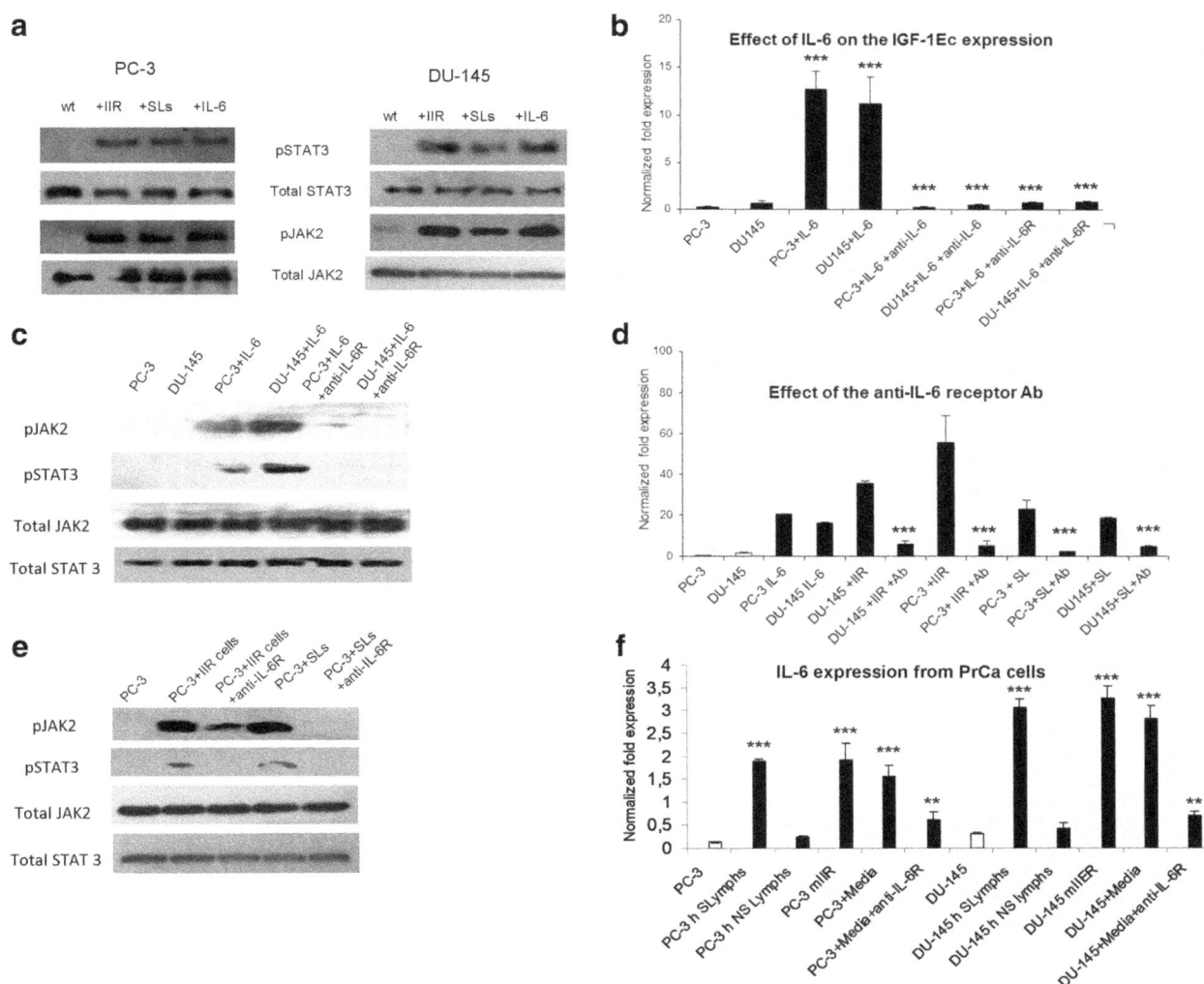

**Fig. 3** Determination of the effect of IL-6 on the IGF-1Ec expression. **a**: Co-incubation of prostate cancer cell lines with the cells of the innate or adaptive immune system (IIR: innate immune response, SL: sensitized lymphocytes) led to JAK2/STAT3 pathway activation as assessed by western blot analysis. **b**: The exogenous administration of 50 nM of IL-6 for 1 h in both prostate cancer cell lines was associated with a significant increase of IGF-1Ec expression in both cell lines (qRT-PCR). This effect was abolished with the addition of anti-IL-6 or anti-IL-6R antibodies. **c**: Treatment of PC-3 and DU-145 cells with IL-6 led to the induction of JAK2 and STAT3 phosphorylation as assessed by western blot analysis. This effect was reversed when these cell lines were treated with the anti-IL-6R antibody. **d**: In both cell lines the IGF-1Ec upregulation resulted after their exposure to the IR cells (innate or adaptive) was reversed when treated with anti-IL-6R antibody (qRT-PCR). **e**: Effect of the anti-IL-6R antibody on the JAK2 and STAT3 phosphorylation induced by the immune system attack (innate or adaptive) on PC-3 cells (western blot analysis). Antibody treatment led to a significant reduction in the phosporylation status of JAK2 and STAT3. Similar results were observed for the DU-145 cells. F: Both prostate cancer cell lines under the attack of the IR (innate or adaptive) were found to express significant amounts of IL-6 (qRT-PCR) compared to the controls. Conditioned media collected from the co-culturing experiments had the same effect on IL-6 expression when introduced in wt prostate cancer cell lines. The IL-6 upregulation was reversed when the cells were treated with the anti IL-6R antibody (**: $p < 0.005$, ***: $p < 0.0005$)

cells, is not able to activate the human IL-6R we examined the IL-6 expression in human prostate cancer cells after co-incubation with mouse IIR cells. Both prostate cancer cell lines (PC-3 and DU-145) were examined for IL-6 secretion as a response to immune attack (innate and adaptive) it was found that both cell lines produced significant IL-6 amounts as a response to immune attack after

48 h as assessed by qRT-PCR ($p = 0.0046$ and $p = 0,0039$ respectively students t test, $n = 3$) (Fig. 3f). In order to determine the mechanism that IL-6 secretion is induced from prostate cancer cells (cell to cell activation or IL-6 secreted from activated cells of the immune system) media was collected 12 h after the initiation of co-incubations of the cells of the human IIR with prostate cancer cell lines. It was

determined that the media obtained from the co-culturing experiments was able to generate the IL-6 production in prostate cancer cells and this effect was abolished when the anti-IL-6R antibody was introduced into the media (Fig. 3f).

Tumors raised from the inoculation of PC-3 and DU-145 cells in SCID mice were examined for the expression of human IL-6 and PEc at different time intervals. Both cell lines give raise to tumors that expressed IL-6 and PEc and that the expression of both factors co-localises and increases proportionally as the tumors progress (Fig. 4).

## Discussion

Recent evidence supports the oncogenic role of the Ec peptide (PEc) in prostate cancer, where PEc has been associated with the induction of cellular proliferation and metastases (Armakolas et al., 2010; Armakolas et al., 2015). Since, in our previous studies, the PEc was artificially introduced into the cancer cells (exogenously or overexpression models) in this study we examine the

condition(s) that prostate cancer cells may secrete PEc physiologically. It was determined that despite the fact that prostate cancer cell lines in in-vitro conditions do not express IGF-1Ec, tumors in SCID mice arising from the same cells do express IGF-1Ec and the IGF-1Ec levels increased as the tumors progressed. Similar seems to be the case in human prostate cancer biopsies where the IGF-1Ec expression levels are significantly associated with tumor stage (the more advanced the tumor the greater the IGF-1Ec expression) (Savvani et al., 2013).

In muscle, IGF-1Ec expression is induced as a response to cellular damage prior to repair (Kandalla et al., 2011). The fact that human tumors are immunogenic (Garg et al., 2015; Galderisi et al., 2010), led to the hypothesis that the immune environment of the host animal may have attacked the xenograft, causing cell damage, leading to PEc secretion. On this ground the effects of the IR (innate and adaptive), in PC-3 and DU-145 cells were investigated, in respect to the IGF-1Ec isoform expression. It was found that both mouse and human cells of the IIR can lead prostate cancer cells to generate IGF-1Ec and to secrete PEc as was determined

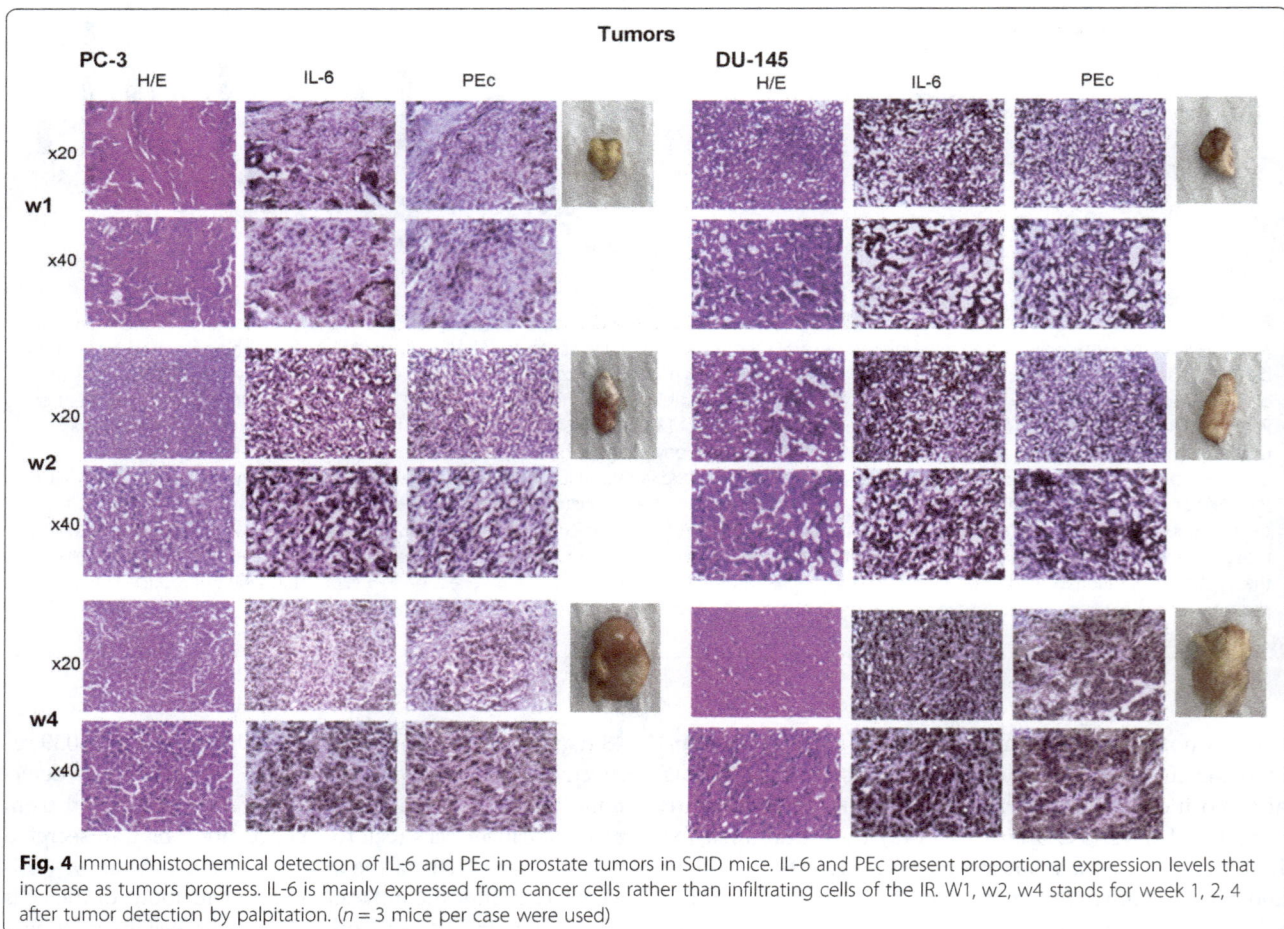

**Fig. 4** Immunohistochemical detection of IL-6 and PEc in prostate tumors in SCID mice. IL-6 and PEc present proportional expression levels that increase as tumors progress. IL-6 is mainly expressed from cancer cells rather than infiltrating cells of the IR. W1, w2, w4 stands for week 1, 2, 4 after tumor detection by palpitation. (n = 3 mice per case were used)

by in vitro co-culturing experiments. In vivo the activation of the IR was examined by monitoring the MIG-1 levels before and after tumor establishment in SCID mice as well as by detecting the mouse CD-45 expressing cells in the tumors. Similar was the case when the prostate cancer cells were co-incubated with human sensitized lymphocytes. Suggesting that the IR that is raised against prostate cancer may lead to the upregulation of IGF-1Ec isoform and to a further extend to PEc secretion.

Previous studies have implicated the action of PEc, in the repair process of the injured muscle via mobilization of satellite/stem cells (Hill et al., 2003). Recent evidence suggests that cancer cell mediated damage by the IR, mobilises Mesenchymal Stem Cells (MSC) to enter tumor prior to generating repair (Galderisi et al., 2010). This process involves chemokines along with other proteins secreted by cancer cells, which attract HMSCs, and increase their migratory activity (Dwyer et al., 2007; Mishra et al., 2008). In the tumor, MSCs may alter the behaviour of the cancer cells and they may differentiate to carcinoma-associated fibroblasts, which are known to be involved in cancer progression (Lin et al., 2008). Thereby, MSC exhibit tissue repair functions and support angiogenesis which simultaneously contributes to promoting the growth of cancer cells

(Karnoub et al., 2007; Mandel et al., 2013). Migration of MSC towards the inflammation site leads to cellular interactions that occur both directly via gap junctions, membrane receptors and nanotubes leading to cell fusion and indirectly via soluble structures and factors (Spaeth et al., 2008).

PEc secreted by prostate cancer cells is capable to mobilize MSC in vitro. In vitro this phenomenon was reversed when the prostate cancer cells under the IR attack were treated with an anti-PEc polyclonal antibody and was abolished when the IGF-1Ec isoform was silenced. In prostate tumors in SCID mice we detected a number of mouse CD-45 negative cells in the tumor and in some instances we also observed fusion of nuclei suggesting repair.

The question raised at this point was how the IR leads to the IGF-1Ec upregulation. Previous studies suggest that the igf-1 gene possesses bSTAT response elements in its structure. Growth Hormone-activated (GH) STAT5B promotes transcription of the IGF-I gene (Fig. 5). STAT1 and STAT3 present a weaker profile of in vitro binding to STAT DNA elements compared to STAT5B in the igf-1 gene, and are less potent inducers of gene transcription (Haque & Sharma, 2006).

The major effectors of the STAT system are cytokines. Cytokine signals are, in general, transient in nature.

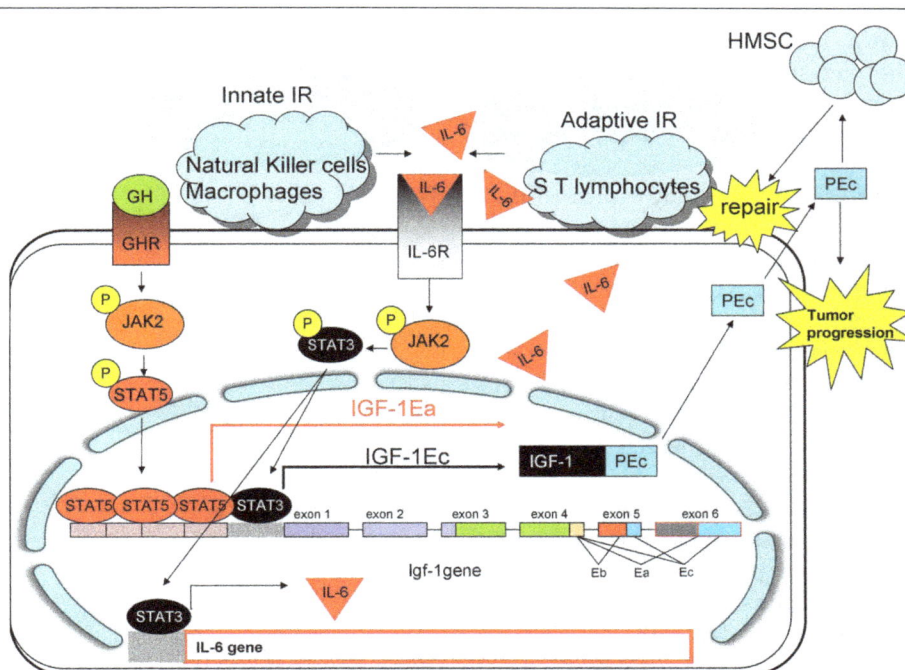

Fig. 5 The effect of the IR on the expression of the IGF-1Ec isoform. GH binding to GHR leads to IGF-1Ea upregulation through JAK2/STA5 pathway. In a similar manner, IL-6 is initially produced by the cells of the immune system attacking prostate tumor.. Binding of IL-6 on IL-6R leads to the upregulation of the IGF-1Ec isoform and to the secretion of PEc as well as to IL-6 secretion from prostate cancer cells, by activating the JAK2/STAT3 pathway. PEc secretion leads to tumor progression and metastases acting in an autocrine and/or paracrine manner and it mobilizes MSC towards the tumor, prior to repair

Therefore, under normal physiological conditions, initiation and attenuation of cytokine signals are tightly controlled via multiple cellular and molecular mechanisms. Aberrant activation of cytokine signalling pathways is, however, found under a variety of patho-physiological conditions including prostate cancer (Haque & Sharma, 2006; Villarino et al., 2015).

Having that in mind, the phosphorylation of the 6 STAT and of 3 JAK proteins that are activated as a response to immune attack was examined. It was determined that the prostate cancer cells treated with the IIR cells or sensitized lymphocytes presented JAK2 and STAT3 phosphorylation. This pathway is activated by IL-6.

Normally IL-6R is expressed only by hepatocytes, neutrophils, monocytes/macrophages and some lymphocytes (Azevedo et al., 2011). Recent evidence suggests that IL-6 may have a crucial role in prostate cancer progression through autocrine on tumor cells or paracrine activity on normal cells in the tumor microenvironment. It has been found that prostate tumor cells produce large amounts of IL-6 and express its receptors, IL-6R (gp80) and gp130, allowing them to respond in an autocrine manner to IL-6 (Mishra et al., 2008; Jones et al., 2001). Both prostate cancer cell lines used in this study possess the IL-6 receptor. Although the exact effects or the mechanisms that IL-6 is involved on prostate cancer cells is not yet known, it has been suggested that IL-6 can modulate the metastatic process as well as the transition from hormone-dependent prostate cancer to castration resistance prostate cancer (Nguyen et al., 2014).

Prostate cancer cells used in this study expressed IL-6 as a response to immune attack that seemed to be associated with the IGF-1Ec upregulation and PEc secretion, through the activation of JAK2/STA3 pathway (Fig. 5). IL-6 expression in cancer cells seems to be initiated by IL-6 produced by the cells of the IR that through IL-6R leads to the production of IGF-1Ec isoform and to the expression of IL-6 through its canonical pathway. The tumor IL-6 is then secreted and generates its positive feedback in an autocrine fashion.

The correlation of IL-6 and PEc is fortified by the fact that both these factors possess similar oncogenic role that is associated with tumor progression and metastases. The fact that the blockade of IL-6 or of the IL-6R lead to PEc downregulation together with the evidence obtained by IHC which indicates that the expression of both of these factors: a) is co-localized in the tumor, b) is proportional and c) it increases as the tumors progress, may be indicative that the oncogenic effect of IL-6 such as the involvement in EMT may be generated through IGF-1Ec isoform and PEc secretion.

## Conclusion

Exogenous IL-6 leads to the production and secretion of IL-6 and PEc from prostate cancer cells and tumors, by activating IL-6R and JAK2/STAT3 pathway. PEc secretion from the tumors, apart from its oncogenic properties, is also associated with the MSC mobilisation and tumor repair. On the other hand IL-6 secretion from the tumor leads to its positive feedback and to the continuous secretion of PEc.

## Additional files

**Additional file 1:** Human Lymphocyte isolation and characterization. Human lymphocytes were isolated from blood and characterized by flow cytometry using the surface markers CD-45 and CD-3 for T lymphocytes (76.75% of the cells) and CD-45 and CD-20 for B lymphocytes (14.18%). Lymphocytes accounted for the 90.93% of the total number of cells isolated. (JPEG 234 kb)

**Additional file 2:** Characterisation of primary human mesenchymal cells. E-cadherin and Vimentin expression as assessed by immunofluorescence staining. The primary isolated human mesenchymal cells expressed Vimentin and they did not express E-cadherin. As a positive control for E-cadherin staining and negative control for Vimentin staining we used the wtPC-3 cells (prostate cancer cells of epithelial origin). (JPEG 184 kb)

**Additional file 3:** Verification of the immune attack on prostate cancer cells. A: Determination of mouse MIG-1 expression using qRT-PCR. Mouse MIG-1 mRNA expression was significantly increased after 6 and 12 hours co-incubation of the cells of the innate immune response (IIR) with wtPC-3 cells as compared to the negative controls ($p < 0.001$ for both time intervals. As a positive control we used SCID mouse white blood cells incubated with IFN γ (20 Units) for 6 hours. (Student's $t$ test, $P < 0.001$, triplicate, error bars refer to s.d ). Lane 1: wtPC-3 cells, 2: SCID mouse white blood cells at 0 hrs and 3: at 6 hours, in tissue culture conditions, 4: MIG-1 expression in SCID mouse blood cells after 6 hours incubation with 20 Units of IFNγ. (Student's $t$ test, $p < 0.01$, triplicate. Error bars refers to s.d). B: Determination of the viable PC-3 or DU-145 cells after co-incubation with cells of the human IIR or with human sensitized lymphocytes (SL), for 48 hours (Trypan blue exclusion assay). Prostate cancer cells presented a significant decrease in every case. (Student's $t$ test, $p < 0.008$, triplicate. Error bars refers to s.d). (NSL: Non-sensitized lymphocytes, IIR: Innate Immune Response, SL: Sensitized Lymphocytes. (JPEG 255 kb)

**Additional file 4:** Effect of the immune response on IGF-1Eb expression. A and B the human innate immune response is associated with significant IGF-1Eb upregulation in prostate cancer cell lines. C, D similar was the case with the human adaptive immune response. E exogenous administration of PEc on prostate cancer cells and PEc overexpression models suggest that IGF-1Eb uprgulation does or does not depend on PEc. (JPEG 157 kb)

**Acknowledgements**
We thank Associate professor Consoulas Chris from Athens Medical School, National and Kapodestrian University of Athens, for the helpful discussions and suggestions. We also thank prof. Perrea Despina for her contribution with the animal house facilities.

**Funding**
Physiology Laboratory, Medical School, National and Kapodestrian University of Athens.

## Authors' contributions

AA: Study design, tumor generation in SCID mice, T cell sensitization, co-culturing experiments, Migration / Invasion assays contribution to the interpretation of the results and to the writing of the paper. DA: Quantitative analysis of the IGF-1 isoforms in the in vitro and in vivo experiments, WB analysis prior to define the pathway leading to the IGF-1Ec generation. LC: qRT-PCR experiments prior to the determination of the effects of the anti IL-6R antibody on IGF-1Ec expression. AN and Ant.A: Isolation and characterization of HMSC. FC: qRT-PCR experiments prior to the determination of the effects of the anti IL-6 antibody on IGF-1Ec expression. TP: IHC, detection of IL-6 and PEc levels in tumors generated in SCID mice, detection of mouse leucocytes in the human tumors, detection of mouse WBC and mouse MSC using mouse centromeric probes in huma tumors in SCID mice (combination of IHC and IF). ATP: Interpretation of all the IHC results. PE: Determination of the effect of anti-IL-6 and anti-IL-6R antibodies on the activation of the JAK-2 STAT3 pathway. SM: Isolation and characterization of human and mouse WBC. SD Help with the qRT-PCR experiments. PD: Contribution to the writing of the paper. PE: Contribution to the writing of the paper. KM: Contribution to the interpretation of the results and to the writing of the paper. All authors read and approved the final manuscript.

## Competing interests

The authors declare that they have no competing interests.

## Author details

[1]Physiology Laboratory, Medical School, National & Kapodistrian University of Athens, 115 27 Goudi-Athens, Greece. [2]Third orthopaedic clinic, KAT General Hospital, 145 61 Kifisia, Attiki, Greece. [3]Oncology Section, Second Department of Internal Medicine, Hippokration Hospital, 115 27 Athens, Greece. [4]Department of Pathology, University of Athens, Medical School, 115 27 Athens, Greece.

## References

Armakolas A, et al. Preferential expression of IGF-1Ec (MGF) transcript in cancerous tissues of human prostate: evidence for a novel and autonomous growth factor activity of MGF E peptide in human prostate cancer cells. Prostate. 2010;70:1233–42.

Armakolas A, et al. Oncogenic role of the Ec peptide of the IGF-1Ec isoform in prostate cancer. Mol Med. 2015;21:167–79.

Armakolas N, Dimakakos A, Armakolas A, Antonopoulos A, Koutsilieris M. Possible role of the Ec peptide of IGF1Ec in cartilage repair. Mol Med Rep. 2016;14:3066–72.

Azevedo A, Cunha V, Teixeira AL, Medeiros R. IL-6/IL-6R as a potential key signaling pathway in prostate cancer development. World J Clin Oncol. 2011;2:384–96.

Bastide C, Bagnis C, Mannoni P, Hassoun J, Bladou F. A nod Scid mouse model to study human prostate cancer. Prostate Cancer Prostatic Dis. 2002;5:311–5.

Blankenstein T, Coulie PG, Gilboa E, Jaffee EM. The determinants of tumour immunogenicity. Nat Rev Cancer. 2012;12:307–13.

Dai Z, Wu F, Yeung EW, Li Y. IGF-IEc expression, regulation and biological function in different tissues. Growth Hormon IGF Res. 2010;20:275–81.

Dwyer RM, et al. Monocyte chemotactic protein-1 secreted by primary breast tumors stimulates migration of mesenchymal stem cells. Clin Cancer Res. 2007;13:5020–7.

Galderisi U, Giordano A, Paggi MG. The bad and the good of mesenchymal stem cells in cancer: boosters of tumor growth and vehicles for targeted delivery of anticancer agents. World J Stem Cells. 2010;2:5–12.

Garg AD, Dudek-Peric AM, Romano E, Agostinis P. Immunogenic cell death. Int J Dev Biol. 2015;59:131–40.

Haabeth OA, et al. Inflammation driven by tumour-specific Th1 cells protects against B-cell cancer. Nat Commun. 2011;2:240.

Haque SJ, Sharma P. Interleukins and STAT signaling. Vitam Horm. 2006;74:165–206.

Hernandez C, Huebener P, Schwabe RF. Damage-associated molecular patterns in cancer: a double-edged sword. Oncogene. 2016;35(46):5931.

Hicks AM, et al. Effector mechanisms of the anti-cancer immune responses of macrophages in SR/CR mice. Cancer immun. 2006;6:1–11.

Hill M, Goldspink G. Expression and splicing of the insulin-like growth factor gene in rodent muscle is associated with muscle satellite (stem) cell activation following local tissue damage. J Physiol. 2003;549:409–18.

Hill M, Wernig A, Goldspink G. Muscle satellite (stem) cell activation during local tissue injury and repair. J Anat. 2003;203:89–99.

Jones SA, Horiuchi S, Topley N, Yamamoto N, Fuller GM. The soluble interleukin 6 receptor: mechanisms of production and implications in disease. FASEB J. 2001;15:43–58.

Kall MA, Hellstrom I, Hellstrom KE. In vitro generation of primary and secondary cytotoxic cell-mediated immune responses to chemically induced mouse sarcomas. Int J Cancer J int Du Cancer. 1976;18:488–97.

Kandalla PK, Goldspink G, Butler-Browne G, Mouly V. Mechano growth factor E peptide (MGF-E), derived from an isoform of IGF-1, activates human muscle progenitor cells and induces an increase in their fusion potential at different ages. Mech Ageing Dev. 2011;132:154–62.

Karnoub AE, et al. Mesenchymal stem cells within tumour stroma promote breast cancer metastasis. Nature. 2007;449:557–63.

Lin SY, et al. The isolation of novel mesenchymal stromal cell chemotactic factors from the conditioned medium of tumor cells. Exp Cell Res. 2008;314:3107–17.

Mandel K, et al. Mesenchymal stem cells directly interact with breast cancer cells and promote tumor cell growth in vitro and in vivo. Stem Cells Dev. 2013;22:3114–27.

Matheny RW Jr, Nindl BC, Adamo ML. Minireview: Mechano-growth factor: a putative product of IGF-I gene expression involved in tissue repair and regeneration. Endocrinology. 2010;151:865–75.

Mavrommatis E, Shioura KM, Los T, Goldspink PH. The E-domain region of mechano-growth factor inhibits cellular apoptosis and preserves cardiac function during myocardial infarction. Mol Cell Biochem. 2013;381:69–83.

Mishra PJ, et al. Carcinoma-associated fibroblast-like differentiation of human mesenchymal stem cells. Cancer Res. 2008;68:4331–9.

Nguyen DP, Li J, Tewari AK. Inflammation and prostate cancer: the role of interleukin 6 (IL-6). BJU Int. 2014;113:986–92.

Philippou A, Maridaki M, Pneumaticos S, Koutsilieris M. The complexity of the IGF1 gene splicing, posttranslational modification and bioactivity. Mol Med. 2014;20:202–14.

Philippou A, et al. Expression of IGF-1 isoforms after exercise-induced muscle damage in humans: characterization of the MGF E peptide actions in vitro. In vivo. 2009;23:567–75.

Savvani A, et al. IGF-IEc expression is associated with advanced clinical and pathological stage of prostate cancer. Anticancer Res. 2013;33:2441–5.

Soleimani M, Nadri S. A protocol for isolation and culture of mesenchymal stem cells from mouse bone marrow. Nat Protoc. 2009;4:102–6.

Spaeth E, Klopp A, Dembinski J, Andreeff M, Marini F. Inflammation and tumor microenvironments: defining the migratory itinerary of mesenchymal stem cells. Gene Ther. 2008;15:730–8.

Stavropoulou A, et al. IGF-1 expression in infarcted myocardium and MGF E peptide actions in rat cardiomyocytes in vitro. Mol Med. 2009;15:127–35.

Varco-Merth B, Rotwein P. Differential effects of STAT proteins on growth hormone-mediated IGF-I gene expression. Am J Physiol Endocrinol Metab. 2014;307:E847–55.

Villarino AV, Kanno Y, Ferdinand JR, O'Shea JJ. Mechanisms of Jak/STAT signaling in immunity and disease. J Immunol. 2015;194:21–7.

# Pharmacological postconditioning with Neuregulin-1 mimics the cardioprotective effects of ischaemic postconditioning via ErbB4-dependent activation of reperfusion injury salvage kinase pathway

# 2

Fuhua Wang[1], Huan Wang[2], Xuejing Liu[2], Haiyi Yu[1], Bo Zuo[1], Zhu Song[1], Ning Wang[1], Wei Huang[2*] and Guisong Wang[1*]

## Abstract

**Background:** The protective effect of Neuregulin-1 (NRG-1) on heart failure is well established. In this study, we assessed whether NRG-1 could protect the heart by mimicking the cardioprotective effects of ischaemic postconditioning (IP).

**Methods:** We used a myocardial reperfusion injury rat model in vivo to compare the cardioprotective effects of NRG-1(3 μg/kg, iv. at the onset of reperfusion) and IP. In Langendorff isolated heart perfusion experiments, we used the erythroblastic leukaemia viral oncogene homolog 4 (ErbB4) inhibitor AG1478, a phosphatidylinositol 3-kinase (PI3K) inhibitor LY294002 and a mitogen-activated protein/extracellular signal regulated kinase (MEK) inhibitor PD98059 to clarify whether the protective effects of NRG-1and IP depend on the NRG-1/ErbB4 signals and the reperfusion injury salvage kinase (RISK) pathway. Infarct size was detected by Evans blue and TTC. Apoptosis was detected by TUNEL assays. The expression of NRG-1/ErbB4 and downstream ERK1/2, AKT, AMPK and p70s6K were detected by western blotting. Hematoxylin/eosin (H&E) staining was used for histological analysis.

**Results:** We found that NRG-1 and IP had similar effects on reducing myocardial infarct size and apoptosis in vivo. NRG-1 heart protein levels were upregulated in the IP group. Phosphorylation of AKT, ERK1/2 and ErbB4 were also increased in both the IP and NRG-1 groups. Furthermore, in Langendorff analyses, the ErbB4 inhibitor AG1478 suppressed the phosphorylation of ErbB4 and the RISK pathway and aggravated myocardial edema and fiber fracture, thereby inhibited the cardioprotective effects in both the IP and NRG-1 groups. For assessment of downstream signals, the PI3K inhibitor LY294002 and the MEK inhibitor PD98059 suppressed the phosphorylation of AKT and ERK1/2 respectively and abolished the cardioprotective effects induced by IP and NRG-1.

(Continued on next page)

* Correspondence: huangwei@bjmu.edu.cn; guisongwang@bjmu.edu.cn
[2]Institute of Cardiovascular Sciences and Key Laboratory of Molecular Cardiovascular Sciences, Ministry of Education, Peking University Health Science Center, 38, XueYuan Road, HaiDian District, Beijing 100191, People's Republic of China
[1]Department of Cardiology, Peking University Third Hospital, Key Laboratory of Cardiovascular Molecular Biology and Regulatory Peptides, Ministry of Health, Key Laboratory of Molecular Cardiovascular Sciences, Ministry of Education. Beijing Key Laboratory of Cardiovascular Receptors Research, 9, HuaYuanBei Road, HaiDian District, Beijing 100191, People's Republic of China

(Continued from previous page)
**Conclusion:** In conclusion, both IP and NRG-1 could reduce infarct size and apoptosis through ErbB4-dependent activation of the RISK pathway in the same model; these results indicated the therapeutic potential of NRG-1 as a pharmacological postconditioning agent against myocardial reperfusion injury.

**Keywords:** Neuregulin-1, Pharmacological postconditioning, Ischaemic postconditioning, Myocardial reperfusion injury, ErbB4

## Background

Acute myocardial infarction (AMI) due to coronary artery occlusion is one of the most common and severe heart diseases in the world (Mozaffarian et al., 2015). Reperfusion of ischaemic myocardium is crucial for salvaging the heart tissue. However, restoration of blood flow could lead to myocardial ischaemia-reperfusion (IR) injury (Ibanez et al., 2015). Ischaemic postconditioning (IP), defined as brief episodes of IR at the onset of reperfusion, is a common strategy to salvage the myocardium suffering from reperfusion injury (Heusch, 2015). The cardioprotective effects of IP rely on activation of the reperfusion injury salvage kinase (RISK) pathway (Hausenloy & Yellon, 2004), which involves phosphatidylinositol 3-kinase/AKT (PI3K/AKT) (Tsang et al., 2004) and extracellular signal-regulated kinase 1/2 (ERK1/2) signalling (Yang et al., 2004). However, IP application is limited to patients with AMI undergoing percutaneous coronary intervention. Therefore, pharmacological approaches that can mimic the cardioprotective effects induced by IP will be more accessible and benefit more patients. Previous studies showed several substances, such as adenosine, bradykinin and opioids, could act as pharmacological postconditioning agents to protect hearts from IR injury. Three major intracellular signal transduction pathways are involved in this protective effects: the eNOS/PKG pathway, the RISK pathway and the survivor activating factor enhancement pathway. However, the cardioprotective effects of these protective factors in clinical settings still remain controversial (Kleinbongard & Heusch, 2015). Therefore, it is still of importance to find more potential cardioprotective factors as pharmacological postconditioning agents.

Neuregulin-1 (NRG-1), a member of the epidermal growth factor (EGF) family (Parodi & Kuhn, 2014), has been shown to play a critical role in the regulation of cardiac development (Odiete et al., 2012) and adult cardiac function (Sawyer & Caggiano, 2011). NRG-1 binds to erythroblastic leukaemia viral oncogene homolog 4(ErbB4), a tyrosine kinase receptor, and induces the conformational changes in ErbB4 that allows dimerization with ErbB2 or ligand-activated ErbB4. These changes provided docking sites for downstream signals that mediates several processes in cardiomyocytes (Odiete et al., 2012). Many studies have shown the potential effects of NRG-1 on heart failure. Administration of NRG-1 improved cardiac function via SERCA2a and cMLCK in a rat heart failure model

(Gu et al., 2010). A phase II clinical trial demonstrated that NRG-1 significantly enhanced cardiac function in patients with chronic heart failure (Gao, 2010). NRG-1 also suppressed apoptosis in injured primary cardiac myocytes through RISK pathway activation (Xu et al., 2014; Jie et al., 2012; Fukazawa, 2003; Liu et al., 2005). In animal experiments, the infarct area induced by IR was increased when NRG-1 was specifically knocked out in the microvascular endothelial cells of mice. This study showed that NRG-1 has an important role against myocardial reperfusion injury in the heart (Hedhli et al., 2011). A recent report demonstrated that exogenous NRG-1 could reduce the infarct size (IS) in a myocardial reperfusion injury in situ model (Ebner et al., 2015). No study to date has detected protective effects of NRG-1 on IR as pharmacological postconditioning agent in a rat model, and comparison of the cardioprotective effects of NRG-1 and IP has not yet performed in the same experimental model. The protective effects of NRG-1 and IP against myocardial reperfusion injury are mediated by the same downstream signalling RISK pathway. Thus, in this study, we compared the protective effects of NRG-1 and IP on IR and also investigated the possible effects of the NRG-1/ErbB signalling pathway on IP. We found that NRG-1 had a similar protective effect in reducing IS compared with IP, and both NRG-1 and IP could reduce apoptosis through ErbB4-dependent activation of the RISK pathway in rat in vivo and the Langendorff model of myocardial reperfusion injury. These findings indicate the therapeutic potential of NRG-1 as a pharmacological postconditioning agent against myocardial reperfusion injury.

## Methods
### Animals
Male adult Sprague-Dawley rats weighing 200–300 g were purchased from the Laboratory Animal Center of Peking University. The Principles of Laboratory Animal Care (NIH publication no. 85–23, revised 1996) were followed, and the experimental protocol was approved by the Animal Care Committee, Peking University Health Science Center.

### Analysis of myocardial reperfusion injury in vivo
*Myocardial reperfusion injury model*
Rats were anaesthetised by sodium pentobarbital (50 mg/kg) through intraperitoneal injection and then ventilated

with a rodent respirator (ALCV9A; Shanghai Alcott Bio-tech Co., Ltd., Shanghai, China) after intubation. A left thoracotomy was performed to open the thorax through the fourth or fifth intercostal space, and the heart was exposed after the ribs were gently distracted. After the pericardium was removed, a 6–0 silk suture was placed under the left anterior descending coronary artery (LAD), and before the suture was tightened, two suture loops were put through the two ends of the suture to reocclude LAD after the ligation. The coronary artery was occluded for 45 min. Ischaemia was confirmed by blanching of the myocardium, dyskinesia of the ischaemic region and ST segment elevation on the ECG. Then, the heart was reper-fused for 24 h by loosening the knot, and this was con-firmed by a marked hyperemic response at reperfusion (Tamareille et al., 2009).

### In vivo experimental protocol

The rats were randomly divided into four groups: (1) CON (control) group, in which the heart was exposed, but the LAD was not occluded; (2) IR (ischaemia reperfusion) group, in which the LAD was occluded for 45 min and re-perfused for 24 h; (3) IP (ischaemic postconditioning) group, in which the LAD was occluded for 45 min, and at the onset of reperfusion, intervention of 6 cycles of 30-s occlusion/30-s reperfusion was performed as the postcon-ditioning treatment, and then the heart was reperfused for 24 h; (4) NRG-1 (IR + NRG-1) group, in which the LAD was occluded for 45 min, and just before reperfusion, re-combinant human NRG-1β2 (3 μg/kg, Prospec, Israel) was intravenously injected via the jugular vein, and the heart was reperfused for 24 h. The dosage of NRG-1 used in this study was chosen based on a previous study (Fang et al., 2010). In the present study, we reperfused the heart for 24 h to observe clear infarct demarcation as shown in previous studies (Liu et al., 2014; King et al., 2014).

### Myocardial reperfusion injury model in Langendorff isolated heart
#### Heart preparation

As previously described (Bell et al., 2011), rats were anaesthetised by sodium pentobarbital (50 mg/kg), and the heart was removed to a Langendorff apparatus and retrogradely perfused through the aorta with the Krebs-Henseleit (K-H) buffer (NaCl 118.5 mM, NaHCO$_3$ 25.0 mM, KCl 4.7 mM, MgSO$_4$ 1.2 mM, KH$_2$PO$_4$ 1.2 mM, glucose 11 mM and CaCl$_2$ 2.5 mM, at pH 7.4 and gassed with 95% O$_2$ and 5% CO$_2$ at 37 °C). With a constant pressure of 70 mmHg, the heart was equili-brated for 20 min.

### Isolated heart experimental protocol

The rats were randomly assigned to six groups: (1) CON (no-intervention) group; (2) IR group, in which the

coronary flow was stopped for 30 min, and then, the heart was reperfused; (3) IP group, in which 6 cycles of 10-s occlusion/10-s reperfusion were performed at the onset of reperfusion, and then the heart was reperfused; (4) IP + AG1478 (an inhibitor of ErbB4) group, in which the same treatment as the IP group was performed, ex-cept 2 μM AG1478 was perfused for 10 min before the reperfusion and lasted for 20 min at the reperfusion period (the dosage of AG1478 was determined according to a previous study (Cai et al., 2016)); (5) NRG-1 group, at the onset of reperfusion, 20 ng/ml NRG-1 was per-fused for 20 min (the dosage of NRG-1 was determined according to a previous study (Ebner et al., 2015)); (6) NRG-1 + AG1478 group, in which the treatment was the same as the NRG-1 group, except 2 μM AG1478 was perfused for 10 min before the reperfu-sion and lasted for 20 min at the reperfusion period. The heart was reperfused for 2 h for TTC staining or 20 min for western blotting.

### Isolated heart experimental protocol-2

The rats were randomly assigned to eight groups: (1) CON (no-intervention) group; (2) IR group, in which the coronary flow was stopped for 30 min, and then, the heart was reperfused; (3) IP group, in which 6 cycles of 10-s occlusion/10-s reperfusion were performed at the onset of reperfusion, and then the heart was reperfused; (4) IP + LY294002 (LY, an inhibitor of PI3K) group, which underwent similar treatment as the IP group, ex-cept 20 μM LY294002 was perfused for 10 min before the reperfusion and lasted for 20 min at the reperfusion period (the dosage of LY294002 was determined accord-ing to a previous study (Tamareille et al., 2009)); (5) IP + PD98059 (PD, an inhibitor of MEK) group, which underwent the same treatment as the IP group, except 20 μM PD98059 was perfused for 10 min before the re-perfusion and lasted for 20 min at the reperfusion period (the dosage of PD98059 was determined according to a previous study (Tamareille et al., 2009)); (6) NRG-1 group, at the onset of reperfusion, 20 ng/ml NRG-1 was perfused for 20 min; (7) NRG-1 + LY294002 group, which underwent the same treatment as the NRG-1 group, except 20 μM LY294002 was perfused for 10 min before the reperfusion and lasted for 20 min at the re-perfusion period; (8) NRG-1 + PD98059 group, which underwent the same treatment as the NRG-1 group, ex-cept 20 μM PD98059 was perfused for 10 min before the reperfusion and lasted for 20 min at the reperfusion period. The heart was reperfused for 2 h for TTC stain-ing or 20 min for western blotting.

### Assessment of IS

The staining was performed as previously described (Xie et al., 2015). At the end of the reperfusion, LAD was ligated again, and the heart was retrogradely infused with Evans blue (Sigma, St. Louis, MO, USA, 0.25% in saline) from the aorta. The non-ischaemic area was stained blue, indicating the area at risk (AR, non-blue region). Then, the heart was frozen at − 20 °C for 30 min and sectioned into 6 slices of 2 mm thickness. The slices were incubated in 1% triphenyltetrazolium chloride (TTC, Sigma, St, Louis, MO, USA) in phosphate buffer (pH 7.4) for 10 min at 37 °C and subsequently soaked in 4% paraformaldehyde for 24 h. TTC staining could differentiate the IS (white region) from the non-infarct AR (red region). In the Langendorff perfusion experiment, rat heart was only stained by TTC without the infusion of Evans blue as described previously (Bell et al., 2011). Non-infarct area of the left ventricle (LV) was stained red. Finally, the slices were arranged from apex to base and digitally photographed. Digital images of the slices were analysed by ImageJ software (NIH, USA) to measure the IS. The final result is expressed as IS/AR% for in vivo results and IS/LV% for Langendorff experiments as previously described (Tamareille et al., 2009).

## Western blotting

At the end of the reperfusion, the LV in the risk area was freeze-clamped in liquid nitrogen before being stored at − 80 °C. Frozen tissue samples were homogenised in RIPA solution, and 80 μg extracted protein was subjected to western blotting. SDS-PAGE and immunoblotting were performed as previously described (Xu et al., 2015). ECL chemiluminescence was used for detection of the bands by an imaging system (molecular imager, ChemiDoc XRS, Bio-Rad, USA), and the densities of the bands were also determined semi-quantitatively using the same system. All protein levels were normalized to that of GAPDH. Primary antibodies used in the experiment were as follows: $^{202}$Thr/$^{204}$Tyr-P-ERK1/2, T-ERK1/2, $^{473}$Ser-P-AKT, T-AKT (pan),$^{389}$Thr-P-p70S6k, p70S6k, $^{172}$Thr-P-AMPK, AMPK (rabbit monoclonal antibodies, Cell Signaling Technology, USA) and caspase 3 antibody (rabbit polyclonal antibody, Cell Signaling Technology, USA); $^{1248}$Tyr-P-ErbB2, ErbB2, $^{1284}$ Tyr-P-ErbB4, T-ErbB4, and NRG-1 (rabbit polyclonal antibodies, Abcam, USA); GAPDH (mouse anti-human monoclonal antibody, Millipore, USA) and appropriate horseradish peroxidase-conjugated secondary antibody (ZSGB-BIO, China).

## Evaluation of apoptosis

Terminal deoxynucleotidyl transferase-mediated dUTP nick end labelling (TUNEL) assays were performed to detect apoptotic cells of the heart tissue sections in the risk area by an in situ cell death detection kit (Roche Applied Science, USA) according to the manufacture's instruction. The nuclei were counted in 10 random fields of an optical microscope (400X, Leica, Germany) for each section, and the results are expressed as a percentage of TUNEL-positive nuclei in the total cell nuclei.

## Histological analysis

After 2 h perfusion, the ischaemic myocardial tissue of the isolated heart was fixed in 4% polyformaldehyde formalin. The paraffin-embedded sections were stained with hematoxylin/eosin (H&E) according to a previous study (Xu et al., 2015). Then the tissue sections were evaluated for histological changes by an optical microscope (400X, Leica, Germany).

## Statistical analysis

All data are presented as the mean ± SEM. Statistical comparisons between the groups were performed using one-way ANOVA followed by Neuman-Keuls post-hoc test or followed by Mann-Whitney test for non-parametric data. The statistical analyses were performed by GraphPad Prism 5.0 (Graph Pad Software, San Diego, CA). A value of $p \leq 0.05$ was considered significant.

## Results

### The equivalent cardioprotective effects of IP and NRG-1 in vivo

After 24 h reperfusion in the IR rat, we compared the cardioprotective effects of IP and NRG-1. The heart slices were stained by Evans blue and TTC, distinguishing the non-ischaemic area (blue region), the area at risk (AR, non-blue region) and IS (white region) (Fig. 1a). The IS/AR% was used to evaluate the damage to the heart as previously described (Xie et al., 2015). Both IP and NRG-1 treatment effectively reduced IS to similar levels compared with the IR group (33.37 ± 2.86% and 36.82 ± 5.04% respectively, vs. 51.87 ± 3.27%, $p < 0.05$; Fig. 1b).

The apoptotic nuclei were stained brown by TUNEL assays. We found that apoptosis increased in the IR group compared to the control group as shown in Fig. 1c-d ($p < 0.001$). The increase of apoptosis induced by myocardial reperfusion injury was suppressed by both IP and NRG-1 treatment (Fig. 1d, $p < 0.01$). Pro-caspase 3 (35 kDa) and its activated fragment cleaved-caspase 3 (17 kDa), as the executor of apoptosis, were assessed by western blotting (Fig. 1e). Cleaved-caspase 3 protein levels were significantly increased in the IR group compared to the control group (Fig. 1f, $p < 0.05$) and decreased in the IP and NRG-1 groups compared with the IR group (Fig. 1f, p < 0.05). Pro-caspase 3 protein levels remained unchanged.

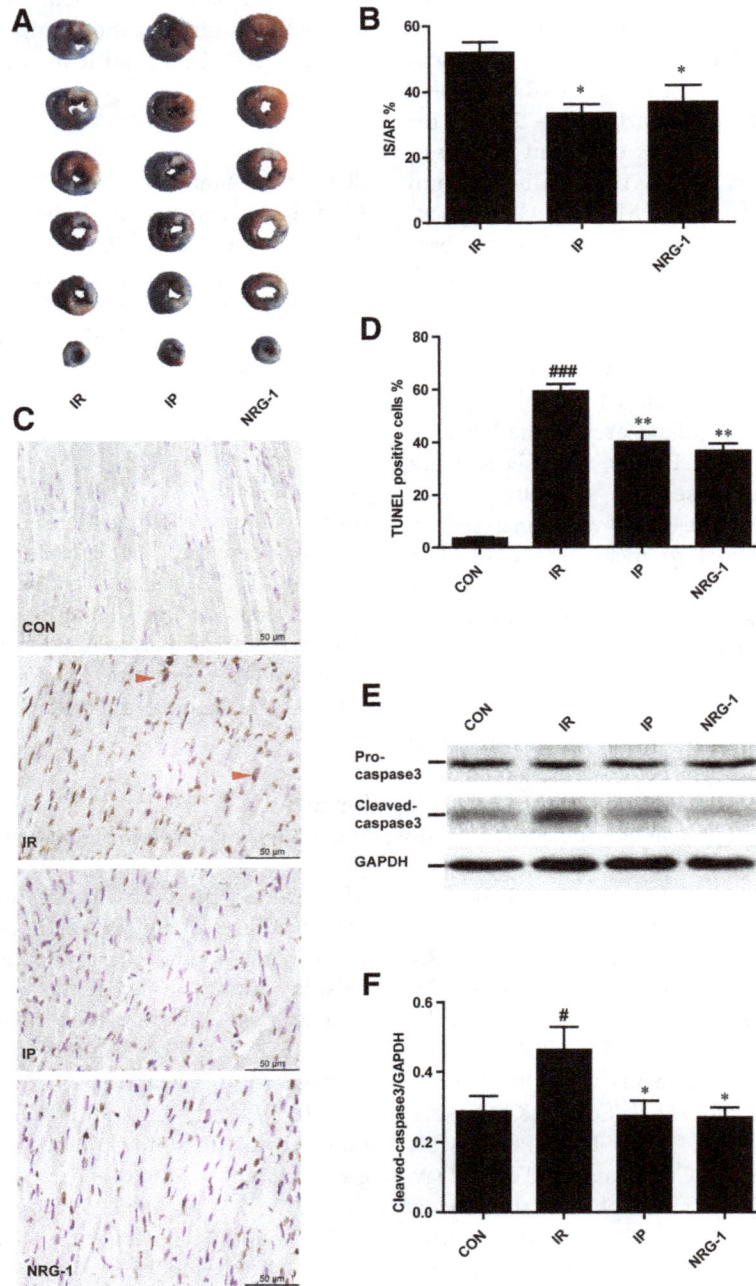

**Fig. 1** Protective effects of both IP and NRG-1 by reducing the IS and apoptosis induced by IR in vivo. (**a**), Representative heart slices stained by Evans blue and TTC. Blue: non-ischaemic area; non-blue: the area at risk (AR); white: infarct size (IS). (**b**), The percentage of infarct size/area at risk (IS/AR%). (**c**), Representative myocardial apoptosis in paraffin sections of the heart at the risk area. The normal cellular nuclei were stained blue by haematoxylin; the apoptotic nuclei were stained brown by TUNEL assay. (**d**), The percentage of TUNEL-positive cells in the total cells. (**e**), Representative protein levels of pro-caspase 3 and cleaved-caspase 3 by western blotting. (**f**), Semi-quantification of cleaved-caspase 3 protein levels normalised to GAPDH. CON: control, IR: ischaemia-reperfusion, IP: ischaemic postconditioning, NRG-1: IR + NRG-1. Data are shown as the mean ± SEM ($n = 6$). #$p < 0.05$, ###$p < 0.001$ vs. CON, *$p < 0.05$, **$p < 0.01$ vs. IR

## Activation of NRG-1/ErbB4 by IP in vivo

To clarify the relationship between IP and NRG-1, we measured the protein expression of NRG-1 (70 kDa), ErbB2 (138 kDa) and ErbB4 (185 kDa) (Fig. 2). After 24 h reperfusion, NRG-1 increased significantly in the IR group compared with control group (Fig. 2b, $p < 0.05$). These results were consistent with a previous study (Fang et al., 2010). A further increase of NRG-1 was

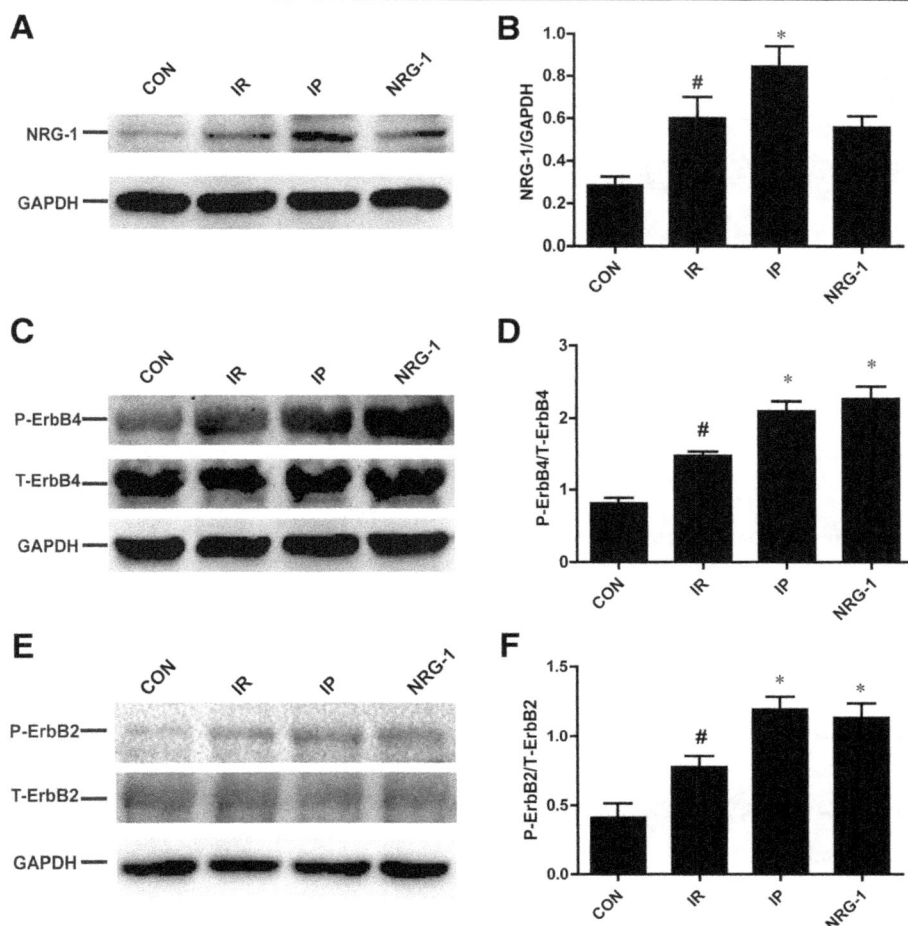

**Fig. 2** Increased NRG-1 and activation of ErbB2/4 by both IP and NRG-1 in vivo. (**a**), Representative protein levels of NRG-1. (**b**), Semi-quantification of protein levels of NRG-1. (**c**), Representative protein levels of P-ErbB4 and T-ErbB4 by western blotting. (**d**), Semi-quantification of the density ratio of P-ErbB4/T-ErbB4. (**e**), Representative protein levels of P-ErbB2 and T-ErbB2. (**f**), Semi-quantification of protein levels of P-ErbB2/T-ErbB2. These protein levels were normalised to GAPDH. CON: control, IR: ischaemia-reperfusion, IP: ischaemic postconditioning, NRG-1: IR + NRG-1. Data are shown as the mean ± SEM ($n = 6$). # $p < 0.05$ vs. CON, *$p < 0.05$ vs. IR

detected in the IP group compared with the IR group (Fig. 2b, $p < 0.05$). ErbB4 is the receptor of NRG-1. Phosphorylation levels of ErbB4 were higher in the IR than in the control group, and the levels were further increased in the NRG-1 group compared to the IR group as expected (Fig. 2d, $p < 0.05$). Interestingly, activation of ErbB4 was also observed in the IP group (Fig. 2d, $p < 0.05$). Total ErbB4 levels remained unchanged in all group. ErbB2 has no direct ligand, but it can be activated by forming a heterodimer with ErbB4 which then triggers the downstream signals. In the NRG-1 and IP group, the phosphorylation of ErbB2 increased significantly compared with the IR group (Fig. 2f, $p < 0.05$).

**Activation of the RISK pathway by IP and NRG-1 in vivo**

The phosphorylation of AKT (60 kDa) and ERK1/2 (44 kDa/42 kDa) was detected by western blotting at the end of 24 h reperfusion as shown in Fig. 4. Following IP or NRG-1 treatment, conspicuous increases in phosphorylation of AKT and ERK1/2 were observed compared with the IR group (Fig. 3b, d). Moreover, there was no significant difference between the IP group and NRG-1 group. The phosphorylation of AMPK (62 kDa) has been showed to play a crucial role in the process of IP. Compared with IR group, the phosphorylation of AMPK was elevated in the IP group, but no significant increase was found with the NRG-1 treatment (Fig. 3e, f).

**The cardioprotective effects of IP were suppressed by the ErbB4 inhibitor ex vivo**

To determine the role of NRG-1 in the IP process, we used the ErbB4 inhibitor AG1478 to block NRG-1 in the Langendorff isolated rat heart perfusion model.

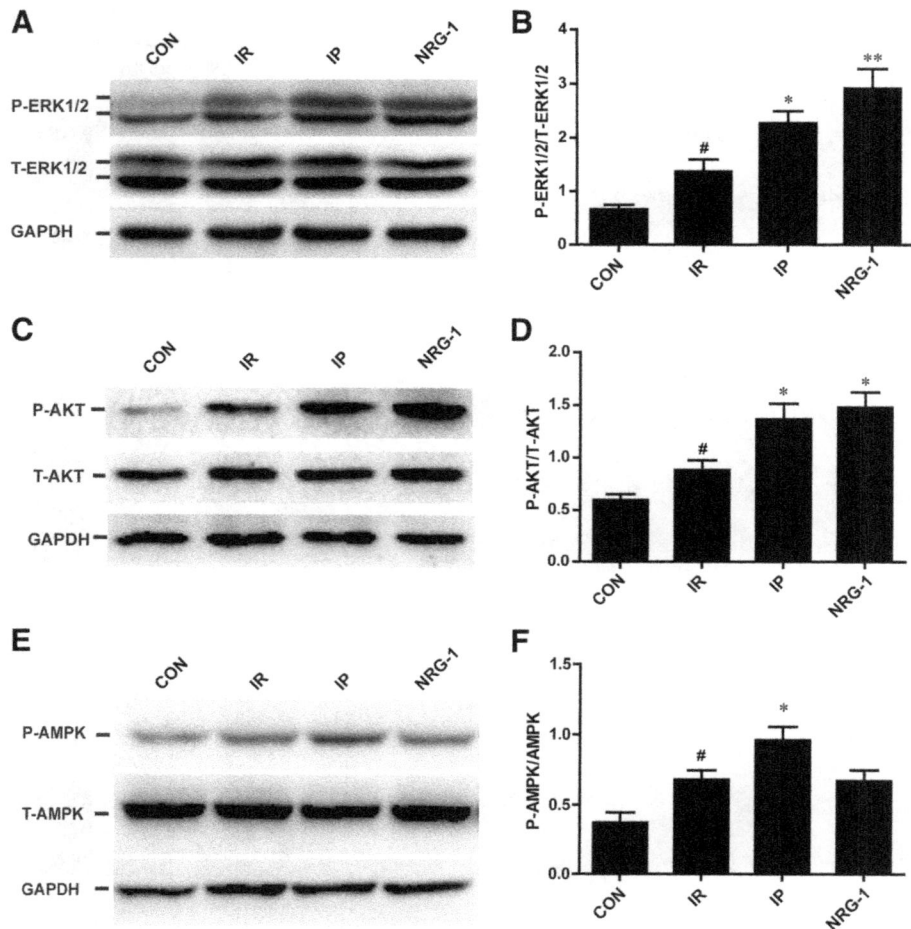

**Fig. 3** Activation of the RISK pathway by IP and NRG-1 in vivo. (**a**), Representative protein levels of P-ERK1/2 and T-ERK1/2 by western blotting. (**b**), Semi-quantification of the density ratio of P-ERK1/2/T-ERK1/2. (**c**), Representative protein levels of P-AKT and T-AKT by western blotting. (**d**), Semi-quantification of the density ratio of P-AKT/T-AKT. (**e**), Representative protein levels of P-AMPK and T-AMPK by western blotting. (**f**), Semi-quantification of the density ratio of P-AMPK/T-AMPK. These protein levels were normalised to GAPDH. CON: control, IR: ischaemia-reperfusion, IP: ischaemic postconditioning, NRG-1: IR + NRG-1. Data are shown as the mean ± SEM (n = 6). #$p < 0.05$ vs. CON; *$p < 0.05$, **$p < 0.01$ vs. IR

After 2 h reperfusion, IS was significantly reduced in the IP and NRG-1 groups compared with the IR group (Fig. 4a, b, $p < 0.05$). The protective effects induced by IP and NRG-1 showed no significant difference. When the ErbB4 inhibitor AG1478 was perfused to the heart, reduction of the IS by IP and NRG-1 treatment was suppressed (Fig. 4b). H&E staining was performed for histological analysis. The myocardial structure in IR group showed irregularly arranged muscle fibers; fracture, degeneration, and necrosis of muscle fibers; severe edema between cells, pyknotic nuclei, and infiltrated inflammatory cells. IP and NRG-1 treatments showed similar effects on reducing the pathological changes of myocytes. AG1478 could suppress the protective effects of IP and NRG-1 on the IR induced pathological changes (Fig. 4c).

## Phosphorylation of ErbB4 and RISK pathway were decreased by the ErbB4 inhibitor ex vivo

To clarify the potential role of ErbB4 in IP, we detected the phosphorylation of ErbB4. The phosphorylation of ErbB4 induced by IP and NRG-1 was significantly suppressed by AG1478 in isolated heart (Fig. 5a). To determine whether ErbB4 plays a role in IP-induced phosphorylation of ERK1/2 and AKT, we reperfused the heart with AG1478 in a Langendorff apparatus. After 20 min reperfusion, the phosphorylation of AKT and ERK1/2 increased substantially after IP and NRG-1 treatment compared with the IR group, consistent with the in vivo study (Fig. 5c-f). Following pretreatment of AG1478, the phosphorylation of ERK1/2 and AKT induced by IP or NRG-1 was reduced considerably compared to the non-AG1478 treated groups (Fig. 5c-f).

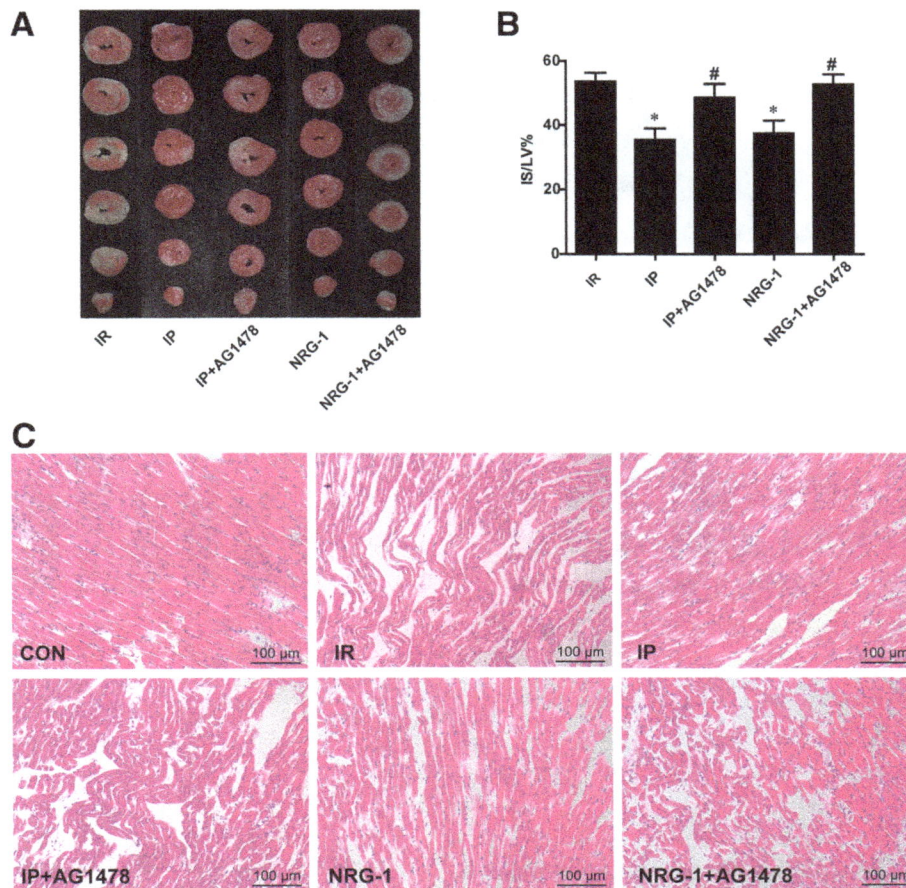

**Fig. 4** Protective effects of IP and NRG-1 were suppressed by the ErbB4 inhibitor AG1478 ex vivo. (**a**), Representative heart slices stained by TTC, red: the ischaemic area, white: infarct area. (**b**), the percentage of infarct size/left ventricle (IS/LV%). (**c**), Histological analysis of heart sections in Langendorff model by hematoxylin and eosin staining. CON: control, IR: ischaemia-reperfusion, IP: ischaemic postconditioning, NRG-1: IR + NRG-1. Data are shown as the mean ± SEM ($n = 6$). *$p < 0.05$ vs. IR; #$p < 0.05$ vs. the same treated group without AG1478

## The cardioprotective effects of IP and NRG-1 were suppressed by PD98059 and LY294002 ex vivo

To determine whether the cardioprotective effects induced by IP and NRG-1depend on RISK pathway activation, we used LY294002 (LY, a PI3K inhibitor) and PD98059 (PD, a MEK inhibitor) to block the phosphorylation of AKT and ERK1/2, respectively, in the Langendorff isolated rat heart perfusion model. After 20 min reperfusion, treatment with LY or PD considerably inhibited the phosphorylation of AKT and ERK1/2 induced by NRG-1 and IP (Fig. 6c-f). In addition to suppression of the RISK pathway, the reduction of IS induced by IP and NRG-1 was reversed by LY and PD (Fig. 6a-b). For downstream signals, we measured the phosphorylation of p70S6K which has been shown to be activated by AKT. P-p70S6K was up regulated in the IP and NRG-1 group than in the IR group. Treatment with LY substantially reduced P-p70S6K induced by IP and NRG-1(Fig. 6g-h).

## Discussion

The present study demonstrated that NRG-1 shows similar cardioprotective effect to those of IP via activation of the NRG-1/ErbB pathway and downstream PI3K-AKT and ERK1/2 signalling, which is termed the RISK pathway. To our knowledge, this is the first study that used a head-to-head comparison of NRG-1 and IP to demonstrate that the NRG-1/ErbB signalling pathway mediates the cardioprotection of IP and the potential use of NRG-1 as a promising agent of pharmacological postconditioning.

The NRG-1/ErbB pathway is considered a compensatory protective mechanism of cardiac injury (Odiete et al., 2012). A recent study indicated that preconditioning with NRG-1 protected the heart from reperfusion injury in an IR rat model (Fang et al., 2010). However, preconditioning with injection of NRG-1 for 20 min before long-term ischaemia is difficult to perform in humans. Pharmacological postconditioning may be an effective

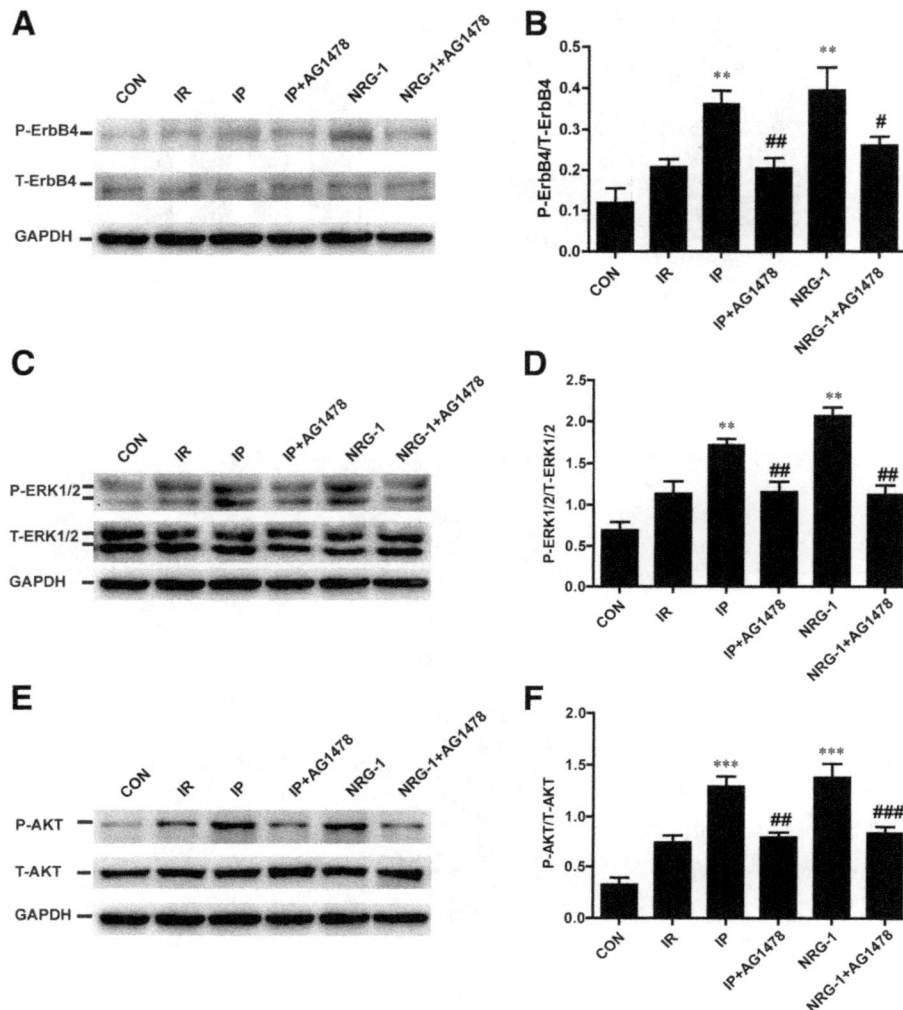

**Fig. 5** The phosphorylation of ErbB4 and the RISK pathway inhibited by AG1478 ex vivo. (**a**), Representative protein levels of P-ErbB4 and T-ErbB4 by western blotting. (**b**), Semi-quantification of the density ratio of P-ErbB4/T-ErbB4. (**c**), Representative protein levels of P-ERK1/2 and T-ERK1/2 by western blotting. (**d**), Semi-quantification of the density ratio of P-ERK1/2/T-ERK1/2. (**e**), Representative protein levels of P-AKT and T-AKT by western blotting. (**f**), Semi-quantification of the density ratio of P-AKT/T-AKT. These protein levels were normalised to GAPDH. CON: control, IR: ischaemia-reperfusion, IP: ischaemic postconditioning, NRG-1: IR + NRG-1. Data are shown as the mean ± SEM ($n = 6$). *$p < 0.05$, **$p < 0.01$, ***$p < 0.001$ vs. IR; #$p < 0.05$, ##$p < 0.01$, ### $p < 0.001$ vs. the same treated group without AG1478

and more applicable therapy. Our study found that postconditioning with injection of NRG-1 simultaneously with reperfusion could reduce IS and apoptosis in the IR rat model in vivo and the Langendorff model. This protective effect of NRG-1 was also confirmed by two studies in mice IR model (Ebner et al., 2015; Ebner et al., 2013). Our results revealed an increase of NRG-1 induced by IR in vivo (Fig. 2), which was described in a previous study indicating the release of NRG-1 from microvascular endothelial cells induced by hypoxia-reoxygenation (Hedhli et al., 2011). Endogenous NRG-1 was insufficient to protect against myocardial reperfusion injury (Fig. 1), but injection of exogenous NRG-1 resulted in increased activation of

downstream signalling pathways compared with that of the IR group (Fig. 3).

The downstream signals of NRG-1 are complicated. After binding with NRG-1, the receptor ErbB4 is phosphorylated by the formation of dimers, and the downstream RISK signalling pathway, including AKT and ERK1/2, is activated. The AKT and ERK1/2 pathway may mediate the effect of NRG-1 signalling on the survival of cardiomyocytes (Odiete et al., 2012). Preconditioning with NRG-1 was found to protect cardiomyocyte from apoptosis by activation of AKT in a rat IR model (Fang et al., 2010). In the present study, we confirmed that postconditioning with NRG-1 could also stimulate the RISK pathway in IR rats in vivo (Fig. 3) and the in

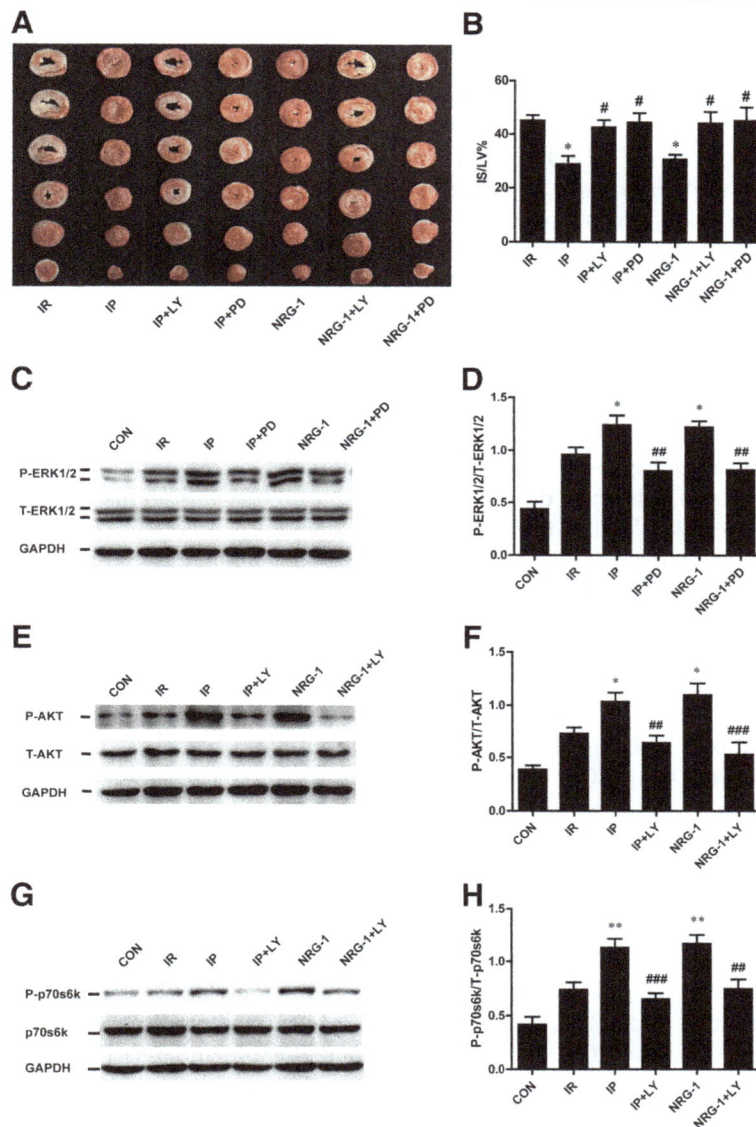

**Fig. 6** Protective effects of IP and NRG-1 abolished by PD980509 and LY294002 ex vivo. (**a**), Representative heart slices stained by TTC, red: the ischaemic area, white: infarct area. (**b**), The percentage of infarct size/left ventricle (IS/LV%). (**c**), Representative protein levels of P-ERK1/2 and T-ERK1/2 by western blotting. (**d**), Semi-quantification of the density ratio of P-ERK1/2/T-ERK1/2. (**e**), Representative protein levels of P-AKT and T-AKT by western blotting. (**f**), Semi-quantification of the density ratio of P-AKT/T-AKT. (**g**), Representative protein levels of P-p70s6k and T-p70s6k by western blotting. (**h**), Semi-quantification of the density ratio of P-p70s6k/T-p70s6k. These protein levels were normalised to GAPDH. CON: control, IR: ischaemia-reperfusion, IP: ischaemic postconditioning, NRG-1: IR + NRG-1, PD: PD98059, LY: LY294002. Data are shown as the mean ± SEM ($n = 6$). *$p < 0.05$, **$p < 0.01$ vs. IR; #$p < 0.05$, ##$p < 0.01$, ###$p < 0.001$ vs. the same treated group without inhibitor

vitro Langendorff model (Fig. 5). and protected cardiomyocytes from apoptosis in vivo (Fig. 1).

Apoptosis plays important roles in myocardial reperfusion injury, and caspase 3 inhibitors could effectively reduce this injury (Hausenloy & Yellon, 2004). IP has been shown to significantly reduce the number of TUNEL-positive cells (Kin et al., 2008) and suppress the activity of caspase 3 (Tian et al., 2011). The anti-apoptotic effects of NRG-1 on cardiomyocytes were identified in many studies and were

assessed on apoptosis induced by $H_2O_2$ (Xu et al., 2014), anthracycline (Fukazawa, 2003) and serum deprivation (Kuramochi et al., 2004). Thus, we explored the anti-apoptotic effect of NRG-1 in an IR rat model. Following treatment with NRG-1, TUNEL-positive cells and cleaved-caspase 3 expression were both reduced significantly compared with those of the IR group, which is similar to the effects of IP. We suggest that NRG-1 might be a promising pharmacological postconditioning agent that significantly suppresses apoptosis induced by IR. The mechanisms of reperfusion injury were complicated, and whether the cardioprotective effect of NRG-1 exclusively relies on the anti-apoptotic effect remains to be evaluated in future studies.

The cardioprotective effect of IP is well established (Heusch, 2015). IP plays an important role in reduction of oxidative stress, inflammation and apoptosis by salvage kinase pathways, including AKT (Tsang et al., 2004), ERK1/2 (Yang et al., 2004), AMPK (Hao et al., 2017), PKC and PKG (Ovize et al., 2010). No activation of AMPK in NRG-1 group suggested AMPK was not involved in the protective effect of NRG-1 (Fig. 3e-f). In this study, we found that NRG-1 and IP had similar anti-apoptotic effects by activation of the RISK pathway in the IR rat model. Increased phosphorylation of ErbB4 was detected in the NRG-1 group compared with the IR group in vivo as expected (Fig. 2). Notably, the activation of ErbB4 was also found in the IP group (Fig. 2). Therefore, we detected the protein levels of NRG-1, the ligand of ErbB4. Our data showed the IP could increase NRG-1 protein expression in the in vivo study. These results suggested that the cardioprotective effect of IP is mediated by the NRG-1/ErbB4 pathway. The shedding of NRG-1, which is regulated by a disintegrin and metalloprotease (ADAM)17/19 (Zhang et al., 2015), may also be a critical part of IP based on a study demonstrating the involvement of ADAM17 in ischaemic preconditioning (Ichikawa et al., 2004). The detailed mechanisms of NRG-1/ErbB4 pathway activation stimulated by postconditioning should be clarified by further investigations.

In the Langendorff experiments, AG1478 could effectively block the activation of NRG-1/ErbB4 pathway after IP treatment, and diminish the activation of the RISK pathway (Fig. 5). These findings suggested that the NRG-1/ErbB4 signalling pathway was involved in IP. AG1478 is not a specific inhibitor of ErbB4, it could also inhibit the activation of EGFR (ErbB1). A previous study showed no activation of EGFR after the incubation of NRG-1 in neonatal rat ventricle myocyte (NRVM) (Fukazawa, 2003). To further clarify the potential role of ErbB4 in IP, we examined the phosphorylation of ErbB4. We found the phosphorylation of ErbB4 was increased by IP and suppressed by AG1478 in isolated heart treated with IP (Fig. 5b). All of these data showed activation of NRG-1/ErbB4 pathway was involved in the protective effects of IP. In isolated cultured cardiomyocytes lacking NRG-1 expression, postconditioning exhibited protective effects against IR injury as well (Sun et al., 2005). NRG-1-independent ErbB4 activation might be involved in protective mechanisms of IP (Forrester et al., 2016). As a mechanical stimulus, IP may be associated with many mechanical and chemical signals. The mechanisms of the NRG-1/ErbB4 signalling pathway activated by IP should be further explored.

To assess the downstream signals, we used LY294002 and PD98059 to block RISK pathway activation and found that the cardioprotective effects induced by NRG-1 and IP were substantially decreased (Fig. 6c-f). Numerous studies have shown that LY can effectively inhibit the effects of NRG-1 and IP by preventing the phosphorylation of AKT, which is consistent with a present study (Tsang et al., 2004; Ebner et al., 2015). p70S6K could be activated by AKT and contributed to the cardioprotective effects (Tsang et al., 2004). Higher level of P-p70S6K was detected in IP and NRG-1 groups than IR group. This result indicated AKT/p70S6K pathway played important role in protective effect of NRG-1 against myocardial reperfusion injury. PD was reported to block the effects of IP by inhibiting the phosphorylation of ERK1/2 (Darling et al., 2005); however, whether PD can block the effects of NRG-1 in a Langendorff model is unknown. In the present study, we found that PD can inhibit the phosphorylation of ERK1/2 induced by NRG-1, which impaired protective effects (Fig. 6c-d).

In this study, we used IR rat models to compare the protective effects of NRG-1 and IP. We know difference between species could lead to different effects of the same drugs (Heusch, 2017). Protective effect of NRG-1 by activation of RISK pathway in patients suffering from myocardial IR injury remained unknown. Whether NRG-1 activated other signalling pathways besides RISK need more investigation. It is difficult to translate the findings in healthy, young animals with acute coronary occlusion/reperfusion to patients of older age, with a variety of co-morbidities and co-medications, suffering from different scenarios of myocardial IR injury. Dosing and timing studies also very important to evaluate the pharmacological effect of NRG-1. Therefore, we need more experiments in different animal models and even larger clinical trials with dosing and timing studies to clarify the protective effect of NRG-1 in patients suffering from myocardial IR injury.

## Conclusion

In conclusion, both NRG-1 and IP have cardioprotective effects by reducing IS and apoptosis through ErbB4-dependent activation of the RISK pathway in a rat myocardial reperfusion injury model. NRG-1 might be a potential pharmacological postconditioning agent for cardioprotection against reperfusion injury.

**Abbreviations**

ADAM: A disintegrin and metalloprotease; AMI: Acute myocardial infarction; AR: the area at risk; CON: Control; EGF: Epidermal growth factor; ErbB4: Erythroblastic leukaemia viral oncogene homolog 4; ERK1/2: Extracellular signal-regulated kinase 1/2; H&E: Hematoxylin/eosin; IP: Ischaemic postconditioning; IR: Ischaemia-reperfusion; IS: Infarct size; K-H: the Krebs-Henseleit; LAD: the left anterior descending coronary artery; LV: the left ventricle; LY: LY294002; MEK: a mitogen-activated protein/extracellular signal regulated kinase; NRG-1: Neuregulin-1; NRVM: Neonatal rat ventricle myocyte; PD: PD98059; PI3K: Phosphatidylinositol 3-kinase; RISK: Reperfusion injury salvage kinase; TTC: Triphenyltetrazolium chloride

## Acknowledgements
We thank the National Natural Science Foundation of the People's Republic of China for supporting the study.

## Funding
This work was supported by the National Natural Science Foundation of the People's Republic of China (81170179, 81070242 and 81470553).

## Authors' contributions
GW, WH conceived and designed the study. FW participated in both the in vivo and in vitro studies and drafted the manuscript. GW, WH and HY helped in drafting the manuscript. HW and XL participated in the in vivo animal studies. BZ, ZS and NW participated in the Langendorff studies. All authors read and approved the final manuscript.

## Competing interests
The authors declare that they have no competing interests.

## References
Bell RM, Mocanu MM, Yellon DM. Retrograde heart perfusion: the Langendorff technique of isolated heart perfusion. J Mol Cell Cardiol. 2011;50:940–50.

Cai MX, et al. Exercise training activates neuregulin 1/ErbB signaling and promotes cardiac repair in a rat myocardial infarction model. Life Sci. 2016;149:1–9.

Darling CE, et al. Postconditioning via stuttering reperfusion limits myocardial infarct size in rabbit hearts: role of ERK1/2. Am J Physiol Heart Circ Physiol. 2005;289:H1618–26.

Ebner B, et al. Uncoupled eNOS annihilates neuregulin-1beta-induced cardioprotection: a novel mechanism in pharmacological postconditioning in myocardial infarction. Mol Cell Biochem. 2013;373:115–23.

Ebner B, et al. In situ postconditioning with neuregulin-1beta is mediated by a PI3K/Akt-dependent pathway. The Canadian journal of cardiology. 2015;31:76–83.

Fang SJ, et al. Neuregulin-1 preconditioning protects the heart against ischemia/reperfusion injury through a PI3K/Akt-dependent mechanism. Chin Med J. 2010;123:3597–604.

Forrester SJ, et al. Epidermal growth factor receptor transactivation: mechanisms, pathophysiology, and potential therapies in the cardiovascular system. Annu Rev Pharmacol Toxicol. 2016;56:627–53.

Fukazawa R. Neuregulin-1 protects ventricular myocytes from anthracycline-induced apoptosis via erbB4-dependent activation of PI3-kinase/Akt. J Mol Cell Cardiol. 2003;35:1473–9.

Gao R, et al. A phase II, randomized, double-blind, multicenter, based on standard therapy, placebo-controlled study of the efficacy and safety of recombinant human neuregulin-1 in patients with chronic heart failure. J Am Coll Cardiol. 2010;55:1907–14.

Gu X, et al. Cardiac functional improvement in rats with myocardial infarction by up-regulating cardiac myosin light chain kinase with neuregulin. Cardiovasc Res. 2010;88:334–43.

Hao M, et al. Myocardial ischemic Postconditioning promotes autophagy against ischemia reperfusion injury via the activation of the nNOS/AMPK/mTOR pathway. Int J Mol Sci. 2017;18

Hausenloy DJ, Yellon DM. New directions for protecting the heart against ischaemia-reperfusion injury: targeting the reperfusion injury salvage kinase (RISK)-pathway. Cardiovasc Res. 2004;61:448–60.

Hedhli N, et al. Endothelium-derived neuregulin protects the heart against ischemic injury. Circulation. 2011;123:2254–62.

Heusch G. Molecular basis of cardioprotection: signal transduction in ischemic pre-, post-, and remote conditioning. Circ Res. 2015;116:674–99.

Heusch G. Critical issues for the translation of Cardioprotection. Circ Res. 2017;120:1477–86.

Ibanez B, Heusch G, Ovize M, Van de Werf F. Evolving therapies for myocardial ischemia/reperfusion injury. J Am Coll Cardiol. 2015;65:1454–71.

Ichikawa Y, et al. The role of ADAM protease in the tyrosine kinase-mediated trigger mechanism of ischemic preconditioning. Cardiovasc Res. 2004;62:167–75.

Jie B, et al. Neuregulin-1 suppresses cardiomyocyte apoptosis by activating PI3K/Akt and inhibiting mitochondrial permeability transition pore. Mol Cell Biochem. 2012;370:35–43.

Kin H, et al. Inhibition of myocardial apoptosis by postconditioning is associated with attenuation of oxidative stress-mediated nuclear factor-kappa B translocation and TNF alpha release. Shock. 2008;29:761–8.

King AL, et al. Hydrogen sulfide cytoprotective signaling is endothelial nitric oxide synthase-nitric oxide dependent. Proc Natl Acad Sci U S A. 2014;111:3182–7.

Kleinbongard P, Heusch G. Extracellular signalling molecules in the ischaemic/reperfused heart - druggable and translatable for cardioprotection? Br J Pharmacol. 2015;172:2010–25.

Kuramochi Y, et al. Cardiac endothelial cells regulate reactive oxygen species-induced cardiomyocyte apoptosis through neuregulin-1beta/erbB4 signaling. J Biol Chem. 2004;279:51141–7.

Liu FF, et al. Heterozygous knockout of neuregulin-1 gene in mice exacerbates doxorubicin-induced heart failure. Am J Physiol Heart Circ Physiol. 2005;289:H660–6.

Liu L, et al. MicroRNA-15b enhances hypoxia/reoxygenation-induced apoptosis of cardiomyocytes via a mitochondrial apoptotic pathway. Apoptosis : an international journal on programmed cell death. 2014;19:19–29.

Mozaffarian D, et al. Heart disease and stroke statistics--2015 update: a report fro the American Heart Association. Circulation. 2015;131:e29–322.

Odiete O, Hill MF, Sawyer DB. Neuregulin in cardiovascular development and disease. Circ Res. 2012;111:1376–85.

Ovize M, et al. Postconditioning and protection from reperfusion injury: where do we stand? Position paper from the working Group of Cellular Biology of the heart of the European society of cardiology. Cardiovasc Res. 2010;87:406–23.

Parodi EM, Kuhn B. Signalling between microvascular endothelium and cardiomyocytes through neuregulin. Cardiovasc Res. 2014;102:194–204.

Sawyer DB, Caggiano A. Neuregulin-1beta for the treatment of systolic heart failure. J Mol Cell Cardiol. 2011;51:501–5.

Sun HY, et al. Hypoxic postconditioning reduces cardiomyocyte loss by inhibiting ROS generation and intracellular Ca2+ overload. Am J Physiol Heart Circ Physiol. 2005;288:H1900–8.

Tamareille S, et al. Myocardial reperfusion injury management: erythropoietin compared with postconditioning. Am J Phys Heart Circ Phys. 2009;297:H2035–43.

Tian Y, et al. Postconditioning inhibits myocardial apoptosis during prolonged reperfusion via a JAK2-STAT3-Bcl-2 pathway. J Biomed Sci. 2011;18:53.

Tsang A, Hausenloy DJ, Mocanu MM, Yellon DM. Postconditioning: a form of "modified reperfusion" protects the myocardium by activating the phosphatidylinositol 3-kinase-Akt pathway. Circ Res. 2004;95:230–2.

Xie L, et al. Depletion of PHD3 protects heart from ischemia/reperfusion injury by inhibiting cardiomyocyte apoptosis. J Mol Cell Cardiol. 2015;80:156–65.

Xu M, et al. Neuregulin-1 protects myocardial cells against H2 O2 -induced apoptosis by regulating endoplasmic reticulum stress. Cell Biochem Funct. 2014;32:464–9.

Xu P, et al. Diet rich in docosahexaenoic acid/Eicosapentaenoic acid robustly ameliorates hepatic steatosis and insulin resistance in seipin deficient lipodystrophy mice. Nutrition & metabolism. 2015;12:58.

Yang X-M, et al. Multiple, brief coronary occlusions during early reperfusion protect rabbit hearts by targeting cell signaling pathways. J Am Coll Cardiol. 2004;44:1103–10.

Zhang P, Shen M, Fernandez-Patron C, Kassiri Z. ADAMs family and relatives in cardiovascular physiology and pathology. J Mol Cell Cardiol. 2015;

# 3

# Serologic features of cohorts with variable genetic risk for systemic lupus erythematosus

Jyotsna Bhattacharya[1], Karalyn Pappas[2], Bahtiyar Toz[3], Cynthia Aranow[1], Meggan Mackay[1], Peter K. Gregersen[4], Ogobara Doumbo[5], Abdel Kader Traore[6], Martin L. Lesser[7], Maureen McMahon[8], Tammy Utset[9], Earl Silverman[10], Deborah Levy[10], William J. McCune[11], Meenakshi Jolly[12], Daniel Wallace[13], Michael Weisman[13], Juanita Romero-Diaz[14] and Betty Diamond[1*]

## Abstract

**Background:** Systemic lupus erythematosus (SLE) is an autoimmune disease with genetic, hormonal, and environmental influences. In Western Europe and North America, individuals of West African descent have a 3–4 fold greater incidence of SLE than Caucasians. Paradoxically, West Africans in sub-Saharan Africa appear to have a low incidence of SLE, and some studies suggest a milder disease with less nephritis. In this study, we analyzed sera from African American female SLE patients and four other cohorts, one with SLE and others with varying degrees of risk for SLE in order to identify serologic factors that might correlate with risk of or protection against SLE.

**Methods:** Our cohorts included West African women with previous malaria infection assumed to be protected from development of SLE, clinically unaffected sisters of SLE patients with high risk of developing SLE, healthy African American women with intermediate risk, healthy Caucasian women with low risk of developing SLE, and women with a diagnosis of SLE. We developed a lupus risk index (LRI) based on titers of IgM and IgG anti-double stranded DNA antibodies and levels of C1q.

**Results:** The risk index was highest in SLE patients; second highest in unaffected sisters of SLE patients; third highest in healthy African-American women and lowest in healthy Caucasian women and malaria-exposed West African women.

**Conclusion:** This risk index may be useful in early interventions to prevent SLE. In addition, it suggests new therapeutic approaches for the treatment of SLE.

## Background

Systemic lupus erythematosus (SLE) is a chronic systemic autoimmune disease characterized by defects in B cell tolerance leading to the production of multiple auto-antibodies. In particular, SLE is characterized by high affinity IgG anti-nuclear autoantibodies including anti-double stranded (ds) DNA antibodies.

Anti-dsDNA antibodies are found in 70% of patients, are pathogenic and are frequently used to monitor disease activity (Pavlovic et al. 2010; Linnik et al. 2005). Published data demonstrate a 'preclinical' period of disease characterized by

the presence of IgG autoantibodies with increasing titers and number of auto- specificities heralding the onset of clinical SLE (Deane and El-Gabalawy 2014; Arbuckle et al. 2003). However, reports of elevated autoantibody titers in first degree relatives suggest that the presence of autoantibodies alone does not confer disease (Ramos et al. 2010).

While the etiology SLE is not known, data suggest that susceptibility requires both a genetic predisposition and environmental triggers. The genetic predisposition is highlighted by the observed familial clustering of SLE and a concordance rate of approximately 30% in identical twins. Over 50 risk alleles for SLE have been identified and disease severity and age of onset relates, in part, to the number of risk alleles present in an individual (Teruel and Alarcon-Riquelme 2016). Disease is 8–10

* Correspondence: bdiamond@northwell.edu
[1]The Feinstein Institute for Medical Research, Center for Autoimmune, Musculoskeletal and Hematopoietic Diseases, 350 Community Dr, Manhasset, NY 11030, USA
Full list of author information is available at the end of the article

times more prevalent in women than men and 3–4 times more prevalent in women of African descent in Europe or North America than in Caucasian women (Gilkeson et al. 2011). In Caribbean populations, an increasing number of African genes rather than genetic admixture is a risk factor for disease (Molokhia et al. 2003; Molokhia and McKeigue 2000). The prevalence of SLE in West African women is not fully established, but several studies have suggested a lower prevalence in African countries (George and Ogunbiyi 2005; McGill and Oyoo 2002; Molokhia et al. 2001). Moreover, disease manifestations appear to be less severe in West African patients, with a lower incidence of renal disease (Zomalheto et al. 2014). It is reasonable to assume that the genetic predisposition to SLE is at least as high in West Africans as in African-Americans and Afro-Caribbeans and the discrepancy in disease prevalence reflects the impact of environmental factors (Molokhia et al. 2001).

Malaria, an endemic infection in sub-Saharan Africa, has long been suggested to mitigate the impact of SLE (Greenwood 1968). That malaria protects against development of SLE has been clearly demonstrated in spontaneously lupus-prone mice (Greenwood et al. 1970). Because it is frequently fatal, it likely has exerted significant pressure on the genome, resulting in the retention of alleles that diminish the severity of infection. Several risk alleles for SLE protect against severe malaria infection. The *FcRllb* risk allele for SLE (T232) leads to a non-functional molecule which cannot move through the plasma membrane to associate with the B cell receptor (Floto et al. 2005). Decreased inhibitory function associated with this risk allele results in increased B cell and myeloid cell activation. While this may increase risk for SLE, it can be beneficial for a response to infection. In humans, *FcRllb* T232 increases phagocytosis of *P. falciparum* by monocyte-derived macrophages in vitro (Clatworthy et al. 2007). Moreover, *FcRllb*-deficient mice are resistant to severe disease following infection with Plasmodium Chabaudi (Clatworthy et al. 2007). Notably, polymorphisms predisposing to low *TNF* levels protect against cerebral malaria. Several lupus-prone strains show reduced levels attributable to a promoter region polymorphism in the *NZB*, *BXSB* and *MRL* strains. (Jiang et al. 1999; Pritchard et al. 2000) and administering *TNF* to these mice can prevent the onset of SLE.

The repertoire of immunocompetent B cells develops as a consequence of tolerance mechanisms that censor a majority of autoreactive B cells during their maturation process. Approximately 75% of immature B cells have an autoreactive BCR compared to 20% of naïve immunocompetent B cells (Hoffman et al. 2016). These B cells are critical for immune homeostasis as they produce IgM antibodies capable of binding to and removing apoptotic debris in a non-immunogenic fashion (Gronwall et al.

2012). Lack of these autoreactive IgM antibodies results in uptake of apoptotic material in dendritic cells (DCs) and DC activation (Ehrenstein et al. 2000). In *NZB/W* lupus-prone mice, production of pathogenic IgG anti-dsDNA autoantibodies coincides with diminished production of IgM autoantibodies, and administration of IgM anti-dsDNA autoantibodies prevents development of renal disease in mice (Werwitzke et al. 2005).

Although malaria infection may protect against the development of SLE in spontaneous murine models of SLE, an association between malarial infection and autoantibodies is well recognized (Daniel-Ribeiro and Zanini 2000). Many of the autoantibodies present in malaria patients are IgM and are not known to be pathogenic (Wozencraft et al. 1990). The ability of IgM autoantibodies to maintain immune quiescence occurs through a C1q dependent mechanism (Gronwall and Silverman 2014).

C1q is a complement component that is important in clearance of apoptotic debris and promotes immune tolerance through regulation of immune cell differentiation and cytokine release (Son et al. 2015). Ninety percent of individuals with severe hereditary C1q deficiency have SLE (Manderson et al. 2004).

We hypothesized that an enhanced ratio of IgG:IgM anti-DNA antibodies and a diminished level of C1q would predispose to SLE. We further hypothesized that exposure to malaria results in increased titers of protective IgM autoantibodies and increases in C1q that retard or prevent onset of SLE in genetically predisposed individuals.

We, therefore, evaluated IgM and IgG anti-dsDNA antibody titers and assessed C1q levels in women with varying risk for SLE based on genetic risk and malaria exposure: African-American SLE patients (SLE); healthy Caucasian women (CHC); healthy African-American women (AAHC); unaffected sisters of SLE patients (SIS); and women from Mali with a history of malaria infection (MAL). We generated a lupus risk index (LRI) based on serum IgG:IgM anti-DNA antibody ratio and C1q level. The a priori hypothesis was that the LRI would be lowest in CHC, then increase through groups MAL, AAHC, SIS, and SLE, in that order. The development of an LRI may prove useful in following at risk individuals over time to identify those that may profit from early intervention and diagnosed SLE patients who might be at risk for an impending flare.

## Methods
### Samples
Serum samples were obtained from 40 Malian women, (MAL) aged 18 to 65. Inclusion criteria included a known history of malaria infection, no history of autoimmune disease or first degree relative with autoimmune disease and no known infection with HIV. Additional serum samples were obtained from 51 SLE patients of African American descent (SLE). All SLE subjects met

1997 ACR revised criteria and were enrolled in the prospective SLE cohort at the Feinstein Institute. Serum samples from 80 healthy African American women (AAHC), age 20 to 68, with no use of immunosuppressive agents in the year prior, and 16 Caucasian healthy controls (CHC), age 28 to 50, were purchased from BioreclamationIVT. Serum from 98 unaffected sisters of SLE patients (SIS), age 14–46, was obtained from the Feinstein Institute SisSLE cohort. The SIS cohort included 67 Caucasian, 11 Hispanics, 7 African-Americans and 12 Asians, (one unknown). The study was approved by the Institutional Review Board at the Northwell Health, Manhasset, NY and the Comité d'Ethique de la FMPOS, Bamako, Mali.

## dsDNA ELISA

To detect IgM and IgG anti-dsDNA antibodies, 96-well plates (Costar, 3690, Corning, Kennenbunk, ME) were coated with calf thymus DNA that had been filtered through a 0.45 um cellulose filter (Millipore, Darmstadt, Germany) to remove ssDNA (#2618, Calbiochem, San Diego, CA) at 2μg/ml in PBS. Plates were dry-coated overnight at 370 C and blocked in 3% FBS/PBS for 1 h at room temperature (RT). Plates were washed 3 times and then incubated with serum samples diluted 1:100 in 0.3% FBS/PBS and assayed in triplicate. Plates were washed 5 times in PBS 0.05% Tween, and then incubated with secondary anti-IgM or IgG alkaline phosphatase conjugated antibodies (SouthernBiotech, Birmingham, AL) diluted 1:000 in 0.3% FBS/PBS for 1 h at 370C, washed 3 times, and developed with alkaline phosphatase substrate (Sigma, St. Louis, MO) at room temperature. Plates were read at 405 nm using a PerkinElmer Victor 3 ELISA reader.

## C1q ELISA

Murine monoclonal anti-human C1q (#A201, Quide San Diego, CA) (25 μl/well of 2μg/ml) in PBS was dry-coated into 96-well polystyrene microtiter plates (Costar, 3690, Corning) overnight at 4 °C. Wells were blocked 3% nonfat dry milk with 50ul/well (# M0841, LabScientific Highlands, NJ) in PBS for 4 h at room temperature. After rinsing the wells three times with PBS-0.05%Tween, 25 μl of serum samples diluted in PBS were added to each well. The serum dilutions were obtained by first making a 1:100 dilution and serially re-diluting this solution until it was 1: 10,000. Samples were incubated overnight at 4 °C. Wells were then washed 3 times with PBS- Tween. Goat antiserum to human C1q (#A301, Quidel) was diluted 1:1000 in 0.3% non-fat milk in PBS and added (25 μl/well) for 2 h at room temperature. After washing 3 times in PBS-Tween, plates were incubated for 1 h at room temperature with rabbit anti-goat IgG antibody conjugated to alkaline phosphatase (#A-4062, Sigma) diluted in 0.3% non-fat milk in PBS at 1:500. The wells were washed 3 times with PBS-

Tween and incubated with 50 μl of alkaline phosphatase substrate (Sigma) in solution (.5 M Na2CO3 and .01 M MgCl2) (check). The absorbance of each well was read at 30 min at 405 nm. The standard curve of purified human C1q was linear in the 2 ng to 250 ng range. Both the standards and serum samples were assayed in triplicate.

## Statistical methods

The primary objective was to compare potential biomarkers of SLE among women grouped by risk for SLE based on race and malaria exposure: healthy Caucasian (CHC) and African American (AAHC) women, African women with past exposure to malaria (MAL), unaffected sisters of lupus patients (SIS), and lupus patients (SLE). Since a high IgG:IgM anti-dsDNA antibody ratio and a low level of C1q are associated with SLE, and a low IgG: IgM anti-dsDNA antibody ratio and high level of C1q are associated with healthy controls, the LRI was calculated by $\frac{IgG}{IgM \times C1q}$. For this analysis, original measurement units were used and plotted on log axis which resulted in data that were consistent with the usual assumptions of normality and equal variance across groups. One-way analysis of variance was used to compare each of these five markers separately across the groups. Upon finding a significant difference, Tukey's method of pairwise comparisons was used, separately for each marker, to determine which groups' means differed from one another on that marker. All statistical tests, including the Tukey test, were performed at the 5% significance level.

## Results
### Anti-dsDNA antibodies

As IgM antibodies precede the generation of IgG antibodies and protect against SLE onset, we assessed IgM anti-DNA antibodies in all 5 cohorts (Fig. 1). Titers were lowest in the SLE, SIS, and AAHC cohorts. Titers were significantly higher in the CHC cohort and highest in the MAL cohort.

We next assessed IgG anti-DNA antibodies in all cohorts (Fig. 2). CHC, AAHC and SIS had similar titers of these antibodies. The MAL cohort exhibited significantly increased IgG anti- dsDNA titers and the SLE cohort exhibited the highest titers.

### IgG:IgM ratio

While significant differences in IgG and IgM anti-DNA titers were present, we reasoned that IgM and IgG antibodies compete for antigen, leading us to ask whether the IgG: IgM ratio was more critical to disease progression than the titer of either alone (Fig. 3). As expected, the SLE cohort had the highest ratio compared to all other cohorts. The MAL, SIS and AAHC cohorts had an intermediate ratio while the CHC cohort had the lowest ratio.

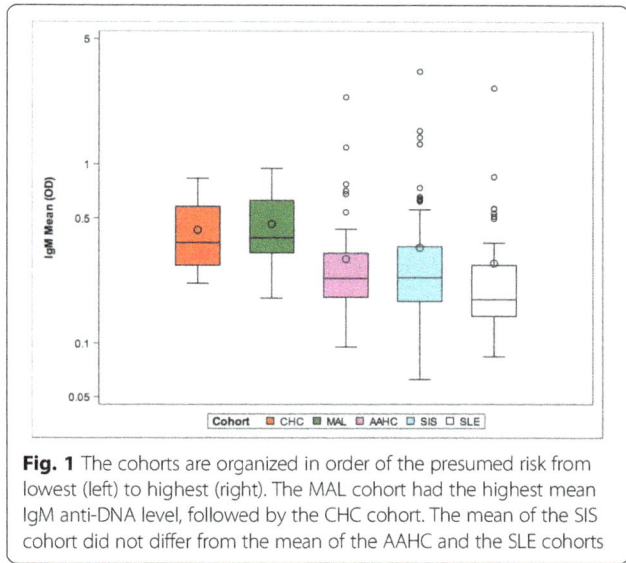

**Fig. 1** The cohorts are organized in order of the presumed risk from lowest (left) to highest (right). The MAL cohort had the highest mean IgM anti-DNA level, followed by the CHC cohort. The mean of the SIS cohort did not differ from the mean of the AAHC and the SLE cohorts

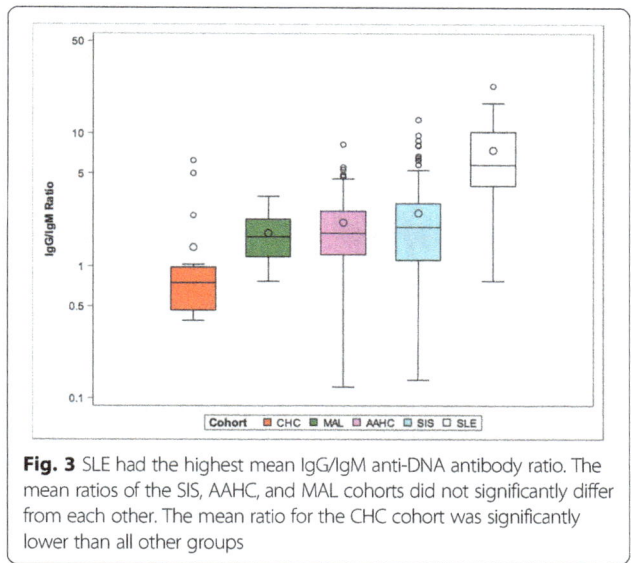

**Fig. 3** SLE had the highest mean IgG/IgM anti-DNA antibody ratio. The mean ratios of the SIS, AAHC, and MAL cohorts did not significantly differ from each other. The mean ratio for the CHC cohort was significantly lower than all other groups

## C1q levels

C1q levels were assessed in all cohorts (Fig. 4). Not only is C1q deficiency among the greatest risk factors for SLE, but C1q inversely correlates with disease activity (Horak et al. 2006). Anti-C1q antibodies have also correlated with disease activity (Bock et al. 2015). C1q levels were lowest in the SLE cohort, slightly higher but still low in the SIS cohort, intermediate within the CHC and AAHC cohorts and highest in individuals exposed to malaria, the MAL cohort.

## Lupus risk index

Based on the putative protection conferred by a low IgG/IgM anti-dsDNA antibody ratio and a high C1q level, the LRI was developed to measure propensity for development of SLE for each individual (Fig. 5). The LRI

was defined as $\frac{IgG}{IgM \times C1q}$ . The SLE patients exhibited the highest mean LRI, followed by the SIS cohort, and then the AAHC cohort, while the CHC and the MAL cohorts exhibited the lowest LRI.

## Discussion

In this study, we examined serologic markers in 5 cohorts with variable risk for SLE to understand pathways that might predispose to or prevent disease onset. As anticipated, we observed high titers of IgM anti-DNA antibodies in the MAL cohort and high titers of IgG anti-DNA antibodies in the SLE cohort. Analysis of the IgG/IgM anti-DNA antibody ratio showed a high ratio in SLE patients, a low ratio in the CHC cohort and intermediate ratios within the SIS, MAL and AAHC cohorts.

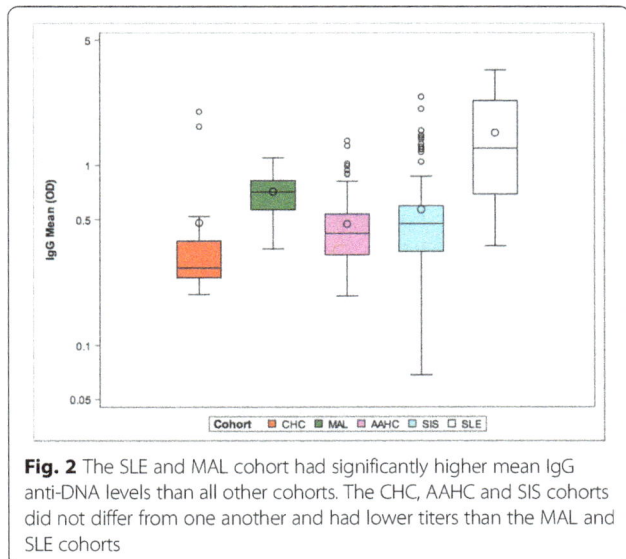

**Fig. 2** The SLE and MAL cohort had significantly higher mean IgG anti-DNA levels than all other cohorts. The CHC, AAHC and SIS cohorts did not differ from one another and had lower titers than the MAL and SLE cohorts

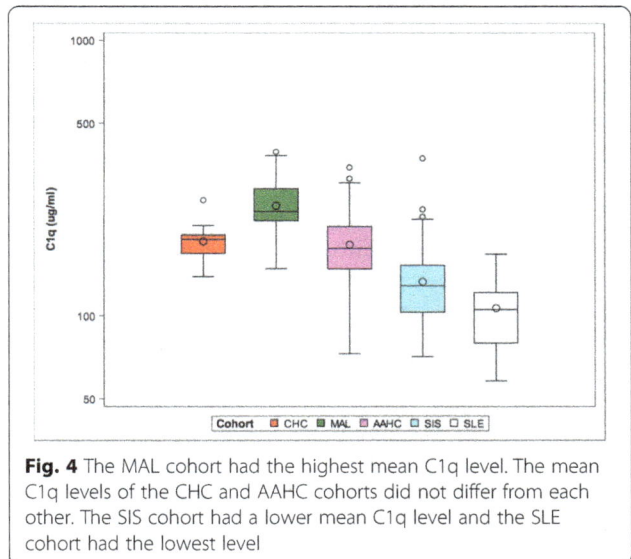

**Fig. 4** The MAL cohort had the highest mean C1q level. The mean C1q levels of the CHC and AAHC cohorts did not differ from each other. The SIS cohort had a lower mean C1q level and the SLE cohort had the lowest level

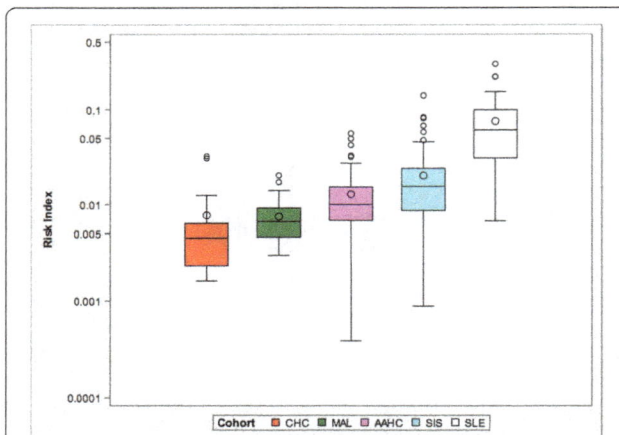

**Fig. 5** All cohorts were significantly different from each other, except the CHC and MAL cohorts which showed no significant difference

The protective properties of IgM antibodies are known. IgM immune complexes engage C1q which will bind LAIR-1, an inhibitory surface receptor on hematopoietic cells (Son and Diamond 2015). IgM precedes IgG anti-dsDNA antibodies in mouse models of SLE and it has been shown in the *NZB/W* model that administration of IgM anti-DNA antibody will delay onset of disease. IgM, especially pentameric IgM, competes with IgG for antigen and thereby diminishes the load of IgG immune complexes including IgG anti-DNA immune complexes that bind to activating Fc receptors on myeloid cells to initiate an inflammatory cascade. Consistent with the model that IgM is protective against autoimmunity and IgG engages inflammatory pathways, mice genetically engineered to secrete IgG but not IgM will develop SLE (Marshak-Rothstein 2006; Boes et al. 2000). Moreover, *B6.Sle1* mice which carry the *sle 1* risk locus from *NZM* mice produce more antigen-specific IgG and total IgG and exhibit enhanced IgM to IgG class switching (Rahman et al. 2007), suggesting that part of the genetic risk for SLE may include a propensity to high IgG levels.

Malaria exposed individuals harbor anti-nuclear antibodies, some of which cross react with malarial antigens. The ANA pattern in malaria is different from patterns observed in SLE, suggesting fine specificity differences, but anti-DNA antibodies have been reported (Hommel et al. 2014; Hirako et al. 2015). That these anti-DNA antibodies are primarily IgM is consistent with reports of high IgM antibodies in response to malarial infection (Pleass et al. 2016; Czajkowsky et al. 2010). Interestingly, the Fulani population in Mali experiences less severe malarial disease than the Dogon population; IgM anti-malarial titers are higher in the Fulani than the Dogon and may in part

account for the less severe disease (Maiga et al. 2013). Why malaria exposure leads to high IgM levels and whether this reflects activation of "innate" B1 or marginal zone B cells or impaired class switching in malaria patients is not known, but may relate to high BAFF levels which are seen in malaria exposed individuals (Scholzen and Sauerwein 2013).

We analyzed serum levels of C1q as low C1q correlates with disease severity and absence of C1q is a strong genetic risk factor for SLE. C1q opsonizes apoptotic cells to remove debris in a non-inflammatory fashion in an IgM-mediated pathway. C1q binds the collagen receptor LAIR-1 through its collagen-like tail to maintain monocyte quiescence and prevent monocyte to DC differentiation (Son et al. 2012). The interaction of C1q with LAIR-1 prevents activation of endosomal TLRs in DCs by nucleic acid ligands. Finally, C1q blocks the transfer of an IFN signature transfer to healthy PBMCs by SLE serum. Thus, IgM antibodies function in conjunction with C1q to mitigate inflammatory pathways.

As expected, C1q levels were diminished in the SLE, and, to a lesser degree, in the SIS cohort. There was no difference between the CHC and AAHC cohorts. C1q levels were highest in the MAL cohort. Mechanisms increasing serum C1q levels are unknown but C1q is produced by anti-inflammatory M2-like macrophages (Fraser et al. 2015). While these have not been specifically shown to be increased in malaria infection, they are increased by helminthic infections (Fairweather and Cihakova 2009). Elevated C1q may also relate to the binding of IgM to Pfem1, a molecule expressed on the membrane of parasite-infected erythrocytes. The interaction of IgM with Pfem prevents the binding of IgM to C1q and may thus raise levels of soluble C1q (Czajkowsky et al. 2010). Based on the IgG:IgM anti-DNA antibody ratio and the C1q level, we generated an LRI. This score confirmed the known risk of SLE; the highest LRI was present in the SLE cohort. Among the non-SLE cohorts, LRI was highest in SIS followed by AAHC, while the CHC and MAL cohorts exhibited the lowest LRI. Although the MAL cohort exhibited relatively high IgG anti-dsDNA antibody titers, the high IgM anti-dsDNA antibody and C1q levels reduced the LRI. These serologic features may contribute to the protection malaria confers against the development of SLE. Understanding how malaria, even when recurrent, blocks the IgM to IgG switch has important therapeutic implications.

## Conclusion

In summary, we have studied populations with different risk for developing SLE to propose a metric to assess that risk. A risk score is as robust as its components are pathophysiologically relevant. DsDNA IgG, IgM and C1q, which are the components of the LRI that we propose, are known to respond to changes in disease activity. A tool such as this that can predict the risk of developing clinical SLE would be useful to assess the effectiveness of early interventions. Therapy with hydroxychloroquine, for example, delays disease onset (Virdis et al. 2015); we would anticipate that its therapeutic effect would be reflected in the LRI. Longitudinal studies, including in our unique sisters cohort are needed to validate our findings. These observations additionally suggest new therapeutic approaches for the treatment of SLE.

## Abbreviations
AAHC: Healthy African American women; CHC: Healthy Caucasian women; LRI: Lupus risk index; MAL: Women from Mali with a history of malaria infection; SIS: Unaffected sisters of SLE patients; SLE: Systemic lupus erythematosus

## Funding
This study was supported by a grant from the Lupus Research Institute and the New York State Department of Health, Empire Clinical Research Investigator Program.

## Authors' contributions
Study conception and design: BD Sample acquisition: CA, MM, OD, AT, PG Analysis and interpretation of data: JB, BT, ML, KP Drafting of manuscript: JB, BD, KP, ML, CA, MM Critical revision: BD. All authors read and approved the final manuscript.

## Competing interests
The authors declare that they have no competing interests.

## Author details
[1]The Feinstein Institute for Medical Research, Center for Autoimmune, Musculoskeletal and Hematopoietic Diseases, 350 Community Dr, Manhasset, NY 11030, USA. [2]Department of Statistical Science, Cornell University, Ithaca, NY, USA. [3]Department of Internal Medicine, Istanbul University, Istanbul, Turkey. [4]The Feinstein Institute for Medical Research, Center for Genomics and Human Genetics, Manhasset, NY, USA. [5]Malaria Research and Training Center, Bamako, Mali. [6]Deputy of the Department of Internal Medicine, University Hospital, Bamako, Mali. [7]The Feinstein Institute for Medical Research, Center of Biostatistics Unit Manhasset, Manhasset, NY, USA. [8]UCLA David Geffen School of Medicine, Los Angeles, CA 90095, USA. [9]University of Chicago Medical Center, Chicago, IL, USA. [10]Hospital for Sick Children, University of Toronto, Toronto, ON M5G 1X8, Canada. [11]University of Michigan, Ann Arbor, Mi 48109, USA. [12]Rush University Medical Center, Chicago, IL 60612, USA. [13]Cedars Sinai Medical Center, Los Angeles, CA 90048, USA. [14]Instituto Nacional de Ciencias Medicas y Nutrician Salvador Zubiran, Mexico City, Mexico.

## References
Arbuckle MR, et al. Development of autoantibodies before the clinical onset of systemic lupus erythematosus. N Engl J Med. 2003;349:1526–33.
Bock M, Heijnen I, Trendelenburg M. Anti-C1q antibodies as a follow-up marker in SLE patients. PLoS One. 2015;10:e0123572.
Boes M, et al. Accelerated development of IgG autoantibodies and autoimmune disease in the absence of secreted IgM. Proc Natl Acad Sci U S A. 2000;97:1184–9.
Clatworthy MR, et al. Systemic lupus erythematosus-associated defects in the inhibitory receptor FcgammaRIIb reduce susceptibility to malaria. Proc Natl Acad Sci U S A. 2007;104:7169–74.

Czajkowsky DM, et al. IgM, Fcμ-receptors, and malarial immune evasion. J Immunol. 2010;184:4597–603.
Daniel-Ribeiro CT, Zanini G. Autoimmunity and malaria: what are they doing together? Acta Trop. 2000;76:205–21.
Deane KD, El-Gabalawy H. Pathogenesis and prevention of rheumatic disease: focus on preclinical RA and SLE. Nat Rev Rheumatol. 2014;10:212–28.
Ehrenstein MR, Cook HT, Neuberger MS. Deficiency in serum immunoglobulin (Ig)M predisposes to development of IgG autoantibodies. J Exp Med. 2000;191:1253–8.
Fairweather D, Cihakova D. Alternatively activated macrophages in infection and autoimmunity. J Autoimmun. 2009;33:222–30.
Floto RA, et al. Loss of function of a lupus-associated FcgammaRIIb polymorphism through exclusion from lipid rafts. Nat Med. 2005;11:1056–8.
Fraser D, Melzer E, Camacho A, Gomez M. Macrophage production of innate immune protein C1q is associated with M2 polarization (INM1P.434). J Immunol. 2015;194:56.11
George A, Ogunbiyi A. Systemic lupus erythematosus: a rarity in West Africa, or a yet to be investigated entity. Lupus. 2005;14:924–5.
Gilkeson G, et al. The United States to Africa lupus prevalence gradient revisited. Lupus. 2011;20:1095–103.
Greenwood BM. Autoimmune disease and parasitic infections in Nigerians. Lancet. 1968;2:380–2.
Greenwood BM, Herrick EM, Voller A. Suppression of autoimmune disease in NZB and (NZB x NZW) F1 hybrid mice by infection with malaria. Nature. 1970;226:266–7.
Gronwall C, Silverman GJ. Natural IgM: beneficial autoantibodies for the controlof inflammatory and autoimmune disease. J Clin Immunol. 2014;34(Suppl 1):S12–21.
Gronwall C, Vas J, Silverman GJ. Protective roles of natural IgM antibodies. Front Immunol. 2012;3:66.
Hirako IC, et al. DNA-containing Immunocomplexes promote Inflammasome assembly and release of pyrogenic cytokines by CD14+ CD16+ CD64high CD32low inflammatory monocytes from malaria patients. MBio. 2015;6:e01605–15.
Hoffman W, Lakkis FG, Chalasani G. B cells, antibodies, and more. Clin J Am Soc Nephrol. 2016;11:137–54.
Hommel B, et al. Chronic malaria revealed by a new fluorescence pattern on the antinuclear autoantibodies test. PLoS One. 2014;9:e88548.
Horak P, et al. C1q complement component and -antibodies reflect SLE activity and kidney involvement. Clin Rheumatol. 2006;25:532–6.
Jiang Y, et al. Genetically determined aberrant down-regulation of FcgammaRIIB1 in germinal center B cells associated with hyper-IgG and IgG autoantibodies in murine systemic lupus erythematosus. Int Immunol. 1999;11:1685–91.
Linnik MD, et al. Relationship between anti-double-stranded DNA antibodies and exacerbation of renal disease in patients with systemic lupus erythematosus. Arthritis Rheum. 2005;52:1129–37.
Maiga B, et al. Human candidate polymorphisms in sympatric ethnic groups differing in malaria susceptibility in Mali. PLoS One. 2013;8:e75675.
Manderson AP, Botto M, Walport MJ. The role of complement in the development of systemic lupus erythematosus. Annu Rev Immunol. 2004;22:431–56.
Marshak-Rothstein A. Toll-like receptors in systemic autoimmune disease. Nat Rev Immunol. 2006;6:823–35.
McGill PE, Oyoo GO. Rheumatic disorders in sub-saharan Africa. East Afr Med J. 2002;79:214–6.
Molokhia M, McKeigue P. Risk for rheumatic disease in relation to ethnicity and admixture. Arthritis Res. 2000;2:115–25.
Molokhia M, McKeigue PM, Cuadrado M, Hughes G. Systemic lupus erythematosus in migrants from West Africa compared with afro-Caribbean people in the UK. Lancet. 2001;357:1414–5.
Molokhia M, et al. Relation of risk of systemic lupus erythematosus to west African admixture in a Caribbean population. Hum Genet. 2003;112:310–8.
Pavlovic M, et al. Pathogenic and epiphenomenal anti-DNA antibodies in SLE. Autoimmune Dis. 2010;2011:462841.
Pleass RJ, Moore SC, Stevenson L, Hviid L. Immunoglobulin M: restrainer of inflammation and mediator of immune evasion by Plasmodium falciparum malaria. Trends Parasitol. 2016;32:108–19.
Pritchard NR, et al. Autoimmune-prone mice share a promoter haplotype associated with reduced expression and function of the fc receptor FcgammaRII. Curr Biol. 2000;10:227–30.
Rahman ZS, et al. Expression of the autoimmune Fcgr2b NZW allele fails to be upregulated in germinal center B cells and is associated with increased IgG production. Genes Immun. 2007;8:604–12.
Ramos PS, Brown EE, Kimberly RP, Langefeld CD. Genetic factors predisposing to systemic lupus erythematosus and lupus nephritis. Semin Nephrol. 2010;30:164–76.

Scholzen A, Sauerwein RW. How malaria modulates memory: activation and
    dysregulation of B cells in Plasmodium infection. Trends Parasitol. 2013;29:
    252–62.
Son M, Diamond B. C1q-mediated repression of human monocytes is regulated
    by leukocyte-associated Ig-like receptor 1 (LAIR-1). Mol Med. 2015;20:559–68.
Son M, Diamond B, Santiago-Schwarz F. Fundamental role of C1q in
    autoimmunity and inflammation. Immunol Res. 2015;63:101–6.
Son M, Santiago-Schwarz F, Al-Abed Y, Diamond B. C1q limits dendritic cell
    differentiation and activation by engaging LAIR-1. Proc Natl Acad Sci U S A.
    2012;109:E3160–7.
Teruel M, Alarcon-Riquelme ME. The genetic basis of systemic lupus
    erythematosus: what are the risk factors and what have we learned.
    J Autoimmun. 2016;74:161–75.
Virdis A, et al. Early treatment with hydroxychloroquine prevents the
    development of endothelial dysfunction in a murine model of systemic
    lupus erythematosus. Arthritis Res Ther. 2015;17:277.
Werwitzke S, et al. Inhibition of lupus disease by anti-double-stranded DNA
    antibodies of the IgM isotype in the (NZB x NZW)F1 mouse. Arthritis Rheum.
    2005;52:3629–38.
Wozencraft AO, Lloyd CM, Staines NA, Griffiths VJ. Role of DNA-binding
    antibodies in kidney pathology associated with murine malaria infections.
    Infect Immun. 1990;58:2156–64.
Zomalheto Z, et al. Pattern of systemic lupus erythematosus in Benin and west
    African patients. La Tunisie Medicale. 2014;92:707–10.

# 4

# Assessment of HIF-1α expression and release following endothelial injury in-vitro and in-vivo

Lamia Heikal[1], Pietro Ghezzi[1], Manuela Mengozzi[1] and Gordon Ferns[1,2]*

## Abstract

**Background:** Endothelial injury is an early and enduring feature of cardiovascular disease. Inflammation and hypoxia may be responsible for this, and are often associated with the up-regulation of several transcriptional factors that include Hypoxia Inducible Factor-1 (HIF-1). Although it has been reported that HIF-1α is detectable in plasma, it is known to be unstable. Our aim was to optimize an assay for HIF-1α to be applied to in vitro and in vivo applications, and to use this assay to assess the release kinetics of HIF-1α following endothelial injury.

**Methods:** An ELISA for the measurement of HIF-1α in cell-culture medium and plasma was optimized, and the assay was used to determine the best conditions for sample collection and storage. The results of the ELISA were validated using Western blotting and immunohistochemistry (IHC). In vitro, a standardized injury was produced in a monolayer of rat aortic endothelial cells (RAECs) and intracellular HIF-1α was measured at intervals over 24 h. In vivo, a rat angioplasty model was used. The right carotid artery was injured using a 2F Fogarty balloon catheter. HIF-1α was measured in the plasma and in the arterial tissue (0, 1, 2, 3 and 5 days post injury).

**Results:** The HIF-1α ELISA had a limit of detection of 2.7 pg/mL and was linear up to 1000 pg/ mL. Between and within-assay, the coefficient of variation values were less than 15%. HIF-1α was unstable in cell lysates and plasma, and it was necessary to add a protease inhibitor immediately after collection, and to store samples at -80 °C prior to analysis. The dynamics of HIF-1α release were different for the in vitro and in vivo models. In vitro, HIF-1α reached maximum concentrations approximately 2 h post injury, whereas peak values in plasma and tissues occurred approximately 2 days post injury, in the balloon injury model.

**Conclusion:** HIF-1α can be measured in plasma, but this requires careful sample collection and storage. The carotid artery balloon injury model is associated with the transient release of HIF-1α into the circulation that probably reflects the hypoxia induced in the artery wall.

**Keywords:** HIF-1α, Injury, Endothelial cells, ELISA, Angioplasty

## Background

Endothelial injury is an early and enduring feature of cardiovascular disease. Inflammation and hypoxia may be partially responsible for this, and are often associated with the up regulation of transcriptional factors that include hypoxia-inducible factor-1 (HIF-1) (Ferns and Heikal 2017).

* Correspondence: G.Ferns@bsms.ac.uk
[1]Brighton and Sussex Medical School Department of Clinical and experimental investigation, University of Sussex, Falmer East Sussex, Brighton BN1 9PS, UK
[2]Brighton and Sussex Medical School Department of Medical Education, Mayfield House, Falmer East Sussex, Brighton BN1 9PH, UK

HIF-1 is a hetero-dimeric transcription factor that consists of an oxygen-regulated α- subunit and a constitutively expressed ß-subunit (Chu and Jones 2016). HIF-1β is expressed in the nucleus and its activity is unaffected by hypoxia, whereas the HIF-1α subunit has a short half-life (5 min) and its stability is regulated by oxygen tension (Gao et al. 2012). Intracellular HIF-1α is unstable under normoxic conditions, being rapidly degraded by prolyl hydroxylase enzymes (Semenza 2014). These enzymes are inactivated under low oxygen levels, explaining why HIF-1α is induced by hypoxia. Some small molecules such as dimethyloxalylglycine (DMOG) can stabilize HIF levels under normoxic conditions by inhibiting prolyl hydroxylase (Zhang et al. 2016). Three distinct HIF-$\alpha$ subunits have been identified (HIF-1$\alpha$, HIF-2$\alpha$ and HIF-3$\alpha$) that have a tissue-specific pattern of expression (Al Okail 2010). HIF-1$\alpha$ and HIF 2$\alpha$ are similar but not identical. HIF-1$\alpha$ is expressed in response to acute hypoxia, whilst HIF-2$\alpha$ is related to chronic responses (Loboda et al. 2012). HIF-1 drives vascular endothelial growth factor (VEGF) expression and angiogenesis while HIF-2 production blocks angiogenesis by inducing the expression of the soluble VEGF receptor-1, sequestering biologically active, free VEGF. It is possible that HIF-2$\alpha$ evolved to regulate the VEGF response to hypoxia and the resultant development of the vascular network (Eubank and Marsh 2011; Eubank et al. 2011; Loboda et al. 2012). Therefore, HIF-1 is a key transcription factor in the adaptive responses to low oxygen (Lambert et al. 2010). HIF-1 is involved in the cellular adaptation to injury, inflammation, infection and cancer (Eubank and Marsh 2011). HIF is also induced by inflammatory cytokines including tumour necrosis factor alpha (TNF-$\alpha$) and interleukin-1$\beta$ (IL-1$\beta$), that increase the accumulation and transcriptional activity of HIF-1$\alpha$ (Gao et al. 2012).

HIF-1 also regulates a variety of other important cellular responses affecting a spectrum of protective/reparative processes including angiogenesis, cell proliferation and survival (Ferns and Heikal 2017; Lambert et al. 2010). It promotes the transcription of more than 100 target genes including several angiogenic factors, apart from VEGF, nitric oxide synthase (the inducible and the endothelial forms), platelet-derived growth factor, and erythropoietin (EPO) (Gao et al. 2012; Natarajan et al. 2007).

Several semi-quantitative methods have been used to estimate HIF-1$\alpha$ levels, for example Western blotting and immunocytochemistry (Karshovska et al. 2007; Srinivasan and Dunn 2011). HIF-1$\alpha$ levels have also been assessed indirectly by quantifying mRNA expression, or by measuring downstream target genes such as VEGF and EPO (Formento et al. 2005; Park et al. 2014).

Due to the need for a more precise method for HIF-1$\alpha$ quantification in biological samples, some quantitative methods have also been developed, that include the enzyme linked immunosorbent assay (ELISA) (Formento et al. 2005). Although it has been reported that HIF-1$\alpha$ is detectable in plasma, (He et al. 2016a) it is unstable and is rapidly degraded under normal oxygen tensions, as discussed above (Park et al. 2014). As a transcription factor, it is normally located within the cell, and there has also been some doubt about its release into plasma (Ferns and Heikal 2017).

Plasma HIF-1$\alpha$ may potentially represent a biomarker of vascular wall hypoxia, or the extent of atherosclerosis. It may also reflect the severity of hypoxia associated with other pathological conditions including some tumours. Hence, there are a number of possible clinical applications for a plasma HIF-1$\alpha$ assay.

Our aim was to optimize an assay for HIF-1$\alpha$ to be applied to in vitro and in vivo studies, and to establish the conditions for sample collection and storage. We then aimed to use the assay to assess the release kinetics of HIF-1$\alpha$ following endothelial injury in vitro and in vivo.

## Methods
All chemicals were from Sigma Aldrich (Dorset, UK), unless otherwise stated.

### Cell culture
Rat aortic endothelial cells (RAECs) were isolated from the aortae of Sprague Dawley rats (male, 2 weeks old) and used between passages 2–5 (Kobayashi et al. 2005). The cells were cultured in Endothelial cell growth medium supplemented with 10% fetal bovine serum (FBS) and Penicillin/Streptomycin (final concentration 100 IU/mL), and were cultured, prior to our experiments, at 37 °C in a humidified atmosphere containing 5% $CO_2$ and 21% $O_2$. When indicated, experiments under hypoxic conditions were performed under 1% $O_2$, 5% $CO_2$ and 94% $N_2$.

### Effect of storage on the HIF-1$\alpha$ stability
Storage time and temperature, and the effects of adding protease inhibitors to the experimental samples were investigated to determine the optimum storage conditions for HIF-1$\alpha$ measurements.

For the effect of temperature, aliquots of samples were taken and maintained at different temperatures (– 80, – 20, 4 and 37 °C). HIF-1$\alpha$ concentrations were determined after 24 h storage using the ELISA as described below.

To determine the effect of storage duration on HIF-1$\alpha$ concentrations, fresh samples were divided into 3 aliquots, and HIF-1$\alpha$ was measured immediately, or after 1 and 2 weeks. Aliquots were stored at -80 °C until analysis.

To assess the requirement for the addition of a protease inhibitor, aliquots from a set of fresh samples were treated with the protease inhibitor, aprotinin (300 nM) (Mosher et al. 2014). These samples were stored for 1 or 2 weeks at -80 °C until they were analyzed.

Linearity, limit of detection and limit of quantification of the assay were determined. Assay precision was assessed by measuring intra and inter-plate replicates with appropriate samples and HIF-1$\alpha$ standards.

### Quantification of HIF-1$\alpha$ after administration of a HIF-1$\alpha$ inducer
Cells were seeded into 24 well plates with a seeding density of $1 \times 10^5$ cell/mL and cultured until 80% confluent. The HIF-1$\alpha$ inducer; DMOG was added at different concentrations ranging from 0 to 500 µM and

incubated for 24 h at 21% $O_2$. Cells incubated in hypoxic conditions (1%$O_2$) were used as a positive control for HIF-1α induction. Cells were then lysed and HIF-1α was measured using the ELISA method. In another set of experiments, cells were similarly treated with different concentrations of DMOG, lysed, and the down-stream effector, VEGF gene expression was measured.

### Scratch assay in vitro injury model

The "scratch assay" is a model of cell/ wound injury, and has been described previously (Heikal et al. 2015). Briefly, a reproducible scratch was produced in the endothelial monolayer, and the cells were then incubated in room air (21% $O_2$) in a 5% $CO_2$ incubator. Cells were then lysed and intracellular HIF-1α assessed. This was evaluated over a period of 24 h using the ELISA.

### Animal studies

Male Sprague Dawley rats (450 g) were used. All animal experiments were performed under UK Home Office approval according to the Animals Scientific Procedures Act, 1986 and subsequent revisions, and conformed to the Guide for the Care and Use of Laboratory Animals published by the National Institutes of Health (NIH Publication No. 85–23, revised 1996). Studies were designed and conducted in accordance with the ARRIVE guidelines (Kilkenny et al. 2010). Rats were acclimatized in home cages for 1 week prior to experimentation with ad libitum access to food and water and on a 12h light-dark cycle.

### Quantification of HIF-1α post DMOG administration

Rats were anesthetized using 2% isoflurane and placed in a supine position. The right carotid artery was exposed and DMOG was applied locally at different concentrations (0–7.5 mg/Kg) on the artery using pluronic gel as the vehicle (30%$w/w$). Three rats were used for each concentration of DMOG. After 24 h, blood was collected from a tail vein, and HIF-1α was measured by ELISA.

Treated animals were culled after 24 h and both the right (treated) and left (untreated) carotid arteries were isolated and snap frozen for PCR analysis.

### Angioplasty in vivo injury model

Injury was induced in the rat's carotid artery using a balloon catheter (for angioplasty) as previously described (Tulis 2007). Briefly, rats (450 g) were anesthetized using 2% isoflurane and placed in a supine position. The right carotid artery was exposed and a 2F Fogarty catheter was used to cause injury. The catheter was inserted into the common carotid artery via the external carotid to cause complete removal of the vascular endothelium from the common carotid artery down to its junction with the aortic arch.

Blood was collected from a tail vein at 0, 1, 2 and 5 days after injury into EDTA containing sample tubes.

Plasma was separated and used for the measurement of HIF-1α using ELISA.

At the end of the experiment, rats were culled. Both the right (treated) and left (untreated) carotid arteries were isolated and snap frozen for PCR analysis.

In another set of experiments culled animals were perfused fixed with PBS followed by 4% paraformaldehyde. Both the right (treated) and left (untreated) carotid arteries were isolated and kept in 4% paraformaldehyde at room temperature for 1 h. Fixed arteries were then placed in a 30% sucrose solution and left overnight after which they were snap frozen in OCT blocks for cryo-sectioning.

### HIF-1α enzyme linked immunosorbent assay (ELISA)

HIF-1α was measured using a commercial ELISA kit (R&D systems/ Biotechne, UK) following the manufacturers' instructions.

a. Standard calibration curves were obtained using HIF-1α protein standards, allowing the limit of detection, limit of quantification and coefficient of variation to be determined.

b. In vitro *samples*: Endothelial cells were lysed in 80 μL lysis buffer (25 mmol/L Tris HCl pH 7. 6, 0.1% SDS, 1% deoxycholate, 1% NP40, 0.5 mol/L EDTA, 40 mmol/L EGTA and protease inhibitors). Lysates were then centrifuged at 11000 $g$ for 15 min at 4 °C and the supernatant was collected. Protein concentrations were quantified using a BCA reagent kit (Pierce Biotechnology). Results were expressed as pg/ mg protein.

c. *Rat plasma*: Blood was collected from the tail vein of each animal and placed into tubes containing EDTA as an anti-coagulant. Blood was kept on ice and centrifuged to separate the plasma, to which a protease inhibitor was immediately added. HIF-1 was then quantified.

### Real time qPCR

The gene expression of vascular endothelial growth factor (VEGF was analysed by quantitative PCR (qPCR). Cells were lysed using TRIzol (Invitrogen, Life Technologies) and RNA was then extracted and purified. RNA quality and concentration were determined using a NanoDrop ND-1000 (NanoDrop Technologies). Reverse transcription and real-time quantitative PCR (qPCR) were carried out on RNA samples for VEGF and β2-microglobulin (a housekeeping gene not affected by changes in oxygen levels), using TaqMan gene expression assays (Applied Biosystems/Life Technologies). For gene expression quantification, the comparative threshold cycle (ΔΔCt) method was used following the manufacturer's instructions. Results were normalized to β2-microglobulin expression and expressed as arbitrary units using one of the normoxic untreated samples as a calibrator.

For the analysis of rat tissue, RNA was extracted and purified from the frozen artery sections using TRIzol (Invitrogen, Life Technologies). RNA quality and concentrations were determined using a NanoDrop ND-1000 (NanoDrop Technologies). Reverse transcription and real-time quantitative PCR (qPCR) were carried out on RNA samples for VEGF and β2-microglobulin as described earlier.

## Western blotting

Western blotting was used to verify the presence of HIF-1α in some samples. Cells were lysed and the protein content of the lysate quantified as previously described (Heikal et al. 2015). Thirty μg of cellular proteins were separated on a 10% SDS-polyacrylamide gel electrophoresis and transferred onto a nitrocellulose membrane (Amersham/ GE Healthcare Life Sciences, Little Chalfont, Buckinghamshire, UK). After blocking with 5% skimmed milk (for HIF-1α detection) or 5% bovine serum albumin; BSA (for GAPDH detection) for 1 h, membranes were incubated with the appropriate primary antibody overnight, followed by HRP-conjugated secondary antibodies for 1 h at room temperature. HIF-1α and GAPDH (loading control) were detected using rabbit anti-HIF-1α (NB100-479, Novus biologicals, UK) and rabbit anti-GAPDH (14C10, Cell Signaling Technology, UK) at 1:500 and 1:1000 respectively and an anti-rabbit secondary antibody (A0545, Sigma Aldrich, UK) at 1:20,000 dilution. Protein bands were visualized by exposing membranes developed with the ECL reagent (Amersham/ GE Healthcare Life Sciences) to chemiluminescence film (Hyperfilm ECL, Amersham/ GE Healthcare Life Sciences). Bands were quantified using Image J software.

## Immunohistochemistry

Snap frozen carotid arteries were embedded in OCT and were cryo-sectioned (5 μm in thickness) and sections placed onto silane-coated slides. Sections were then washed with PBS and blocked using 10% donkey serum and 0.3% Triton X-100 for 1 h a room temperature, they were incubated with mouse anti-HIF-1α at 1:50 dilution in 1% donkey serum at 4 °C overnight. Donkey anti-mouse IgG-FITC (sc-2099, Santa Cruz Biotechnology, Germany) (1:100 dilution each) was the secondary antibodies used to detect HIF-1 (green stain). For comparing HIF-1α expression in different sections, instrument (fluorescence microscope) settings were kept constant for all sections using uninjured arteries as the control. In another set of experiments, cryo-sliced carotid artery sections were used to visualize endothelial cells (ECs) and smooth muscle cells post injury. Arteries were stained with rabbit anti-CD31 (NB100-2284, Novus biologicals, UK) at 1:50 dilution and mouse anti-alpha smooth muscle actin at 1:50 dilution (NB2-33006, Novus biologicals, UK) followed by Alexafluor 647 conjugated anti-rabbit secondary antibody (red stain) and FITC-conjugated anti-mouse secondary antibody (green stain) respectively at 1:200 dilution each. Cellular nuclei were stained with Prolong® Gold anti-fade reagent with DAPI (P36941, Life technologies, UK). Images were obtained using a fluorescence microscope (Leica CTR 5000).

## Statistical analysis

All data were analyzed using Graph Pad Prism 4 software. Differences in treatment were tested for significance using one-way analysis of variance (ANOVA) followed by a Bonferroni correction for multiple comparisons post-hoc test.

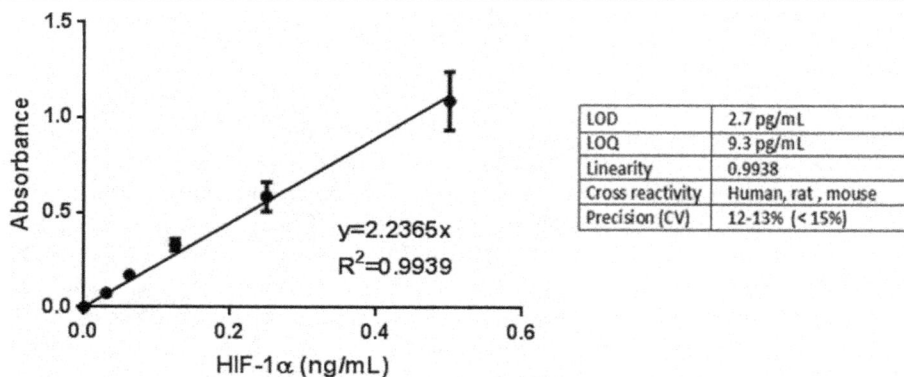

| LOD | 2.7 pg/mL |
| LOQ | 9.3 pg/mL |
| Linearity | 0.9938 |
| Cross reactivity | Human, rat , mouse |
| Precision (CV) | 12-13% (< 15%) |

$y = 2.2365x$
$R^2 = 0.9939$

**Fig. 1** Calibration curve for standard HIF-1α aprotein at concentration range (0–500 ng/mL) using ELISA assay for protein quantification. The calibration curve was used to determine linearity, the limit of detection and quantification as well as inter and intra variability of the assay. Each point represents the mean ± SEM of 6 independent experiments

# Results

## Reliability of the ELISA assay for the quantification of HIF-1α in biological samples

Figure 1 shows the results of a typical standard curve using standard recombinant HIF-1α. The assay was linear between 0 and 1000 pg/ mL ($r = 0.99$). The method was sensitive, with a detection limit of 2.7 pg/ mL. The ELISA had an intra and inter-assay coefficient of variation of < 15% and an accuracy of 99.4% ± 8.3%.

The results of the HIF-1α measurement using the ELISA assay were compared with the findings using the conventional semi-quantitative assay; Western blot. The Western blot in Fig. 2a shows a specific band for the recombinant HIF-1α standard protein at a molecular weight of approximately130 kDa with a band intensity that was concentration dependent and detectable in the range used (6–200 ng/mL). When cell lysates were analyzed by Western blot, we could detect a specific band for HIF-1α at the molecular weight of 130 kDa in addition to a faint degradation band at 80 kDa. (Lidgren et al. 2005; Srinivasan and Dunn 2011) A stronger signal of the higher molecular weight band was detected in cells cultured for 24 in hypoxia. GAPDH was used as a loading control showing a band in each cell lysate at molecular weight 40 kDa.

## Temperature, storage time and presence of protease inhibitors are critical for the stability of HIF-1α

Figure 3a shows the detection of HIF-1α by ELISA in cell lysates kept for 24 h at different temperatures. Storage at -80 °C appears essential for the optimal preservation of the protein. In the experiment shown in Fig. 3b, samples were kept at -80 °C for prolonged periods of time, with and without aprotinin. It is very clear that a protease inhibitor is essential for preventing the degradation of HIF-1α in the stored samples. Other protease inhibitors such as Complete Mini protease inhibitor cocktail (Roche) were tested and showed similar protection against HIF-1α degradation (data not shown).

## Measurement of HIF-1α in cell lysates and plasma samples

HIF-1α was detected in cell lysates treated with DMOG. HIF-1α was measured in cell lysates using the optimized sample collection discussed in the previous section. HIF-1α was induced using DMOG. DMOG caused a significant increase HIF-1α levels when incubated with RAECs for 2 h at a concentration of 100 µM (Fig. 4a) and resulted in transcriptional activation of HIF-1α target genes, increasing the expression of VEGF gene 3–4 fold (Fig. 4b).

## HIF-1α is increased in cell lysate in an in vitro injury model

The kinetics of HIF-1α release was investigated in the scratch assay model. HIF-1α concentrations in the lysate reached a maximum at approximately 2 h post injury, after which they gradually returned to baseline (Fig. 5a). This pattern of HIF-1α levels was mirrored by changes in VEGF gene expression (Fig. 5b).

## Circulating HIF-1α in rats treated with DMOG

HIF-1α was increased in plasma after treatment of the carotid artery with DMOG applied locally at a concentration ranging from 0 and 7.5 mg/Kg in a dose-dependent fashion (Fig. 6a). VEGF gene expression in the treated carotid arteries was consistent with the increased levels of plasma HIF-1α following DMOG administration, but there was no increase in the contralateral, untreated artery (Fig. 6b).

## Circulating HIF-1α after in vivo arterial injury

The kinetics of HIF-1α release was then measured in a rat model of carotid angioplasty, using the optimised conditions for plasma sample collection and storage, prior to analysis using the ELISA method. HIF-1α release reached a maximum at approximately 2 days after injury, and then fell over the next 5 days, but remained above baseline (Fig. 7a). In a separate experiment, we looked at the effect of adding proteinase inhibitors to the blood immediately after collection before plasma

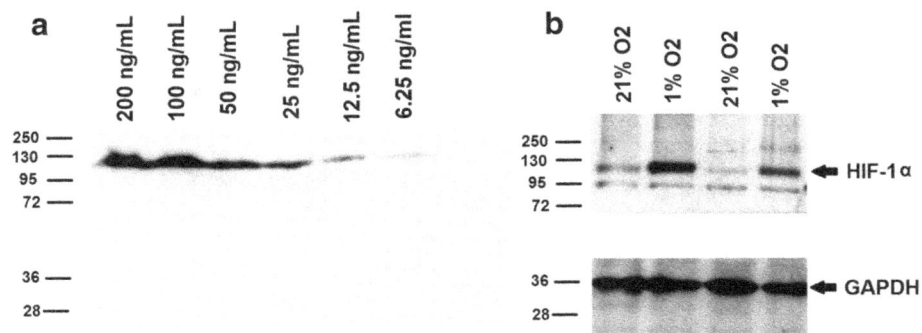

Fig. 2 Western blot analysis of HIF-1α. a Different concentrations of HIF-1α standard protein and b cell lysates from the cells cultured in 21% or 1% O₂. HIF-1α standards and in cell lysates showed a band at a molecular weight of approximately 130 kDa. GAPDH (loading control) showed a band at a molecular weight of approximately 36 kDa. Numbers on the left indicate the migration of molecular weight standards

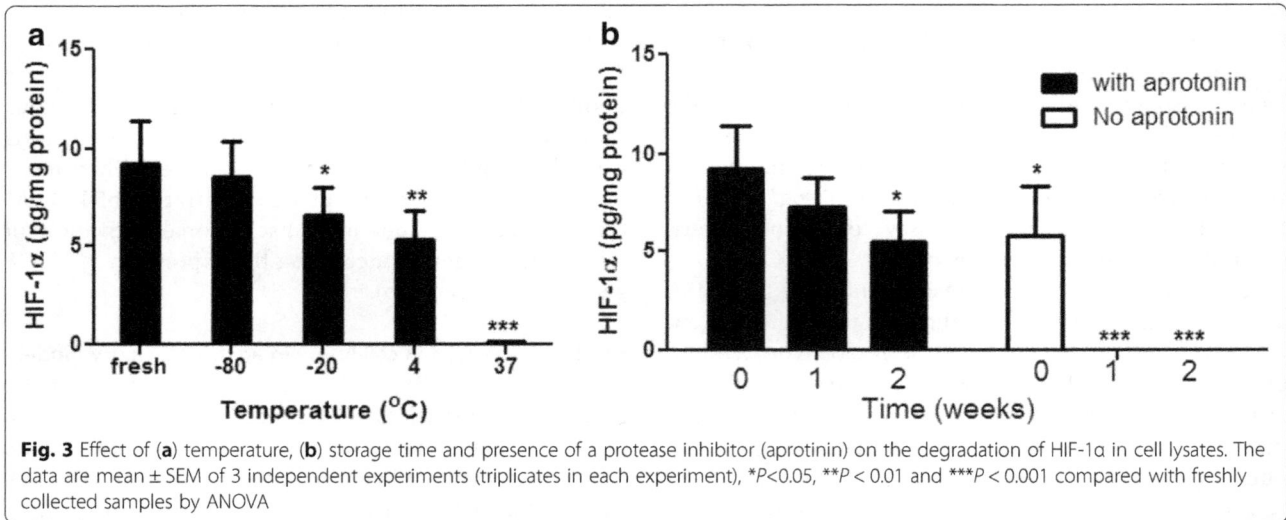

**Fig. 3** Effect of (**a**) temperature, (**b**) storage time and presence of a protease inhibitor (aprotinin) on the degradation of HIF-1α in cell lysates. The data are mean ± SEM of 3 independent experiments (triplicates in each experiment), *$P<0.05$, **$P < 0.01$ and ***$P < 0.001$ compared with freshly collected samples by ANOVA

separation. This has been done by spiking the blood with HIF-1α protein (0.6 ng/mL). Blood samples were then split where protease inhibitor was added to one group after which plasma was separated. In the other group, plasma was separated first prior to the addition of protease inhibitor. Samples were then stored for 48 h prior to analysis. This showed that there was no significant difference between adding the protease inhibitor to the blood immediately after collection or to the plasma after separation and found that this was equally effective. Blood samples were kept on ice after collection and plasma was separated rapidly. Although adding the inhibitor immediately to the blood rather than after plasma separation did not increase the recovery of HIF-1α further (See Additional file 1), this may be more practical in a clinical setting. An increase in local VEGF gene expression in the carotid artery was only observed in

injured arteries reaching a maximum level at 2 days after injury, consistent with changes in plasma HIF-1α, and falling to baseline by the fifth day after injury. Uninjured contralateral arteries from the same rats showed no change in VEGF gene expression (Fig. 7b).

### HIF-1α localization

Tissue HIF-1α levels were also assessed in the injured carotid arteries using immunohistochemistry. An increase was observed in the smooth muscle cells that was maximal 2 days after injury (Fig. 8c) and still detectable at 5 days (Fig. 8d). HIF-1α was co-localised in the smooth muscle cells after injury.

### Discussion

A reliable and sensitive HIF-1α ELISA was established and used to assess the stability of HIF-1α in plasma and

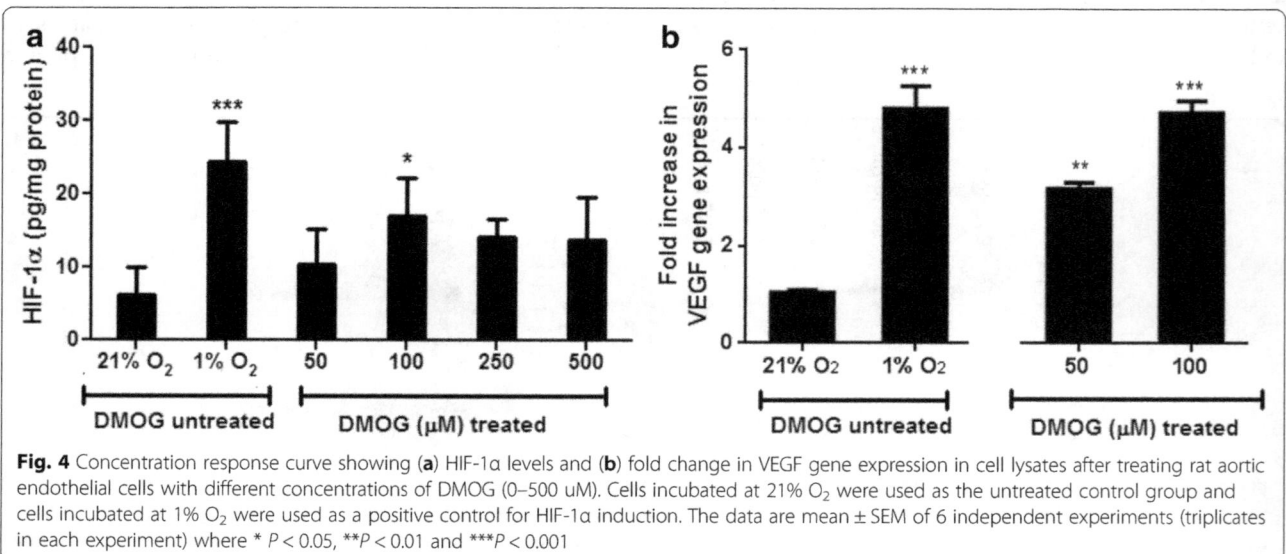

**Fig. 4** Concentration response curve showing (**a**) HIF-1α levels and (**b**) fold change in VEGF gene expression in cell lysates after treating rat aortic endothelial cells with different concentrations of DMOG (0–500 uM). Cells incubated at 21% $O_2$ were used as the untreated control group and cells incubated at 1% $O_2$ were used as a positive control for HIF-1α induction. The data are mean ± SEM of 6 independent experiments (triplicates in each experiment) where * $P < 0.05$, **$P < 0.01$ and ***$P < 0.001$

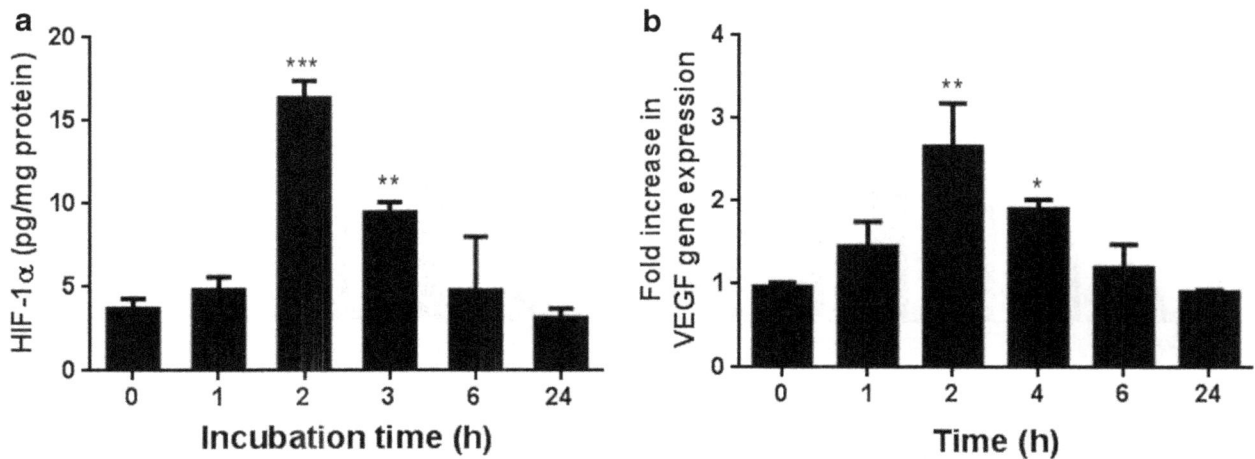

**Fig. 5** Time course of the levels of intracellular HIF-1α (**a**) and VEGF mRNA (**b**) after a scratch assay in vitro. HIF-1α was measured by ELISA and VEGF mRNA by qPCR. HIF-1α levels are expressed as pg/mg protein and VEGF mRNA levels as arbitrary units versus the uninjured samples. Data are the mean ± SEM of 6 samples. $*P < 0.05$, $P** < 0.01$ and $***P < 0.001$

tissue culture medium. Samples could be stored for several days at -80 °C but required the addition of aprotinin. HIF-1α was released following endothelial injury in vitro and in vivo, in the balloon injury model in the rat.

Hypoxia has important effects on intermediary metabolism, cholesterol disposal, and the inflammatory response, and promotes changes in the cellular and extracellular composition of the artery wall that may impact on the response to injury and atherosclerosis. HIF and its down-stream effector gene products have been increasingly recognized for their key role in regulating a wide-spectrum of cellular events, including angiogenesis, cell proliferation, apoptosis and protective response to limit tissue damage (Imtiyaz and Simon 2010; Walshe and D'Amore 2008). There is also increasing evidence that HIF-1α plays a critical role in an early cardioprotective response (Ke and Costa 2006; Tekin et al. 2010), whilst HIF-2α mediates a delayed cardio protective effect, playing an important role in adapting the cells to

chronic hypoxia and injury (Bautista et al. 2009; Ong and Hausenloy 2012). Therefore measurement of HIF-1α rather than HIF-2α may be useful for the assessment of acute disease severity and prognosis.

### The measurement of HIF-1α in plasma and cells

Although HIF-1α is known to be unstable, there have been previous reports of the measurement of HIF-1α in plasma in man and in rats (He et al. 2016b; Li et al. 2015; Xu et al. 2016). However the description of the sample collection and storage procedures are poorly reported in these studies. In this current paper we have confirmed that HIF-1α is indeed unstable, and that careful collection procedures are essential to prevent its degradation. We found that blood samples and cell lysates can be stored for up to two weeks at -80 °C in the presence of protease inhibitors. Whilst we used aprotinin at a final concentration of 300 nM, we found that other protease inhibitors such

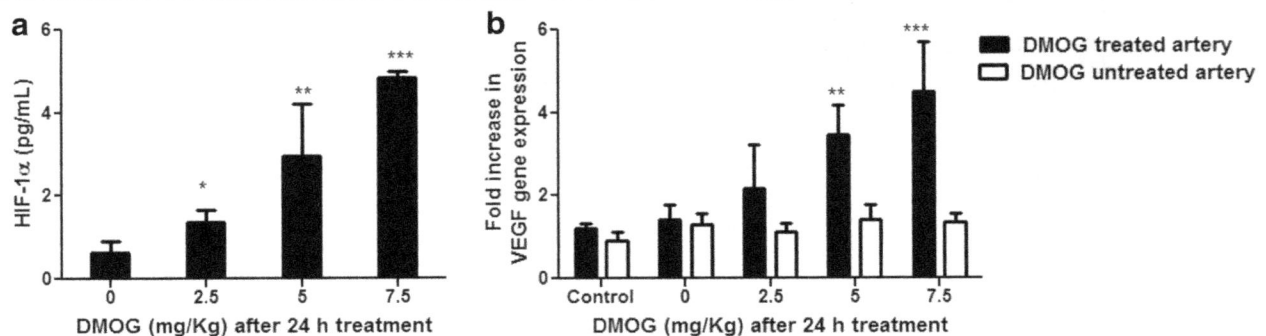

**Fig. 6** Induction of plasma HIF-1α (**a**) and VEGF gene expression in the carotid artery tissue (**b**) after local application of DMOG (0–7.5 mg/Kg) as arbitrary units versus the uninjured samples. Data are the mean ± SEM ($n = 6$), $*P < 0.05$, $**P < 0.01$, $***P < 0.001$

**Fig. 7 a** Increase in plasma HIF-1α in a rat angioplasty model. Plasma levels of HIF-1α, measured by ELISA, increased after injury, reaching a maximum after 48 h. (**b**) VEGF mRNA levels in the injured carotid and the contralateral carotid of the same rats as arbitrary units versus the uninjured samples. Data are mean ± SEM ($n = 6$). *$P < 0.05$, ** $P < 0.01$ and *** $P < 0.001$

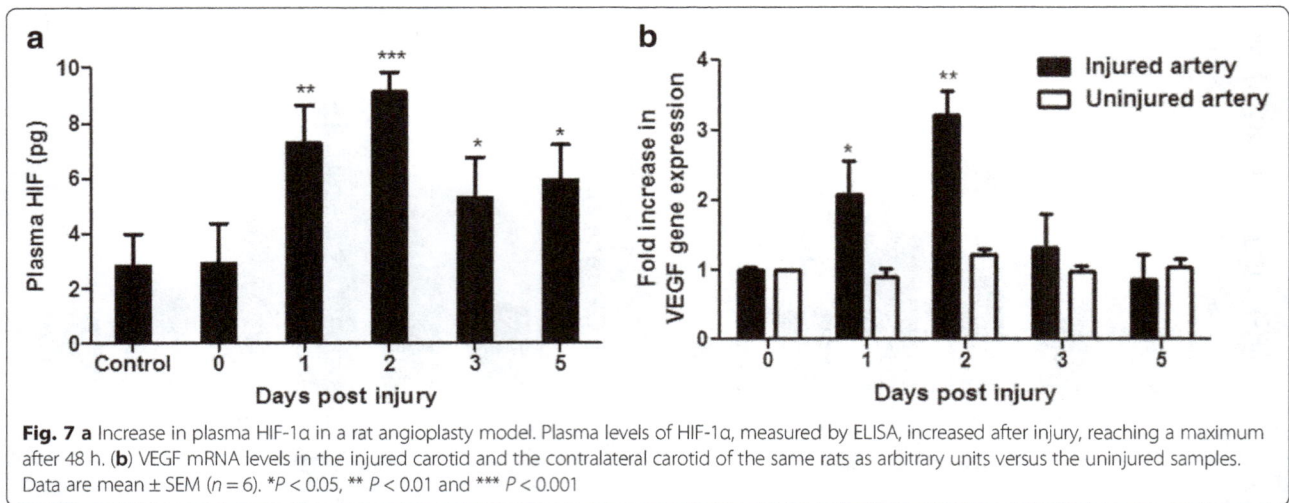

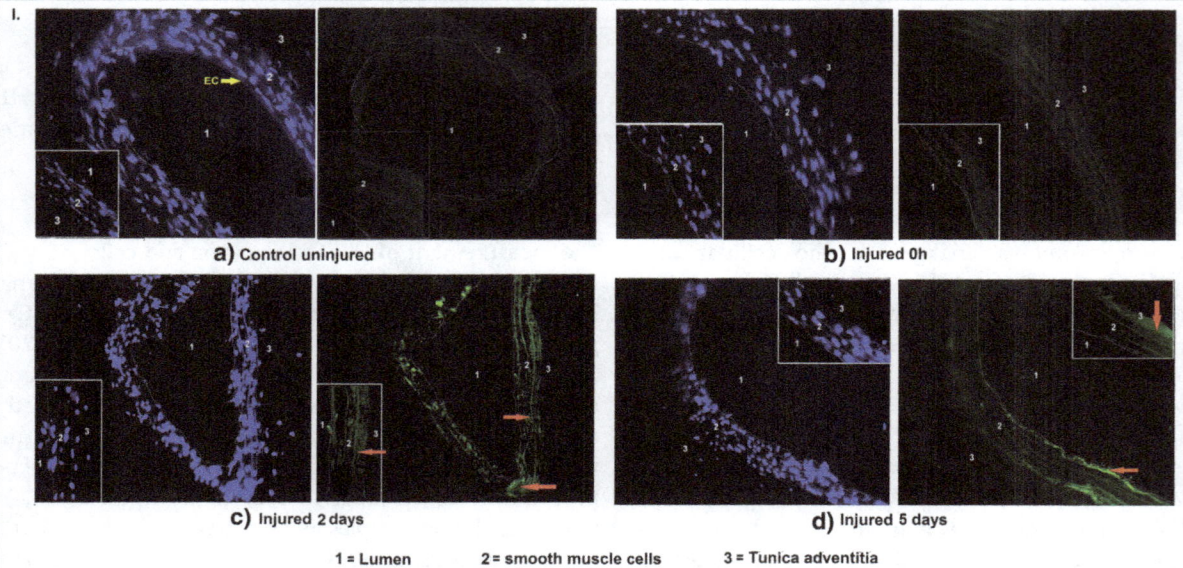

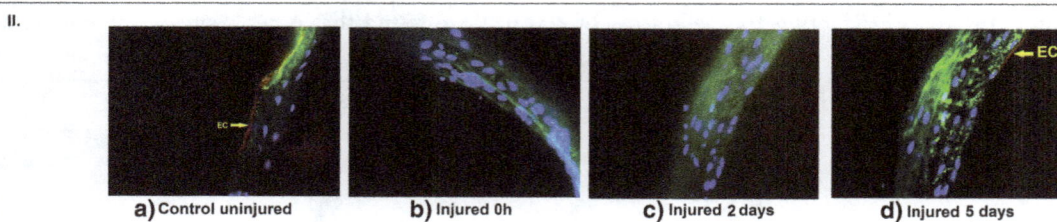

**Fig. 8** Panel I represents immunohistochemistry of (**a**) untreated carotid arteries and injured carotid arteries (**b**) immediately after injury (**c**) 2 days post injury and (**d**) 5 days post injury using a Leica CTR 5000 fluorescence microscope. Arteries were stained with mouse anti-HIF-1α and followed by FITC-conjugated anti-mouse secondary antibody (green stain) to visualize HIF-1α. Nuclei were stained with DAPI (Blue stain). 1 represents the lumen, 2 represents the smooth muscle cells and 3 represents the Tunica adventitia. Images shown are at 40× magnification and 63× magnification (inset images). Red arrows indicate the localization of HIF-1α expression in the smooth muscle cells. Panel II represents the staining of endothelial cells (EC) and smooth muscle cells (SMCs). The yellow arrow indicates EC layer in control (uninjured) arteries which is removed post injury and starts to regenerate 5 days post injury. Arteries were stained with rabbit anti-CD31 and mouse anti-alpha smooth muscle actin followed by Alexafluor 647 conjugated anti-rabbit secondary antibody (red stain) and FITC-conjugated anti-mouse secondary antibody (green stain) to visualize EC and SMCs respectively

as Complete Mini protease inhibitor cocktail tablets (Roche) have a similar effect (data not shown).

The HIF-1α ELISA was robust, of adequate sensitivity and precision for use in biological samples. The values obtained using the ELISA were consistent with Western blot analysis using different HIF-1α antibodies. The measurement of HIF-1α in the in vitro studies was also consistent with expectations: hypoxia and a known HIF-1α inducer increased intracellular HIF-1α levels and down-stream VEGF expression. HIF-1α is involved in regulating the expression of VEGF, which is one of the most potent proangiogenic growth factors (Song et al. 2017). The expression of VEGF was measured to confirm that the levels of HIF-1α in the biological samples were sufficient to cause down-stream signalling.

We observed that there was a transient increase in the expression of HIF-1α and VEGF in a model of rat aortic endothelial cell (RAECs) injury in vitro. The rapid increase in HIF-1α levels from injured RAECs reached a peak level at approximately 2 h post injury in the scratch model. This occurred under normoxic conditions and in the absence of inflammatory cells showing that HIF-1α is directly involved in the adaptive response to cell injury.

### HIF-1α and vascular injury

vIn vivo, DMOG, applied locally to a rat carotid artery, caused a systemic increase in plasma HIF-1α that peaked at 2 days, and was approximately 3-fold higher than baseline values. This was associated with an upregulation of the local, but not the contralateral VEGF arterial tissue expression. HIF-1α appears to be an important mediator of the pro-atherogenic cellular response to hypoxia and is up-regulated in inflammatory and hypoxic areas of carotid arteries in simple and complex lesions from patients with carotid artery disease. In vascular smooth muscle cells, HIF-1α can be activated under normoxic conditions by platelet products such as platelet derived growth factor and thrombin (Gorlach et al. 2001). In the rat carotid balloon injury model, platelets are deposited on the injured artery within minutes of injury, and that they are important in the subsequent formation of the neo-intima (Fingerle et al. 1989). In a murine model of vascular injury, HIF-1α expression was shown to be increased in the smooth muscle cells of the tunica media, as early as 1 day after injury, HIF-1α mRNA expression was induced at 6 h after injury, and its inhibition by the local application of HIF-1α -siRNA reduced neo-intimal area by 49% and significantly decreased the neo-intimal smooth muscle cells content. HIF-1α expression therefore appears to be directly involved in the formation of the neo-intima after vascular injury (Karshovska et al. 2007).

## Conclusions

It is possible to measure HIF-1α in biological samples using an ELISA assay, although careful sample preparation and storage is essential. This may be of value in conditions in which tissue hypoxia may play a role, including cancer, cardiovascular disease and pulmonary disease.

HIF-1α is rapidly up-regulated in an in vitro, wound-healing model, the scratch assay, even in the absence of hypoxia. It is therefore likely to play an important role in orchestrating the response to injury.

The up-regulation of HIF-1α expression and release was more sustained in the rat balloon injury model, where plasma HIF-1α reached its peak concentrations 2 days post injury. The differences in the kinetics of HIF-1α expression and release for the in vitro and in vivo models could be due to the complexity of the in vivo model. The latter model involves several cell types, including VSMS, platelets and inflammatory cells; these may interact to stimulate pathways that could lead to a more sustained HIF release that may have implications for conditions such as coronary atherosclerosis, restenosis and stroke.

## Additional file

**Additional file 1: Figure S1**. Effect of adding the protease inhibitor; aprotinin on HIF-1α levels in plasma when added directly to the blood after collection versus addition to the plasma after separation. Blood was spiked with HIF-1α protein (0.6 ng/mL). Blood samples were then split into two groups where the protease inhibitor was added to one group after which plasma was separated. In the other group, plasma was separated first prior to the addition of protease inhibitor. Data represented are the mean ± SEM of 3 rats (triplicate of each). (DOCX 23 kb)

### Abbreviations
DMOG: Dimethyloxalylglycine; ELISA: Enzyme linked immunosorbent assay; HIF-1α: Hypoxia inducible factor-1 alpha; RAECs: Rat aortic endothelial cells; VEGF: Vascular endothelial growth factor

### Acknowledgements
I would like to acknowledge Willie-Henri Quah, a Junior research associate medical students who did some of the preliminary work for this study.

### Funding
This work has been funded by Brighton and Sussex Medical School.

### Authors' contributions
GF, LH and PG designed the research study. LH performed the research. MM provided help and advice on the ELISA experiments. LH analyzed the data. LH, GF and PG wrote the manuscript. All authors contributed to editorial changes in the manuscript. All authors read and approved the final manuscript.

### Competing interests
The authors declare they have no competing interests as defined by *Molecular Medicine*, or other interests that might be perceived to influence the results and discussion reported in this paper.

## References

Al Okail MS. Cobalt chloride, a chemical inducer of hypoxia-inducible factor-1 alpha in U251 human glioblastoma cell line. Journal of Saudi Chemical Society. 2010;14:197–201. https://doi.org/10.1016/j.jscs.2010.02.005.

Bautista L, Castro MJ, López-Barneo J, Castellano A. Hypoxia inducible factor-2α stabilization and maxi-K+ channel β1-subunit gene repression by hypoxia in cardiac myocytes. Role in preconditioning. Circ Res. 2009;104:1364–72. https://doi.org/10.1161/circresaha.108.190645.

Chu HX, Jones NM. Changes in hypoxia-inducible Factor-1 (HIF-1) and regulatory prolyl hydroxylase (PHD) enzymes following hypoxic-ischemic injury in the neonatal rat. Neurochem Res. 2016;41:515–22. https://doi.org/10.1007/s11064-015-1641-y.

Eubank TD, Marsh CB. HIFs: a-cute answer to inflammation? Blood. 2011;118:485–7. https://doi.org/10.1182/blood-2011-05-355164.

Eubank TD, Roda JM, Liu HW, O'Neil T, Marsh CB. Opposing roles for HIF-1 alpha and HIF-2 alpha in the regulation of angiogenesis by mononuclear phagocytes. Blood. 2011;117:323–32. https://doi.org/10.1182/blood-2010-01-261792.

Ferns GAA, Heikal L. Hypoxia in Atherogenesis. Angiology. 2017;68:472–93. https://doi.org/10.1177/0003319716662423.

Fingerle J, Johnson R, Clowes AW, Majesky MW, Reidy MA. Role of platelets in smooth muscle cell proliferation and migration after vascular injury in rat carotid artery. Proc Natl Acad Sci U S A. 1989;86:8412–6. https://doi.org/10.1073/pnas.86.21.8412.

Formento JL, Berra E, Ferrua B, Magné N, Simos G, Brahimi-Horn C, Pouysségur J, Milano G. Enzyme-Linked Immunosorbent Assay for Pharmacological Studies Targeting Hypoxia-Inducible Factor 1α. Clinical and Diagnostic Laboratory Immunology. 2005;12:660–4. https://doi.org/10.1128/CDLI.12.5.660-664.2005.

Gao LG, Chen Q, Zhou XL, Fan L. The role of hypoxia-inducible factor 1 in atherosclerosis. J Clin Pathol. 2012;65:872–6. https://doi.org/10.1136/jclinpath-2012-200828.

Gorlach A, Diebold I, Schini-Kerth VB, Berchner-Pfannschmidt U, Roth U, Brandes RP, Kietzmann T, Busse R. Thrombin activates the hypoxia-inducible factor-1 signaling pathway in vascular smooth muscle cells role of the p22(phox)-containing NADPH oxidase. Circ Res. 2001;89:47–54. https://doi.org/10.1161/hh1301.092678.

He J, Hu Y, Hu M, Zhang S, Li B. The relationship between the preoperative plasma level of HIF-1α and clinic pathological features, prognosis in non-small cell lung cancer. Sci Rep. 2016a;6:20586. https://doi.org/10.1038/srep20586.

He JB, Hu Y, Hu MM, Zhang SY, Li BL. The relationship between the preoperative plasma level of HIF-1 alpha and clinic pathological features, prognosis in non-small cell lung cancer. Sci Rep. 2016b;6 https://doi.org/10.1038/srep20586.

Heikal L, Ghezzi P, Mengozzi M, Ferns G. Low oxygen tension primes aortic endothelial cells to the reparative effect of tissue-protective cytokines. Mol Med. 2015;21:709–16.

Imtiyaz HZ, Simon MC. Hypoxia-inducible factors as essential regulators of inflammation. Curr Top Microbiol Immunol. 2010;345:105–20. https://doi.org/10.1007/82_2010_74.

Karshovska E, Zernecke A, Sevilmis G, Millet A, Hristov M, Cohen CD, Schmid H, Krotz F, Sohn HY, Klauss V, et al. Expression of HIF-1 alpha in injured arteries controls SDF-1 alpha-mediated neointima formation in apolipoprotein E-deficient mice. Arteriosclerosis Thrombosis and Vascular Biology. 2007;27:2540–7. https://doi.org/10.1161/atvbaha.107.151050.

Ke QD, Costa M. Hypoxia-inducible factor-1 (HIF-1). Mol Pharmacol. 2006;70:1469–80. https://doi.org/10.1124/mol.106.027029.

Kilkenny C, Browne WJ, Cuthill IC, Emerson M, Altman DG. Improving bioscience research reporting: the ARRIVE guidelines for reporting animal research. PLoS Biol. 2010;8:e1000412. https://doi.org/10.1371/journal.pbio.1000412.

Kobayashi M, Inoue K, Warabi E, Minami T, Kodama T. A simple method of isolating mouse aortic endothelial cells. J Atheroscler Thromb. 2005;12:138–42. https://doi.org/10.5551/jat.12.138.

Lambert CM, Roy M, Robitaille GA, Richard DE, Bonnet S. HIF-1 inhibition decreases systemic vascular remodelling diseases by promoting apoptosis through a hexokinase 2-dependent mechanism. Cardiovasc Res. 2010;88:196–204. https://doi.org/10.1093/cvr/cvq152.

Li WL, Wang KJ, Liu ZW, Ding WG. HIF-1 alpha change in serum and callus during fracture healing in ovariectomized mice. Int J Clin Exp Pathol. 2015;8:117–26.

Lidgren A, Hedberg Y, Grankvist K, Rasmuson T, Vasko J, Ljungberg B. The expression of hypoxia-inducible factor 1α is a favorable independent prognostic factor in renal cell carcinoma. Clin Cancer Res. 2005;11:1129–35.

Loboda A, Jozkowicz A, Dulak J. HIF-1 versus HIF-2 - is one more important than the other? Vasc Pharmacol. 2012;56:245–51. https://doi.org/10.1016/j.vph.2012.02.006.

Mosher RA, Coetzee JF, Allen PS, Havel JA, Griffith GR, Wang C. Effects of sample handling methods on substance P concentrations and immunoreactivity in bovine blood samples. Am J Vet Res. 2014;75:109–16. https://doi.org/10.2460/ajvr.75.2.109.

Natarajan R, Salloum FN, Fisher BJ, Ownby ED, Kukreja RC, Fowler AA. Activation of hypoxia-inducible factor-1 via prolyl-4 hydroxylase-2 gene silencing attenuates acute inflammatory responses in postischemic myocardium. Am J Phys Heart Circ Phys. 2007;293:H1571–80. https://doi.org/10.1152/ajpheart.00291.2007.

Ong S-G, Hausenloy DJ. Hypoxia-inducible factor as a therapeutic target for cardioprotection. Pharmacol Ther. 2012;136:69–81. https://doi.org/10.1016/j.pharmthera.2012.07.005.

Park SR, Kinders RJ, Khin S, Hollingshead M, Antony S, Parchment RE, Tomaszewski JE, Kummar S, Doroshow JH. Validation of a hypoxia-inducible factor-1α specimen collection procedure and quantitative ELISA in solid tumor tissues. Anal Biochem. 2014;459:1–11. https://doi.org/10.1016/j.ab.2014.04.025.

Semenza GL. Hypoxia-inducible factor 1 and cardiovascular disease. In: Julius D, editor. Annual review of physiology, vol. 76; 2014. p. 39–56.

Song SL, Xiao XY, Guo D, Mo LQ, Bu C, Ye WB, Den QW, Liu ST, Yang XX. Protective effects of Paeoniflorin against AOPP-induced oxidative injury in HUVECs by blocking the ROS-HIF-1 alpha/VEGF pathway. Phytomedicine. 2017;34:115–26. https://doi.org/10.1016/j.phymed.2017.08.010.

Srinivasan S, Dunn JF. Stabilization of hypoxia-inducible factor-1α in buffer containing cobalt chloride for western blot analysis. Anal Biochem. 2011;416:120–2. https://doi.org/10.1016/j.ab.2011.04.037.

Tekin D, Dursun AD, Xi L. Hypoxia inducible factor 1 (HIF-1) and cardioprotection. Acta Pharmacol Sin. 2010;31:1085–94. https://doi.org/10.1038/aps.2010.132.

Tulis DA. Rat carotid artery balloon injury model. Methods in molecular medicine. 2007;139:1.

Walshe TE, D'Amore PA. The role of hypoxia in vascular injury and repair. Annual Review of Pathology: Mechanisms of Disease. 2008;3:615–43. https://doi.org/10.1146/annurev.pathmechdis.3.121806.151501.

Xu M, Zhang Y, Tang L, Huang H. Concentration analysis of hypoxia-inducible factor-1 alpha and vascular endothelial growth factor in patients with aortic aneurysm at different stages and its clinical significance. Cell Mol Biol. 2016;62:73–6.

Zhang S, Ma K, Liu YW, Pan XB, Chen QM, Qi L, Li SJ. Stabilization of hypoxia-inducible factor by DMOG inhibits development of chronic hypoxia-induced right ventricular remodeling. J Cardiovasc Pharmacol. 2016;67:68–75. https://doi.org/10.1097/fjc.0000000000000315.

# 5

# AEG-1 is involved in hypoxia-induced autophagy and decreases chemosensitivity in T-cell lymphoma

Jiaqin Yan[1], Junhui Zhang[2], Xudong Zhang[1], Xin Li[1], Ling Li[1], Zhaoming Li[1], Renyin Chen[3], Lei Zhang[1], Jingjing Wu[1], Xinhua Wang[1], Zhenchang Sun[1], Xiaorui Fu[1], Yu Chang[1], Feifei Nan[1], Hui Yu[1], Xiaolong Wu[1], Xiaoyan Feng[1], Wencai Li[3] and Mingzhi Zhang[1]*

## Abstract

**Background:** This study was to examine the link between astrocyte elevated gene-1 (AEG-1) and hypoxia induced-chemoresistance in T-cell non-Hodgkin's lymphoma (T-NHL), as well as the underlying molecular mechanisms.

**Methods:** Expression of AEG-1, LC3-II, and Beclin-1 were initially examined in human T-NHL tissues ($n = 30$) and normal lymph node tissues ($n = 16$) using western blot, real-time PCR and immunohistochemistry. Western blot was also performed to analyze the expression of AEG-1, LC3-II, and Beclin-1 in T-NHL cells (Hut-78 and Jurkat cells) under normoxia and hypoxia. Additionally, the proliferation and apoptosis of Hut-78 cells exposed to different concentration of Adriamycin (ADM) in normoxia and hypoxia were evaluated by MTT and Annexin-V FITC/PI staining assay. Finally, the effects of AEG-1 on Hut-78 cells exposed to ADM in hypoxia were assessed by MTT and Annexin-V FITC/PI staining assay, and 3-MA (autophagy inhibitor) was further used to determine the underlying mechanism.

**Results:** AEG-1, LC3-II and Beclin-1 expression were significantly increased in T-NHL tissues compared with normal tissues. Incubation of Hut-78 and Jurkat cells in hypoxia obviously increased AEG-1, LC3-II and Beclin-1 expression. Hypoxia induced proliferation and reduced apoptosis of Hut-78 cells exposed to ADM. AEG-1 overexpression further increased proliferation and decreased apoptosis of Hut-78 cells exposed to ADM in hypoxia. Moreover, overexpression of AEG-1 significantly inversed 3-MA induced-changes in cell proliferation and apoptosis of Hut-78 cells exposed to ADM in hypoxia.

**Conclusions:** This study suggested that AEG-1 is associated with hypoxia-induced T-NHL chemoresistance via regulating autophagy, uncovering a novel target against hypoxia-induced T-NHL chemoresistance.

**Keywords:** Astrocyte elevated gene-1 (AEG-1), T-cell non-Hodgkin's lymphoma (T-NHL), Hypoxia, Autophagy, Chemosensitivity

## Background

The lymphoma, a type of blood cancer, is roughly classified as Hodgkin's lymphoma (HD) and non-Hodgkin's lymphoma (NHL), and NHL represents the most common malignancy (Hadzipecova et al., 2007). T-cell lymphoma (T-NHL) accounts for approximately 15% of NHL in the United States (Tian et al., 2016). Currently, chemotherapy still remains the major choice for the treatment of T-NHL, especially at the advanced stages, but T-NHL is not that sensitive to conventional chemotherapy (R et al., 1987). These chemotherapy options ultimately yield poor outcomes in T-NHL patients, mainly resulted from the chemoresistance development of T-NHL. Actually, more than 90% of deaths from cancer are associated with drug resistance and metastasis (Ahmad et al., 2012).

* Correspondence: mingzhi_zhang@sohu.com
[1]Department of Oncology, The First Affiliated Hospital, Zhengzhou University, No. 1 Jianshe East Road, Zhengzhou, Henan 450052, People's Republic of China
Full list of author information is available at the end of the article

Hypoxia is a common characteristic in solid tumors (Zhang et al., 2016a). Hypoxic environment triggers various adaptive responses in hepatocellular carcinoma (HCC) to survival in tough environment, and it provides a strong selective pressure for the survival of HCC, which results in the "survival of the fittest" and elimination of the inferior (Bogaerts et al., 2015; Zhang et al., 2016b). Reports also revealed that HCC cells in hypoxia are more resistant to chemotherapy than the cells growing in normoxia (Bogaerts et al., 2015; Zhang et al., 2016b; Lionel et al., 2012). Hypoxia in the tumor microenvironment is the major cause of drug resistance in cancer chemotherapy (Cosse & Michiels, 2008), but the mechanism by which hypoxia induces drug resistance in tumors is unclear. Several studies have shown that this process is mediated by autophagy. Song et al. (Song et al., 2009) found that autophagy was a protective way to participate in HCC chemotherapy resistance under hypoxic conditions, and chemotherapy induced-cell death in hypoxia was less than that in normoxia. They also observed that autophagy was significantly increased in hypoxia, and inhibition of autophagy by 3-MA or RNA interference increased cell death and improved drug resistance. In normoxia, antitumor drug 4-HPR resulted in cell death by inducing the apoptosis; while in hypoxia, 4-HPR induced autophagy, and 3-MA or chloroquine further enhanced apoptosis and reduced the survival of cells exposed to 4-HPR, suggesting that autophagy can prevent tumor cell death and may induce hypoxia-induced drug resistance to 4-HPR (Liu et al., 2011; XW et al., 2010). These studies fully demonstrate that autophagy is involved in the process of resistance induced by hypoxia.

Astrocyte elevated gene-1 (AEG-1) was initially cloned as neuropathology related gene in primary human embryos astrocytes in 2002 (Kang, 2002). Several researches have demonstrated the important role of AEG-1 in the progression of different tumors, including proliferation, metastasis, chemoresistance, and angiogenesis (Chang et al., 2016; X M & KK, 2013). Autophagy can be reflected by monitoring the accumulation of autophagy marker LC3- II. Silencing AEG-1 in a variety of tumor cell lines reduced LC3- II accumulation and restored chemosensitivity (Bhutia et al., 2010; Zou et al., 2016; Xie & Zhong, 2016). Besides, hypoxia inducible factor (HIF-1α) promoted AEG-1 expression by binding to the AEG-1 promoter (Zhao et al., 2017). However, it is unclear whether AEG1 participates in the regulation of autophagy and chemoresistance induced by hypoxia in T-NHL.

## Methods
### Tissue samples
Patients who were diagnosed with T-NHL at The First Affiliated Hospital of Zhengzhou University were included

in the study after obtaining their oral and written informed consent. The biopsy specimens of patients ($n = 30$) were prepared by the Department of Clinical Pathology for paraffin-embedded tumor tissue sections. The control group consisted of 16 samples of lymph node that were obtained from normal lymph nodes in the disused tissues after standard operations, and the candidates were excluded from all kinds of tumors. This study was reviewed and approved by the Ethics Committee of the Medical Faculty at the First Affiliated Hospital of Zhengzhou University (Scientific Research-2017-LW-73).

### Cell culture and treatment
T-NHL cell lines (Hut-78 and Jurkat) were obtained from the Cell Bank of Chinese Academy of Science (Shanghai, China). Cells were cultured in RPMI-1640 medium supplemented with 10% heat-inactivated FBS (fetal bovine serum), 50 U/ml penicillin and 50 U/ml streptomycin (Sigma-Aldrich, St. Louis, MO, USA) at 37 °C in a humidified atmosphere containing 5% CO2.

Hypoxia treatment was performed by placing the cells in a sealed chamber (Thermo Forma) filled with mixture gases of 1% O2, 5% CO2, and 94% N2.

### Plasmid construction and cell transfection
The pcDNA3.1 vector was purchased from Invitrogen (USA). PcDNA3.1-AEG-1, a plasmid containing AEG-1, was constructed by Invitrogen (USA). The plasmid constructs carrying siRNA against AEG-1 and HIF-1α were designed and constructed as previously described (Yan et al., 2012) . Hut-78 and Jurkat cells were seeded in six-well plates at a density of $1 \times 10^6$ cells per well. Subsequently, the transfection was performed by Lipofectamine™ 2000 (Invitrogen, USA) according to the manufacturer's instructions. The stable transfection cells were verified for RT-PCR and western blot analysis.

### Immunohistochemical assay
Standard immunoperoxidase procedures were used to visualize AEG-1 and LC3-II expression, as previously described (Yan et al., 2012). Briefly, paraffin sections were deparaffinized in xylene, followed by a graded series of alcohols (100, 95 and 75%) and re-hydrated in water followed by Tris-buffered saline. Following antigen retrieval, slides were incubated with 3% $H_2O_2$ to prevent endogenous peroxidase. Then slides were blocked with 5% normal serum and incubated with anti-AEG-1 and anti- LC3-II antibody. After washing, the tissue sections were treated with biotinylated anti-rabbit secondary antibody (Zymed Laboratories Inc., South San Francisco, CA, USA), followed by further incubation with streptavidin-horseradish peroxidase complex (Zymed). Tissue sections were then

immersed in 3, 3′-diaminobenzidine and counterstained with 10% Mayer's hematoxylin, dehydrated and mounted.

### RNA extraction, reverse transcription and real-time PCR

Total-RNA from cultured cells was extracted using the TRIzol reagent according to the manufacturer's instructions. The cDNA synthesis was performed in accordance with the protocol of the Takara Reverse Transcription System for real-time PCR [Takara Biotechnology (Dalian) Co., Ltd., China] with 2 μg RNA and reverse transcription performed with random primers. Real-time PCR primers were designed according to http://www.ncbi.nlm.nih.gov. The sequences of the PCR primers used were as follows: AEG-1, forward 5′-CGGTACCCCGGCTGGGTGAT-3′ and reverse 5′-CTCCTCCG CTTTTTGCGGGC-3′; HIF-1α, forward 5′-GTCGGACAGCCTCACCAAACAG AG C-3′and reverse 5′-GTTAACTTGATCCAAAGCT CTGAG-3′; GAPDH, forward 5′-CGGAGTCAACGGAT TTGGTCGTATTGG-3′ and reverse 5′-GCTCCTGGA AGA TGGTGATGGGATTTCC-3′. Real-time PCR analysis was carried out on a LightCycler real-time PCR instrument using SYBR Green I kit (Tiangen Biotech Co., Ltd., Beijing, China) according to the manufacturer's instructions. Each reaction was carried out in triplicate. Data were analyzed using the $2^{-\Delta\Delta Ct}$ method as described elsewhere (Fan et al., 2005).

### Western blotting assay

Total proteins were extracted by lysing cells in buffer (50 mM Tris pH 7.4, 150 mM NaCl, 0.5% NP-40, 50 mM NaF, 1 mM $Na_3VO_4$, 1 mM phenylmethylsulfonyl fluoride, 25 mg/ml leupeptin and 25 mg/ml aprotinin). The lysates were cleared by centrifugation and the supernatants were collected. Proteins were extracted using the protein extraction kit following the manufacturer's instructions. Protein concentration was determined using protein assay reagent (Bio-Rad, Hercules, CA, USA). Equal amounts of protein were separated on SDS-PAGE, transferred to PVDF membranes, incubated with antibodies against AEG-1, HIF-1α, LC3-I, LC3-II, Beclin-1, and GAPDH, followed by incubation with the secondary antibodies. The membrane was then washed three times and visualized with diaminobenzidine. Quantification of the proteins was detected with the ECL system (Pierce Biotechnology Inc., Rockford, IL, USA). Each value represents the mean of triple experiments, and is presented as the relative density of protein bands normalized to GAPDH.

### MTT cell viability assay

MTT assay was carried out as previously described (Yan et al., 2012). Cells were seeded in a 96-well plate at a concentration of $2.5 \times 10^4$/ml (100 μl/well). Six parallel wells were assigned to each group. Then, 20 μl/well of 5 mg/ml MTT (3-(4,5-dimethylthiazol-2-yl)-2,5-diphenyl-tetrazolium bromide) was added at different time after seeding and were then incubated for another 4 h. The supernatant was removed and the product converted from MTT was dissolved by adding 150 μl/well dimethylsulfoxide (DMSO). The plate was gently shaken for 15 min at room temperature and an enzyme-linked immunosorbent assay reader was used to measure the absorbance of each well at 570 nm.

### Annexin V-FITC flow cytometric analysis

Annexin V-FITC apoptosis detection kit (BD Biosciences, San Jose, CA, USA) was adopted to detect early apoptosis, as previously described (Yan et al., 2012). Briefly, after culturing for 48 h, each group of cells was harvested, washed twice with pre-chilled PBS and resuspended in binding buffer (HEPES-NaOH 10 mM pH 7.4, 144 mM NaCl and 25 mM $CaCl_2$) at a concentration of $1 \times 10^6$ cells/ml. One hundred microliters of this solution ($1 \times 10^5$ cells) was mixed with 5 μl of Annexin V-FITC and 5 μl of PI (BD Biosciences) according to the manufacturer's instructions. The mixed solution was gently vortexed and incubated in the dark at room temperature (25 °C) for 15 min. Four hundred microliters of 1X dilution buffer were added to each tube and cell apoptosis analysis was performed by flow cytometry (BD FACSCalibur) within 1 h. At least 10,000 events were recorded and represented as dot plots.

### Statistical analysis

The SPSS13.0 software (SPSS, Inc., Chicago, IL, USA) was used for all statistical analyses, and results are expressed as mean ± SEM. The comparison between two groups was evaluated by Student's t test; the comparison between multiple groups was performed using one-way analysis of variance (ANOVA), followed by the Tukey's test. Results were considered statistically significant at $P < 0.05$.

## Results

### AEG-1, LC3-II, Beclin-1, and HIF-1α are significantly up-regulated in T-NHL tissues

To examine the expression of AEG-1 in T-NHL, tumor tissues ($n = 30$) and normal lymph node tissues ($n = 16$) were first employed and analyzed by RT-PCR and western blot. AEG-1 expression was significantly up-regulated in tumor tissues compared with normal tissues, both in mRNA (Fig. 1a) and protein levels (Fig. 1b). Western blot analysis also revealed the elevated levels of autophagy-related markers LC3-II and Beclin-1 in T-NHL tissues (Fig. 1b). Additionally, HIF-1α level was also elevated in T-NHL tissues (Fig. 1b). Immunohistochemical staining further confirmed high levels of AEG-1 and LC3-II in T-NHL tissues, which were rarely detected in normal tissues (Fig. 1c).

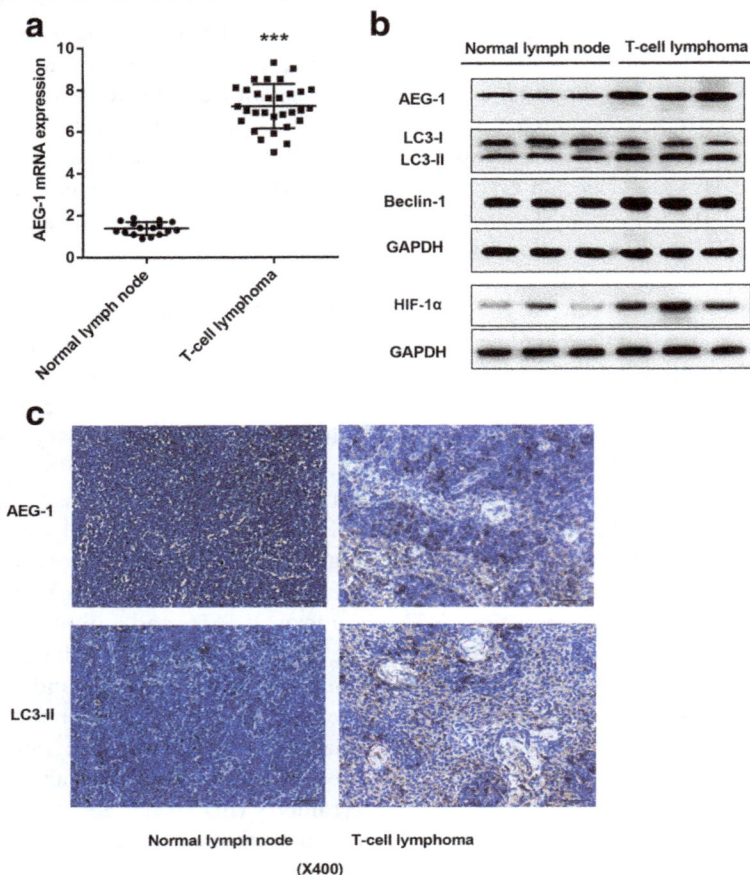

**Fig. 1** Relative expression of AEG-1, Beclin-1 and LC3-II in T-NHL tissues and normal lymphoid tissues. **a** Detection of AEG-1 in 30 T-NHL tissues and 16 normal lymphoid tissues using RT-PCR. **b** Expression of AEG-1, Beclin-1, LC3-I, LC3-II and HIF-1α were detected by western blot. **c** AEG-1 and LC3-II were detected by immunohistochemical assay. Bar = 20 μm. ***$p < 0.001$, T-NHL tissues vs. normal lymphoid tissues

## Hypoxia triggers expression of AEG-1, LC3-II and Beclin-1 in T-NHL cells

To understand the effects of hypoxia on AEG-1 expression and autophagy in T-NHL, we detected the expression of AEG-1, LC3-II and Beclin-1 in hypoxia via western blot assay. Jurkat and Hut-78 cells were incubated in normoxia or hypoxia for 0, 12, 24, 48 and 72 h, respectively. The expression of AEG-1, LC3-II and Beclin-1 was much higher in hypoxia than normoxia at 12, 24, 48 and 72 h, both in Jurkat (Fig. 2a) and Hut-78 (Fig. 2b) cells. Quantitation analysis of western blot further confirmed up-regulated expression of AEG-1 (Fig. 2c), LC3-II (Fig. 2d) and Beclin-1 (Fig. 2e) as well as LC3-II/LC3-I ratio (Fig. 2f) in hypoxia, but not in normoxia in Jurkat cells. Similar results were also observed in Hut-78 cells (Fig. 2g-j). Additionally, the positive control for authophagy under starvation conditions further demonstrated that hypoxia induced authophagy in T-NHL cells through the detection of LC3-I, LC3-II and Beclin-1 expression (Additional file 1).

## Knocking down HIF-1α inhibits expression of AEG-1, LC3-II and Beclin-1 in T-NHL cells under hypoxia

Transcriptional factor HIF-1α is a master regulator upon hypoxia, and it has been reported that HIF-1α promoted AEG-1 expression by binding to its promoter (Zhao et al., 2017). Here, to further elucidate the detailed role of HIF-1α in T-NHL under hypoxia, HIF-1α was first silenced in Jurkat (Fig. 3a) and Hut-78 (Fig. 3b) cells, and RT-PCR was performed to assess transfection efficiency. Moreover, western blot results revealed that AEG-1, LC3-II and Beclin-1 expression as well as LC3-II/LC3-I ratio were remarkably decreased in Jurkat cells transfected with HIF-1α siRNA under hypoxia (Fig. 3c-e). Similarly, under the hypoxic condition, Hut-78 cells transfected with HIF-1α siRNA exhibited the same trend (Fig. 3f-h).

## AEG-1 reduces chemosensitivity of Hut-78 cells under hypoxia

Hut-78 cells were first treated with different doses of ADM under normoxia and hypoxia for 24 h. MTT assay

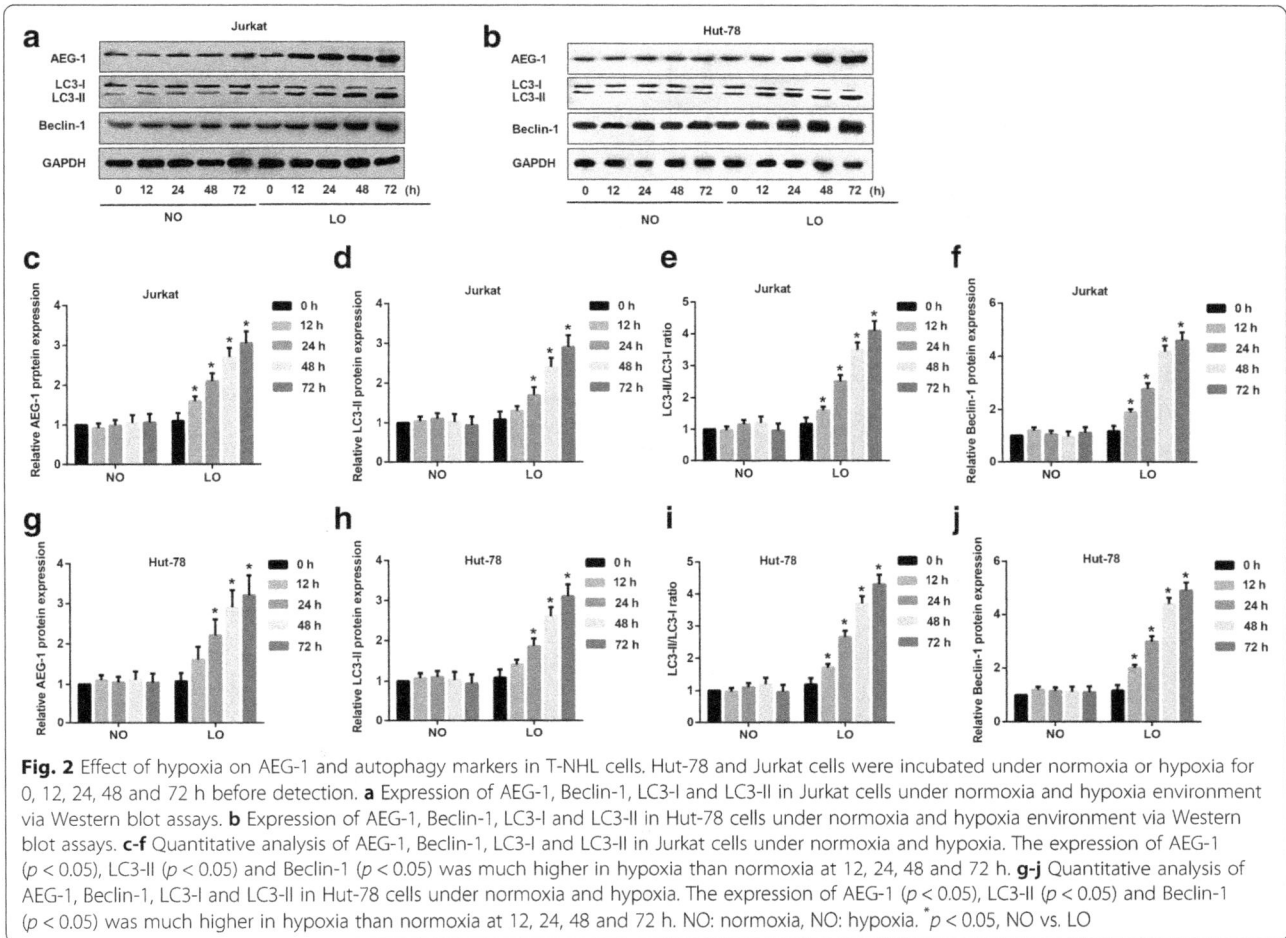

**Fig. 2** Effect of hypoxia on AEG-1 and autophagy markers in T-NHL cells. Hut-78 and Jurkat cells were incubated under normoxia or hypoxia for 0, 12, 24, 48 and 72 h before detection. **a** Expression of AEG-1, Beclin-1, LC3-I and LC3-II in Jurkat cells under normoxia and hypoxia environment via Western blot assays. **b** Expression of AEG-1, Beclin-1, LC3-I and LC3-II in Hut-78 cells under normoxia and hypoxia environment via Western blot assays. **c-f** Quantitative analysis of AEG-1, Beclin-1, LC3-I and LC3-II in Jurkat cells under normoxia and hypoxia. The expression of AEG-1 ($p < 0.05$), LC3-II ($p < 0.05$) and Beclin-1 ($p < 0.05$) was much higher in hypoxia than normoxia at 12, 24, 48 and 72 h. **g-j** Quantitative analysis of AEG-1, Beclin-1, LC3-I and LC3-II in Hut-78 cells under normoxia and hypoxia. The expression of AEG-1 ($p < 0.05$), LC3-II ($p < 0.05$) and Beclin-1 ($p < 0.05$) was much higher in hypoxia than normoxia at 12, 24, 48 and 72 h. NO: normoxia, NO: hypoxia. $^*p < 0.05$, NO vs. LO

revealed that ADM dose-dependently decreased cell viability both in normoxia and hypoxia, while cell viability in hypoxia was much higher than that in normoxia (Fig. 4a). In contrast, cell apoptosis was significantly increased in a dose-dependent manner both in normoxia and hypoxia, but the apoptosis of cells incubated in hypoxia was signally decreased compared with that in normoxia (Fig. 4b). These results indicated that hypoxia attenuated the response of Hut-78 cells to ADM. Then RT-PCR was performed to assess the transfection efficiency of pcDNA3.1-AEG-1 and AEG-1 siRNA in Hut-78 cells. AEG-1 expression was significantly increased in cells transfected with pcDNA3.1-AEG-1, but that was significantly decreased in cells transfected with AEG-1 siRNA (Fig. 4c). Besides, western blot revealed that AEG-1 overexpression markedly up-regulated Beclin-1 expression and LC3-II/LC3-I ratio, but those were significantly down-regulated in cells transfected with AEG-1 siRNA, both in normoxia and hypoxia (Fig. 4d). In contrast, p62 expression was markedly down-regulated in cells with AEG-1 overexpression, but AEG-1 siRNA significantly up-regulated p62 expression, both in normoxia

and hypoxia (Fig. 4d). Especially, Beclin-1 expression and LC3-II/LC3-I ratio in hypoxia were prominently increased, while p62 expression in hypoxia were prominently decreased in comparison to normoxia (Fig. 4d). Further, under hypoxic conditions, AEG-1 overexpression signally enhanced the viability of Hut-78 cells following ADM treatment (Fig. 4e), while cell apoptosis was noteworthy reduced (Fig. 4f). These results indicated that AEG-1 blunted sensitivity of Hut-78 cells to ADM in hypoxia.

## AEG-1 reduces chemosensitivity of Hut-78 cells by promoting autophagy under hypoxia

To illuminate the underlying mechanisms by which AEG-1 reduced the response of Hut-78 cells to ADM in hypoxia, 3-MA (10 mM, autophagy inhibitor) was employed (Nakanishi et al., 2016). MTT assay showed that inhibition of autophagy under hypoxia significantly decreased cell viability after ADM treatment, while AEG-1 partly improved the inhibition of cell viability by 3-MA (Fig. 5a). AEG-1 also significantly reversed the

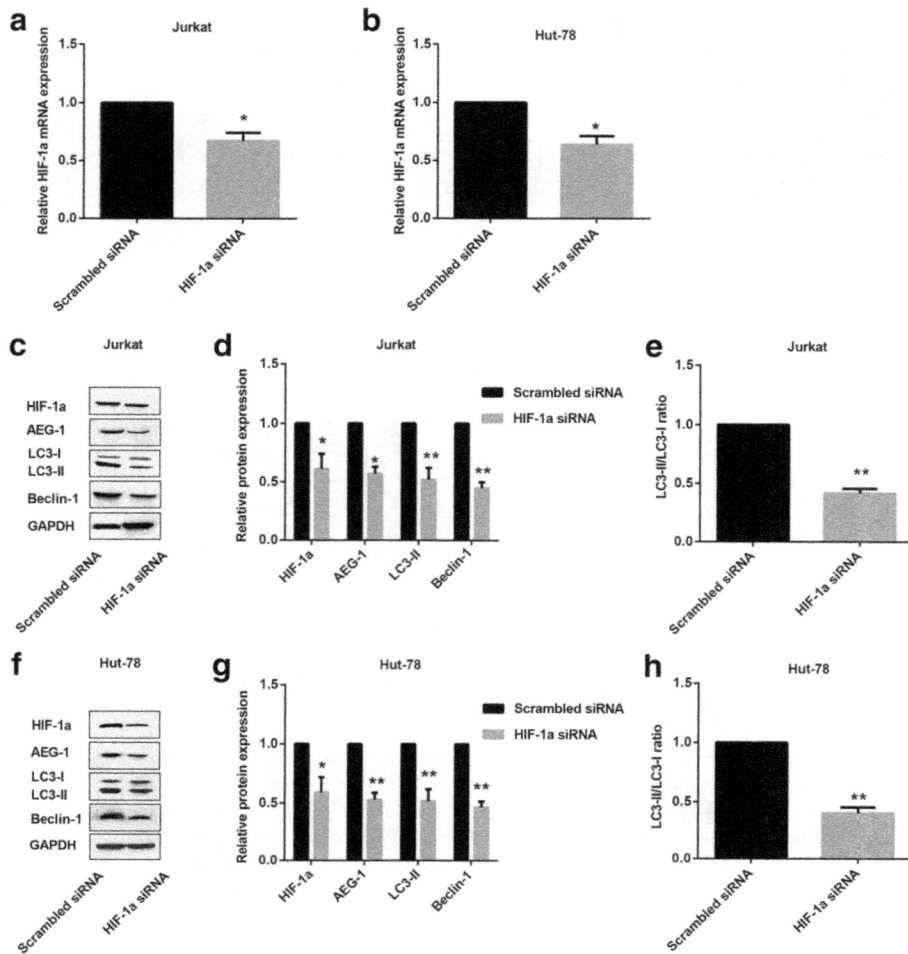

**Fig. 3** Effect of HIF-1α on AEG-1 and autophagy markers in T-NHL cells exposed to hypoxia. HIF-1α siRNA and the negative control (Scrambled siRNA) were transfected into Hut-78 and Jurkat cells, respectively. The mRNA expression of HIF-1α in Jurkat cells (**a**, $p < 0.05$) and Hut-78 cells (**b**, $p < 0.05$) were measured with RT-PCR. **c** Expression of HIF-1α, AEG-1, Beclin-1, LC3-I and LC3-II in Jurkat cells were detected by western blot. **d** Quantitative analysis of HIF-1α ($p < 0.05$), AEG-1 ($p < 0.05$), Beclin-1 ($p < 0.01$) and LC3-II ($p < 0.01$) in Jurkat cells. **e** Quantitative analysis of ratio of LC3-II/LC3-I ($p < 0.01$) in Jurkat cells. **f** Expression of HIF-1α, AEG-1, Beclin-1, LC3-I and LC3-II in Hut-78 cells were detected by western blot. **g** Quantitative analysis of HIF-1α ($p < 0.05$), AEG-1 ($p < 0.01$), Beclin-1 ($p < 0.01$) and LC3-II ($p < 0.01$) in Hut-78 cells. **h** Quantitative analysis of ratio of LC3-II/LC3-I ($p < 0.01$) in Hut-78 cells. $^*p < 0.05$, $^{**}p < 0.01$. HIF-1α siRNA vs.Scrambled siRNA

up-regulation of cell apoptosis induced by 3-MA in Hut-78 cells exposed to ADM under hypoxia (Fig. 5b).

## Discussion

Increasing evidence suggests that AEG-1 acts as an oncogene and is involved in many aspects of tumorigenesis, including protection from serum starvation-induced apoptosis, promoted tumor growth, angiogenesis and migration (Emdad et al., 2009; Emdad et al., 2007). High expression of AEG-1 has been reported in ovarian cancer tissues compared to normal ovarian tissues (Blanco et al., 2011). Besides, microarray analysis also confirmed that AEG-1 is associated with the regulation of chemoresistance (Meng et al., 2013). Actually, AEG-1 has been verified to be up-regulated in T-NHL and is associated

with tumor growth in our previous study (Yan et al., 2012), but its effect on chemosensitivity in T-NHL is not understood.

The present study found that AEG-1 expression was remarkably increased in T-NHL specimens, which has been reported in our previous study (Yan et al., 2012). Besides, LC3-II and Beclin-1 were also remarkably increased in T-NHL specimens. In addition, AEG-1, LC3-II, and Beclin-1 were obviously induced in T-NHL cells in hypoxia. Hypoxia is also an important factor in promoting drug resistance. It can also be obtained that hypoxia blunted the response of Hut-78 cells to ADM, and overexpression of AEG-1 further enhanced the resistance of Hut-78 cells to ADM in hypoxia, as evidenced by cell viability and apoptosis assays. Above

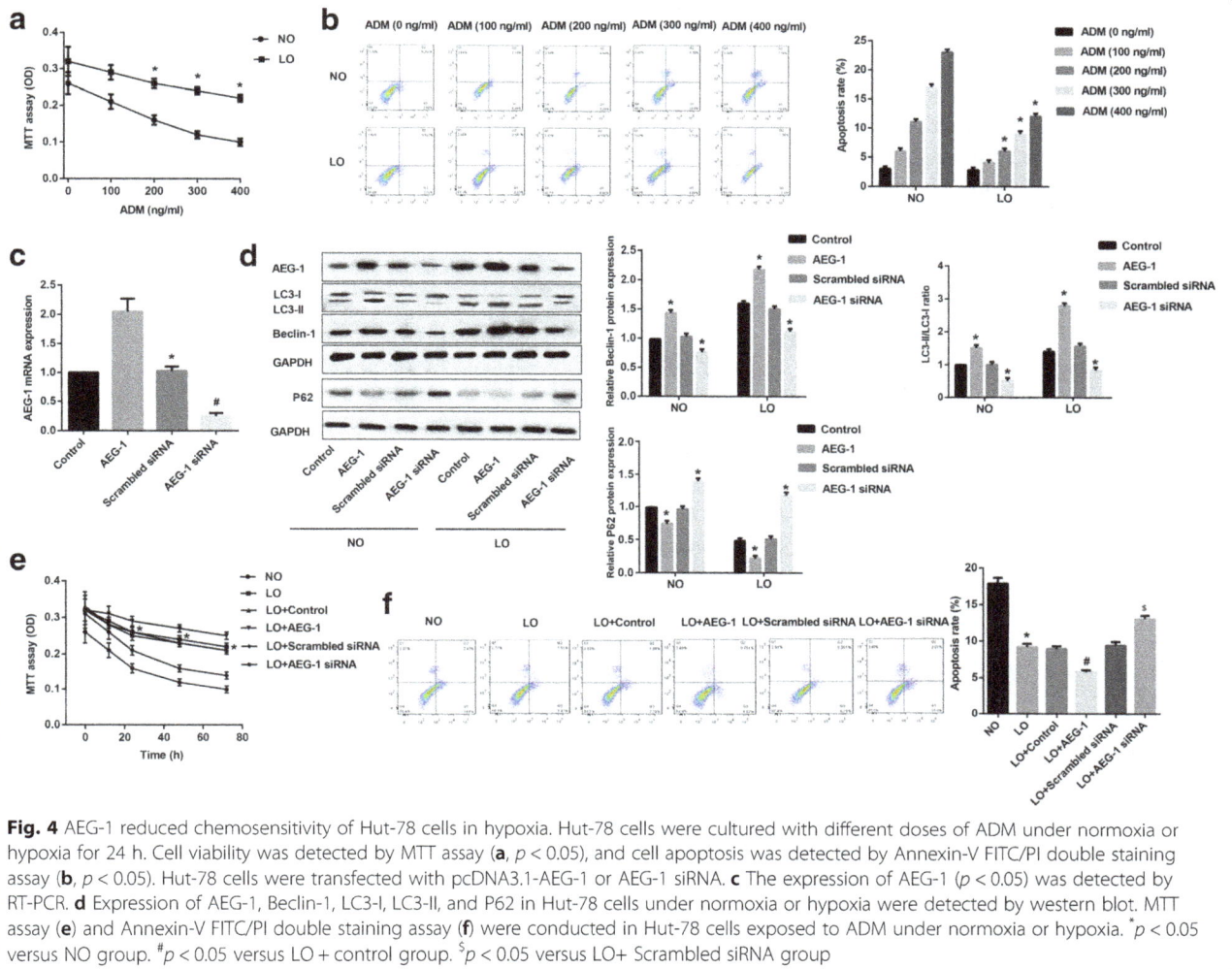

**Fig. 4** AEG-1 reduced chemosensitivity of Hut-78 cells in hypoxia. Hut-78 cells were cultured with different doses of ADM under normoxia or hypoxia for 24 h. Cell viability was detected by MTT assay (**a**, $p < 0.05$), and cell apoptosis was detected by Annexin-V FITC/PI double staining assay (**b**, $p < 0.05$). Hut-78 cells were transfected with pcDNA3.1-AEG-1 or AEG-1 siRNA. **c** The expression of AEG-1 ($p < 0.05$) was detected by RT-PCR. **d** Expression of AEG-1, Beclin-1, LC3-I, LC3-II, and P62 in Hut-78 cells under normoxia or hypoxia were detected by western blot. MTT assay (**e**) and Annexin-V FITC/PI double staining assay (**f**) were conducted in Hut-78 cells exposed to ADM under normoxia or hypoxia. $^*p < 0.05$ versus NO group. $^\#p < 0.05$ versus LO + control group. $^\$p < 0.05$ versus LO+ Scrambled siRNA group

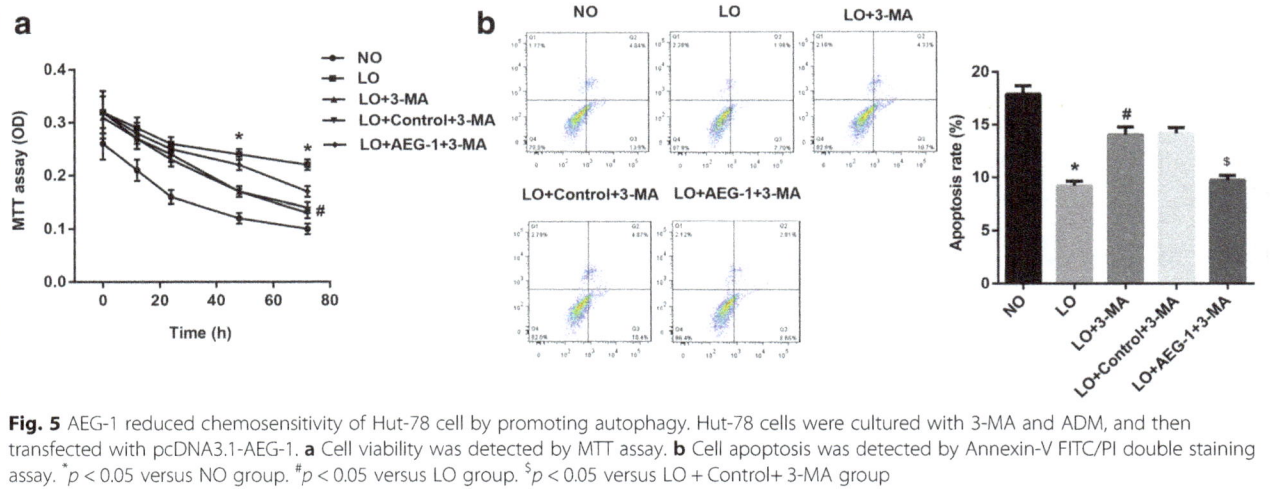

**Fig. 5** AEG-1 reduced chemosensitivity of Hut-78 cell by promoting autophagy. Hut-78 cells were cultured with 3-MA and ADM, and then transfected with pcDNA3.1-AEG-1. **a** Cell viability was detected by MTT assay. **b** Cell apoptosis was detected by Annexin-V FITC/PI double staining assay. $^*p < 0.05$ versus NO group. $^\#p < 0.05$ versus LO group. $^\$p < 0.05$ versus LO + Control+ 3-MA group

results indicated that AEG-1 was largely responsible for chemoresistance of Hut-78 cells in hypoxia, which was in accordance with the results observed in hepatocellular carcinoma (HCC) (Xie & Zhong, 2016).

In addition, we also proposed a mechanism by which AEG-1 enhanced chemoresistance of Hut-78 cells in hypoxia. A large amount of studies have demonstrated that autophagy plays a vital role in hypoxia-induced drug resistance (Liu et al., 2010; Ko et al., 2012; Rzymski et al., 2009). Thus, to illuminate the specific role of autophagy in chemoresistance of Hut-78 cells exposed to hypoxia, 3-MA (autophagic inhibitor) was selected. We found that inhibition of autophagy under hypoxia attenuated the cell viability and increased the apoptosis rate of Hut-78 cells, further, AEG-1 partially abolished the effect of 3-MA on the response of Hut-78 cells to ADM in hypoxia as revealed by MTT and apoptosis assays, indicating that AEG-1 reduced chemosensitivity of Hut-78 cells by inducing autophagy. It was reported that activation of autophagy inhibits tumor metastasis through the induction of HIF-1α (Indelicato et al., 2010). Previous studies have confirmed that hypoxia can induce autophagy through at least three pathways including activating transcription factor4, hypoxia-inducible factor1 and AMP-activated protein kinase (Liu et al., 2010; Rzymski et al., 2009; Kim et al., 2011). Actually, we also observed that the inhibition of HIF-1α significantly down-regulated AEG-1, LC3-II, Beclin-1 expression, and LC3-II/LC3-I ratio in T-NHL cells exposed to hypoxia. Unfortunately, the detail relationship between HIF-1α and AEG-1 in chemoresistance of Hut-78 cells exposed to hypoxia is not clear, which needs further investigation.

## Conclusion

In this paper, our data presents evidence that AEG-1, LC3-II, Beclin-1, and HIF-1α are significantly up-regulated in T-NHL tissues, and hypoxia triggers AEG-1, LC3-II and Beclin-1 expression in T-NHL cells (Hut-78 and Jurkat cells). AEG-1 also reduces chemosensitivity of Hut-78 cells in hypoxia. Further, AEG-1 enhances chemoresistance of Hut-78 cells exposed to hypoxia by promoting autophagy. This study contributes to the target therapy against the drug resistance in T-NHL.

## Additional file

**Additional file 1:** Hut-78 and Jurkat cells were incubated under normoxia, hypoxia or starvation environment for 48 h before detection. a Western blot assays and quantitative analysis of AEG-1, Beclin-1, and LC3-II in Jurkat cells under normoxia, hypoxia or starvation environment. b Quantitative analysis of LC3-II/LC3-I ratio in Jurkat cells under normoxia, hypoxia or starvation environment. The expression of AEG-1 (p < 0.05), LC3-II (p < 0.05), Beclin-1 (p < 0.05) and LC3-II/LC3-I ratio (p<0.05) was much higher in hypoxia or starvation environment than normoxia in Jurkat cells. c Western blot assays

and quantitative analysis of AEG-1, Beclin-1, and LC3-II in Hut-78 cells under normoxia, hypoxia or starvation environment. d Quantitative analysis of LC3-II/LC3-I ratio in Hut-78 cells under normoxia, hypoxia or starvation environment. The expression of AEG-1 (p < 0.05), LC3-II (p < 0.05), Beclin-1 (p < 0.05) and LC3-II/LC3-I ratio (p<0.05) was much higher in hypoxia or starvation environment than normoxia in Hut-78 cells. NO: normoxia, NO: hypoxia. *p < 0.05, NO vs. LO or starvation. (TIF 574 kb)

### Abbreviations
ADM: Adriamycin; AEG-1: Astrocyte elevated gene-1; ANOVA: One-way analysis of variance; DMSO: Dimethylsulfoxide; GAPDH: Glyceraldehyde-3-phosphate dehydrogenase; HCC: Hepatocellular carcinoma; HD: Hodgkin's lymphoma; HIF-1α: Hypoxia inducible factor; NHL: Non-Hodgkin's lymphoma; T-NHL: T-cell non-Hodgkin's lymphoma

### Authors' contributions
YJQ and ZJH designed the project; ZJH, ZXD, LX, LL, LZM, CRY, ZL performed the experiments; WJJ, WXH, SZC, FXR, CY, NFF, YH, WXL interpreted and analyzed the data; FXY, LWC, ZMZ drafted the manuscript. All authors have approved the submitted version and agree to be personally accountable for the contributions and for ensuring that questions related to the accuracy or integrity of any part of the work.

### Competing interests
The authors declare that they have no competing interests.

### Author details
[1]Department of Oncology, The First Affiliated Hospital, Zhengzhou University, No. 1 Jianshe East Road, Zhengzhou, Henan 450052, People's Republic of China. [2]Department of Otorhinolaryngology, The Third Affiliated Hospital of Zhengzhou University, Zhengzhou, Henan 450052, People's Republic of China. [3]Department of pathology, The First Affiliated Hospital, Zhengzhou University, Zhengzhou, Henan 450052, People's Republic of China.

### References
Ahmad A, Sakr WA, Rahman KM. Novel targets for detection of cancer and their modulation by chemopreventive natural compounds. Front Biosci. 2012;4:410–25.

Bhutia SK, et al. Astrocyte elevated gene-1 induces protective autophagy. Proc Natl Acad Sci U S A. 2010;107:22243.

Blanco MA, et al. Identification of staphylococcal nuclease domain-containing 1 (SND1) as a Metadherin-interacting protein with metastasis-promoting functions. J Biol Chem. 2011;286:19982–92.

Bogaerts E, et al. Time-dependent effect of hypoxia on tumor progression and liver progenitor cell markers in primary liver tumors. PLoS One. 2015;10:e0119555.

Chang Y, et al. Lentivirus-mediated knockdown of astrocyte elevated Gene-1 inhibits growth and induces apoptosis through MAPK pathways in human retinoblastoma cells. PLoS One. 2016;11:e0148763.

Cosse JP, Michiels C. Tumour hypoxia affects the responsiveness of cancer cells to chemotherapy and promotes cancer progression. Anti Cancer Agents Med Chem. 2008;8:790.

Emdad L, et al. Astrocyte elevated gene-1: recent insights into a novel gene involved in tumor progression, metastasis and neurodegeneration. Pharmacol Ther. 2007;114:155–70.

Emdad L, et al. Astrocyte elevated gene-1 (AEG-1) functions as an oncogene and regulates angiogenesis. Proc Natl Acad Sci U S A. 2009;106:21300.

Fan B, Wang YX, Yao T, Zhu YC. p38 mitogen-activated protein kinase mediates hypoxia-induced vascular endothelial growth factor release in human endothelial cells. Acta Pharmacol Sin. 2005;57:13–20.

Hadzipecova L, Petrusevska G, Stojanovic A. Non-Hodgkin's lymphomas: immunologic prognostic studies. Prilozi. 2007;28:39–55.

Indelicato M, et al. Role of hypoxia and autophagy in MDA-MB-231 invasiveness. J Cell Physiol. 2010;223:359–68.

Kang D. Identification and cloning of human astrocyte genes displaying elevated expression after infection with HIV-1 or exposure to HIV-1 envelope glycoprotein by rapid subtraction hybridization, RaSH. Oncogene. 2002;21:3592–602.

Kim J, Kundu M, Viollet B, Guan KL. AMPK and mTOR regulate autophagy through direct phosphorylation of Ulk1. Nat Cell Biol. 2011;13:132.

Ko YH, Cho YS, Won HS, Jeon EK, Hong YS. Possible role of autophagy inhibition in hypoxia-induced chemoresistance of pancreatic cancer cells. J Clin Oncol. 2012;30:224.

Lionel F, et al. TMEM45A is essential for hypoxia-induced chemoresistance in breast and liver cancer cells. BMC Cancer. 2012;12:391.

Liu D, Yang Y, Liu Q, Wang J. Inhibition of autophagy by 3-MA potentiates cisplatin-induced apoptosis in esophageal squamous cell carcinoma cells. Med Oncol. 2011;28:105–11.

Liu X-W, et al. HIF-1α-dependent autophagy protects HeLa cells from fenretinide (4-HPR)-induced apoptosis in hypoxia ☆. Pharmacol Res. 2010;62:416.

Meng X, Thiel KW, Leslie KK. Drug resistance mediated by AEG-1/MTDH/LYRIC. Adv Cancer Res. 2013;120:135.

Nakanishi T, et al. Autophagy is associated with cucurbitacin D-induced apoptosis in human T cell leukemia cells. Med Oncol. 2016;33:1–8.

R E, et al. Treatment of cutaneous T-cell lymphoma by extracorporeal photochemotherapy. Preliminary results N Engl J Med. 1987;316:297–303.

Rzymski T, Milani M, Singleton DC, Harris AL. Role of ATF4 in regulation of autophagy and resistance to drugs and hypoxia. Cell Cycle. 2009;8:3838–47.

Song J, et al. Hypoxia-induced autophagy contributes to the chemoresistance of hepatocellular carcinoma cells. Autophagy. 2009;5:1131.

Tian YY, et al. Restoration of microRNA-373 suppresses growth of human T-cell lymphoma cells by repressing CCND1. Eur Rev Med Pharmacol Sci. 2016;20:4435.

X M KWT, KK L. Drug resistance mediated by AEG-1/MTDH/LYRIC. Adv Cancer Res. 2013;120:135–57.

Xie Y, Zhong DW. AEG-1 is associated with hypoxia-induced hepatocellular carcinoma chemoresistance via regulating PI3K/AKT/HIF-1alpha/MDR-1 pathway. EXCLI J. 2016;15:745–57.

XW L, et al. HIF-1α-dependent autophagy protects HeLa cells from fenretinide (4-HPR)-induced apoptosis in hypoxia. Pharmacological Research the Official Journal of the Italian Pharmacological. Society. 2010;62:416–25.

Yan J, Zhang M, Chen Q, Zhang X. Expression of AEG-1 in human T-cell lymphoma enhances the risk of progression. Oncol Rep. 2012;28:2107–14.

Zhang J, et al. Hypoxia attenuates Hsp90 inhibitor 17-DMAG-induced cyclin B1 accumulation in hepatocellular carcinoma cells. Cell Stress Chaperones. 2016a;21:339–48.

Zhang J, et al. Hypoxia attenuates Hsp90 inhibitor 17-DMAG-induced cyclin B1 accumulation in hepatocellular carcinoma cells. Cell Stress Chaperones. 2016b;21:1–10.

Zhao T, et al. HIF-1α binding to AEG-1 promoter induced upregulated AEG-1 expression associated with metastasis in ovarian cancer. Cancer Medicine. 2017;6:1072–81.

Zou M, et al. AEG-1/MTDH-activated autophagy enhances human malignant glioma susceptibility to TGF-β1-triggered epithelial-mesenchymal transition. Oncotarget. 2016;7:13122–38.

# 6

# Identification of ethyl pyruvate as a NLRP3 inflammasome inhibitor that preserves mitochondrial integrity

Sujun Li[1†], Fang Liang[1†], Kevin Kwan[2†], Yiting Tang[3,4], Xiangyu Wang[1,4], Youzhou Tang[1], Jianhua Li[2], Huan Yang[2], Sangeeta S. Chavan[2], Haichao Wang[5], Ulf Andersson[6], Ben Lu[1,4*] and Kevin J. Tracey[2*]

## Abstract

**Background:** The NLRP3 inflammasome, a cytosolic complex that mediates the maturation of IL-1β and IL-18 as well as the release of high mobility group box 1 (HMGB1), contributes to the lethality of endotoxic shock. Ethyl pyruvate (EP) was previously shown to inhibit HMGB1 release and promote survival during endotoxemia and experimental sepsis. However, the underlying protective mechanism remains elusive.

**Result:** EP dose-dependently inhibited the ATP-, nigericin-, alum-, and silica-induced caspase-1 activation and HMGB1 release in mouse macrophages. EP failed to inhibit DNA transfection- or Salmonella Typhimurium-induced caspase-1 activation and HMGB1 release. Mechanistically, EP significantly attenuated mitochondrial damage and cytoplasmic translocation of mitochondrial DNA, a known NLRP3 ligand, without influencing the potassium efflux, the lysosomal rupture or the production of mitochondrial reactive oxygen species (mtROS).

**Conclusion:** Ethyl pyruvate acts as a novel NLRP3 inflammasome inhibitor that preserves the integrity of mitochondria during inflammation.

**Keywords:** Ethyl pyruvate, The NLRP3 inflammasomes, Mitochondrial damage, HMGB1, Interleukin-1beta

## Background

Macrophages, the cells at the front line of defense against infection, express pattern-recognition receptors (PRRs) to detect various inflammatory motifs. PRRs include the membrane-bound Toll-like receptors (TLRs) and NOD-like receptors (NLRs), which scan foreign invaders or sterile tissue damages for pathogen-associated (PAMPs) or damage-associated (DAMPs) molecular patterns. Many NLR family member have been reported to exhibit inflammasome activity in vitro. For instance, NLR family, pyrin domain containing 3 (NLRP3) acts as danger sentinel that self-oligomerize via homotypic NACHT domain interactions to form high-molecular weight complexes that trigger caspase-1 autoactivation (Schroder & Tschopp, 2010).

The NLRP3 inflammasome, an intracellular protein complex consisting of NLRP3, ASC and Caspase-1, controls the activation of caspase-1 and the maturation of the pro-inflammatory cytokines interleukin (IL)-1β and IL-18 (Mariathasan et al., 2006). Accumulated evidence show that the NLRP3 inflammasome also mediates the release of high mobility group box 1 (HMGB1), a late mediator of lethal sepsis, and contributes to the pathogenesis of septic shock (Lu et al., 2012; Lamkanfi et al., 2010; Qin et al., 2006; Rittirsch et al., 2008; Wang et al., 2004; Wang et al., 1999). HMGB1 is an evolutionarily conserved and abundantly expressed nuclear and cytoplasmic protein. Under the physiological condition, HMGB1 predominantly locates in the nucleus due to its two nuclear location sequences (NLSs) in most cell types (Lu et al., 2012; Andersson & Tracey, 2011). Infectious

* Correspondence: xybenlu@csu.edu.cn; kjtracey@northwell.edu
[†]Equal contributors
[1]Department of Hematology and Key Laboratory of non-resolving inflammation and cancer of Human Province, The 3rd Xiangya Hospital, Central South University, Changsha, Hunan province 410000, People's Republic of China
[2]Laboratory of Biomedical Science, Feinstein Institute for Medical Research, 350 Community Drive, Manhasset, NY 11030, USA
[4]Key Laboratory of Medical Genetics, School of Biological Science and Technology, Central South University, Changsha, Hunan province 410000, People's Republic of China
Full list of author information is available at the end of the article

agents or molecules released from damaged cells, such as lipopolysaccharide (LPS), a major cell wall component of gram negative bacteria, ATP or monosodium uric acid crystal (MSU) could induce the translocation of HMGB1 from the nucleus to the cytoplasm and the subsequent release of HMGB1 (Lu et al., 2012; Andersson & Tracey, 2011). Extracellular HMGB1 exerts a variety of biological function by engaging multiple receptors. Though the released HMGB1 might facilitate tissue repair during sterile injury, excessive accumulation of extracellular HMGB1 in tissue or circulation contributes importantly to the pathogenesis of many inflammatory or autoimmune diseases, such as sepsis and colitis (Andersson & Tracey, 2011). Notably, genetic deletion of NLRP3 or ASC, two essential components of the NLRP3 inflammasome, blocked LPS-, ATP- or MSU-induced HMGB1 release in cultured macrophages or during endotoxemia (Lamkanfi et al., 2010). Accordingly, the deletion of NLRP3 or ASC confers significant protection against lethal endotoxemia (Mariathasan et al., 2006; Mariathasan et al., 2004). Neutralizing the extracellular HMGB1 using anti-HMGB1 monoclonal antibodies significantly increased the survival during lethal endotoxemia or bacterial sepsis (Lamkanfi et al., 2010; Qin et al., 2006; Wang et al., 1999). These findings establish a critical role of the NLRP3 inflammasome - HMGB1 axis in endotoxemia and sepsis.

We and others previously found that ethyl pyruvate, a metabolite derivative, confers significant protection against experimental sepsis- and endotoxemia-induced lethality, and markedly attenuates the disease severity of experimental colitis (Ulloa et al., 2002; Miyaji et al., 2003; Davé et al., 2009). These studies also show that ethyl pyruvate inhibits LPS-induced HMGB1 release from cultured macrophages and during endotoxemia (Ulloa et al., 2002). However, the underlying mechanism by which ethyl pyruvate inhibits HMGB1 release remains unclear. Early works have shown that EP could work as an anti-inflammatory agent. (Yang et al., 2016) Besides, We and others previously show that inflammasome activation could trigger HMGB1 release in vitro and in vivo (Lu et al., 2012; Lamkanfi et al., 2010). Considering pathogenic known role of the NLRP3 inflammasome in endotoxic shock (Mariathasan et al., 2006; Mariathasan et al., 2004), together with EP's anti-inflammatory effect, here we postulate that ethyl pyruvate might inhibit HMGB1 release and thus play a protective role in sepsis- and endotoxemia-induced lethality by inhibiting the NLRP3 inflammasome activation.

## Methods
### Reagents
Ultra-pure LPS and the NLRP3 inflammasome agonists ATP, Nigericin, Nano-SiO$_2$, Alum Crystals were obtained from Invivogen (San Diego, California). Ethyl pyruvate (EP) was purchased from ThermoFisher Scientific(Shanghai, China). Anti-mouse IL-1β (AF-401-NA) was from R&D and anti-mouse caspase-1 (sc-514) was from Santa Cruz. Mouse HMGB1 mAb IgG2b 2G7 (noncommercial antibody), originally from Critical Therapeutic Inc. (Boston, MA, USA) is available upon request. Acridine orange was purchased from SigmaAldrich (St. Louis, MO). MitoSox™ was purchased from ThermoFisher Scientific (Shanghai, China), and JC-1 from Beyotime (C2006). Mitochondrial isolation and purification kits were from QIAGEN (Hilden, Germany). Murine macrophage colony-stimulating factor (GM-CSF) and human macrophage colony-stimulating factor (M-CSF) were purchased from PEPROTECH (New Jersey, USA).

### Cell preparation and stimulation
#### Peritoneal mouse macrophages
Peritoneal mouse macrophages C57BL/6 mice were isolated in 10% sucrose solution following bilateral injection of 1 ml of thioglycolate bilaterally 3 days prior. Cells were cultured in RPMI medium 1640 supplemented with 10% FBS, 100 U/mL penicillin, and 100 μg/mL streptomycin. One million peritoneal macrophages, plated in 12-well plates, were primed with ultra-pure LPS (1 μg/ml) for 3 h in the presence or the absence of EP (1 and 5 mM), and then stimulated with ATP(5 mM, 30 min), Nigericin (10 μM,1 h), Nano-SiO2 (10μg/ml, 6h) or Alum Crystals (20μg/ml, 6h). For Salmonella infection, wild-type S. typhimurium was grown overnight in Luria–Bertani (LB) broth, then reinoculated at a dilution of 1:100 and grown to mid-exponential phase (3 h) to induce expression of the Salmonella pathogenicity island 1 type III secretion system. To minimize the involvement of NLRP3 inflammasome activation during Salmonella infection, unprimed macrophages were infected with wild-type S. typhimurium (m.o.i. is from 5 to 100). The supernatant samples were collected 1 h after infection. To study AIM2 inflammasome activation, macrophages were transfected with random DNA using Lipofectamine 2000 at a concentration of 1 mg DNA plus 3.5 ml lipofectamine 2000 per ml. The supernatant samples were collected 6 h after transfection.

#### Human macrophages
Primary blood mononuclear cells were isolated by density-gradient centrifugation. Then cells were collected and cultured in RPMI 1640 medium with 10% heat-inactivated human serum. After 2 h incubation at 37 °C, Adherent cells were detached with 10 mM EDTA, and then re-suspended ($10^6$ cells/ml) in medium

supplemented with human macrophage colony-stimulating factor (20 ng/ml), and cultured for 7 d.

### Human acute monocytic leukemia cell lines (THP-1)

Human acute monocytic leukemia cell lines (THP-1)were cultured in RPMI medium 1640 supplemented with 10% FBS, 100 U/mL penicillin, and 100 µg/mL streptomycin. When cells were 70% confluence, treatment was carried out in RPMI medium 1640.

### Cytotoxicity assay

Cell supernatants were analyzed using a lactate dehydrogenase (LDH) cytotoxicity assay kit purchased from TAKARA (California, USA) per manufacture recommendations.

### Elisa

Levels of IL-1β, and TNF-α in the culture medium were determined using quantitative ELISA kits (R & D Systems, Minneapolis, MN, USA) and HMGB1 (IBL International) according to the manufacturer's instructions.

### Western-blot analysis

Supernatant and cell lysates were analyzed using western blot for caspase-1 p10, IL-1β, and HMGB1 release. Proteins from cell-free supernatants were extracted by methanol/chloroform precipitation as previously described. Briefly, cell culture supernatants were precipitated by the addition of an equal volume of methanol and 0.25 volumes of chloroform, then were vortexed and centrifuged for 10 min at 20,000 g. The upper phase was discarded and 500 µl methanol was added to the interphase. This mixture was centrifuged for 10 min at 20,000 g and the protein pellet was dried at 55 °C, re-suspended in Laemmli buffer and boiled for 5 min at 99 °C. Cell extracts were prepared as described previously (Wang et al., 2004). Samples were separated by 4–20% SDS-PAGE or 4–20% native-PAGE and were transferred onto PVDF membranes. The relative band intensity was quantified by using the NIH image 1.59 software to determine HMGB1 levels regarding standard curves generated with purified HMGB1 as described previously.

### Intracellular K+ concentration detection

Cells were washed twice with 0.9% Nacl and collected after appropriate treatments. Then, $1 \times 106$ cells from each group were resuspended in 300ul ddH2O. Then the cells were subjected to there Freeze/thaw cycles. Supernatant were collected and used for potassium measurement. Potassium in these samples are assessed by a automatic biochemical analyser (ABBOTT ARCHITECT C16000).

### Flow cytometry analysis

Mitochondrial ROS production, lysosomal rupture and mitochondrial membrane potential were assessed by flow cytometry. Briefly, to measure Mitochondrial ROS production, cells were primed with ultra-pure LPS (1 µg/ml) for 3 h in the presence of EP (5 mM), followed by treatment with ATP (5 mM,30 min) or Nigericin (10 µM,1 h). Staining treated cells with MitoSOX™ (2.5 µM) for 15 min at 37 °C. For lysosomal rupture measuring, Peritoneal mouse macrophageswere primed with ultra-pure LPS (1 µg/ml) for 3 h in the presence of EP (5 mM), and then stained with Acridine Orange (1µg/ml) for 30 min.After staining, stimulated cells with Alum (20µg/ml) or Nano-SiO$_2$(10µg/ml) 6 h. After treatment, cells were collected and quickly transferred on ice for FACS analysis. To determine mitochondrial potential-dependent damage, cells were stained with JC-1 according to the manufacturer's protocol. Cells were then monitored and analyzed by a flow cytometer (FACS Verse, BD Biosciences).

### Mitochondrial DNA release assay

$1 \times 10^7$ peritoneal macrophages were homogenized with a TB syringe, and then were subjected to centrifugation at 2000 g for 10 min at 4 °C. Protein concentration and volume of the supernatant were normalized, followed by centrifugation at 6000 g for 10 min at 4 °C to produce a supernatant corresponding to the cytosolic fraction. DNA was isolated from 200 µl of the cytosolic fraction using a QIAamp DNA Minikit purchased from QIAGEN (Hilden, Germany). The levels of mtDNA encoding cytochrome c oxidase 1 were measured by quantitative real-time PCR with same volume of the DNA solution. The following primers were used: mouse cytochrome c oxidaseI forward, 5′-GCCCCAGATATAGCATTCCC-3′, and reverse, 5′-GTTCATCCTGTTCCTGCTCC-3′.

### Electron microscopy (EM)

Electron micrographs of mitochondria in LPS-primed THP-1 cells were taken after incubation with ATP or nigericin for 15 min in the presence or the absence of ethyl pyruvate (5 mM) using HITACHITransmissionElectronMicroscopeH7700 (HITACHI, Japan). Objects were magnified 15 thousand times and macrographs of mitochondria were collected by gatan ORIUS CCD CAMERA.

### Statistical analysis

Data in the figures and text are expressed as mean ± SEM of at least three independent experiments ($n$ = 3–6). Significance of difference between groups was determined by two-tailed Students $t$-test. A $p$ value < 0.05 was considered statistically significant.

## Results

### Ethyl pyruvate inhibits NLRP3 agonists-induced inflammasome activation in mouse macrophages

To determine whether ethyl pyruvate (EP) inhibits the NLRP3 inflammasome activation, LPS-primed mouse peritoneal macrophages were stimulated with ATP in the presence or the absence of different concentrations of EP. EP exposure dose-dependently inhibited ATP-induced activation of caspase-1, cleavage of pro-IL-1β and HMGB1 release (Fig. 1a). Addition of EP failed to inhibit the expression of pro-IL-1β in the cell lysate (Fig. 1a), indicating that the inhibition of IL-1β production by EP is due to the suppression of inflammasome activation, rather than LPS-induced priming. Further, we observed that EP dose-dependently inhibited ATP-induced pyroptosis in LPS-primed mouse peritoneal macrophages, as showed by LDH assay (Fig. 1b).

To test whether EP inhibits the NLRP3 inflammasome activation induced by NLRP3 agonists other than ATP, LPS-primed mouse peritoneal macrophages were stimulated with nigericin, a known potassium ionophore in the presence of absence of different concentrations of EP. Notably, EP exposure significantly inhibited IL-1β expression at the concentration of 5 mM. EP slightly inhibited TNF at the concentration of 5 mM, suggesting that EP more specifically inhibits NLRP3-dependent cytokine release (Fig. 1c). Furthermore, EP dose-dependently inhibits IL-1β production and pyroptosis in LPS-primed mouse peritoneal macrophages induced by silica and Alum crystal (Fig. 1d). Intriguingly, EP showed weaker inhibitory effect in crystals-induced NLRP3 inflammasome activation than that induced by ATP or NIG. Taken together, these results indicate that EP inhibits the NLRP3 inflammasome activation in mouse macrophages.

### Ethyl pyruvate specifically inhibits the NLRP3 inflammasome activation

To address the specificity of EP in inhibiting the NLRP3 inflammasome activation, we next investigated whether EP inhibits the activation of AIM2 or NLRC4 inflammasome. Mouse peritoneal macrophages were either primed

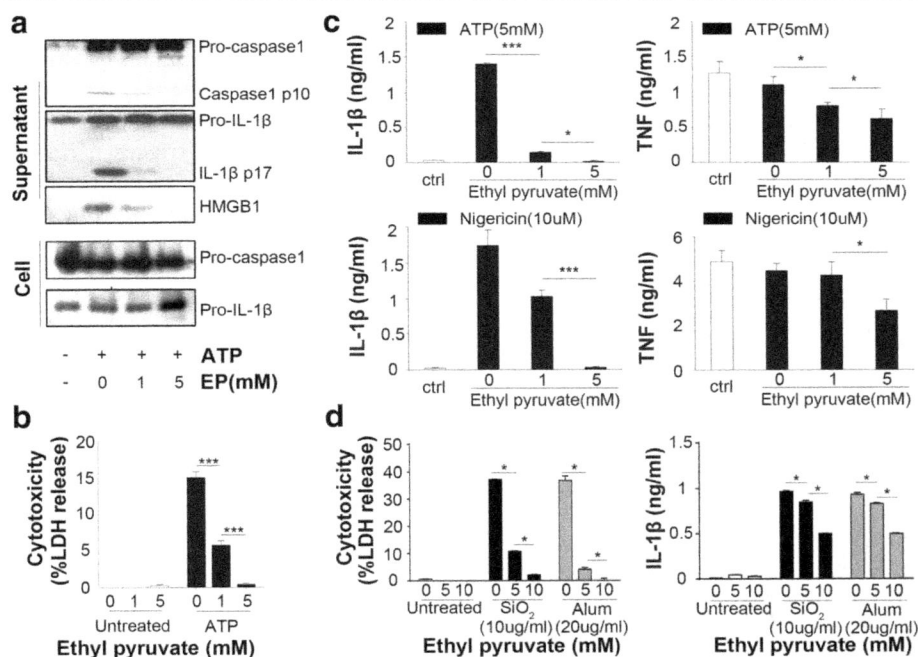

**Fig. 1** Ethyl pyruvate inhibits NLRP3 agonists-induced inflammasome activation in mouse macrophages. **a** Peritoneal mouse macrophages were primed with ultra-pure LPS (1 μg/ml) for 3 h. in the presence or the absence of EP (1 or 5 mM), and then stimulated with ATP (5 mM) for 30 min. The pro-caspase1, cleavage of caspase-1 and Pro-IL-1β, IL-1β and the release of HMGB1 in supernatants and expression of pro-caspase1, pro-IL-1β in cell were assessed by Western-blot. **b** Peritoneal mouse macrophages were primed with ultra-pure LPS (1 μg/ml) for 3 h. in the presence or the absence of EP (1 or 5 mM), and then stimulated with ATP (5 mM) for 30 min. Cytotoxicity was assessed by lactate dehydrogenase (LDH) assay. **c** Peritoneal mouse macrophages were primed with ultra-pure LPS (1 μg/ml) for 3 h. in the presence or the absence of EP (1 or 5 mM), and then stimulated with ATP (5 mM) or nigericin (10 μM) for 30 min. Levels of IL-1β and TNF-α in the culture medium were determined by ELISA. **d** Peritoneal mouse macrophages were primed with ultra-pure LPS (1 μg/ml) for 3 h. with or without EP (5 or 10 mM), and then stimulated with alum (20 μg/ml) or silica (10 μg/ml) 6h. Cytotoxicity was analyzed by LDH assay and IL-1β level was determined by ELISA. Results are means ± SEM ($n = 3$). *$p < 0.05$; **$p < 0.01$; ***$p < 0.001$

with LPS and then stimulated with nigericin, or directly stimulated with salmonella typhimurium (ST), a known NLRC4 inflammasome agonist (Mariathasan et al., 2004), or transfected with poly(dA-dT). poly(dA-dT) (hereafter termed poly (dA: dT)), a known AIM2 inflammasome agonist (Hornung et al., 2009; Fernandes-Alnemri et al., 2009). Consistently, EP exposure dose-dependently inhibited HMGB1 release in nigericin-treated macrophages. However, the addition of EP failed to inhibit caspase-1 activation and HMGB1 release induced by salmonella typhimurium infection or poly(dA:dT) transfection (Fig. 2a-b). These results indicate that EP specifically inhibits the NLRP3 inflammasome activation.

## Inhibition of NLRP3 activation by EP is independent of potassium efflux

A role of potassium (K⁺) efflux in NLRP3 activation has been proposed since several NLRP3 activators including ATP, NIG, MSU and particulate matters like silica and Alum crystal trigger the efflux of K⁺ and preventing K⁺ efflux blocks inflammasome activation induced by NLRP3 agonists (Muñoz-Planillo et al., 2013; He et al., 2016). Therefore, we next determined whether EP inhibits the NLRP3 inflammasome activation through regulating the K⁺ efflux. To test this possibility, LPS-primed mouse peritoneal macrophages were stimulated with ATP or nigericin in the presence or the absence of different concentrations of EP. EP exposure dose-dependently inhibited ATP- or NIG-induced cytotoxicity (%) (Fig. 3b) and IL-1β release (Fig. 3c) whereas failed to affect K⁺ efflux (Fig. 3a). Thus, Inhibition of NLRP3 activation by EP is independent of potassium efflux.

## Inhibition of NLRP3 activation by EP is independent of lysosomal rupture

It has been proposed that lysosomal rupture mediates the NLRP3 inflammasome activation induced by particulate matters, such as silica and Alum crystal (Hornung et al., 2008; Halle et al., 2008). Since EP inhibits the NLRP3 inflammasome activation induced by particulate matters including silica and alum crystal, we investigated whether EP inhibits the NLRP3 inflammasome activation through regulating the lysosomal rupture. To test this possibility, LPS-primed mouse peritoneal macrophages were stimulated with silica or Alum crystal in the presence or the absence of different concentrations of EP, and lysosomal rupture was assessed by flow cytometry. Surprisingly, EP exposure failed to prevent, but instead promoted silica- or Alum-induced lysosomal rupture (Fig. 4a), although EP dose-dependently inhibited silica- or Alum-induced cytotoxicity (Fig. 4b). Therefore, inhibition of NLRP3 activation by EP is independent of lysosomal rupture.

## Ethyl pyruvate inhibits NLRP3 agonists-induced mitochondrial damage

In addition to K⁺ efflux and lysosomal rupture, accumulated evidence show that mitochondrial damage is critical for the NLRP3 inflammasome activation (Zhou et al., 2011; Nakahira et al., 2011; Shimada et al., 2012; Zhong et al., 2016). To test whether ethyl pyruvate prevents NLRP3 agonists-triggered mitochondrial damage, we directly assessed mitochondrial integrity in human acute monocytic leukemia cell lines (THP-1) using electron microscopy (EM). Whereas nigericin, and to a

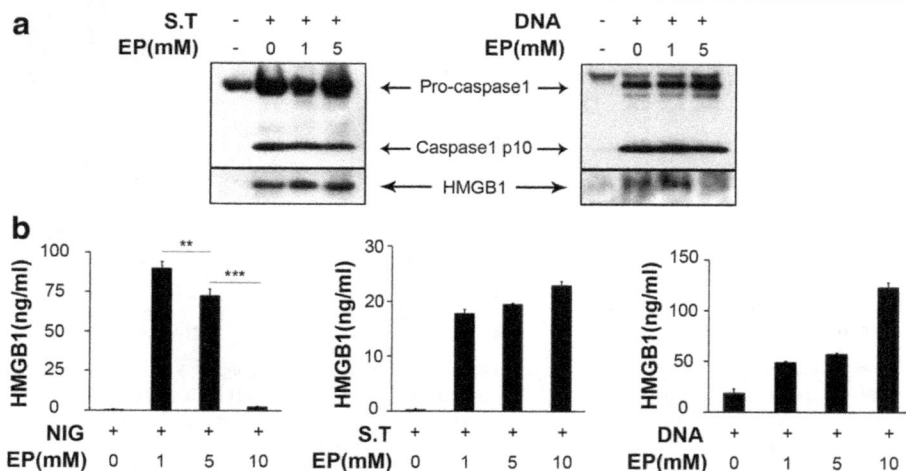

Fig. 2 Ethyl pyruvate specifically inhibits the NLRP3 inflammasome activation. For Salmonella infection, unprimed macrophages were infected with wild-type S. typhimurium and the supernatant samples were collected 1 h after infection. For the AIM2 inflammasome activation, macrophages were transfected with DNA using Lipofectamine 2000 and the supernatant samples were collected 6 h after transfection. **a** Pro-caspase1, caspase1 and HMGB1 release were assessed by Western-blot. **b** Supernatant levels of HMGB1were determined by ELISA. Results are means ± SEM (n = 3). *p < 0.05; **p < 0.01; ***p < 0.001

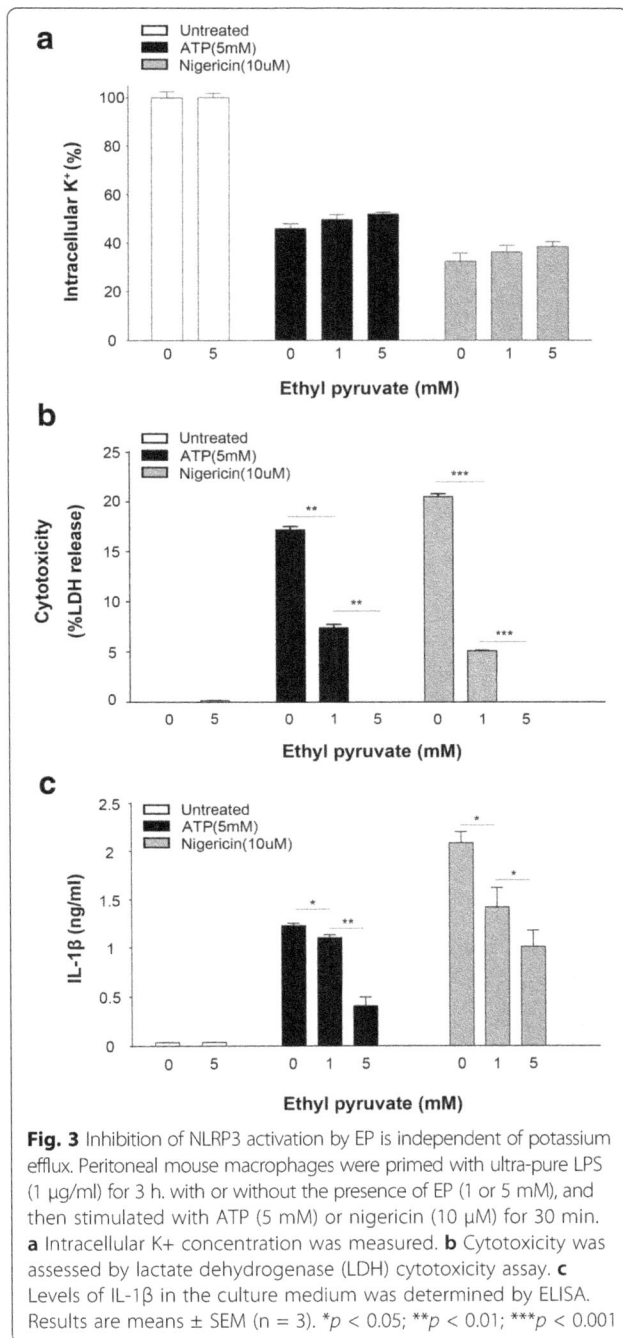

**Fig. 3** Inhibition of NLRP3 activation by EP is independent of potassium efflux. Peritoneal mouse macrophages were primed with ultra-pure LPS (1 μg/ml) for 3 h. with or without the presence of EP (1 or 5 mM), and then stimulated with ATP (5 mM) or nigericin (10 μM) for 30 min. **a** Intracellular K+ concentration was measured. **b** Cytotoxicity was assessed by lactate dehydrogenase (LDH) cytotoxicity assay. **c** Levels of IL-1β in the culture medium was determined by ELISA. Results are means ± SEM (n = 3). *$p < 0.05$; **$p < 0.01$; ***$p < 0.001$

green fluorecence increased when mitochondrial damage occurs. EP could reduce the proportion of mitochondrial damaged cells (Fig. 5c), in accordance with the results by electron microscopy.

Early studies indicate that mitochondrial DNA (mtDNA) release into the cytoplasm is highly linked to the NLRP3 inflammasome activation. Oxidized mtDNA was reported to function as a direct NLRP3 ligand that induces the assembly and activation of the NLRP3 inflammasome (Shimada et al., 2012). Accordingly, we reasoned that EP might prevent mtDNA release into the cytoplasm. To test this hypothesis, mouse macrophages were stimulated with ATP or nigericin in the presence or the absence of EP. The cytoplasmic fraction was analyzed for mtDNA levels using qPCR with primers for cytochrome C oxidase-1 gene. Indeed, EP inhibits ATP- or nigericin-induced mtDNA release into the cytoplasm (Fig. 5d). These results suggest that the mechanisms by which EP inhibits the NLRP3 inflammasome activation, are at least in part, through the inhibition of mitochondrial damage.

### Ethyl pyruvate does not inhibit NLRP3 agonists-induced mtROS production

Early studies indicate that mitochondrial reactive oxygen species (mtROS) production contributes to mitochondrial damage and the NLRP3 inflammasome activation (Zhou et al., 2011). Accordingly, we next tested whether EP inhibits NLRP3 agonists-induced mtROS production in mouse macrophages. A robust mtROS generation was detected when treated with ATP while little mtROS was induced when treated with nigericin. Notably, EP did not inhibit mtROS production in these cells as measured by flow cytometry (Fig. 6). Together with the finding that EP inhibits NLRP3 agonists-induced mitochondrial damage, these observations suggest that the mechanism through which EP prevents mitochondrial damage and the NLRP3 inflammasome activation is independent of mtROS production.

### Ethyl pyruvate inhibits NLRP3 agonists-induced inflammasome activation in human macrophages

We finally examined whether EP inhibits the NLRP3 inflammasome activation in human macrophages. ATP stimulation of LPS-primed human macrophages rapidly induced IL-1β secretion, which was dose-dependently inhibited by EP (Fig. 7a). In contrast, addition of EP at 1 and 5 mM failed to attenuate LPS-induced production of non-NLRP3 inflammasome dependent cytokines, such as IL-6 or TNF production (Fig. 7b). This suggests that EP inhibits the NLRP3 inflammation activation in both murine and human macrophages.

lesser extent, ATP induced accumulation of many highly damaged, electron-dense mitochondria, this effect was strongly inhibited by ethyl pyruvate in the concentration of 5 mM (Fig. 5a-b). To futher confirm the finding that EP significantly relieves mitochondrial damage, we employed JC-1, a dye used to detect the mitochondrial membrane potentialmeasure and assess mitochondrial integrity. The JC-1 red fluorecence decreased and JC-1

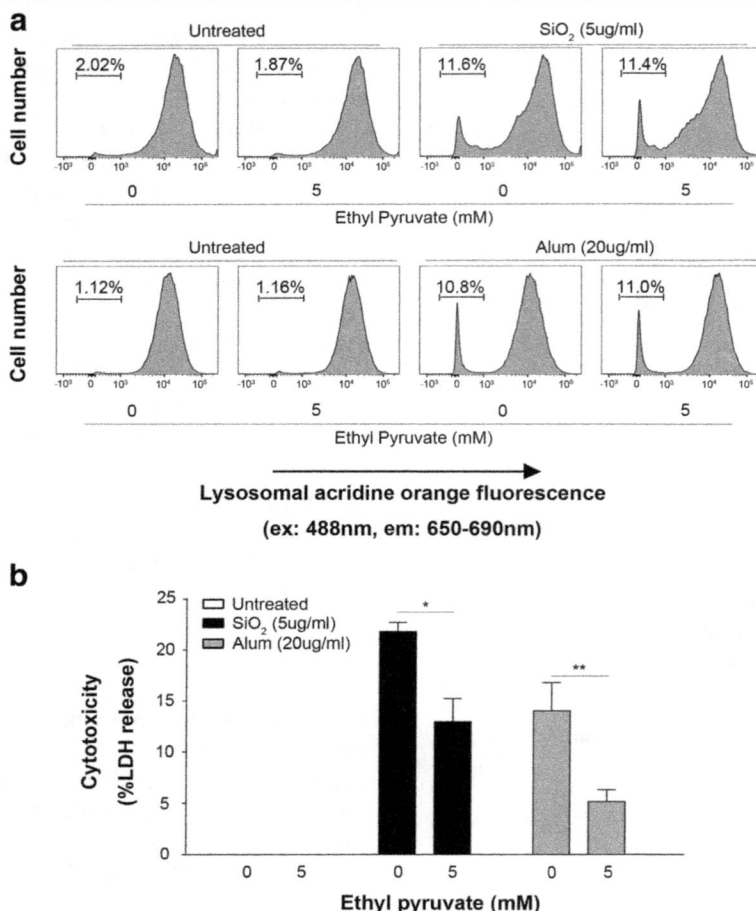

**Fig. 4** Inhibition of NLRP3 activation by EP is independent of lysosomal rupture. Peritoneal mouse macrophages were primed with ultra-pure LPS (1 μg/ml) for 3 h. in the presence or the absence of 5 mM EP, and then stained with acridine orange (1 μg/ml) for 30 min at 37 °C. Cells were then stimulated by alum (20 μg/ml) or silica (10 μg/ml) 6h. **a** After stimulation, cells were analyzed by flow cytometry for lysosomal acridine orange fluorescence. **b** Cytotoxicity was assessed using LDH assay. Results are means ± SEM (n = 3). *$p < 0.05$; **$p < 0.01$; ***$p < 0.001$

## Discussion

Ethyl pyruvate is a small molecule and a food additive that exerts anti-inflammatory effect. We and others previously show that treatment with ethyl pyruvate is able to ameliorate systemic inflammation and prevents multiple organ dysfunctions in a number of disorders, including endotoxemia, bacterial sepsis, acute pancreatitis, alcoholic liver injury, acute respiratory distress syndrome, acute viral myocarditis and acute kidney injury. However, the underlying mechanisms by which ethyl pyruvate attenuates systemic inflammation remain elusive. In this study, we first show that ethyl pyruvate inhibits NLRP3 agonists-induced inflammasome activation through preventing mitochondrial damage. Interestingly, ethyl pyruvate neither inhibits the activation of AIM2 or NLRC4 inflammasome nor affects the inflammatory responses that are not related to the inflammasome activity.

The NLRP3 inflammasome is an intracellular protein complex comprised of NLRP3, ASC and caspase-1. Upon stimulation by a variety of endogenous or exogenous danger signals, these inflammasome components rapidly assemble into the active NLRP3 inflammasome, cumulating in the maturation of IL-1β and IL-18, as well as pyroptosis, a lytic form of programmed cell death (Strowig et al., 2012). The NLRP3 inflammasome importantly orchestrates host innate immune responses to infections or sterile injuries. Deregulated NLRP3 inflammasome activity, however, contributes to the pathogenesis of a number of human diseases or life-threatening conditions, such as endotoxemia, sepsis, alcoholic liver injury, colitis and acute kidney injury. Together with findings in current study, these observations could explain why ethyl pyruvate is able to confer protection in various diseases or life-threatening conditions. It is noteworthy that ethyl pyruvate is well-known to inhibit HMGB1 release from active

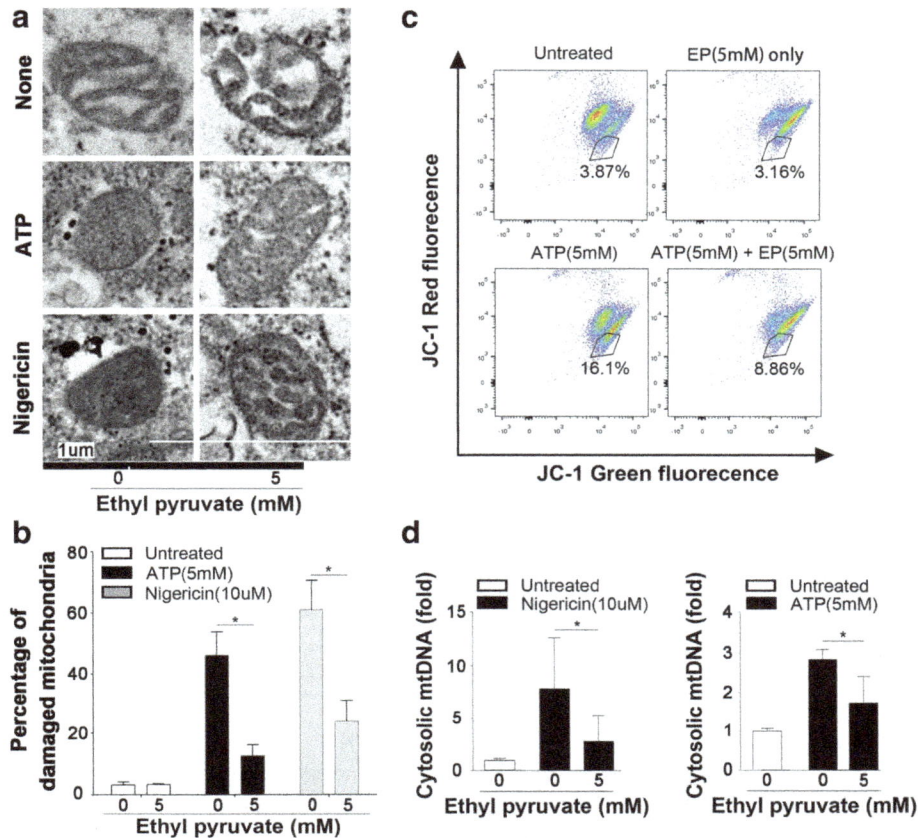

**Fig. 5** Ethyl pyruvate inhibits NLRP3 agonists-induced mitochondrial damage. **a** Electron micrographs of mitochondria in LPS-primed THP-1 cells after incubation with ATP (5 mM) or nigericin (10 μM) for 15 min in the presence or the absence of ethyl pyruvate (5 mM). Shown in panel A are representative images of normal, partially damaged, or heavily damaged mitochondria. Scale bars, 1 um. **b** Quantification of damaged mitochondria in (a). Results are means ± SEM (n = 6). **c** Mouse macrophages were primed with LPS or LPS + EP, followed by treatment with ATP (5 mM, 20 min). Cells were stained with JC-1 and analyzed by a flow cytometer. Cells in the gate represent mitochondrial depolarization or mitochondrial damage. **d** mtDNA release from LPS-primed mouse peritoneal macrophages after stimulation of ATP (5 mM) or nigericin (10 μM) for 30 min in the presence or the absence of ethyl pyruvate (5 mM). Results are means ± SEM (n = 3). *p < 0.05; **p < 0.01; ***p < 0.001

immune cells or in inflammatory diseases (Ulloa et al., 2002; Miyaji et al., 2003; Davé et al., 2009). HMGB1 is a proinflammatory mediator that contributes to the pathogenesis of many disorders, including sepsis and colitis. We and others recently found that the release of HMGB1 is an important downstream event of inflammasome activation (Nakahira et al., 2011; Groß et al., 2016). Neutralizing extracellular HMGB1 with monoclonal antibodies confers considerate protection against Caspase-1/Caspase-11-mediated lethality during endotoxemia (Lamkanfi et al., 2010). Consistent with these findings, we observed in this study that ethyl pyruvate dose-dependently inhibits the NLRP3 agonists-induced HMGB1 release.

Though the NLRP3 inflammasome has been extensively studied due to its important roles in immune responses and diseases, how various endogenous or exogenous danger signals activate the NLRP3 inflammasome still remains largely unknown. In recent years, several cellular events have been proposed to be the

triggers for the NLRP3 inflammasome activation. These include potassium efflux, lysosomal rupture, mitochondrial reactive oxygen species (ROS) production and mitochondrial damage. Potassium efflux could be induced by most NLRP3 stimuli, and therefore has been proposed to be the common pathway for the NLRP3 inflammasome activation. However, ethyl pyruvate has no detectable effect on the ATP- or nigericin-induced potassium efflux at the concentration, when it could completely abolish ATP- or nigericin-induced inflammasome activation. These observations suggest that ethyl pyruvate inhibits the NLRP3 inflammasome activation through affecting the downstream signal of potassium efflux. Disruption of the lysosomal membrane, caused by phagocytosis of particulate matter such as silica or Alum crystals, could also activate the NLRP3 inflammasome. Though ethyl pyruvate could effectively inhibit silica- or Alum-induced inflammasome activation, it barely affects the phagosomal rupture-induced by silica- or Alum. Further, we also noticed that ethyl pyruvate

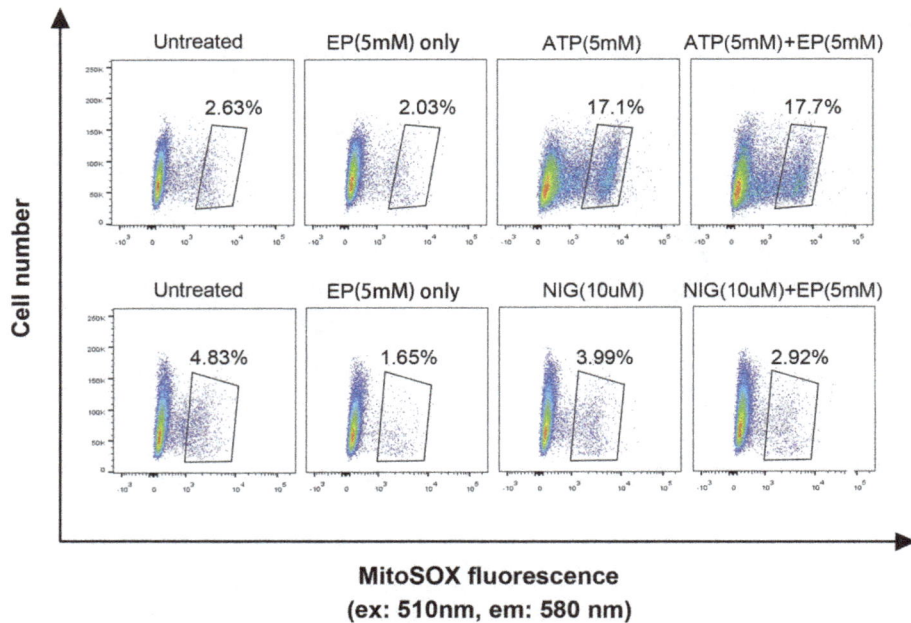

**Fig. 6** Ethyl pyruvate does not inhibit NLRP3 agonists-induced mtROS production. MtROS levels were determined by MitoSOX staining of LPS-primed human acute monocytic leukemia cell lines (THP-1) after stimulation with ATP (5 mM) or nigericin (10 μM) in the presence or the absence of 5 mM EP

fails to inhibit ATP-induced mitochondrial ROS production. A number of studies demonstrate that mitochondrial ROS is critical for the NLRP3 inflammasome activation (Zhou et al., 2011; Nakahira et al., 2011; Groß et al., 2016). However, some other studies indicate that mitochondrial ROS is dispensable for the activation of NLRP3 inflammasome (Muñoz-Planillo et al., 2013; Bauernfeind et al., 2011; Won

et al., 2013). One explanation for the discrepancy is that mitochondrial ROS activate the NLRP3 inflammasome in the context-dependent manner, which suggests that the downstream events of mitochondrial ROS might be the actual trigger for the NLRP3 inflammasome activation.

Excessive mitochondrial ROS could lead to mitochondrial damage. Accumulated evidences show an essential

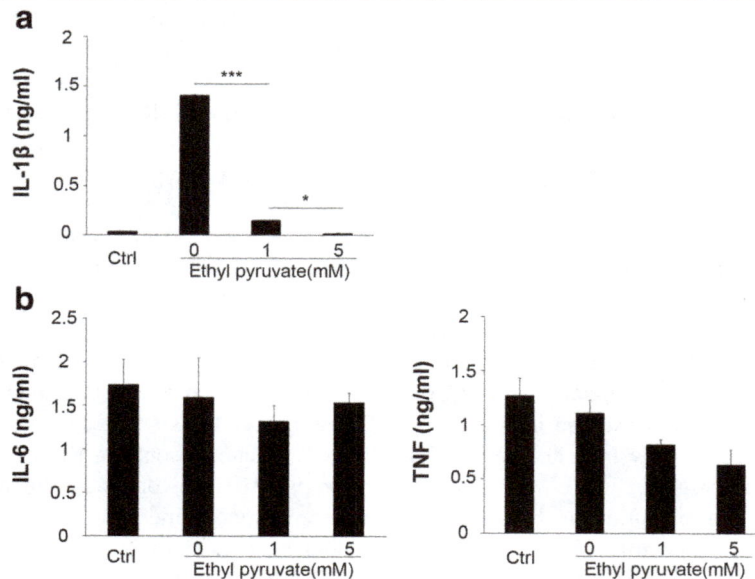

**Fig. 7** Ethyl pyruvate inhibits NLRP3 agonists-induced inflammasome activation in human macrophages. Human macrophages were primed with ultra-pure LPS (1 μg/ml) for 3 h. in the presence or the absence of EP (1 or 5 mM), and then stimulated with ATP (5 mM) for 30 min. **a** IL-1β level and (**b**) IL-6, TNF production were determined by ELISA. Results are means ± SEM (n = 3). *$p < 0.05$; **$p < 0.01$; ***$p < 0.001$

role of mitochondrial damage in the NLRP3 inflammasome activation (Zhong et al., 2016; Wang et al., 2014; Shimada et al., 2012; Iyer et al., 2013). Iyer et al. show that the cytosolic oxidized mitochondrial DNA released by damaged mitochondria serve as NLRP3 ligands and could induce the NLRP3 inflammasome activation (Shimada et al., 2012). Another study demonstrates that the cardiolipins exposed on the surface of damaged mitochondria can directly bind NLRP3 and play critical roles in the activation of NLRP3 inflammasome (Iyer et al., 2013). As show in current study, ethyl pyruvate prevents mitochondrial damage and inhibits the release of mitochondrial DNA into the cytosol in NLRP3 agonist-stimulated macrophages. Though whether cytosolic oxidized mitochondrial DNA is a bona fide NLRP3 ligand requires further investigation, our findings suggest that ethyl pyruvate inhibits the NLRP3 inflammasome activation, at least in part, through preventing mitochondrial damage.

## Conclusion

Together, our findings establish ethyl pyruvate as a novel NLRP3 inhibitor and unravel the mechanisms by which this metabolite derivative exerts anti-inflammatory effect in various types of diseases or illnesses, such as sepsis, alcoholic liver injury, and acute kidney injury. Mechanistically, ethyl pyruvate inhibits the NLRP3 inflammasome activation, at least in part, by reducing mitochondrial damage.

### Acknowledgements

The authors thank clinical laboratory and central lab of Xiangya Hospital for intracellular K+ concentration detection, Flow cytometry analysis and Electron Microscopy. This work was supported in part by grants from The National Natural Science Foundation of China (81470345, 81422027, 81400149 and 81700127), and China Post Doctor Science Foundation.

### Funding

This work was supported in part by grants from The National Natural Science Foundation of China (81470345, 81422027, 81400149 and 81700127), and China Post Doctor Science Foundation.

### Authors' contributions

BL and KJT conceived the project and designed experiments; SL and FL designed experiments, performed the experiments, analyzed the data and wrote the paper; KK performed the experiments, analyzed the data; YT supervised the study; XW, YT, JL, HY, SSC, HW and UA performed the experiments.

### Competing interests

The authors declare that they have no competing interests.

### Author details

[1]Department of Hematology and Key Laboratory of non-resolving inflammation and cancer of Human Province, The 3rd Xiangya Hospital, Central South University, Changsha, Hunan province 410000, People's Republic of China. [2]Laboratory of Biomedical Science, Feinstein Institute for Medical Research, 350 Community Drive, Manhasset, NY 11030, USA. [3]Department of Physiology, School of Basic medical research, Central South University, Changsha, Hunan province, People's Republic of China. [4]Key Laboratory of Medical Genetics, School of Biological Science and Technology, Central South University, Changsha, Hunan province 410000, People's Republic of China. [5]Department of Emergency Medicine, North Shore University Hospital, Manhasset, NY 11030, USA. [6]Department of Women's and Children's Health, Karolinska Institute, 171 76 Stockholm, Sweden.

### References

Andersson U, Tracey KJ. HMGB1 is a therapeutic target for sterile inflammation and infection. Annu Rev Immunol. 2011;29:139–62.

Bauernfeind F, et al. Cutting edge: reactive oxygen species inhibitors block priming, but not activation, of the NLRP3 inflammasome. J Immunol. 2011; 187(2):613–7.

Davé SH, et al. Ethyl pyruvate decreases HMGB1 release and ameliorates murine colitis. J Leukoc Biol. 2009;86(3):633–43.

Fernandes-Alnemri T, Yu JW, Datta P, Wu J, Alnemri ES. AIM2 activates the inflammasome and cell death in response to cytoplasmic DNA. Nature. 2009; 458(7237):509–13.

Groß CJ, et al. K+ efflux-independent NLRP3 Inflammasome activation by small molecules targeting mitochondria. Immunity. 2016;45(4):761–73.

Halle A, et al. The NALP3 inflammasome is involved in the innate immune response to amyloid-beta. Nat Immunol. 2008;9:857–65.

He Y, Zeng MY, Yang D, Motro B, Núñez G. NEK7 is an essential mediator of NLRP3 activation downstream of potassium efflux. Nature. 2016; 530(7590):354–7.

Hornung V, et al. Silica crystals and aluminum salts activate the NALP3 inflammasome through phagosomal destabilization. Nat Immunol. 2008;9:847–56.

Hornung V, et al. AIM2 recognizes cytosolic dsDNA and forms caspase-1-activating inflammasome with ASC. Nature. 2009;458(7237):514–8.

Iyer SS, et al. Mitochondrial cardiolipin is required for Nlrp3 inflammasome activation. Immunity. 2013;39(2):311–23.

Lamkanfi M, et al. Inflammasome-dependent release of the alarmin HMGB1 in endotoxemia. J Immunol. 2010;185:4385–92.

Lu B, et al. Novel role of PKR in inflammasome activation and HMGB1 release. Nature. 2012;488:670–4.

Mariathasan S, et al. Differential activation of the inflammasome by caspase-1 adaptors ASC and Ipaf. Nature. 2004;430:213–8.

Mariathasan S, et al. Cryopyrin activates the inflammasome in response to toxins and ATP. Nature. 2006;440:228–32.

Miyaji T, et al. Ethyl pyruvate decreases sepsis-induced acute renal failure and multiple organ damage in aged mice. Kidney Int. 2003;64(5):1620–31.

Muñoz-Planillo R, et al. K+ efflux is the common trigger of NLRP3 inflammasome activation by bacterial toxins and particulate matter. Immunity. 2013;38(6): 1142–53.

Nakahira K, et al. Autophagy proteins regulate innate immune responses by inhibiting the release of mitochondrial DNA mediated by the NALP3 inflammasome. Nat Immunol. 2011;12(3):222–30.

Qin S, et al. Role of HMGB1 in apoptosis-mediated sepsis lethality. J Exp Med. 2006;203:1637–42.

Rittirsch D, et al. Functional roles for C5a receptors in sepsis. Nat Med. 2008; 14:551–7.

Schroder K, Tschopp J. The inflammasomes. Cell. 2010;140(6):821–32.

Shimada K, et al. Oxidized mitochondrial DNA activates the NLRP3 inflammasome during apoptosis. Immunity. 2012;36(3):401–14.

Strowig T, Henao-Mejia J, Elinav E, Flavell R. Inflammasomes in health and disease. Nature. 2012;481(7381):278–86.

Ulloa L, et al. Ethyl pyruvate prevents lethality in mice with established lethal sepsis and systemic inflammation. Proc Natl Acad Sci U S A. 2002;99(19): 12351–6.

Wang H, et al. HMG-1 as a late mediator of endotoxin lethality in mice. Science. 1999;285:248–51.

Wang H, et al. Cholinergic agonists inhibit HMGB1 release and improve survival in experimental sepsis. Nat Med. 2004;10:1216–21.

Wang X, et al. RNA viruses promote activation of the NLRP3 inflammasome through a RIP1-RIP3-DRP1 signaling pathway. Nat Immunol. 2014;15(12): 1126–33.

Won J-H, et al. Rotenone-induced impairment of mitochondrial electron transport chain confers a selective priming signal for NLRP3 Inflammasome activation. J Biol Chem. 2013;290(45):27425–37.

Yang R, Zhu S, Tonnessen TI. Ethyl pyruvate is a novel anti-inflammatory agent to treat multiple inflammatory organ injuries. J Inflamm. 2016;13:37.

Zhong Z, et al. NF-κB restricts Inflammasome activation via elimination of damaged mitochondria. Cell. 2016;164(5):896–910.

Zhou R, Yazdi AS, Menu P, Tschopp J. A role for mitochondria in NLRP3 inflammasome activation. Nature. 2011;469(7329):221–5.

# 7

# Trans-heterozygosity for mutations enhances the risk of recurrent/chronic pancreatitis in patients with cystic fibrosis

Valentina Maria Sofia[1], Cecilia Surace[1], Vito Terlizzi[2], Letizia Da Sacco[3], Federico Alghisi[4], Antonella Angiolillo[5], Cesare Braggion[2], Natalia Cirilli[6], Carla Colombo[7], Antonella Di Lullo[8,9], Rita Padoan[10], Serena Quattrucci[11], Valeria Raia[12], Giuseppe Tuccio[13], Federica Zarrilli[14], Anna Cristina Tomaiuolo[1], Antonio Novelli[1], Vincenzina Lucidi[4], Marco Lucarelli[15,16], Giuseppe Castaldo[8,17†] and Adriano Angioni[1*†]

## Abstract

**Background:** Recurrent (RP) and chronic pancreatitis (CP) may complicate Cystic Fibrosis (CF). It is still unknown if mutations in genes involved in the intrapancreatic activation of trypsin (IPAT) or in the pancreatic secretion pathway (PSP) may enhance the risk for RP/CP in patients with CF.

**Methods:** We enrolled: 48 patients affected by CF complicated by RP/CP and, as controls 35 patients with CF without pancreatitis and 80 unrelated healthy subjects. We tested a panel of 8 genes involved in the IPAT, i.e. *PRSS1, PRSS2, SPINK1, CTRC, CASR, CFTR, CTSB* and *KRT8* and 23 additional genes implicated in the PSP.

**Results:** We found 14/48 patients (29.2%) with mutations in genes involved in IPAT in the group of CF patients with RP/CP, while mutations in such genes were found in 2/35 (5.7%) patients with CF without pancreatitis and in 3/80 (3.8%) healthy subjects ($p < 0.001$). Thus, we found mutations in 12 genes of the PSP in 11/48 (22.9%) patients with CF and RP/CP. Overall, 19/48 (39.6%) patients with CF and RP/CP showed one or more mutations in the genes involved in the IPAT and in the PSP while such figure was 4/35 (11.4%) for patients with CF without pancreatitis and 11/80 (13.7%) for healthy controls ($p < 0.001$).

**Conclusions:** The trans-heterozygous association between *CFTR* mutations in genes involved in the pathways of pancreatic enzyme activation and the pancreatic secretion may be risk factors for the development of recurrent or chronic pancreatitis in patients with CF.

**Keywords:** Cystic fibrosis, Recurrent/chronic pancreatitis, *CFTR* gene, Trypsin, Pancreatic pathways, Trans-heterozogosity

## Background

Cystic Fibrosis (CF) is the most common inherited autosomal recessive disease in Caucasians. It is caused by defects in the CF *transmembrane conductance regulator (CFTR)* gene, which encodes a cAMP-regulated chloride channel. Defects in the CFTR protein cause abnormal chloride transport across the apical membranes of epithelial cells in the airways, pancreas, intestine, vas deferens, and sweat glands leading to progressive lung disease, pancreatic dysfunction, male infertility, and elevated sweat electrolytes, respectively (Castellani & Assael, 2017). About 85% of individuals affected by CF suffer from pancreatic insufficiency (PI), in most cases since the birth. However, 15% of the patients retain pancreatic sufficiency (PS) that permits adequate digestion (Walkowiak et al., 2008). About 85% of individuals affected by CF suffer from pancreatic insufficiency (PI), in most cases since the birth. However, 15% of the patients retain pancreatic sufficiency (PS) that permits adequate digestion (Walkowiak et al., 2008).

Recurrent pancreatitis (RP) and chronic pancreatitis (CP) may complicate CF. It was firstly mentioned by Shwachman et al. in 1975 (Shwachman et al., 1975).

* Correspondence: adriano.angioni@opbg.net
†Giuseppe Castaldo and Adriano Angioni contributed equally to this work.
[1]Laboratory of Medical Genetics Unit, "Bambino Gesù" Children's Hospital, IRCCS, Viale di San Paolo 15, 00146 Rome, Italy
Full list of author information is available at the end of the article

They reported, in a period of 20 years in 2000 patients with CF, 10 cases of pancreatitis (0.5%), all with PS. Currently, a frequency of recurrent/chronic pancreatitis between 17% (Durno et al., 2002) and 22% (Ooi et al., 2011) is estimated in patients with CF.

The dysfunction of the CFTR protein has a role in the pathogenesis of pancreatitis because it causes the impaired secretory function of pancreatic duct cells and the altered flow of digestive pro-enzymes into the duodenum triggering recurrent episodes of pancreatitis that in some patients may evolve to chronic pancreatitis (Walkowiak et al., 2008; Lew et al., 2017). This complication is more frequent in patients with CF and PS (that frequently have at least one class IV-V CFTR mutation), in which pancreatic acinar islets still produce pancreatic enzymes that may be prematurely activated within the pancreas. Recurrent/chronic pancreatitis has been observed also independently by the development of CF. In fact, Bishop et al. showed a frequency up to 30% of RP/CP in subjects carrying only one *CFTR* mutation in the absence of any sign of CF (Bishop et al., 2005). However, only a small percentage of patients with *CFTR* mutations or with CF experience RP or CP, suggesting that other risk factors must be involved (Walkowiak et al., 2008).

In fact, in addition to *CFTR*, patients with idiopathic recurrent or chronic pancreatitis have been investigated for other genes related to the premature intra-pancreatic activation of trypsin pathway. The first gene related to pancreatitis was the cationic trypsinogen gene *protease serine 1* (*PRSS1*) in 1996: a gain of function missense mutation i.e., the R122H, was identified as a risk factor for CP (Whitcomb et al., 1996). In the following years, loss-of-function variants in the *pancreatic secretory trypsin inhibitor* (*SPINK1*) (Chen et al., 2000), *calcium-sensing receptor* (*CASR*) (Felderbauer et al., 2003) and *chymotrypsinogen C* (*CTRC*) (Szmola & Sahin-Toth, 2007) genes, firmly established the pivotal role of prematurely activated trypsin within the pancreas in the etiology of pancreatitis. Moreover, our group demonstrated that mutations in several dozens of genes bearing to six different pancreatic pathways represent risk factors for recurrent/chronic pancreatitis (Sofia et al., 2016) reinforcing the concept that trans-heterozygous mutations in different genes are involved in the pathogenesis of idiopathic pancreatitis.

Interestingly, we described trans-heterozygosity for mutations in different genes also in a patient with CF and RP that was compound heterozygous for the [delta]F508 and G91G *CFTR* mutations and had a pathogenic mutation in the *CTRC* gene (Tomaiuolo et al., 2015).

Thus, to better define the role of trans-heterozygosity for mutations in different genes as a risk factor for RP/CP in patients with CF, in this study we investigated a cohort of CF patients with RP/CP in comparison to patients with

CF without pancreatitis and to healthy subjects to compare the frequency of mutations in a panel of genes related to the intra-pancreatic activation of trypsin (IPAT) and a group of other genes related to pancreatic secretion pathways (PSP) previously reported to contribute to to the pathogenesis of pancreatitis (Sofia et al., 2016).

## Methods
### Patients
The informed consent was obtained from all patients or from the parents or guardians of minors. The study was approved by the Ethical Committee (Scientific Board of "Bambino Gesù" Children's Hospital, IRCCS, Rome, Italy) and was conducted in accordance with the Helsinki Declaration.

We enrolled 48 unselected patients affected by CF complicated by RP or CP recruited through a multi-centric study involving 9 Italian CF centres. The main data (i.e., age at diagnosis of CF, age at diagnosis of RP/CP, *CFTR* genotype and pancreatic status) are reported in Table 2. As control populations, we studied 35 unselected patients with CF without symptoms or history of pancreatitis (see Table 3 for the data of age at diagnosis of CF, *CFTR* genotype and pancreatic status) and 80 unrelated, adult healthy subjects of the same ethnic group of the patients with CF (i.e., Italian from at least two generations) whose DNA samples and anonymized clinical data (in particular absence of CF and of any pancreatic disorder) were available, in the biological bank of our Institution.

The diagnosis of CF was done according to the international criteria (Farrell et al., 2017). Pancreatic sufficiency in patients with CF was defined on the basis of two values of faecal pancreatic elastase > 200 mg/g measured in subjects free from acute gastrointestinal events (Walkowiak et al., 2016) or on the basis of normal 72-h fecal fat balance (Walkowiak et al., 2008). Recurrent pancreatitis was diagnosed in patients that had at least two episodes of acute pancreatitis (at a distance of at least six months after the resolution of the previous episode) each one with abdominal pain (once excluded other causes) in association with the increase of serum lipase (at least 2X the upper reference limit) and/or imaging evidence (e.g., pancreatic edema, hemorrhage or necrosis) (Morinville et al., 2012; Kumar et al., 2016). Chronic pancreatitis was diagnosed according to the M-ANNHEIM criteria (Schneider et al., 2007) in patients in which instrumental analysis revealed calcifications or characteristic ductal changes. All the patients with CP had a positive anamnesis for episodes of recurrent pancreatitis.

### Next-generation targeted sequencing of pancreatic genes
Targeted resequencing was performed using a uniquely customized design TruSeq Custom Amplicon Low Input

technology (Illumina, San Diego, CA) with the MiSeq sequencing platform (Illumina). This technology is a fully integrated DNA-to-data solution, including online probe design and ordering through the Illumina website, sequencing assay, automated data analysis, and offline software for reviewing results. Online probe design was performed by entering target genomic regions into Design Studio software (Illumina). We designed a panel of eight genes included in IPAT genes (Sofia et al., 2016; Chen & Férec, 2009; Mahurkar et al., 2006; Cavestro et al., 2003): *CFTR* (NM_000492.3), *SPINK1* (NM_003122.3), *PRSS1* (NM_002769.4), *protease, serine 2* (*PRSS2*) (NM_002770.2), *CTRC* (NM_007272.2), *CASR* (NM_001178065.1), *cathepsin B* (*CTSB*) (NM_147780.2) and *keratin 8* (*KRT8*) (NM_002273). The sequence of these genes was obtained consulting the University of California, Santa Cruz, Genome Browser Home (https://genome.ucsc.edu/cgi-bin/hgGateway, last accessed October 2015) with a coverage of 100%. MiSeq system provides fully integrated on-instrument data analysis software. Each single variant reported in the vCard output file was evaluated for the coverage and the Q score and visualized via Integrative Genomics Viewer (Thorvaldosdottir et al., 2013; Robinson et al., 2011). All mutations identified by MiSeq Reporter were validated by Sanger sequencing using standard protocols.

In the second step, we selected the genes encoding proteins related to the pancreatic activation of zymogens (Sofia et al., 2016). Such genes were selected among the genes annotated in the "Pancreatic Secretion Pathway" (map04972), available in the KEGG database (Kanehisa et al., 2014). The 23 genes selected were classified into four groups according to the activity of the encoded protein or their role in the pathogenesis of pancreatitis: (i) genes encoding proteins involved in pancreatic secretion and ion homeostasis (*PPY, F2RL1, TMPRSS15, SCL4A2, SLC4A4, SLC26A3, CPB1, CLPS*) (Berni Canani et al., 2010; Sharma et al., 2005; Stevens et al., 2004; Multigner et al., 1985); (ii) genes encoding proteins involved in calcium ($Ca^{2+}$) signalling and zymogen granules exocytosis (*PRKCD, ITPR3, GP2, TRPC3, STIM1, ATP2C2, TRPV1, TRPV5, TRPV6, PIK3CG*) (Jin et al., 2015; Williams, 2008; Ramnath et al., 2010; Lupia et al., 2004); (iii) genes encoding proteins involved in autophagy (*HSP90AA1, LAMP2, MAP1LC3B*) (Willemer et al., 1989; Gukovskaya & Gukovsky, 2012; Fortunato & Kroemer, 2009) and (iv) autoimmune pancreatitis-related genes (*CA4, ABCF1*) (Ohmuraya & Yamamura, 2008). To search mutations in such genes, we used the targeted resequencing performed by a uniquely customized design: TruSeq Custom Amplicon Low Input Kit (Illumina) with the MiSeq sequencing platform (Illumina). The probe design (locus-specific oligos) was carried out by entering the target genomic regions into Design Studio software

(Illumina). The design was performed over a cumulative target region of 99.328 bp and generated a panel of 677 amplicons with a coverage of 100% of the cumulative region. Library preparation and sequencing runs have been performed according to the manufacturer's procedure. Only the *PRSS2* gene was analyzed by Sanger sequencing because its genomic sequence was updated in the University of California Santa Cruz (UCSC) genome database after the design of the resequencing panel.

**Data and bioinformatic analysis**

The MiSeq Reporter software, a data analysis software included in the MiSeq system, performs secondary analysis on the base calls and quality score (Qscore) generated by the Real-Time Analysis software during the sequencing run and provides a list of all detected variants compared with the reference genome (*Homo sapiens*, hg19, build 37.2). Each single variant reported in the output file was evaluated for the coverage and the Qscore and visualized via the Integrative Genome Viewer (Thorvaldosdottir et al., 2013). Based on the guidelines of the American College of Medical Genetics and Genomics (Rehm et al., 2013), all regions that had been sequenced with a sequencing depth < 30 were considered not suitable for the analysis. Furthermore, we established a minimum threshold in Qscore of 30 (base call accuracy of 99.9%). All identified variants were analyzed with bioinformatic softwares evaluating the impact of change in amino-acidic structure on protein functionality with several parameters, and we filtered all variants to retain those alterations with a high disease-causing potential. We used four tools based on different parameters: PolyPhen-2 (Adzhubei et al., 2010), Align-GVGD (Mathe et al., 2006; Hicks et al., 2011), DNA SIFT (Ng & Henikoff, 2001) and MutationTaster (Schwarz et al., 2010). To facilitate the analysis of the potential splicing mutations, we used Human Splicing Finder to predict the effects of mutations on splicing signals or motifs in any human sequence (Desmet et al., 2009). Sanger sequencing using standard protocols validated the variants that have been predicted as "damaging" by at least three tools. For each of these mutations we assessed the frequency in the general population reported by the ExAC (Exome Aggregation Consortium) tool.

**Results**

All individuals from the three groups, i.e., patients with CF and RP/CP ($n = 48$), patients with CF and without pancreatitis ($n = 35$) and healthy subjects ($n = 80$) were investigated for mutations in the 8 genes encoding proteins involved in IPAT and in the 23 genes encoding proteins involved in the PSP (Table 1). All the 48 patients with CF and RP/CP (Table 2) and the 35 with CF

**Table 1** Number and % of subjects with mutations in IPAT genes; PSP genes and at least one gene (IPAT & PSP) in: patients with CF and recurrent/chronic pancreatitis (RP/CP); patients with CF without pancreatitis and healthy subjects

| | n of cases | IPAT | PSP | IPAT & PSP |
|---|---|---|---|---|
| CF and RP/CP | 48 | 14 (29.2) | 11 (22.9) | 19 (39.6) |
| CF without pancreatitis | 35 | 2 (5.7) | 3 (8.5) | 4 (11.4) |
| healthy subjects | 80 | 3 (3.8) | 8 (10) | 11 (13.7) |
| Chi square and (p) | | 20.4 ($p < 0.001$) | 4.39 ($p = 0.11$) | 14.5 ($p < 0.001$) |

without pancreatitis (Table 3) had a pathological sweat test (i.e., $> 60$ mEq/L) with the exception of a patient with CF without pancreatitis that had a value of 53 mEq/L, and all patients from both the groups had two *CFTR* mutations with the exception of a patient with CF and RP in which only one mutation was known. Among the 48 patients with CF and RP/CP we found 39 patients (81.2%) with PS and 9 patients with PI (18.8%); these figures were 13/33 (30.4%) and 20 (69.6%), respectively, among the patients with CF without pancreatitis ($p < 0.001$).

As shown in Table 1 and Fig. 1a, in the group of patients with CF and RP/CP we found 14/48 patients (29.2%) with mutations in IPAT genes, while mutations in such genes were found in 2/35 (5.7%) patients with CF without pancreatitis (Table 1 and Fig. 1b) and in 3/80 (3.8%) healthy subjects (Table 1 and Fig. 1c) (chi square: 20.4, $p < 0.001$).

Going to the type of mutations in IPAT genes in the patients with CF and RP/CP: 2 were heterozygous for a splicing mutation in *PRSS1* in *cis*, 4 patients were heterozygous for *CTRC* mutations, 3 patients were heterozygous for *PRSS2* mutations, 2 patients were heterozygous for *CASR* mutations and 2 patients were heterozygous for *KRT8* mutations; 1 patient had a splicing mutation in *PRSS1* and a missense mutation in *KRT8* (Table 2). All these mutations were absent in our controls and were found with a frequency $< 1\%$ in the general population as annotated in the ExAC tool (Additional file 1: Table S1). While, the 2 patients with CF without pancreatitis had, in IPAT genes, a heterozygous *PRSS1/PRSS2* hybrid mutation and a heterozygous missense mutation of *CTRC*, respectively (Table 3). Finally, the three healthy subjects had all a heterozygous missense mutation in the *KRT8*, *CASR* and *SPINK1* genes, respectively (Table 4).

Thus, all individuals from the three groups were studied for mutations in the 23 genes encoding proteins of PSP. In the group of patients with CF and RP/CP (Fig. 1a, Table 1, Table 2), the analysis revealed mutations in 11/48 (22.9%) patients. While, as shown in Fig. 1b and c and in Tables 3 and 4, mutations in such genes were found in 3/35 (8.5%) patients with CF without pancreatitis and in 8/80 (10%) healthy subjects (chi square: 4.39; $p = 0.11$).

Going to the type of mutations, of the 11 patients with CF and RP/CP (Table 2) 7 patients showed heterozygous mutations, 1 displayed a homozygous mutation and 3 patients were trans-heterozygous for mutations in more than one gene. Finally (Table 2 and Additional file 1: Table S1), in this group of patients, we found 13 missense mutations in 12 genes encoding proteins of PSP: (i) *SLC4A2*, *TMPRSS15*, *SLC26A3* and *SLC4A4* genes encoding proteins involved in pancreatic secretion and ion homeostasis; (ii) *TRPV1*, *TRPV5*, *TRPV6*, *PIK3CG*, *PRKCD* and *ATP2C2* genes encoding proteins involved in calcium ($Ca^{2+}$) signalling and zymogen granules exocytosis and (iii) *MAP1LC3B*, *LAMP2* genes encoding proteins involved in autophagy. One nonsense homozygous mutation was found in *TRPV1*. All these mutations were not present in the 35 CF patients without pancreatitis and in the 80 healthy subjects (Table 2 and Additional file 1: Table S1).

Among the 35 patients with CF without pancreatitis (Table 3), one patient was trans-heterozygous for mutations in the genes of both panels and 2 patients had mutations only in the genes of the PSP. In the cohort of healthy controls (Table 4), we found 7 individuals with variants in at least one gene of the PSP.

All the mutations found in patients and controls had a frequency $< 1\%$ in the general population (data not shown).

Finally, 19/48 (39.6%) patients with CF and RP/CP had mutations in at least one gene of the IPAT or PSP pathway. While, this is true for 4/35 (11.4%) patients with CF without CP and for 11/80 (13.7%) healthy subjects, chi square: 14.5, $p < 0.001$ (Fig. 1 and Table 1). Additional file 1: Table S1 reports a summary of all gene mutations found in the three groups of subjects studied.

## Discussion

Our study confirms that the occurrence of RP/CP is more frequent in patients with CF and PS (Walkowiak et al., 2008) and demonstrates that patients with CF and RP/CP have a significantly higher frequency of mutations in genes encoding proteins that may promote the auto-activation of pancreatic proenzymes or regulate pancreatic secretion. The small number of cases precluded clinical comparison between patients bearing mutations and those *wild-type* for all genes tested. Thus,

**Table 2** Sweat chloride (mmol/L, SC), pancreatic status, age at CF and pancreatitis diagnosis, *CFTR* genotype and mutations in genes related to intra-pancreatic activation of trypsin (IPAT) and pancreatic secretion pathway (PSP) genes in 48 patients with CF and recurrent/chronic pancreatitis

| ID | SC | Pancreatic status | Diagnosis of CF (Age) | RP/CP onset | *CFTR* genotype | IPAT genes | PSP genes |
|---|---|---|---|---|---|---|---|
| 1 | 117 | S | 19 Y | 5 Y | [delta]F508/c.2657 + 5G > A | / | / |
| 2 | 77 | S | 20 Y | 35 Y | N1303 K/P205S | / | / |
| 3 | 90 | S | 5 M | 10 Y | G85E/c.489 + 1G > T | / | *TRPV1*: c.755C > T (P252L) |
| 4 | 109 | S | 3 M | 17 Y | G542X/c.2657 + 5G > A | / | *SLC4A2*: c.299G > T (R109L); *TRPV6*: c.806C > T (T269 M) |
| 5 | 77 | I | 2 M | 8 M | [delta]F508/I1027T | / | *PIK3CG*: c.1613C > T (P538L); *TMPRSS15*: c.935C > T (T312I) |
| 6 | 84 | S | 14 Y | 26 Y | R347P/R347P | / | / |
| 7 | 100 | S | 2 M | 4 Y | c.2657 + 5G > A/c.2657 + 5G > A | / | / |
| 8 | 62 | S | 16 Y | 16 Y | [delta]F508/D110H | / | / |
| 9 | 109 | S | 1 M | 3 Y | N1303 K/c.2657 + 5G > A | / | / |
| 10 | 80 | S | 7 M | 19 Y | c.2657 + 5G > A/L1077P | / | / |
| 11 | 63 | S | 9 Y | 24 Y | W1282X/R347P | / | / |
| 12 | 92 | S | 4 M | 11 Y | [delta]F508/D579G | / | / |
| 13 | 66 | S | 1 M | 3 Y | c.579 + 1G > T/D1152H | / | / |
| 14 | 74 | S | 43 Y | 10 Y | [delta]F508/D1152H | PRSS1: c.[592-11C > T;c.592-8C > T] | / |
| 15 | 67 | S | 46 Y | 12 Y | [delta]F508/D1152H | PRSS1: c.[592-11C > T;c.592-8C > T] | / |
| 16 | 60 | S | 10 Y | 2 Y | S1297 fs*5/D993G | / | / |
| 17 | 90 | S | 1 Y | 4 Y | [delta]F508/I1000_A1004del | / | / |
| 18 | 85 | I | 5 M | 3 Y | [delta]F508/G85E | CTRC: c.514A > G (K172E) | *TRPV1*: c.1261C > T (R421X)• |
| 19 | 106 | S | 12 Y | 8 Y | N1303 K/D579G | / | / |
| 20 | 76 | I | 9 Y | 18 Y | [delta]F508/I1234V | / | / |
| 21 | 78 | S | 11 Y | 9 Y | [delta]F508/G91G | CTRC: c. 703G > A (V235I) | *PRKCD*: c.1501G > T (G501 W); *MAP1LC3B*: c.73G > C (E25Q) |
| 22 | 73 | S | 1 Y | 3 Y | [delta]F508/S1255P | / | / |
| 23 | 73 | I | 27 Y | 34 Y | Q220*/(V562I;A1006E) | PRSS2: c.292A > T (K98X) | SLC26A3: c.2276C > A (P759Q) |
| 24 | 88 | S | 1 Y | 17 Y | [delta]F508/D1152H | PRSS2: c.689C > T (T230I) | SLC4A4: c.976A > G (I326V) |
| 25 | 101 | I | 4 M | 9 Y | 1717-1G > A/R334W | PRSS2: c.571G > A (G191R) | ATP2C2: c.2381G > A (R794Q) |
| 26 | 100 | I | 1 M | 10 Y | 1717-1G > A/R334W | / | / |
| 27 | 79 | S | 25 Y | na | N1303 K/R334W | / | / |
| 28 | 103 | S | 21 Y | 21 Y | N1303 K/R334W | / | LAMP2: c.586A > T (T196S) |
| 29 | 64 | S | 4 Y | 25 Y | R553X /2789 + 5G > A | KRT8: c.184G > T (G62C) | / |
| 30 | 93 | S | 2 M | 6 Y | 2789 + 5G > A/2789 + 5G > A | / | / |
| 31 | 110 | S | 4 Y | 4 Y | [delta]F508/2789 + 5G > A | CTRC: c.649G > A (G217S) | / |
| 32 | 76 | S | 16 Y | na | D614G/((TG)11 T5;V562I;A1006E) | / | / |
| 33 | 75 | S | 50 Y | na | [delta]F508/un | *CTRC: c.514A > G (K172E)* | / |
| 34 | 69 | I | 3 M | 14 Y | N1303 K/H139R | / | / |

**Table 2** Sweat chloride (mmol/L, SC), pancreatic status, age at CF and pancreatitis diagnosis, *CFTR* genotype and mutations in genes related to intra-pancreatic activation of trypsin (IPAT) and pancreatic secretion pathway (PSP) genes in 48 patients with CF and recurrent/chronic pancreatitis *(Continued)*

| ID | SC | Pancreatic status | Diagnosis of CF (Age) | RP/CP onset | *CFTR* genotype | IPAT genes | PSP genes |
|---|---|---|---|---|---|---|---|
| 35 | 119 | S | 4 M | 23 Y | N1303 K/G85E | / | / |
| 36 | 64 | S | 17 Y | 49 Y | S549R(A > C)/R334L | / | / |
| 37 | 68 | S | 36 Y | 24 Y | [delta]F508/R334L | / | / |
| 38 | 73 | S | 3 M | 14 Y | L997F/L320 V | / | *TRPV1: c.1781C > T (A594V)* |
| 39 | 65 | I | 5 M | 5 M | [delta]F508/D110H | *KRT8: c.1073C > T (A358V)* | / |
| 40 | 110 | S | 17 Y | 32 Y | [delta]F508/S945 L | / | / |
| 41 | 81 | S | 35 Y | 40 Y | [delta]F508/2789 + 5G > A | *KRT8: c.184G > T (G62C); PRSS1: c.592-24C > T* | / |
| 42 | 82 | S | 14 Y | 28 Y | R347P/R347P | / | / |
| 43 | 91 | S | 25 Y | 30 Y | [delta]F508/2789 + 5G > A | / | / |
| 44 | 114 | S | 7 Y | 23 Y | [delta]F508/2789 + 5G > A | / | / |
| 45 | 116 | S | 1 M | 19 Y | [delta]F508/3272-26A > G | / | / |
| 46 | 84 | S | na | 43 Y | R1066H/T501I | / | / |
| 47 | 76 | I | 3 M | na | [delta]F508/S549 N | *CASR: c.445G > A (V149I)* | *TRPV5: c.1726G > A (A576T)* |
| 48 | 60 | S | 16 Y | 30 Y | [delta]F508/E193K | *CASR: c.565A > G (N189D)* | / |

All mutations in IPAT and PSP genes were heterozygous with the exception of the c.1261C > T mutation in the *TRPV1* gene (*) that was homozygous
S sufficiency, I insufficiency, M months, Y years, *na* not available, *un* unknown

the trans-heterozygosity for mutations in the *CFTR* and in other genes represents a risk factor for pancreatitis even in patients with CF, as we recently demonstrated for patients with idiopathic RP/CP (Sofia et al., 2016).

Among the genes encoding proteins involved in the premature activation of trypsin, we found mutations in 14 patients with CF and RP/CP in *PRSS1*, *PRSS2*, *CTRC*, *CASR* and *KRT8* genes. Eight of such mutations were known as pathogenic, while for other 6 mutations, three bioinformatic tools predicted a pathogenic effect and the ExAC tool reported the absence or the very low frequency in the general population. Going in detail, we found two mutations in *PRSS1*: the first is the [c.592-11C > T;c.592-8C > T] complex allele was found in two siblings. Keiles et al. (Keiles & Kammesheidt, 2006) described the same complex allele in an 18-years old woman with pancreatitis; she also carried the T908 N *CFTR* mutation. Furthermore, the *PRSS1* splicing mutation c.592-24C > T previously described in two siblings with CP (Singhi et al., 2014) was found in a patient with the *CFTR* genotype [delta]F508/2789 + 5G > A. The patient carried also a *KRT8* mutation.

Thus, we found three mutations in *PRSS2*. The T230I and K98X mutations are novel. The T230I was reported as pathogenic by the three bioinformatic tools; the K98X is a nonsense mutation causing an early stop codon. The third mutation in *PRSS2* gene, i.e., the G191R, had been

analysed by Witt et al. (Witt et al., 2006). They demonstrated that the recombinant G191R protein showed a complete loss of trypsin activity owing to the introduction of a new tryptic cleavage site rendering the enzyme hypersensitive to autocatalytic proteolysis. Furthermore, we found three missense mutations in *CTRC*. The K172E was identified in two patients. Masson et al. described the K172E mutation in a patient with idiopathic chronic pancreatitis (Masson et al., 2008). Thus, in two other patients with the *CFTR* [delta]F508/G91G and [delta]F508/2789 + 5G > A genotype we identified the *CTRC* V235I and G217S missense mutations, respectively. Rosendahl et al. investigated the functional consequences of these two *CTRC* missense mutations through transient transfections in HEK 293 T cells (Rosendahl et al., 2008). They demonstrated that the G217S causes a loss-of-function of the *CTRC* protein, whereas the V235I results in normal or slightly reduced function, respectively. Moreover, data observed in another report suggest a role for the V235I mutation in triggering the pancreatic phenotype in a patient with CF (Tomaiuolo et al., 2015). Rosendahl identified the G217S mutation also in a healthy control and similarly, in our study we found it in a patient with CF without RP/CP thus, we cannot conclude on the pathogenic role of such mutation.

In addition, we found two missense mutations in *CASR*: the V149I and the N189D; both the mutations

**Table 3** Sweat chloride (mmol/L, SC), genotype of *CFTR*, intra-pancreatic activation of trypsin (IPAT) and pancreatic secretion pathway (PSP) genes in patients with CF without chronic pancreatitis

| N | SC | Pancreatic status | Diagnosis of CF (Age) | *CFTR* genotype | IPAT genes (mutations) | PSP genes (mutations) |
|---|----|-----|------|------|------|------|
| 1 | 93 | S | 25 Y | [delta]F508/ [delta]F508 | / | / |
| 2 | 98 | I | 14 Y | F311 L/ M348 K/ W1145X | / | *TRPV1*: c.381C > A (C127X) |
| 3 | 97 | S | 6 Y | [delta]F508/ [delta]F508 | / | / |
| 4 | 87 | I | 6 M | [delta]F508 / c.2046_2047insA | PRSS1/PRSS2 hybrid | *ATP2C2*: c.643G > T (D215Y) |
| 5 | 76 | S | 3 M | G542X/ N1303 K | / | / |
| 6 | 73 | S | 33 Y | [delta]F508 / V562I/ A1006E | / | / |
| 7 | 62 | S | 3 M | S977F/ N1303 K | / | / |
| 8 | 92 | S | 9 Y | G85E/ R334L | / | / |
| 9 | 76 | I | 9 M | [delta]F508/I1234V | / | / |
| 10 | 85 | I | 0 M | N1303 K/L1077P | / | / |
| 11 | 70 | S | 1 M | G542X/2184insA | / | / |
| 12 | 53 | S | 3 Y | [delta]F508/P5L | / | / |
| 13 | 79 | I | 10 Y | R347P/P5L | / | / |
| 14 | 135 | I | 4 M | [delta]F508/2789 + 5G > A | / | / |
| 15 | 99 | I | 10 M | [delta]F508/S549R | / | / |
| 16 | 60 | I | 2 M | [delta]F508/991delC | / | / |
| 17 | 87 | I | 11 Y | R709X/ L1077P | / | / |
| 18 | 79 | S | 4 Y | [delta]F508/ I1234V | | / |
| 19 | 142 | S | 0 M | Q39X/ CFTRdele4–11 | / | / |
| 20 | 98 | S | 4 M | [delta]F508/CFTRdele2 | | / |
| 21 | 98 | I | 5 Y | [delta]F508/ Q685PfsX4 | CTRC: c.649G > A (G217S) | / |
| 22 | 81 | I | 3 Y | [delta]F508/T338I | / | / |
| 23 | 80 | I | 2 M | [delta]F508/P5L | / | / |
| 24 | 65 | I | 2 M | G178R/ CFTRdup19 | / | / |
| 25 | 90 | I | 1 M | [delta]F508 L732X | / | / |
| 26 | 78 | I | 2 M | [delta]F508/G542X | / | / |
| 27 | 100 | I | 1 M | [delta]F508/2789 + 5G > A | / | / |
| 28 | 61 | I | 1 M | [delta]F508/N1303 K | / | / |
| 29 | 86 | I | 3 M | 2789 + G > A/2789 + G > A | / | / |
| 30 | 96 | I | 0 M | [delta]F508/N1303 K | / | / |
| 31 | 100 | S | 1 Y | [delta]F508/E193K | / | / |
| 32 | 70 | I | 6 M | [delta]F508/N1303 K | / | / |
| 33 | 111 | I | 46 Y | [delta]F508/N1303 K | / | / |
| 34 | 68 | I | 0 M | [delta]F508/4040delA | / | / |
| 35 | 100 | S | 33 Y | [delta]F508/ [delta]F508 | / | TRPV1: c.1790C > T (T597 M) |

*Het* heterozygous, *na* not available

*S* sufficiency, *I* insufficienc, *na* not available. All mutations in IPAT and in PSP genes were heterozygous

were considered pathogenic by bioinformatic tools and by the very low frequency in the general population.

Finally, we found two missense mutations in *KRT8*. The G62C was identified in two PS patients: the first case had the R553X/2789 + 5G > A *CFTR* genotype and the second had the [delta]F508/2789 + 5G > A *CFTR* genotype in addition to the c.592-24C > T mutation in *PRSS1*. Initially, the *KRT8* G62C mutation was considered pathogenic by Cavestro and coworkers (Cavestro et al., 2003). Later, Witt et al. observed that the frequency of the mutation did not differ between patients with acute or chronic pancreatitis, pancreatic adenocarcinoma and control individuals (Witt et al., 2006). Also in our study, this mutation was found in a healthy subject. Thus, we

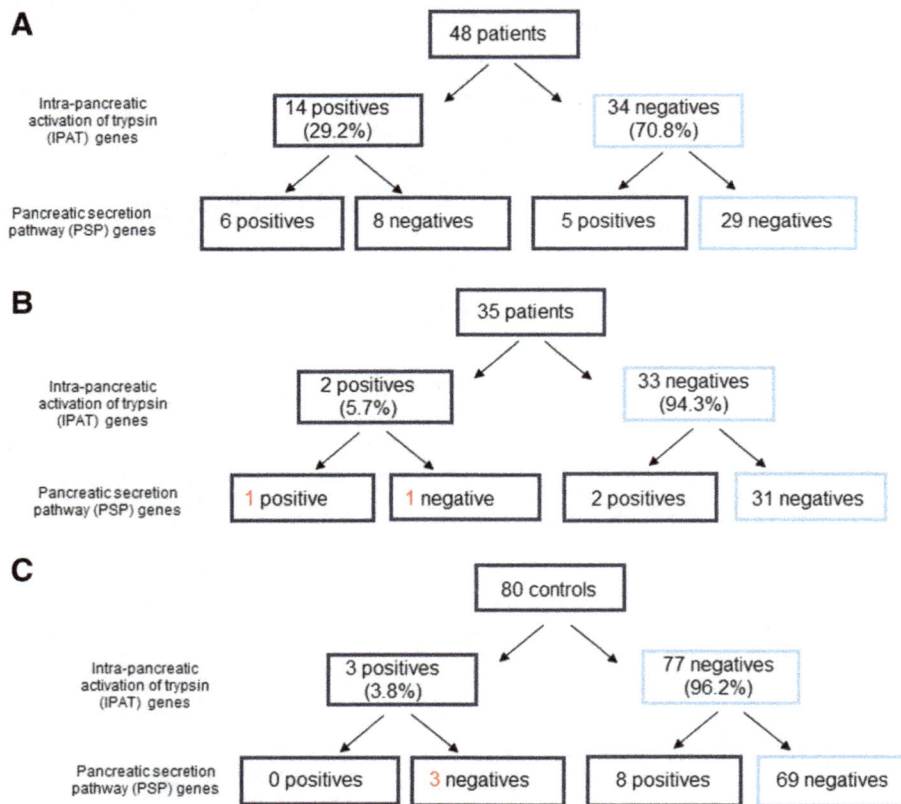

**Fig. 1** Flowchart of the results of molecular analysis in 48 patients affected by CF and recurrent/chronic pancreatitis (**a**), in 35 patients with CF and without pancreatitis (**b**) and in 80 healthy subjects (**c**)

cannot conclude on the pathogenic role of such mutation. Finally, the *KRT8* A358V novel mutation was identified in a patient with the [delta]F508/D110H *CFTR* genotype and we speculate on its pathogenetic role on the basis of the bioinformatic prediction and of its absence in alleles from the general population. Interestingly, in a recent study it was demonstrated an interaction between KRT8 and the CFTR protein that could influence the function of CFTR (Treiber et al., 2006).

All the genes discussed so far are involved in the premature intra-pancreatic activation of trypsin. This pathway plays a pivotal role in triggering the activation cascade

**Table 4** Genotype of *CFTR* and mutations in intra-pancreatic activation of trypsin (IPAT) and pancreatic secretion pathway (PSP) genes in in healthy controls

| Patient ID | IPAT genes | PSP genes |
| --- | --- | --- |
| ID-823 | / | *ITPR3*: c.2755G > T (G919C) |
| ID-1156 | / | *SLC4A4*: c.2528C > T (A843V) |
| ID-55 | / | *TRPV5*: c.256G > C (A86P) |
| ID-96 | / | *ATP2C2*: c.629C > T (T210 M) |
| ID-181 | *KRT8*: c.184G > T (G62C) | / |
| ID-182 | / | *TRPV5*: c.1490 T > C (M497 T) |
| ID-183 | / | *SLC4A4*: c.1805A > G (K602R); *TRPV5*: c.1490 T > C (M497 T) |
| ID-252 | *CASR*: c.1672G > T (A558S) | / |
| ID-508 | / | *ITPR3*: c.1574C > G (P525R) |
| ID-663 | / | *ITPR3*: c.1244 T > C (L415P) |
| ID-352 | *SPINK1*: c.101A > G (N34S) | / |

All mutations in IPAT and in PSP genes were heterozygous

of all pancreatic digestive zymogens caused by the breaking of the interactions of these proteins in pancreas leading to injury of acinar cells and consequently recurrent attacks of pancreatitis (Sofia et al., 2016; Chen & Férec, 2009).

Moving to patients with CF without pancreatitis, we found two cases with mutations IPAT genes: a patient had the *PRSS1/PRSS2* hybrid and a the *CTRC* G217S, a mutation previously identified in a normal subject by Rosendahl et al. (Rosendahl et al., 2008). In healthy subjects, we identified three individuals with mutations in *SPINK1*, *CASR* and *KRT8* genes. The N34S mutation identified in *SPINK1* was described by Threadgold et al. as a variation associated with a familial pattern of idiopathic chronic pancreatitis (Threadgold et al., 2002). Actually, it is considered not disease causing being found in normal control too with an average prevalence of 2.5% and an allele frequency of 1.25% (Premchandar & s, 2017). The missense A558S identified in *CASR* is a novel mutation considered potentially pathogenic by bioinformatic analysis despite a frequency of about 1% in the general population, while the *KRT8* G62C mutation found in another healthy control was identified also in healthy subjects by Witt et al. (Witt et al., 2006).

All mutations found in the second group of 23 genes PSP in the three groups of subjects were classified as possibly damaging by the three bioinformatic tools and all but two had a frequency in the general population < 0.1%. However, even if there is a trend of higher frequency of such mutations in patients with CF and RP/CP as compared to the patients with CF without pancreatitis and to healthy controls, the difference is not significant. To be noted that 6 out of 14 patients affected by CF with RP/CP with mutations in genes encoding proteins potentially involved in premature intra-pancreatic activation of trypsin also have mutations in genes of the pancreatic secretion pathway, in particular those belonging to the $Ca^{2+}$ signalling, pancreatic secretion and autophagy pathways, further reinforcing the concept that trans-heterozygous mutations in different genes may have a synergic effect in the pathogenesis of RP/CP.

## Conclusions

Our data strongly suggest that the trans-heterozygosity for mutations in CFTR and in genes encoding proteins involved in IPAT and PSP may enhance the risk for RP/CP in patients with CF, as we previously demonstrated in subjects with idiopathic RP/CP (Sofia et al., 2016). Further studies are called, to define if patients with trans-heteroygous mutations have a more severe outcome of pancreatitis (the small number of cases limited such evaluation in the present study) and functional studies are necessary to elucidate the pathogenetic mechanism of pancreatitis in patients bearing mutated genes/proteins.

## Additional file

> **Additional file 1: Table S1.** List of mutations in genes involved in the intrapancreatic activation of trypsin (IPAT) and pancreatic secretion pathway (PSP) and allelic frequency (%) in the three groups of subjects studied (A: CF with RP; B: CF without RP; C: healthy controls) and D: in the general population. (ExAC tool). (DOCX 17 kb)

### Abbreviations
CF: cystic fibrosis; CFTR: cystic fibrosis transmembrane conductance regulator; CP: chronic pancreatitis; IPAT: intra-pancreatic activation of trypsin; PI: pancreatic insufficiency; PS: pancreatic sufficiency; PSP: pancreatic secretion pathways; RP: recurrent pancreatitis

### Acknowledgements
We acknowledge the Ministero della Salute (Rome, Italy) L.548/93 for the regional research funding quote of years 2007–15.
We acknowledge the Società Italiana per lo studio della Fibrosi Cistica (SIFC) that stimulated this multicentric study. We are also grateful to Dr. Gianfranco Savoldi for his precious suggestions in reviewing genetic data.

### Authors' contributions
The manuscript was written by GC and Adriano Angioni. VMS and CS performed NGS of pancreatic genes, variants analysis and validation, interpretation of the data and revised critically the manuscript. LDS contributed to design of pancreatic gene panel and data analysis. VMS, CS, and ACT contributed to experimental performance and data interpretation. VT, FA, Antonella Angiolillo, CB, NC, CC, ADL, RP, SQ, VR, GT, FZ, VL, and ML recruited patients, collected biological samples, and performed clinical evaluations. Antonella Angiolillo, NC, RP, AN, VL, and ML revised critically the manuscript. GC and Adriano Angioni had a main role in conception and design, analyses, interpretation of the data and revised critically the manuscript. All authors read and approved the final manuscript.

### Competing interests
The authors declare they have no competing interests or other interests that might be perceived to influence the results and discussion reported in this paper.

### Author details
[1]Laboratory of Medical Genetics Unit, "Bambino Gesù" Children's Hospital, IRCCS, Viale di San Paolo 15, 00146 Rome, Italy. [2]Department of Pediatrics, Tuscany Regional Centre for Cystic Fibrosis, Anna Meyer Children's Hospital, Florence, Italy. [3]Multifactorial Diseases and Complex Phenotypes Research Area, "Bambino Gesù" Children's Hospital, IRCCS, Rome, Italy. [4]Cystic Fibrosis Unit, "Bambino Gesù" Children's Hospital, IRCCS, Rome, Italy. [5]Department of Medicine and Health Sciences "Vincenzo Tiberio", University of Molise, Campobasso, Italy. [6]Regional Cystic Fibrosis Centre, United Hospitals, Mother – Child Department, Ancona, Italy. [7]Cystic Fibrosis Regional Centre (Lombardia), IRCCS Ca' Granda Foundation, University of Milan, Milan, Italy. [8]CEINGE-Biotecnologie Avanzate, Naples, Italy. [9]Department of Neuroscience, ORL Section, University of Naples Federico II, Naples, Italy. [10]Cystic Fibrosis Support Centre, Pediatric Department, Children's Hospital, ASST Spedali Civili, Brescia, Italy. [11]Cystic Fibrosis Regional Centre (Lazio), Sapienza University and Policlinico Umberto I, Rome, Italy. [12]Cystic Fibrosis Regional Centre (Campania), Department of Medical Transalational Sciences, Section of Pediatrics, University of Naples Federico II, Naples, Italy. [13]Cystic Fibrosis Regional Centre, Soverato Hospital, Catanzaro, Italy. [14]Department of Biosciences and Territory, University of Molise, Isernia, Italy. [15]Department of Cellular Biotechnologies and Hematology, Sapienza University of Rome,

Rome, Italy. [16]Pasteur Institute, Cenci Bolognetti Foundation, Sapienza University of Rome, Rome, Italy. [17]Department of Molecular Medicine and Biotechnologies, University of Naples Federico II, Naples, Italy.

## References

Adzhubei IA, et al. A method and server for predicting damaging missense mutations. Nat Methods. 2010;7:248–9.

Berni Canani R, Terrin G, Cardillo G, Tomaiuolo R, Castaldo G. Congenital diarrheal disorders: improved understanding of gene defects is leading to advances in intestinal physiology and clinical management. J Pediatr Gastroenterol Nutr. 2010;50:360–6.

Bishop MD, et al. The cystic fibrosis transmembrane conductance regulator gene and ion channel function in patients with idiopathic pancreatitis. Hum Genet. 2005;118:372–81.

Castellani C, Assael BM. Cystic fibrosis: a clinical view. Cell Mol Life Sci. 2017;74:129–40.

Cavestro GM, et al. Association of keratin 8 gene mutation with chronic pancreatitis. Dig Liver Dis. 2003;35:416–20.

Chen JM, Férec C. Chronic pancreatitis: genetics and pathogenesis. Annu Rev Genomics Hum Genet. 2009;10:63–87.

Chen JM, Mercier B, Audrezet MP, Férec C. Mutational analysis of the human pancreatic secretory trypsin inhibitor (PSTI) gene in hereditary and sporadic chronic pancreatitis. J Med Genet. 2000;37:67–9.

Desmet FO, et al. Human splicing finder: an online bioinformatics tool to predict splicing signals. Nucleic Acids Res. 2009;37:e67.

Durno C, Corey M, Zielenski J, Tullis E, Tsui LC, Durie P. Genotype and phenotype correlations in patients with cystic fibrosis and pancreatitis. Gastroenterology. 2002;123:1857–64.

Farrell PM, et al. Diagnosis of cystic fibrosis: consensus guidelines from the Cystic Fibrosis Foundation. J Pediatr. 2017;181:1–58.

Felderbauer P, et al. A novel mutation of the calcium sensing receptor gene is associated with chronic pancreatitis in a family with heterozygous SPINK1 mutations. BMC Gastroenterol. 2003;3:34–41.

Fortunato F, Kroemer G. Impaired autophagosome-lysosome fusion in the pathogenesis of pancreatitis. Autophagy. 2009;5:850–3.

Gukovskaya AS, Gukovsky I. Autophagy and pancreatitis. Am J Physiol Gastrointest Liver Physiol. 2012;303:G993–1003.

Hicks S, Wheeler DA, Plon SE, Kimmel M. Prediction of missense mutation functionality depends on both the algorithm and sequence alignment employed. Hum Mutat. 2011;32:661–8.

Jin CX, Hayakawa T, Ko SB, Ishiguro H, Kitagawa M. Pancreatic stone protein/regenerating protein family in pancreatic and gastrointestinal diseases. Intern Med. 2015;50:1507–16.

Kanehisa M, Goto S, Sato Y, Furumichi M, Tanabe M. Data, information, knowledge and principle: back to metabolism in KEGG. Nucleic Acids Res. 2014;42:D199–205.

Keiles S, Kammesheidt A. Identification of CFTR, PRSS1, and SPINK1 mutations in 381 patients with pancreatitis. Pancreas. 2006;33:221–7.

Kumar S, Ooi CY, Werlin S, Abu-El-Haija M, Barth B, Bellin MD, et al. Pediatric acute recurrent and chronic pancreatitis: lessons from INSPPIRE. JAMA Pediatr. 2016;170:562–9.

Lew D, Afghani E, Pandol S. Chronic Pancreatitis: Current Status and Challenges for Prevention and Treatment. Dig Dis Sci. 2017;62:1702–12.

Lupia E, et al. Ablation of phosphoinositide 3-kinase-gamma reduces the severity of acute pancreatitis. Am J Pathol. 2004;165:2003–11.

Mahurkar S, et al. Association of cathepsin B gene polymorphisms with tropical calcific pancreatitis. Gut. 2006;55:1270–5.

Masson E, Chen JM, Scotet V, Le Maréchal C, Férec C. Association of rare chymotrypsinogen C (CTRC) gene variations in patients with idiopathic chronic pancreatitis. Hum Genet. 2008;123:83–91.

Mathe E, et al. Computational approaches for predicting the biological effect of p53 missense mutations: a comparison of three sequence analysis based methods. Nucleic Acids Res. 2006;34:1317–25.

Morinville VD, Husain SZ, Bai H, Barth B, Alhosh R, Durie PR, et al. Definitions of pediatric pancreatitis and survey of present clinical practices. J Pediatr Gastroenterol Nutr. 2012;55:261–5.

Multigner L, Sarles H, Lombardo D, De Caro A. Pancreatic stone protein. II. Implication in stone formation during the course of chronic calcifying pancreatitis. Gastroenterology. 1985;89:387–91.

Ng PC, Henikoff S. Predicting deleterious amino acid substitutions. Genome Res. 2001;11:863–74.

Ohmuraya M, Yamamura K. Autophagy and acute pancreatitis: a novel autophagy theory for trypsinogen activation. Autophagy. 2008;4:1060–2.

Ooi CY, Dorfman R, Cipolli M, Gonska T, Castellani C, Keenan K, et al. Type of CFTR mutation determines risk of pancreatitis in patients with cystic fibrosis. Gastroenterology. 2011;140:153–61.

Premchandar A, et al. New insights into interactions between the nucleotide-binding domain of CFTR and keratin 8. Protein Sci. 2017;26:343–54.

Ramnath RD, Sun J, Bhatia M. PKC delta mediates pro-inflammatory responses in a mouse model of caerulein-induced acute pancreatitis. J Mol Med. 2010;88:1055–63.

Rehm HL, et al. ACMG clinical laboratory standards for next-generation sequencing. Genet Med. 2013;15:733–47.

Robinson JT, et al. Integrative genomics viewer. Nat Biotechnol. 2011;29:24–6.

Rosendahl J, et al. Chymotrypsin C (CTRC) variants that diminish activity or secretion are associated with chronic pancreatitis. Nat Genet. 2008;40:78–82.

Schneider A, Löhr JM, Singer MV. The M-ANNHEIM classification of chronic pancreatitis: introduction of a unifying classification system based on a review of previous classifications of the disease. J Gastroenterol. 2007;42:101–19.

Schwarz JM, Rodelsperger C, Schuelke M, Seelow D. Mutation taster evaluates disease-causing potential of sequence alterations. Nat Methods. 2010;7:575–6.

Sharma A, et al. Protection against acute pancreatitis by activation of protease-activated receptor-2. Am J Physiol Gastrointest Liver Physiol. 2005;288:G388–95.

Shwachman H, Lebenthal E, Khaw KT. Recurrent acute pancreatitis in patients with cystic fibrosis with normal pancreatic enzymes. Pediatrics. 1975;55:86–95.

Singhi AD, et al. The histopathology of PRSS1 hereditary pancreatitis. Am J Surg Pathol. 2014;38:346–53.

Sofia VM, et al. Extensive molecular analysis suggested the strong genetic heterogeneity of idiopathic chronic pancreatitis. Mol Med. 2016;26:300–9.

Stevens T, Conwell DL, Zuccaro G. Pathogenesis of chronic pancreatitis: an evidence-based review of past theories and recent developments. Am J Gastroenterol. 2004;99:2256–70.

Szmola R, Sahin-Toth M. Chymotrypsin C (caldecrin) promotes degradation of human cationic trypsin: identity with Rinderknecht's enzyme Y. Proc Natl Acad Sci U S A. 2007;104:11227–32.

Thorvaldsdottir H, Robinson JT, Mesirov JP. Integrative genomics viewer (IGV): high-performance genomics data visualization and exploration. Brief Bioinform. 2013;14:178–92.

Threadgold J, et al. The N34S mutation of SPINK1 (PSTI) is associated with a familial pattern of idiopathic chronic pancreatitis but does not cause the disease. Gut. 2002;50:675–81.

Tomaiuolo AC, et al. Relationship between CFTR and CTRC variants and the clinical phenotype in late-onset cystic fibrosis disease with chronic pancreatitis. J Mol Diagn. 2015;17:171–8.

Treiber M, et al. Keratin 8 sequence variants in patients with pancreatitis and pancreatic cancer. J Mol Med. 2006;84:1015–22.

Walkowiak J, Glapa A, Nowak JK, Bober L, Rohovyk N, Wenska-Chyży E, et al. Pancreatic Elastase-1 Quick Test for rapid assessment of pancreatic status in cystic fibrosis patients. J Cyst Fibros. 2016;15:664–8.

Walkowiak J, Lisowska A, Blaszczyński M. The changing face of the exocrine pancreas in cystic fibrosis: pancreatic sufficiency, pancreatitis and genotype. Eur J Gastroenterol Hepatol. 2008;20:157–60.

Whitcomb DC, et al. Hereditary pancreatitis is caused by a mutation in the cationic trypsinogen gene. Nat Genet. 1996;14:141–5.

Willemer S, Kloppel G, Kern HF, Adler G. Immunocytochemical and morphometric analysis of acinar zymogen granules in human acute pancreatitis. Virchows Arch A Pathol Anat Histopathol. 1989;415:115–23.

Williams JA. Receptor-mediated signal transduction pathways and the regulation of pancreatic acinar cell function. Curr Opin Gastroenterol. 2008;24:573–9.

Witt H, et al. A degradation-sensitive anionic trypsinogen (PRSS2) variant protects against chronic pancreatitis. Nat Genet. 2006;38:668–73.

# 8

# Enrichment of B cell receptor signaling and epidermal growth factor receptor pathways in monoclonal gammopathy of undetermined significance: a genome-wide genetic interaction study

Subhayan Chattopadhyay[1,2*†] (iD), Hauke Thomsen[1†], Miguel Inacio da Silva Filho[1], Niels Weinhold[3,4], Per Hoffmann[5,6], Markus M. Nöthen[5,7], Arendt Marina[8], Karl-Heinz Jöckel[8], Börge Schmidt[8], Sonali Pechlivanis[8], Christian Langer[9], Hartmut Goldschmidt[3,10], Kari Hemminki[1,11] and Asta Försti[1,11]

## Abstract

**Background:** Recent identification of 10 germline variants predisposing to monoclonal gammopathy of undetermined significance (MGUS) explicates genetic dependency of this asymptomatic precursor condition with multiple myeloma (MM). Yet much of genetic burden as well as functional links remain unexplained. We propose a workflow to expand the search for susceptibility loci with genome-wide interaction and for subsequent identification of genetic clusters and pathways.

**Methods:** Polygenic interaction analysis on 243 cases/1285 controls identified 14 paired risk loci belonging to unique chromosomal bands which were then replicated in two independent sets (case only study, 82 individuals; case/control study 236 cases/ 2484 controls). Further investigation on gene-set enrichment, regulatory pathway and genetic network was carried out with stand-alone in silico tools separately for both interaction and genome-wide association study-detected risk loci.

**Results:** Intronic-PREX1 (20q13.13), a reported locus predisposing to MM was confirmed to have contribution to excess MGUS risk in interaction with SETBP1, a well-established candidate predisposing to myeloid malignancies. Pathway enrichment showed B cell receptor signaling pathway ($P < 5.3 \times 10^{-3}$) downstream to allograft rejection pathway ($P < 5.6 \times 10^{-4}$) and autoimmune thyroid disease pathway ($P < 9.3 \times 10^{-4}$) as well as epidermal growth factor receptor regulation pathway ($P < 2.4 \times 10^{-2}$) to be differentially regulated. Oncogene ALK and CDH2 were also identified to be moderately interacting with rs10251201 and rs16966921, two previously reported risk loci for MGUS.

**Conclusions:** We described novel pathways and variants potentially causal for MGUS. The methodology thus proposed to facilitate our search streamlines risk locus-based interaction, genetic network and pathway enrichment analyses.

**Keywords:** MGUS, MM, Genome-wide interaction, Pathway, Network, B-cell signaling, EGFR signaling

* Correspondence: s.chattopadhyay@dkfz-heidelberg.de
†Subhayan Chattopadhyay and Hauke Thomsen contributed equally to this work.
[1]Division of Molecular Genetic Epidemiology, German Cancer Research Center (DKFZ), Im Neuenheimer Feld 580, 69120 Heidelberg, Germany
[2]Faculty of Medicine, University of Heidelberg, Heidelberg, Germany
Full list of author information is available at the end of the article

## Background

Monoclonal gammopathy of undetermined significance (MGUS) is a premalignant phase of multiple myeloma (MM) and the most common plasma cell dyscrasia present in as high as 3.2% of general population below 50 years of age and up to 5.3% for population aged 70 years or older (Kyle et al. 2018). At an approximate annual rate of 1% MGUS progresses to MM, lympho-plasmacytic lymphoma/ Waldenström macroglobuline-mia or amyloid light chain amyloidosis (AL amyloidosis) (Kyle et al. 2006; Dispenzieri et al. 2010). Apart from the knowledge of familial clustering from population studies, there has not been much development in deciphering the genetic architecture of MGUS (Greenberg et al. 2012; Frank et al. 2016; Landgren et al. 2009). Of late, 17 risk loci have been found predisposing to MM among which 9 are supposed to share association with MGUS (Mitchell et al. 2016; Thomsen et al. 2017; Weinhold et al. 2014; Greenberg et al. 2013).

A GWAS from our group on 243 German individuals with MGUS has recently discovered 10 susceptibility loci with varying degree of significance (Thomsen et al. 2017). GWAS on a genetic heterogeneous disorder such as MGUS would possibly be subject to 'missing herit-ability' which asserts, an association study can account for merely a small proportion of true causal genetic vari-ations due to low detection power (Manolio et al. 2009). Linear interactions on paired single nucleotide polymor-phisms (SNPs) can thus be used to inflate genomic reso-lution of test space and find novel risk locus pairs which otherwise would remain undetected. In a case/control approach statistical interaction models explain extra additive effects due to co-occurrences of two variants on top of the fixed effects (Cordell 2009). We use an un-biased statistic with high convergence rate, and observe increased detection power for genome-wide interacting pairs (Wellek and Ziegler 2009). Gene-set enrichment along with genome-wide pathway analysis that measures association of a phenotype to a predefined genetic clus-ter has become rather common in extending biological understanding of differentially regulated pathways affect-ing quantitative traits and phenotype variation (Rama-nan et al. 2012; Khatri et al. 2012). This approach of mapping cancer susceptibility regions and detection of novel pathways in site-specific cancers has opened opportunities to new therapeutic approaches (Yi et al. 2017; Lee and Gyu Song 2015). Here we report a case/control interaction study on a discovery population of 243 MGUS cases and 1285 controls. The findings are subsequently supported by a case-only interaction study on 82 cases and finally confirmed with case/control interaction analysis on another population of 236 cases and 2484 controls. We pursue pathway enrichment ana-lysis on a subsequent stage, based on both our current

interaction study and the previous GWAS. To this end we use three in silico tools to discover novel pathways, corresponding genetic loci and clusters predisposing to MGUS taking into account significance of previously detected risk loci.

## Methods

### Ethics

Collection of samples and clinicopathological informa-tion from subjects was undertaken with the relevant ethical board approvals in accordance with the tenets of the Declaration of Helsinki. All subjects provided written informed consent. Ethical approval was obtained from Ethics committee of medicine faculty, University of Hei-delberg, Heidelberg, Germany.

### Datasets

The University Clinic of Heidelberg and the University Clinic Ulm discovered 243 MGUS cases among which 114 (47%) were males with a mean age at diagnosis of 62 years, SD ± 11 years. The Ig isotype distribution was 72% IgG, 12% IgA, and 16% other Ig isotypes (Thomsen et al. 2017; Weinhold et al. 2014). These MGUS cases were identified during diagnostic work-up of a different unrelated disease. Out of the 243 cases, two developed MM within 3 years after sampling and 46 individuals were seen only at the time of sampling. IgM MGUS cases were excluded from the Heidelberg/Ulm cohort. For replication, 236/82 MGUS patients were identified for case-control/case-only replication in Essen within the Heinz -Nixdorf Recall (HNR) study (Schmermund et al. 2002). About 61% of the replication set were males with the mean age at diagnosis of 64 years, SD ± 9 years. Detection of MGUS was based on internationally accepted criteria (Criteria for the classification of mono-clonal gammopathies 2003): monoclonal protein concen-tration less than 30 g/l, less than 10% monoclonal plasma cells in bone marrow, normal plasma calcium and kidney function and no bone destruction or anemia. The reference population for the Heidelberg/Ulm set consisted of 1285 German individuals from the HNR study of whom 59% were males with a mean age at sampling of 60 years, SD ± 8 years (Schmermund et al. 2002). The reference population for the Essen set was also recruited within the HNR study, adding up to 2484 individuals, not overlapping with the reference popula-tion for the Heidelberg set.

Illumina HumanOmniExpress-12v1.1 chip arrays were used for genotyping the Heidelberg/Ulm MGUS set and the corresponding control set was genotyped using the Illumina HumanOmniExpress-12v.1.0 chip array (Schmer-mund et al. 2002). The Essen set was genotyped using six different chips: 365 (15 cases, 350 controls) were geno-typed on Illumina HumanCoreExome-12v1−1 chip arrays,

1491 (82 cases, 1409 controls) on Illumina HumanCore Exome-12 v1–0 chip arrays, 133 (119 cases, 14 controls) on Illumina Human660W Quad_v1 chip arrays, 811 (45 cases, 766 controls) on Illumina Human Omni-Quad V.1 chip arrays and 1385 (82 cases, 1303 controls) on Illumina HumanOmniExpress-12v.1.0 chip arrays (Additional file 1). The amount of overlaps among the SNPs genotyped is reported in Additional file 2. Quality control assessment for genotyping has previously been described and all variants and samples considered for the final analysis passed the predefined thresholds (Broderick et al. 2011; Chubb et al. 2013).

## Quality control of GWAS samples

We excluded SNPs with less than 1% minor allele frequency, and also if the call rate was less than 99% in cases and controls. Genotype distribution in controls was tested for Hardy-Weinberg equilibrium with a $\chi2$ test with 1 degree of freedom or Fisher's exact test and SNPs with $P$ value lower than $10^{-5}$ was removed. This stringent quality control filtering produced 489,555 autosomal SNPs from Heidelberg/Ulm GWAS set for further analysis common to all of the 243 cases and 1285 controls and also 82 HNR samples (cases) genotyped on the same array. Application of similar quality control protocol rendered 195,490 autosomal SNPs present in 236 cases and 2484 controls of Essen GWAS set.

## Statistical and bioinformatics analysis

### Genome-wide case-control interaction analysis with CASSI and INTERSNP

Statistical analyses were performed with R version 3.3.1, CASSI version 3, and INTERSNP v1.15 (Table 1). All pairwise combinations of post-quality controlled selected SNPs from Heidelberg/Ulm GWAS were tested for interactions on genome-wide scale. The interaction term of a pairwise fixed effects logistic regression model involving binary regressors may be interpreted to be the ratio of the odds ratios of association between alleles in cases to the odds ratios of association between alleles in controls. Hence the odds ratio of association between

alleles in cases will be equal to that of the population interaction odds ratio given the odds ratio of association between alleles in controls are equal to 1. Epistasis enforces a logistic regression with linearity assumption among the fixed single marker effects and interaction effect of the two markers (Karkkainen et al. 2015; Purcell et al. 2007). This includes all 489,555 SNPs and approximately N = $1.2 \times 10^{11}$ interactions. However, linkage disequilibrium (LD) among the SNPs, if not taken into account in argument space, possibly renders a large portion of tests redundant which destabilizes the test statistic. To avoid this deflation of test power, we employed Wellek-Ziegler statistic which promises high variance stability and unbiased estimate on the condition of Hardy-Weinberg equilibrium conformity (Wellek and Ziegler 2009). CASSI Genome-Wide Interaction Analysis software is used to this end and we benefit from the computational efficiency thus achieved. Interaction test in CASSI (–wz) was applied with default initial pruning on single marker association $P$ value at $10^{-3}$ level of significance which decreases the computational burden (Ueki and Cordell 2012). This step selected $2.8 \times 10^7$ SNP pairs to be tested for interaction. For replication of interactions in the discovery set, reanalysis with full log-linear model was obtained with INTERSNP which selects a user-predefined number of top single marker hits as candidate SNPs for subsequent interaction tests. On a predefined level of 5000 selections, INTERSNP produced approximately N = $1.25 \times 10^7$ variant pairs (Herold et al. 2009).

### Case-only analysis with CASSI

We chose the additional smaller cohort of 82 individuals with MGUS for a validation study and adopt a case-only approach. Case-only approach in SNP – SNP interaction studies answers the question of association (or correlation) between alleles of two loci irrespective of phenotypic categorization. Assuming the general population (control group) is devoid of any correlation between the specific loci, the case-only approach ensures evidence of gene-gene functional pair interactions with higher power

**Table 1** Overview of tools and different subsequent protocols in use. Study designs enlist three stages of analysis

| Tool in use | Statistic used | Statistical model in use | Default pre-selection criteria for interaction test | Study design | No. of tests performed | Bonferroni adjusted genome-wide level of significance (< 1% FDR) | No. of risk loci pairs discovered |
|---|---|---|---|---|---|---|---|
| CASSI | Wellek-Zeigler statistic | Logistic regression; fixed effects weighted model | Single marker test $P$ value $< 10^{-3}$ | Discovery study | $2.8 \times 10^7$ | $5 \times 10^{-10}$ | 561 |
| | | | | Follow up study | $4.4 \times 10^5$ | $5 \times 10^{-10}$ | 352 |
| | | | | Replication study | $8.2 \times 10^6$ | $5 \times 10^{-10}$ | 23 |
| INTERSNP | Chi square statistic | Full log-linear model | Top 5000 variants of single marker test | Discovery study | $1.25 \times 10^7$ | $8 \times 10^{-10}$ | none |

*FDR* false discovery rate

in detection due to reduced number of multiple testing. As the risk loci are tested against each other rather than a reference set, allelic co-occurrence indicates bi-allelic interaction jointly predisposing phenotype changes (Ueki and Cordell 2012). However, case-only approach makes a quite strong assumption of no apparent genetic correlation among controls which is difficult to justify under the effects of LD which calls for cautious investigation of the results which further needs to be tested against a control population as reference to avoid misinterpretation due to the assumption. Case-only interaction test with CASSI with Wellek-Ziegler statistics (–wz-cc-only) on post quality-controlled SNPs rendered transformed Fisher's Z statistics on $4.4 \times 10^5$ out of a total of $1.2 \times 10^{11}$ interaction pairs. We re-observed 31 genome-wide significant pairs from the discovery set. The number of overlaps detected between the two tested interaction population sets with high power extracted from the case-only set ensured viability of the replication GWAS data being used for replication (Wu et al. 2010).

### Case-control replication study with CASSI

The Essen GWAS data consisting of 236 cases and 2484 controls was chosen for the case-control replication of the results obtained. The interaction tests for replication were performed similarly as explained before using Wellek-Ziegler statistic. Approximately $N = 8.2 \times 10^6$ tests were performed among the 195,490 SNPs after application of initial quality control. Among the quality-controlled SNPs from the Essen GWAS, we observed 188,198 overlaps with that of the Heidelberg/Ulm discovery GWAS. With approximately 35% cross table commonality we do not expect to see chance findings overlapping with high significance which takes care of the 'winner's curse' (Shi et al. 2016; Poirier et al. 2015; Jiang and Yu 2016).

### Network analysis with STRING

Two-locus epistasis evidence is verified by network construction with the in silico tool STRING. It is a web-based data repository dedicated to protein-protein interactions among 2.5 million proteins among 630 organisms including mammalians (version 8.0) (Jensen et al. 2009). Scores for each of the interacting protein pair is computed with combined scores integrating discovery probabilities from different sources adjusting for arbitrary false positives. Subsequently pathway enrichment is performed with the background repository for the interaction identified loci.

### Gene prioritization and pathway analysis of the MGUS GWAS

Due to LD, causal regulatory elements often remain unidentified in genome-wide association studies. To gain biological insight, pathway analysis via gene-set enrichment is traditionally carried out to integrate signals from different sentinel variants and linked SNPs. We applied three tools designed for biological interpretation of GWAS: Pathway Scoring Algorithm (PASCAL), Data-driven Expression Prioritized Integration for Complex Traits (DEPICT) and Meta-Analysis Gene Set Enrichment of Variant Associations (MAGENTA). PASCAL is a pathway analysis tool developed for association summary statistics for variants annotated to genes. PASCAL uses maximum of chi-squares (MOCS) or sum of chi-squares (SOCS) statistics with null distribution as Gamma with varying degrees of freedom (Lamparter et al. 2016). Although pathway scoring was performed using both MOCS and SOCS statistics, the results were comparable and SOCS produced deflated significance levels with similar order as of that by MOCS. With empirical sampling and subsequent supervised clustering according to the significance levels introduced by single marker association tests, it utilizes the idea of gene fusions i.e. clusters of correlated genes, for which the variants are in LD. We performed gene set enrichment analysis (GSEA) using single marker $P$ values from our published GWAS on MGUS and SNPs were mapped to closest genes searched 20 kb upstream and downstream from the gene. However, SNPs, corresponding to several genes responsible for regulating a single pathway, if they were in LD, were used to cluster the corresponding genes as single genetic entities for the given pathway and were called 'gene fusions'. Kyoto encyclopedia of genes and genomes (KEGG), REACTOME and BioCarta libraries were used for pathway enrichment.

For further investigation of the distinguished pathways, we used DEPICT, a gene prioritization, tissue enrichment and pathway analysis tool for biological interpretation of GWASs distributed by Broad institute, which employs Python shell script on a Java platform for efficiency (Pers et al. 2015). This framework is built on sophisticated predictive modeling employing guilt by association on reconstituted gene sets to perform gene prioritization and GSEA (van Rheenen et al. 2016). Depict derives enrichment analysis viability from 77,840 gene expression datasets. We used DEPICT's gene set knowledge base derived from Gene ontology (GO), Ensembl, The Mammalian Phenotype (MP), KEGG and REACTOME and followed analogous analyses.

Literature on pathway analysis with MAGENTA is populous (Koster et al. 2014; Wang et al. 2012; Duncan et al. 2014). We executed GSEA in MAGENTA from MATLAB platform as a replication tool. For pathway analysis, single marker association $P$ values and chromosomal regions were annotated to genes corresponding to a pre-existing chromosomal range and enrichment computation was applied on non-confounders (Segrè et al. 2010; Shim et al. 2015). Pathway annotations were extracted in back end from GO, KEGG, Protein Analysis through Evolutionary Relationships (PANTHER), BioCarta and REACTOME databases. Across the three platforms thus used to prioritize pathways, $p$ values are pooled subject to a total overlap and are combined using empirical Brown's method. Traditionally p values thus analyzed are assumed to be dependent and thus the method applied provided a conservative restriction. All additional analyses were performed with R version 3.3.1.

## Results

### Genome-wide interaction analysis identifies 23 variant pairs

Two machine level in silico tools, CASSI and INTERSNP were employed to explore curated genome-wide interaction on a set of 243 German individuals diagnosed with MGUS in a case-control design. Among the 489,555 genotyped post-quality control SNPs, a brute search algorithm required $1.2 \times 10^{11}$ tests at a whole-genome scale to perform a multivariate log-linear association test. However, CASSI restricted the runs to approximately $2.8 \times 10^7$ overall tests at the system-defined single marker association test threshold of $P = 10^{-3}$. As approximately $2.8 \times 10^7$ tests were performed, Bonferroni corrected level of global threshold of significance was determined to be $5 \times 10^{-10}$ which restricts the family-wise error rate (FWER) at 1% (Table 1). Selection of chance findings over significant variants was thus avoided by applying Bonferroni correction for multiple testing. At this empirically determined $P < 5 \times 10^{-10}$, CASSI reported 561 significant variant pairs. The top ranked interaction (rs12471071 [2q37] - rs1385453 [9p24]) from the discovery set had a Wellek-Zeigler (W-Z) $P = 4.19 \times 10^{-13}$ and a simple logistic regression $P = 8.67 \times 10^{-11}$ (Additional file 3). Although the CASSI algorithm detected several common variant SNP pairs to be genome-wide significant, previous researches demonstrate that such findings were often subject to false discovery.

Interaction tests in INTERSNP were employed according to subjective pre-selection of the 5000 most significantly associated SNPs from the single marker tests ($P = 2.47 \times 10^{-3}$) which restricted the number of tests performed to an approximate $1.25 \times 10^7$ pairs. Subsequently, 693 unique interaction pairs were identified at $5 \times 10^{-5}$ significance level where none of the observations reached genome-wide threshold of approximate $8 \times 10^{-10}$ calculated taking Bonferroni correction into account on 99% confidence level. The top interaction was found to be between rs10099120 and rs3738270 with $P = 9.05 \times 10^{-8}$ and we note, rs10099120 is located in the intronic region of RALYL and rs3738270 corresponds to a missense mutation on IGFN1 (Additional file 4). Overall 52 common variant pairs were co-discovered for both INTERSNP and CASSI.

A follow-up case-only analysis by CASSI on the 82 cases genotyped, rendered approximately $4.4 \times 10^5$ overall tests after initial single marker test shrinkage similar to that described above. The most significant interaction (rs4433825 [16p13] - rs2295179 [20p12]) showed a case-only $P = 3.35 \times 10^{-24}$ against W-Z case-control $P = 1.5 \times 10^{-12}$. At $5 \times 10^{-10}$ level we detected 352 variant pairs replicated in the discovery set with varying levels of significance (Additional file 5). The order of significance observed in the follow-up analysis is consistent with the literature of case-only studies bolstering higher detection power due to the inherent mathematical assumption although we decided not to interpret the results as evidence of functional relation between variants due to the difference in number of overlapping SNP pairs tested with the discovery set. As the single marker pre-selection criteria prunes significant number of SNPs, the observed overlaps are ensured to have presumably higher individual fixed effects which is devoid of the hypotheses (Ueki and Cordell 2012). Nonetheless it confirms viability of the case-control replication study with a larger genetically overlapping sample(s).

Next, we evaluated W-Z interactions by CASSI in the case-control replication set consisting $8.2 \times 10^6$ test pairs with an inflation factor of 1.0151 (Additional file 6). We were able to replicate 23 out of all 561 genome-wide significant variant pairs of the discovery set which are annotated to same chromosomal regions (Table 2, Fig. 1). The top interaction was found among variants annotated to TNC and CRYL1 corresponding to 9q33 and 13q12 (rs10118040 – rs7337130, W-Z $P = 6.9 \times 10^{-11}$ and rs1330368 – rs7337231, W-Z $P = 2.48 \times 10^{-8}$, respectively). Among the 23 replications, 14 were unique regions and there were 5 regions with multiple unique interactions. Interestingly, SETBP1 and PREX1 interaction at 18q12 and 20q13 were represented by 6 SNP-SNP pairwise overlaps with LD coefficient of $r^2 < 0.2$ between SNPs belonging to corresponding regions. The locus at 20q13 has already been identified as a predisposing locus for MM and as an expression and methylation quantitative trait locus at PREX1 without affecting an active promoter site (Mitchell et al. 2016). SETBP1 is a well-established candidate gene harboring somatic mutation in various myeloid malignancies including secondary acute myeloid leukemia (sAML) and chronic myelomonocytic leukemia (CMML) (Makishima et al. 2013). Previously our group had identified 10 common variant risk loci for MGUS (Thomsen et al. 2017), among which two SNPs showed noteworthy interactions in our analysis: rs10251201 (7p21, GLCCI1) with rs1104869 (2p23, ALK), W-Z $P = 8.75 \times 10^{-7}$ and rs16966921 (18q12, GALNT1) with rs8092870 (18q12, CDH2), W-Z P =

**Table 2** Summary results for identified risk loci pair overlaps

| Gene1 | Chr1 | Gene2 | Chr2 | Discovery set | | | | | | | |
|---|---|---|---|---|---|---|---|---|---|---|---|
| | | | | SNP1 (Risk allele) | Position (hg19,bp) | MAF | SNP2 (Risk allele) | Position (hg19,bp) | MAF | WZ P-value | OR (95% CI) |
| TNC | 9q33.1 | CRYL1 | 13q12.11 | rs10118040 (T) | 117,879,414 | 0.40 | rs7337130 (C) | 21,021,343 | 0.31 | 6.91E-11 | 2.64 (1.91-3.65) |
| SETBP1 | 18q12.3 | PREX1 | 20q13.13 | rs12959213 (C) | 42,769,020 | 0.41 | rs6066791 (T) | 47,251,687 | 0.26 | 7.07E-11 | 2.39 (1.75-3.25) |
| SETBP1 | 18q12.3 | PREX1 | 20q13.13 | rs12959213 (C) | 42,769,020 | 0.41 | rs6066791 (T) | 47,251,687 | 0.26 | 7.07E-11 | 2.39 (1.75-3.25) |
| ERBB4 | 2q34 | RORA | 15q22.2 | rs1546717 (G) | 212,902,339 | 0.10 | rs1159814 (A) | 61,431,996 | 0.41 | 9.07E-11 | 5.03 (2.89-8.77) |
| PARK2 | 6q26 | C14orf177 | 14q32.2 | rs6455744 (T) | 162,060,468 | 0.38 | rs7359146 (C) | 99,084,602 | 0.14 | 1.12E-10 | 2.92 (1.96-4.33) |
| ETNK1 | 12p12.1 | TMC2 | 20p13 | rs2467112 (C) | 23,071,644 | 0.19 | rs1028441 (T) | 2,600,186 | 0.24 | 1.20E-10 | 3.24 (2.12-4.95) |
| aLOC646784 / HFM1 | 1p22.2 | LOC647259 | 13q21.1 | rs674135 (G) | 91,675,675 | 0.26 | rs4146191 (A) | 62,872,965 | 0.47 | 1.44E-10 | 2.61 (1.89-3.60) |
| ERBB4 | 2q34 | PTPRD | 9p23 | rs1437919 (A) | 212,110,840 | 0.23 | rs10978043 (G) | 9,860,402 | 0.19 | 2.64E-10 | 3.38 (2.19-5.22) |
| AUTS2 | 7p11.22 | HS6ST3 | 13q32.1 | rs1011780 (A) | 70,124,648 | 0.28 | rs9556582 (G) | 97,040,531 | 0.46 | 2.68E-10 | 2.40 (1.75-3.29) |
| SETBP1 | 18q12.3 | PREX1 | 20q13.13 | rs12959213 (C) | 42,769,020 | 0.41 | rs4810836 (T) | 47,228,931 | 0.25 | 3.04E-10 | 2.40 (1.75-3.25) |
| SETBP1 | 18q12.3 | PREX1 | 20q13.13 | rs12959213 (C) | 42,769,020 | 0.41 | rs4810836 (T) | 47,228,931 | 0.25 | 3.04E-10 | 2.40 (1.75-3.25) |
| CNTN4 | 3p26.3 | FAM19A1 | 3p14.1 | rs2619566 (C) | 2,624,938 | 0.12 | rs1032376 (A) | 68,317,975 | 0.19 | 3.28E-10 | 4.66 (2.71-8.02) |
| CNTN4 | 3p26.3 | FAM19A1 | 3p14.1 | rs2619566 (G) | 2,624,938 | 0.12 | rs1032376 (A) | 68,317,975 | 0.19 | 3.28E-10 | 4.66 (2.71-8.02) |
| TNC | 9q33.1 | CRYL1 | 9q33.1 | rs2071520 (T) | 117,880,792 | 0.32 | rs7337130 (C) | 21,021,343 | 0.31 | 3.50E-10 | 2.80 (1.99-3.15) |
| CSMD1 | 8p23.2 | LOC392301 | 9q13 | rs1700112 (G) | 4,097,418 | 0.41 | rs410684 (A) | 31,673,588 | 0.42 | 3.84E-10 | 2.16 (1.62-2.87) |
| CSMD1 | 8p23.2 | LOC392301 | 9q13 | rs1700112 (G) | 4,097,418 | 0.41 | rs410684 (A) | 31,673,588 | 0.42 | 3.84E-10 | 2.16 (1.62-2.87) |
| ERBB4 | 2q34 | LOC729802 | 9p23 | rs1437919 (A) | 212,110,840 | 0.23 | rs7851513 (G) | 9,842,176 | 0.19 | 3.92E-10 | 3.10 (2.05-4.69) |
| KHDRBS3 | 8q24.23 | KSR2 | 12q24.23 | rs4909494 (C) | 136,646,548 | 0.46 | rs10774941 (T) | 118,037,655 | 0.27 | 4.22E-10 | 2.51 (1.83-3.45) |
| SETBP1 | 18q12.3 | PREX1 | 20q13.13 | rs12959213 (C) | 42,769,020 | 0.41 | rs6095212 (T) | 47,233,383 | 0.25 | 4.25E-10 | 2.39 (1.75-3.25) |
| SETBP1 | 18q12.3 | PREX1 | 20q13.13 | rs12959213 (C) | 42,769,020 | 0.41 | rs6095212 (T) | 47,233,383 | 0.25 | 4.25E-10 | 2.39 (1.75-3.25) |
| MAN1A1 | 6q22.31 | FRMD4A | 10p13 | rs808034 (A) | 119,467,743 | 0.39 | rs789761 (C) | 14,137,678 | 0.48 | 4.72E-10 | 0.46 (0.34-0.61) |
| BNC2 | 9p22.3 | CDH13 | 16q23.3 | rs7867771 (T) | 16,314,909 | 0.28 | rs11149564 (C) | 83,441,027 | 0.44 | 4.82E-10 | 2.20 (1.62-3.00) |
| DAOA | 13q33.2 | TOM1L1 | 17q22 | rs5012127 (G) | 105,119,100 | 0.17 | rs4793773 (A) | 52,646,414 | 0.27 | 4.89E-10 | 2.81 (1.88-4.02) |

**Table 2** Summary results for identified risk loci pair overlaps *(Continued)*

| Gene1 | Replication set SNP1 (Risk allele) | Position (hg19,bp) | MAF | SNP2 (Risk allele) | Position (hg19,bp) | MAF | WZ P value | OR (95% CI) |
|---|---|---|---|---|---|---|---|---|
| TNC | rs1330368 (A) | 117,821,026 | 0.48 | rs7337231 (G) | 20,896,618 | 0.49 | 2.48E-08 | 1.05 (0.96–1.14) |
| SETBP1 | rs11082429 (G) | 42,743,790 | 0.44 | rs170536 (A) | 46,878,722 | 0.32 | 4.25E-08 | 1.01 (0.93–1.09) |
| SETBP1 | rs1376230 (T) | 42,703,052 | 0.35 | rs6063251 (C) | 47,015,157 | 0.43 | 6.37E-07 | 1.03 (0.94–1.11) |
| ERBB4 | rs6745249 (G) | 213,130,571 | 0.48 | rs974065 (A) | 60,952,440 | 0.34 | 1.06E-10 | 1.13 (1.04–1.22) |
| PARK2 | rs6927285 (G) | 162,010,329 | 0.43 | rs8022922 (A) | 98,987,292 | 0.44 | 1.23E-14 | 1.06 (0.98–1.14) |
| ETNK1 | rs7313039 (C) | 23,091,130 | 0.47 | rs6050256 (T) | 2,554,907 | 0.48 | 2.04E-07 | 1.05 (0.97–1.14) |
| ªLOC646784 / HFM1 | rs7416823 (T) | 157,386,394 | 0.31 | rs428328 (C) | 63,110,606 | 0.41 | 2.24E-09 | 1.05 (0.96–1.13) |
| ERBB4 | rs6747637 (G) | 212,406,789 | 0.45 | rs4427223 (A) | 10,663,815 | 0.48 | 7.35E-14 | 1.01 (0.93–1.09) |
| AUTS2 | rs10267303 (T) | 70,082,913 | 0.47 | rs12876541 (C) | 97,304,003 | 0.44 | 3.33E-08 | 1.06 (0.97–1.14) |
| SETBP1 | rs11082429 (G) | 42,743,790 | 0.44 | rs170536 (A) | 46,878,722 | 0.32 | 4.25E-08 | 0.98 (0.90–1.06) |
| SETBP1 | rs1376230 (T) | 42,703,052 | 0.35 | rs6063251 (C) | 47,015,157 | 0.43 | 6.37E-07 | 0.97 (0.89–1.05) |
| CNTN4 | rs1499133 (C) | 2,952,214 | 0.41 | rs7610023 (T) | 68,123,731 | 0.40 | 4.14E-09 | 1.05 (0.97–1.14) |
| CNTN4 | rs1178491 (G) | 2,342,825 | 0.36 | rs6549098 (A) | 68,323,280 | 0.40 | 2.83E-08 | 0.98 (0.90–1.06) |
| TNC | rs1330368 (A) | 117,821,026 | 0.48 | rs7337231 (G) | 20,896,618 | 0.49 | 2.48E-08 | 0.96 (0.89–1.04) |
| CSMD1 | rs2740939 (C) | 3,872,513 | 0.48 | rs7853053 (T) | 32,211,402 | 0.49 | 2.04E-16 | 1.04 (0.95–1.12) |
| CSMD1 | rs2740929 (C) | 3,879,918 | 0.49 | rs7853053 (T) | 32,211,402 | 0.49 | 3.81E-10 | 1.04 (0.95–1.12) |
| ERBB4 | rs6747637 (G) | 212,406,789 | 0.45 | rs4427223 (A) | 10,663,815 | 0.48 | 7.35E-14 | 0.92 (0.85–0.99) |
| KHDRBS3 | rs16905387 (G) | 136,539,132 | 0.42 | rs7972142 (A) | 118,211,046 | 0.44 | 3.97E-13 | 1.05 (0.96–1.13) |
| SETBP1 | rs11082429 (G) | 42,743,790 | 0.44 | rs170536 (A) | 46,878,722 | 0.32 | 4.25E-08 | 1.04 (0.96–1.12) |
| SETBP1 | rs1376230 (T) | 42,703,052 | 0.35 | rs6063251 (C) | 47,015,157 | 0.43 | 6.37E-07 | 1.03 (0.95–1.11) |
| MAN1A1 | rs1295392 (G) | 119,676,177 | 0.45 | rs751498 (A) | 13,929,130 | 0.47 | 1.25E-09 | 1.05 (0.96–1.14) |
| BNC2 | rs1415471 (A) | 16,656,653 | 0.44 | rs7194615 (G) | 82,769,498 | 0.44 | 1.07E-08 | 1.02 (0.94–1.09) |
| DAOA | rs3015345 (A) | 105,860,621 | 0.45 | rs8070668 (G) | 52,991,636 | 0.38 | 6.06E-10 | 1.05 (0.97–1.14) |

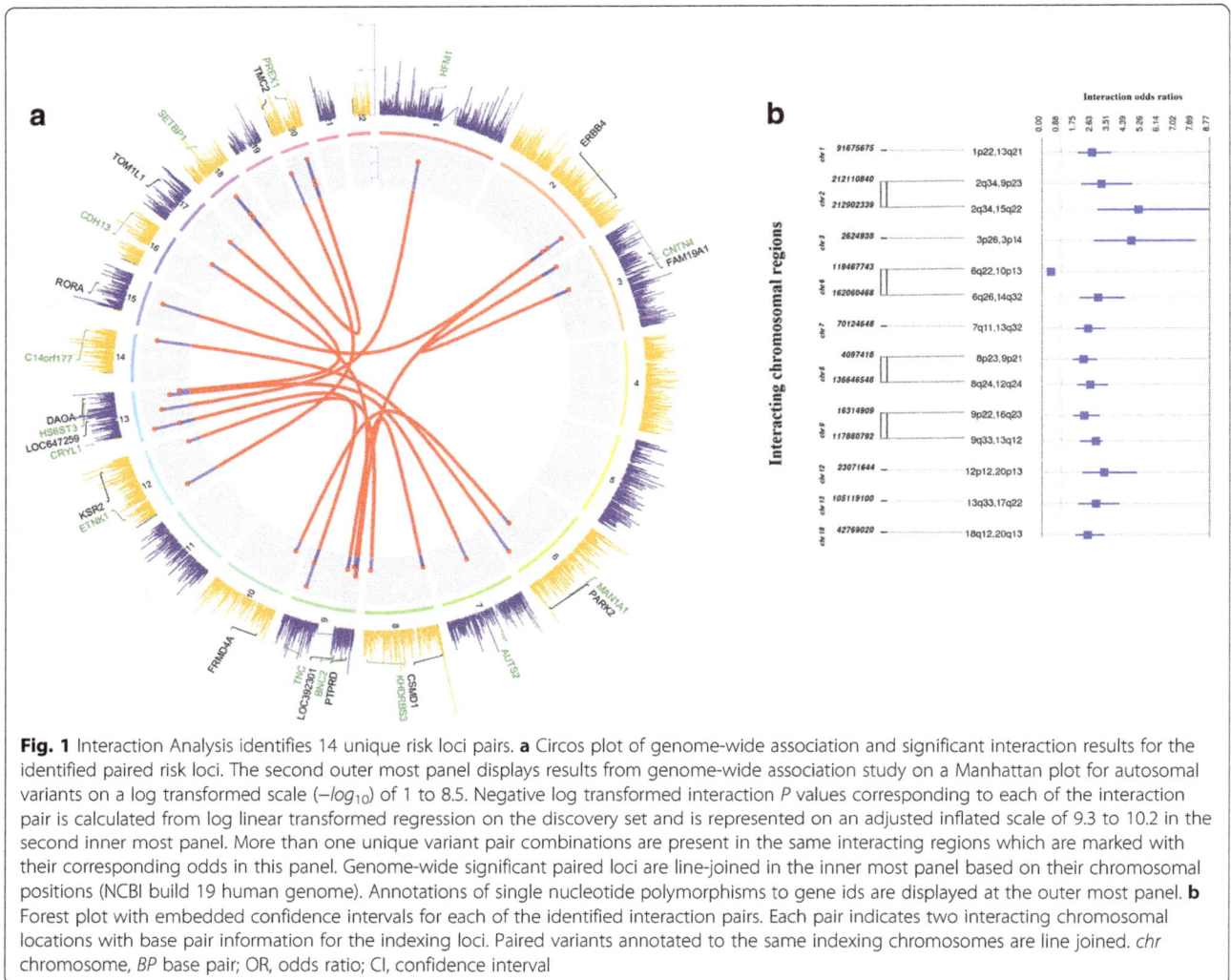

**Fig. 1** Interaction Analysis identifies 14 unique risk loci pairs. **a** Circos plot of genome-wide association and significant interaction results for the identified paired risk loci. The second outer most panel displays results from genome-wide association study on a Manhattan plot for autosomal variants on a log transformed scale ($-log_{10}$) of 1 to 8.5. Negative log transformed interaction $P$ values corresponding to each of the interaction pair is calculated from log linear transformed regression on the discovery set and is represented on an adjusted inflated scale of 9.3 to 10.2 in the second inner most panel. More than one unique variant pair combinations are present in the same interacting regions which are marked with their corresponding odds in this panel. Genome-wide significant paired loci are line-joined in the inner most panel based on their chromosomal positions (NCBI build 19 human genome). Annotations of single nucleotide polymorphisms to gene ids are displayed at the outer most panel. **b** Forest plot with embedded confidence intervals for each of the identified interaction pairs. Each pair indicates two interacting chromosomal locations with base pair information for the indexing loci. Paired variants annotated to the same indexing chromosomes are line joined. *chr* chromosome, *BP* base pair; OR, odds ratio; CI, confidence interval

$1.71 \times 10^{-7}$. Although both the latter two SNPs are located at 18q12, they are not in LD ( $r^2 < 0.2$ ).

### ErbB signaling and B cell receptor signaling are enriched based on genetic network analysis

A partnership dependence structure of functional network was constructed with the risk variants from the final overlapping set subject to identifiable annotation from the interaction analyses. Twenty-six such reconstituted genes were used as nodes which together with first order interacting genes created scaffolding for further enrichment analysis (Fig. 2). Thirty-six potentially differentially regulated pathways were identified (Additional file 7). Among them were 18 enriched pathways at 0.01 level of significance, with as many as 5 gene nodes downstream to KEGG ErbB signaling pathway ($P = 7.09 \times 10^{-5}$) and 3 gene nodes downstream to KEGG B cell receptor signaling pathway ($P = 5.32 \times 10^{-3}$) were found to be the two most significant pathways.

### GSEA and pathway analysis confirms enrichment of ErbB cascade and detects pathways upstream to B cell receptor signaling in the MGUS GWAS

Similar to genome wide-association and interaction studies, pathway enrichment for MGUS is still unexplored in literature due to obvious limitations regarding caveats in identification and inclusion of adequate MGUS cases. We identified 65 enriched pathways at 95% confidence (19 at 99%) employing PASCAL (Additional file 8). For confirmation of our results we employed MAGENTA on the same set and detected 111 functionally enriched pathways significant at 95% level (22 at 99%) (Additional file 9). Although 28 overlapping pathways between the two algorithms used were discovered with a combined corrected $P < 0.025$ (Additional file 10), we wanted to extend our search introducing more detection power with curated microarray data. Further gene set enrichment analysis (GSEA) and pathway enrichment with DEPICT identified 99 pathways at the suggestive threshold of $10^{-5}$ (4 at

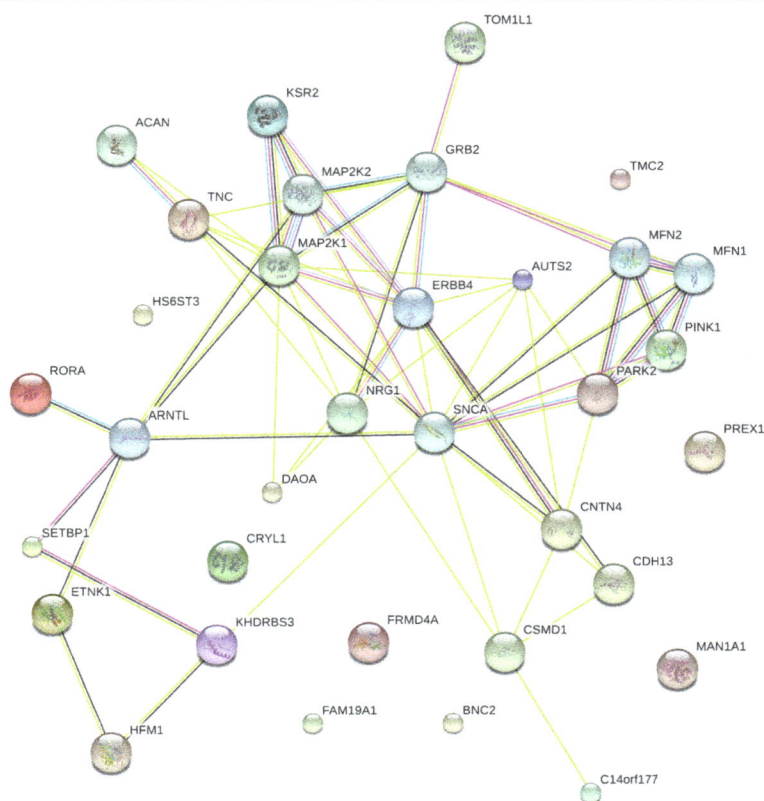

**Fig. 2** Genetic Interaction network. A network of 26 identified genes annotated to risk loci with added predicted genes in interaction. All nodes represent first order interaction. Colored edges convey status of predicted network edge correspondingly cyan, curated database; magenta, experimentally determined; forest green, gene neighborhood; red, gene fusion; navy blue, gene co-occurrence; lawn green, text mining; black, co-expression; lavender indigo, protein homology. Node color signifies protein functionality. Additional nodes are considered based on prediction score ≥ 0.9 (for more details, refer to STRING data base)

genome-wide threshold of $5 \times 10^{-8}$) (Additional file 11). With a combined analysis throughout the three algorithms, we observe 9 pathways with varying levels of significance (Table 3). Among the overlapping pathways, KEGG allograft rejection pathway (combined $P = 1.60 \times 10^{-6}$) and KEGG autoimmune thyroid disease pathway (combined $P = 5.41 \times 10^{-6}$), both related to B cell receptor signaling pathway, were the two most significant ones. Thus we determine that the B-cell receptor signaling pathway and EGFR regulatory pathway are present in both the interaction and genome-wide association study-oriented pathway analyses with statistical significance.

**Table 3** Combined results of gene set enrichment analysis from MAGENTA, PASCAL and DEPICT. Pathways are pooled from several repositories which are enlisted with data base. $P$ values from PASCAL, DEPICT and MAGENTA are corrected for multiple testing

| Data base | Pathway | PASCAL P value | DEPICT P value | MAGENTA P value | *Combined P value |
|---|---|---|---|---|---|
| KEGG | Allograft rejection | 0.083 | 0.001 | 0.005 | 5.62E-04 |
| KEGG | Autoimmune thyroid disease | 0.043 | 0.001 | 0.022 | 9.30E-04 |
| KEGG | Glycosaminoglycan biosynthesis keratan sulfate | 0.008 | 0.171 | 0.036 | 9.89E-03 |
| REACTOME | Platelet aggregation plug formation | 0.044 | 0.952 | 0.005 | 2.28E-02 |
| REACTOME | EGFR downregulation | 0.776 | 0.951 | 0.003 | 2.45E-02 |
| REACTOME | Integrin cell surface interactions | 0.16 | 0.396 | 0.011 | 4.51E-02 |
| KEGG | Dorso ventral axis formation | 0.151 | 0.233 | 0.022 | 4.78E-02 |
| REACTOME | P130CAS linkage to MAPK signaling for integrins | 0.035 | 0.988 | 0.032 | 4.85E-02 |

*Pooled p values are combined using empirical Brown's method assuming dependency across test hypotheses

## Discussion

Here we investigated MGUS, the preliminary phase of the lymphoproliferative neoplasm MM, assuming biological evidence of genetic burden to be spread across the whole genome spectrum. Performing genome-wide interaction analysis with case/control and case-only data together with subsequent follow-ups, our design essentially narrows down brute-force search to rather sizable genomic regions. Extending from the methodology developed by Ueki and colleagues for systematic implementation of Wellek – Zeigler statistics in interaction tests (Ueki and Cordell 2012), we propose a workflow to integrate statistical findings with biological knowledge base. Streamlining detection of risk loci with enriched protein-protein interacting networks to discover differentially regulated novel pathways facilitates understanding of disease mechanisms and congregates statistical evidence with biologically interpretable information.

Rather than simple bi-allelic association estimated with a dichotomous logistic model, we employed Pearson's product-moment correlation coefficient $r^2$ for association test. In simple linear association models, loss in precision is surmountable subject to non-conformity to Hardy-Weinberg equilibrium, especially while estimating for variant pairs in high LD. Wellek and Zeigler established genotype-based estimator of pearsonian r to be unbiased and circumstantial loss in information for unphased genotypes to be considerably lower than the haplotype-based estimators (Wellek and Ziegler 2009). Hence, we used genotype-based W-Z statistic, which employs a variance stabilizing Fisher's z transformation and produces robust estimates with high convergence rate.

Literature recognizes statistical interaction and functional interaction among genes/proteins exclusively, as the former stands for genetic association and the latter signifies biological process dependency. Thus, translation of statistical evidence to interpretable genetic functional involvement is of utmost importance. Creating node-based protein networks with STRING enabled us to visualize statistical clusters of genes in inter-play among the interacting genomic loci and observe the enriched biological processes that confer to them relating small genetic hubs created by clusters of genes specific to pathways. Consequently, we executed gene-prioritization and enrichment analysis accumulating tests in the previously published MGUS GWAS data from three different algorithms, PASCAL, MAGENTA and DEPICT, that engage different repositories. Observed overlaps therefore served as strong evidence connecting interacting common variant loci to the pathways via genetic networks.

We detected KEGG allograft rejection (hsa05330) and autoimmune thyroid disease (hsa05320) pathways with highest combined power from all three GWAS enrichment algorithms. Conspicuously B cell receptor signaling which is enriched in our genetic network is also downstream to both of the pathways. This pathway is shown to be dependent on mitogen-activated protein kinase signaling (MAPK), phosphatidylinositol-3 kinase and protein kinase B signaling (PI3K-Akt), nuclear factor κB signaling (NF-κB) and calcium signaling pathways. It is also dependent on adhesion molecule induced mechanisms that mediate immune tolerance in T cell receptor signaling cascade. Detection of ErbB signaling (hsa04012) in genetic network enrichment is also supported by detection of EGFR downregulation pathway from our pathway analysis. We identified ErbB4 (HER4) to be a high-risk locus interacting with 15q22 and 9p23. ErbB4 is one of the four epidermal growth factor receptor (EGFR) family members with tyrosine kinase activity. In both cancerous and non-cancerous cells, EGFR plays a crucial role in controlling key cellular pathways influencing cell proliferation, differentiation and development through MAPK and PI3K/Akt pathways and overexpression of which is associated to multiple cancer types (Yarden and Sliwkowski 2001). *PTPRD* has been characterized as a tumor suppressor gene in MM and a homozygous deletion in PTPRD encoding locus is known to modulate phosphorylation of STAT3 that promotes IL6 signaling (Lohr et al. 2014). Whereas, RORα is a regulator of circadian clock, responsible for cytokine secretion especially interleukins (Paiva et al. n.d.). Contextually, with a mechanistic aggression, circulating MM tumor cells undergo circadian rhythm dependent selective egression. Circadian rhythm was one of the suggestively selected enriched pathways encompassing the genetic network (Additional file 7, $p = 1.38 \times 10^{-2}$). Involvement of HER4 in cancer has yet not been comprehensively addressed, although it has been shown to be overexpressed in colorectal cancer and postulated to promote carcinogenesis in general (Lau et al. 2014; Williams et al. n.d.).

We find rs10251201, one of the previously identified risk loci for MGUS with moderate significance, annotated to 36 kb 5′ to GLCCT1 in interaction with rs1104869 mapping to an intronic region of an oncogene, anaplastic lymphoma receptor tyrosine kinase (ALK). Notably ALK amplification, mutations and especially chromosomal rearrangements have been found in several cancers (Chiarle et al. 2008). Another previously identified MGUS risk locus (rs16966921) annotated to GALNT1 was shown in our data to have moderately significant interaction with (rs8092870) annotated to cadherin 2 (CDH2), an adhesion molecule and downstream target of FGFR3 signaling pathway (Takehara et al. 2015). Cell adhesion is an integral part of cell surface interaction and is of two major types: cell-to-cell and cell-to-extracellular matrix (ECM). Cadherin family cell adhesion molecules play important roles in the formation and functions of cell-cell adhesions. CDH2 is associated with several neoplasias and has been reported to be overexpressed in MM co-existing with the t(4,14) translocation (Dring et al. 2004). Interestingly, we also identified a novel risk locus on another cadherin gene, CDH13 in an interaction with 9p22. CDH13 is not involved in cell-cell adhesion, but protects vascular endothelial cells from apoptosis due to oxidative stress and is found to be hypermethylated in myeloid leukemia, B-cell lymphomas among several other cancers (Andreeva and Kutuzov 2010).

At cell-ECM adhesions, the major transmembrane proteins are integrin heterodimers. Several integrins, including integrin-$\beta$1, $-\beta$7 and $-\alpha$8 have been shown to play a role in MM cell adhesion, migration, invasion, bone marrow homing and drug resistance. We observed REACTOME integrin cell surface interactions pathway as a comparably significant hit from all three of our pathway analyses. Our assumption of interplay between cell adhesion and integrin pathways is also supported by the discovery of the REACTOME platelet aggregation (plug information) pathway, a crucial adhesion mechanism not only in normal hemostasis but also in pathophysiological processes such as inflammation, immune-mediated host defense and cancer metastasis. Integrin-$\alpha$IIb$\beta$3 plays a key role in platelet adhesion and aggregation (Ruggeri and Mendolicchio 2007).

Functional epistasis traditionally derives its appeal on the assumption of polygenic risk where genes in ensemble are supposed to accumulate larger deregulating impact than considered individually. Although direct aggregation of interaction test and enrichment analysis may seem tempting following a step-wise implementation procedure, caveats due to low statistical power render it unfeasible. Hence, a major limitation of this study is the low case numbers which mostly is due to the scarcity of identifiable individuals. MGUS being an asymptomatic condition, studies are dependent on indirect diagnosis in its entirety. We admit that detection power of our analysis is marginally compromised accounting for stringent selection criteria since pairwise interaction algorithms require large statistical power to avoid high false discovery rate and that may result subsequent rejection of false negative results. However, we have minimized this loss of information by analyzing gene set and pathway enrichment on GWAS summary statistics parallel to the interaction test. Fang et al. 2017 have recently proposed such a procedure on building pathway map based on linear interaction model. Although to make the later analysis viable, their study proposes selection of risk loci at a very nominal level of significance (Fang et al. 2017). Unfortunately, this rather permissive selection criterion makes their proposed BridGE algorithm unreliable as it may allow a large proportion of false positive findings. This calls for further careful inspection in the statistics to achieve robustness in inference.

## Conclusion

In summary, we developed a method that unifies variant pair interaction with genetic networks and pathway enrichment. We also discovered evidence which supports that several signaling cascades including B cell receptor, epidermal growth receptor and cell adhesion related pathways play a role and are regulated via several interacting loci in development of MGUS that possibly explicates its further progression to MM.

## Additional files

**Additional file 1:** Top interactions from W-Z discovery set interaction test compared with simple logistic linear interaction test (brute force epistasis). Description: SNP1 and SNP2 are the two SNP candidates of a pair from the discovery population belonging to chromosomes denote by Chr1 and Chr2; gene1 and gene2 are the corresponding genes annotated to SNP1 and SNP2, respectively. W-Z P value is Wellek Ziegler test p-value. (DOCX 22 kb)

**Additional file 2:** Top interactions from W-Z case-only test in confirmation set. Description: SNP1 and SNP2 are the two corresponding SNP candidates of a pair from the case-only population belonging to chromosomes denote by Chr1 and Chr2; gene1 and gene2 are the corresponding genes annotated to SNP1 and SNP2, respectively. W-Z P value is Wellek Ziegler case-only test p-value; BP is base pair. (DOCX 21 kb)

**Additional file 3:** Top interactions from W-Z interaction test on the replication set. Description: SNP1 and SNP2 are the two SNP candidates of a pair from the replication set population belonging to chromosomes denote by Chr1 and Chr2; gene1 and gene2 are the corresponding genes annotated to SNP1 and SNP2, respectively. W-Z P value is Wellek Ziegler case-control test p-value; BP is base pair. (DOCX 22 kb)

**Additional file 4:** Overlapped interactions from INTERSNP and CASSI W-Z interaction tests on discovery set. Description: SNP1 and SNP2 are the two SNP candidates of a pair from the discovery set population belonging to chromosomes denote by Chr1 and Chr2; gene1 and gene2 are the corresponding genes annotated to SNP1(s) and SNP2(s), respectively. W-Z P value is Wellek Ziegler case-control test p-value from CASSI and INTERSNP P value is full log-linear test p-value from INTERSNP; BP is base pair. IN: INTERSNP; CAS: CASSI. (DOCX 22 kb)

**Additional file 5:** Gene set enrichment analysis in genetic network with STRING. Description: Based on the indexing nodes and the additional predicted first order interacting m=nodes, STRING performs enrichment analysis on several molecular, biological, cellular process related pathway analysis with Gene Onltology (GO) and KEGG database. All tests are performed with guilt by association assumption and P values are corrected for multiple testing. A protein-protein enrichment index is reported with analysis depicting level of confidence in the detected enriched processes which is reported to be 0.0039 (significant at 5% level). (DOCX 21 kb)

**Additional file 6:** PASCAL gene set enrichment analysis results at 1% level of significance. (DOCX 20 kb)

**Additional file 7:** MAGENTA gene set enrichment analysis results at 1% level of significance. (DOCX 20 kb)

**Additional file 8:** All detected pathways mutually discovered in both MAGENTA and PASCAL at a 5% level of combined significance. (DOCX 21 kb)

**Additional file 9:** DEPICT gene set enrichment analysis results at Bonferroni corrected genome wide significance level. (DOCX 18 kb)

**Additional file 10:** Summary of Illumina bead chips used for genotyping different batches of cases and controls. (DOCX 19 kb)

**Additional file 11:** Number of overlaps in number of SNPs prior quality control between different chips used in genotyping. Chip numbers are defined in Additional file 10. (DOCX 19 kb)

## Abbreviations
CMML: Chronic myelomonocytic leukemia; EGFR: Epidermal growth factor receptor; FWER: Family wise error rate; GO: Gene ontology; GSEA: Gene set enrichment analysis; HNR: Heinz Nixdorf-Recall; KEGG: Kyoto encyclopedia of genes and genomes; LD: Linkage disequilibrium; MGUS: Monoclonal gammopathy of undetermined significance; MM: Multiple myeloma; MOCS: Maximum of chi-square; MP: Mammalian Phenotype; PANTHER: Protein Analysis through Evolutionary Relationships; sAML: Secondary acute myeloid leukemia; SNP: Single nucleotide polymorphism; SOCS: Sum of chi-square; W-Z: Wellek-Zeigler

## Funding
We would like to thank Deutsche Krebshilfe, the Dietmar Hopp Foundation, the German Ministry of Education and Science (BMBF: CLIOMMICS (01ZX1309)), Multiple Myeloma Research Foundation and the Harald Hupper Foundation for providing funding for this study. K-H J was supported by the Heinz Nixdorf Foundation (Germany), the Ministerium für Innovation, Wissenschaft und Forschung des Landes Nordrhein-Westfalen and the Faculty of Medicine University Duisburg-Essen.

## Authors' contributions
SC, HT, and MIdSF analyzed the data; NW, CL and HG provided the Heidelberg and Ulm MGUS samples and patient data; K-H J, AM, BS and SP provided the Essen samples and patient data; PH and MMN were responsible for the GWAS; HT, KH and AF designed the study; SC wrote the first draft of the manuscript; HT and AF critically reviewed the manuscript; all authors read and accepted the final version of the manuscript.

## Competing interests
The authors declare that they have no competing interests.

## Author details
[1]Division of Molecular Genetic Epidemiology, German Cancer Research Center (DKFZ), Im Neuenheimer Feld 580, 69120 Heidelberg, Germany. [2]Faculty of Medicine, University of Heidelberg, Heidelberg, Germany. [3]Department of Internal Medicine V, University of Heidelberg, Heidelberg, Germany. [4]Myeloma Institute, University of Arkansas for Medical Sciences, Little Rock, AR, USA. [5]Institute of Human Genetics, University of Bonn, Bonn, Germany. [6]Department of Biomedicine, University of Basel, Basel, Switzerland. [7]Department of Genomics, Life & Brain Research Center, University of Bonn, Bonn, Germany. [8]Institute for Medical Informatics, Biometry and Epidemiology, University Hospital Essen, University of Duisburg-Essen, Essen, Germany. [9]Department of Internal Medicine III, University of Ulm, Ulm, Germany. [10]National Centre of Tumor Diseases, Heidelberg, Germany. [11]Center for Primary Health Care Research, Lund University, Malmö, Sweden.

## References
Andreeva AV, Kutuzov MA. Cadherin 13 in cancer. Genes Chromosom Cancer. 2010;49(9):775–90.

Broderick P, Chubb D, Johnson DC, Weinhold N, Forsti A, Lloyd A, Olver B, Ma YP, Dobbins SE, Walker BA, et al. Common variation at 3p22.1 and 7p15.3 influences multiple myeloma risk. Nat Genet. 2011;44(1):58–61.

Chiarle R, Voena C, Ambrogio C, Piva R, Inghirami G. The anaplastic lymphoma kinase in the pathogenesis of cancer. Nat Rev Cancer. 2008;8(1):11–23.

Chubb D, Weinhold N, Broderick P, Chen B, Johnson DC, Forsti A, Vijayakrishnan J, Migliorini G, Dobbins SE, Holroyd A, et al. Common variation at 3q26.2, 6p21.33, 17p11.2 and 22q13.1 influences multiple myeloma risk. Nat Genet. 2013;45(10):1221–5.

Cordell HJ. Detecting gene-gene interactions that underlie human diseases. Nat Rev Genet. 2009;10(6):392–404.

Criteria for the classification of monoclonal gammopathies. Multiple myeloma and related disorders: a report of the international myeloma working group. Br J Haematol. 2003;121(5):749–57.

Dispenzieri A, Katzmann JA, Kyle RA, Larson DR, Melton LJ 3rd, Colby CL, Therneau TM, Clark R, Kumar SK, Bradwell A, et al. Prevalence and risk of progression of light-chain monoclonal gammopathy of undetermined significance: a retrospective population-based cohort study. Lancet (London, England). 2010;375(9727):1721–8.

Dring AM, Davies FE, Fenton JAL, Roddam PL, Scott K, Gonzalez D, Rollinson S, Rawstron AC, Rees-Unwin KS, Li C, et al. A global expression-based analysis of the consequences of the t(4;14) translocation in myeloma. Clin Cancer Res. 2004;10(17):5692.

Duncan LE, Holmans PA, Lee PH, O'Dushlaine CT, Kirby AW, Smoller JW, Öngür D, Cohen BM. Pathway analyses implicate glial cells in schizophrenia. PLoS One. 2014;9(2):e89441.

Fang G, Wang W, Paunic V, Heydari H, Costanzo M, et al. Discovering genetic interactions bridging pathways in genome-wide association studies. bioRxiv 182741. (2017). https://doi.org/10.1101/182741.

Frank C, Fallah M, Chen T, Mai EK, Sundquist J, Forsti A, Hemminki K. Search for familial clustering of multiple myeloma with any cancer. Leukemia. 2016; 30(3):627–32.

Greenberg AJ, Lee AM, Serie DJ, McDonnell SK, Cerhan JR, Liebow M, Larson DR, Colby CL, Norman AD, Kyle RA, et al. Single-nucleotide polymorphism rs1052501 associated with monoclonal gammopathy of undetermined significance and multiple myeloma. Leukemia. 2013;27(2):515–6.

Greenberg AJ, Rajkumar SV, Vachon CM. Familial monoclonal gammopathy of undetermined significance and multiple myeloma: epidemiology, risk factors, and biological characteristics. Blood. 2012;119(23):5359–66.

Herold C, Steffens M, Brockschmidt FF, Baur MP, Becker T. INTERSNP: genome-wide interaction analysis guided by a priori information. Bioinformatics. 2009; 25(24):3275–81.

Jensen LJ, Kuhn M, Stark M, Chaffron S, Creevey C, Muller J, Doerks T, Julien P, Roth A, Simonovic M, et al. STRING 8—a global view on proteins and their functional interactions in 630 organisms. Nucleic Acids Res. 2009;37(Database issue):D412–6.

Jiang W, Yu W. Power estimation and sample size determination for replication studies of genome-wide association studies. BMC Genomics. 2016;17(Suppl 1):3.

Karkkainen HP, Li Z, Sillanpaa MJ. An efficient genome-wide multilocus epistasis search. Genetics. 2015;201(3):865–70.

Khatri P, Sirota M, Butte AJ. Ten years of pathway analysis: current approaches and outstanding challenges. PLoS Comput Biol. 2012;8(2):e1002375.

Koster R, Mitra N, D'Andrea K, Vardhanabhuti S, Chung CC, Wang Z, Loren Erickson R, Vaughn DJ, Litchfield K, Rahman N, et al. Pathway-based analysis of GWAs data identifies association of sex determination genes with susceptibility to testicular germ cell tumors. Hum Mol Genet. 2014;23(22):6061–8.

Kyle RA, Larson DR, Therneau TM, Dispenzieri A, Kumar S, Cerhan JR, Rajkumar SV. Long-term follow-up of monoclonal Gammopathy of undetermined significance. N Engl J Med. 2018;378(3):241–9.

Kyle RA, Therneau TM, Rajkumar SV, Larson DR, Plevak MF, Offord JR, Dispenzieri A, Katzmann JA, Melton LJ 3rd. Prevalence of monoclonal gammopathy of undetermined significance. N Engl J Med. 2006;354(13):1362–9.

Lamparter D, Marbach D, Rueedi R, Kutalik Z, Bergmann S. Fast and rigorous computation of gene and Pathway scores from SNP-based summary statistics. PLoS Comput Biol. 2016;12(1):e1004714.

Landgren O, Kristinsson SY, Goldin LR, Caporaso NE, Blimark C, Mellqvist UH, Wahlin A, Bjorkholm M, Turesson I. Risk of plasma cell and lymphoproliferative disorders among 14621 first-degree relatives of 4458 patients with monoclonal gammopathy of undetermined significance in Sweden. Blood. 2009;114(4):791–5.

Lau C, Killian KJ, Samuels Y, Rudloff U: ERBB4 Mutation Analysis: Emerging Molecular Target for Melanoma Treatment. In: Thurin M., Marincola F. (eds) Molecular Diagnostics for Melanoma. Methods in Molecular Biology (Methods and Protocols). Totowa: Humana Press. 2014; 1102.

Lee YH, Gyu Song G. Genome-wide pathway analysis in pancreatic cancer. J Buon. 2015;20(6):1565–75.

Lohr JG, Stojanov P, Carter SL, Cruz-Gordillo P, Lawrence MS, Auclair D, Sougnez C, Knoechel B, Gould J, Saksena G, et al. Widespread genetic heterogeneity in multiple myeloma: implications for targeted therapy. Cancer Cell. 2014; 25(1):91–101.

Makishima H, Yoshida K, Nguyen N, Przychodzen B, Sanada M, Okuno Y, Ng KP, Gudmundsson KO, Vishwakarma BA, Jerez A, et al. Somatic SETBP1 mutations in myeloid malignancies. Nat Genet. 2013;45(8):942–6.

Manolio TA, Collins FS, Cox NJ, Goldstein DB, Hindorff LA, Hunter DJ, McCarthy MI, Ramos EM, Cardon LR, Chakravarti A, et al. Finding the missing heritability of complex diseases. Nature. 2009;461(7265):747–53.

Mitchell JS, Li N, Weinhold N, Forsti A, Ali M, van Duin M, Thorleifsson G, Johnson DC, Chen B, Halvarsson BM, et al. Genome-wide association study identifies multiple susceptibility loci for multiple myeloma. Nat Commun. 2016;7:12050.

Paiva B, Paino T, Sayagues JM, Garayoa M, San-Segundo L, Martín M, Mota I, Sanchez ML, Bárcena P, Aires-Mejia I, Corchete L, Jimenez C, Garcia-Sanz R, Gutierrez NC, Ocio EM, Mateos MV, Vidriales MB, Orfao A, San Miguel JF, et al: Detailed characterization of multiple myeloma circulating tumor cells shows unique phenotypic, cytogenetic, functional, and circadian distribution profile. (1528–0020 (Electronic)). n.d.

Pers TH, Karjalainen JM, Chan Y, Westra H-J, Wood AR, Yang J, Lui JC, Vedantam S, Gustafsson S, Esko T et al: Biological interpretation of genome-wide association studies using predicted gene functions. 2015, 6:5890.

Poirier JG, Faye LL, Dimitromanolakis A, Paterson AD, Sun L, Bull SB. Resampling to address the Winner's curse in genetic association analysis of time to event. Genet Epidemiol. 2015;39(7):518–28.

Purcell S, Neale B, Todd-Brown K, Thomas L, Ferreira MA, Bender D, Maller J, Sklar P, de Bakker PI, Daly MJ, et al. PLINK: a tool set for whole-genome association and population-based linkage analyses. Am J Hum Genet. 2007;81(3):559–75.

Ramanan VK, Shen L, Moore JH, Saykin AJ. Pathway analysis of genomic data: concepts, methods, and prospects for future development. Trends Genet. 2012;28(7):323–32.

Ruggeri ZM, Mendolicchio GL. Adhesion mechanisms in platelet function. Circ Res. 2007;100(12):1673–85.

Schmermund A, Mohlenkamp S, Stang A, Gronemeyer D, Seibel R, Hirche H, Mann K, Siffert W, Lauterbach K, Siegrist J, et al. Assessment of clinically silent atherosclerotic disease and established and novel risk factors for predicting myocardial infarction and cardiac death in healthy middle-aged subjects: rationale and design of the Heinz Nixdorf RECALL study. Risk factors, evaluation of coronary calcium and lifestyle. Am Heart J. 2002;144(2):212–8.

Segrè AV, Consortium D, Investigators M, Groop L, Mootha VK, Daly MJ, Altshuler D. Common inherited variation in mitochondrial genes is not enriched for associations with type 2 diabetes or related glycemic traits. PLoS Genet. 2010;6(8):e1001058.

Shi J, Park JH, Duan J, Berndt ST, Moy W, Yu K, Song L, Wheeler W, Hua X, Silverman D, et al. Winner's curse correction and variable Thresholding improve performance of polygenic risk modeling based on genome-wide association study summary-level data. PLoS Genet. 2016;12(12):e1006493.

Shim U, Kim HN, Lee H, Oh JY, Sung YA, Kim HL. Pathway analysis based on a genome-wide association study of polycystic ovary syndrome. PLoS One. 2015;10(8):e0136609.

Takehara T, Teramura T, Onodera Y, Frampton J, Fukuda K. Cdh2 stabilizes FGFR1 and contributes to primed-state pluripotency in mouse epiblast stem cells. Scientific Reports. 2015;5(1).

Thomsen H, Campo C, Weinhold N, Filho MI, Pour L, Gregora E, Vodicka P, Vodickova L, Hoffmann P, Nöthen MM, Jöckel KH, Langer C, Hajek R, Goldschmidt H, Hemminki K, Försti A. Genomewide association study on monoclonal gammopathy of unknown significance (MGUS). Eur J Haematol. 2017;99(1):70–9.

Ueki M, Cordell HJ. Improved statistics for genome-wide interaction analysis. PLoS Genet. 2012;8(4):e1002625.

van Rheenen W, Shatunov A, Dekker AM, McLaughlin RL, Diekstra FP, Pulit SL, van der Spek RAA, Vosa U, de Jong S, Robinson MR, et al. Genome-wide association analyses identify new risk variants and the genetic architecture of amyotrophic lateral sclerosis. Nat Genet. 2016;48(9):1043–8.

Wang J, Gao F, Liu Z, Qiao M, Niu X, Zhang K-Q, Huang X. Pathway and molecular mechanisms for malachite green biodegradation in Exiguobacterium sp. MG2. PLoS One. 2012;7(12):e51808.

Weinhold N, Johnson DC, Rawstron AC, Forsti A, Doughty C, Vijayakrishnan J, Broderick P, Dahir NB, Begum DB, Hosking FJ, et al. Inherited genetic susceptibility to monoclonal gammopathy of unknown significance. Blood. 2014;123(16):2513–7. quiz 2593

Wellek S, Ziegler A. A genotype-based approach to assessing the association between single nucleotide polymorphisms. Hum Hered. 2009;67(2):128–39.

Williams CS, Bernard JK, Demory Beckler M, Almohazey D, Washington MK, Smith JJ, Frey MR: ERBB4 is over-expressed in human colon cancer and enhances cellular transformation. (1460–2180 (Electronic)). n.d.

Wu X, Dong H, Luo L, Zhu Y, Peng G, Reveille JD, Xiong M. A novel statistic for genome-wide interaction analysis. PLoS Genet. 2010;6(9):e1001131.

Yarden Y, Sliwkowski MX. Untangling the ErbB signalling network. Nat Rev Mol Cell Biol. 2001;2(2):127–37.

Yi S, Lin S, Li Y, Zhao W, Mills GB, Sahni N. Functional variomics and network perturbation: connecting genotype to phenotype in cancer. Nat Rev Genet. 2017;18(7):395–410.

# 9

# Different sulfonylureas induce the apoptosis of proximal tubular epithelial cell differently via closing K$_{ATP}$ channel

Rui Zhang[1†], Xiaojun Zhou[1†], Xue Shen[3], Tianyue Xie[3], Chunmei Xu[1], Zhiwei Zou[2], Jianjun Dong[2,4*] and Lin Liao[1,5*]

## Abstract

**Background:** Sulfonylureas (SUs) are widely prescribed for the treatment of type 2 diabetes (T2DM). Sulfonylurea receptors (SURs) are their main functional receptors. These receptors are also found in kidney, especially the tubular cells. However, the effects of SUs on renal proximal tubular epithelial cells (PTECs) were unclear.

**Methods:** Three commonly used SUs were included in this study to investigate if different SUs have different effects on the apoptosis of PTECs. HK-2 cells were exposed to SUs for 24 h prior to exposure to 30 mM glucose, the apoptosis rate was evaluated by Annexin/PI flow cytometry. Bcl-2, Bax and the ratio of LC3II to LC3I were also studied by western blot in vitro. Diazoxide was used to evaluate the role of K$_{ATP}$ channel in SUs-induced apoptosis of PTECs. A Student's t-test was used to assess significance for data within two groups.

**Results:** Treatment with glibenclamide aggravated the apoptosis of HK-2 cells in high-glucose, as indicated by a significant decrease in the expression of Bcl-2 and increase in Bax. Additionally, the decreased LC3II/LC3I reflects that the autophagy was inhibited by glibenclamide. Similar but less pronounced change was found in glimepiride group, however, nearly opposite effects were found in gliclazide group. Further, the effects of glibenclamide on apoptosis promotion and the decreased LC3II/LC3I were ameliorated obviously by treatment with 100uM diazoxide. The potential protection effect of gliclazide was also inhibited after opening the K$_{ATP}$ channel.

**Conclusion:** Our results suggest that, the effects of glibenclamide and glimepiride on PTECs apoptosis, especially the former, were achieved in part by closing the K$_{ATP}$ channel. In contrast to glibenclamide and glimepiride, therapeutic concentrations of gliclazide showed an inhibitory effect on apoptosis of PTECs, which may have a benefit in the preservation of functional PTECs mass.

**Keywords:** Diabetes kidney disease, Proximal tubular epithelial cells, ATP-dependent potassium channel, Glibenclamide, Glimepiride, Gliclazide

## Background

Sulfonylureas (SUs) is one of the most commonly prescribed class of drugs for treatment of type 2 diabetes mellitus (T2DM) (Tahrani et al. 2016). SUs binds to their receptors (sulfonylurea receptor, SUR), which are subunit of the ATP-dependent potassium (K$_{ATP}$) channel, thus closing the K$_{ATP}$ channel in pancreatic β-cells,

resulting in insulin secretion and decreases blood glucose (Gribble & Reimann, 2003).

Diabetic kidney disease (DKD) is one of the major microvascular complications of diabetes (Zoja et al. 2015). Glomerulopathy associated with diffuse or nodular glomerulosclerosis was originally deemed as the main pathologic change (Ilatovskaya et al. 2015). Researchers have recently come to appreciate the key role played by proximal renal tubules in DKD (Wakino et al. 2015; De Nicola et al. 2014). Studies show that one-third of diabetic patients with microalbuminuria having no or minimal glomerular changes, only proximal tubular lesions (Singh et al. 2008). Tubulopathy, especially the apoptosis of proximal

* Correspondence: dongjianjun@sdu.edu.cn; cwc_ll@sdu.edu.cn
†Rui Zhang and Xiaojun Zhou contributed equally to this work.
[2]Department of Endocrinology, Qilu Hospital of Shandong University, Jinan, Shandong, China
[1]Department of Endocrinology, Shandong Provincial Qianfoshan Hospital, Shandong University, Jinan, Shandong, China
Full list of author information is available at the end of the article

tubular epithelial cells (PTECs), is shown to play an important role in DKD, which occurs earlier than glomerulopathy (Magri & Fava, 2011; Tojo & Kinugasa, 2012; Barzilay et al. 2013).

The effects of SUs on DKD have been thought to be due to their indirect effects via their ability to decrease blood glucose (Giannico et al 2007). Few studies have examined whether SUs have direct effects on the kidney. SURs are present in a wide variety of extra-pancreatic tissues (Gribble & Reimann, 2003). Investigations indicated that SUR2, one common subtype of SUR, is located in PTECs (Zhou et al. 2008; Szamosfalvi et al. 2002). Hence, it is conceivable that SUs could act directly on the PTECs. As a $K_{ATP}$ channel blocker, SUs close the $K_{ATP}$ channels, leading to membrane depolarization and opening of voltage-operated $Ca^{2+}$ channels, which further cause $Ca^{2+}$ influx, and intracellular rise of $Ca^{2+}$. This process may subsequently induce $Ca^{2+}$-dependent-apoptosis (Efanova et al. 1998). Several studies have shown that the opening of the $K_{ATP}$ channel is renoprotective (Shiraishi et al. 2014; Assad et al. 2009; Zhang et al. 2013). So, SUs might have detrimental effects on kidney, which is a concern in clinical practice.

The aim of our present study was to explore the effects of three widely prescribed SUs (glibenclamide, glimepiride and gliclazide) on the apoptosis of PTECs, an important progress in the development of DKD. To determine whether these SUs could be differentiated with regard to their effects on the apoptosis of PTECs and to analyze their possible underlying molecular mechanisms. Our results showed that glibenclamide and glimepiride, especial the former, promotes the apoptosis of PTECs through interacting with $K_{ATP}$ channels. These pro-apoptosis effects of glibenclamide and glimepiride are mediated, at least in part, via downregulation of autophagy activity in renal tubular cells. To the contrary, gliclazide showed an inhibitory effect on apoptosis of PTECs.

## Methods
### Cell culture
Human proximal tubular epithelial cells (Ryan et al. 1994) (HK-2, American Type Cell Collection, Rockville, MD) were cultured in the RPMI 1640 medium containing 10% fetal bovine serum (Gibco, USA), 11.1 mM glucose, 100 U/ml penicillin and 100 µg/ml streptomycin(Sigma, St. Louis, MO) at 37 °C, 5% $CO_2$ and 95% humidity. The culture medium was replaced with fresh medium every 2–3 days and expanded to new culture plates when the cell reach approximately 80% confluence.

### Antibodies, drugs and reagents
Antibodies in the study were from the following sources: anti-Bcl-2 and anti-Bax (polyclonal) from Proteintech Group(Chicago, IL), anti-LC3(Mono) from Cell Signaling Technology(Beverly, MA), anti-β-actin from Sigma(St. Louis, MO). All secondary antibodies (polyclonal) were from Jackson ImmunoResearch Laboratories Inc. (West Grove, PA). Glibenclamide, glimepiride, gliclazide and diazoxide (DZ, a $K_{ATP}$ channel opener) were all purchased from Sigma (St. Louis. MO, U.S.A). They were dissolved in dimethyl sulfoxide (DMSO) and stored at – 80 °C until use. Solutions of SUs as well as DZ were prepared fresh each day. Controls were performed in the presence of appropriate concentration of solvent (DMSO). Unless indicated, other reagents were from Sigma (St. Louis. MO).

To investigate the effects of the three SUs in HG-induced tubular epithelial cell apoptosis, the HK-2 cells were treated with these SUs for 24 h prior to exposure to 30 mM glucose for 24 h. To further investigate the role of $K_{ATP}$ channels in this process, the HK-2 cells were treated with 100uM DZ for 24 h prior to exposure to SUs and 30 mM glucose.

### Cell viability assay
The HK-2 cells were seeded in 96-well plates at a concentration of $5 \times 10^3$ Cells/ml and incubated at 37 °C. CCK-8 assay was employed to assess the viability of the cells. After being subjected to the above-mentioned treatments, the cells were washed with phosphate-buffered saline (PBS), and 10ul CCK-8 solution at 10% dilution was added to each well, and the plate was then incubated for approximately 24 h in an incubator. The absorbance at 450 nm was assayed using a microplate reader (Molecular Devices, Sunnyvale, CA, USA). The mean of the optical density (OD) of 3 wells in the indicated groups were used to calculate the percentage of cell viability according to the following formula: cell viability (%) = ($OD_{treatment\ group}$/$OD_{control\ group}$) × 100. The experiment was repeated 5 times.

### Apoptosis determination
The cells were incubated with 5 µl of Annexin V and 5 µl of propidium iodide (PI) for 15 min at room temperature in dark, according to the manufacturer's instruction (BD Biosciences, SanJose, CA), and then subjected to flow cytometry to measure the apoptosis rate (%).

### Western blot analysis
Protein concentrations in cell extracts were determined (BioRad, Richmond, California, USA). Equal amounts of protein fractions of lysates were resolved over SDS-PAGE gels, transferred to PVDF membranes. After blocking with skim milk, membranes were incubated with anti-LC3I, LC3II, Bcl-2 and Bax. Corresponding secondary antibody were used. The peroxidase activity was detected by chemiluminescence using the ECL detection system. Optical density of the bands was quantified by densitometric analysis using ImageJ software (National Institutes of Health, USA). β-actin (#3700, Cell Signaling Technology) was used as an internal control.

## Statistical analysis

All statistical analyses were performed using Statistical Product and Service Solutions (SPSS) 19.0 software (from IBM). A Student's t-test was used to assess significance for data within two groups. All data are presented as the means ± SEM, and significance was set at $P < 0.05$.

## Results

### Effect of SUs on human proximal tubule epithelial cell viability

Our results revealed that SUs exposure led to a dose-dependent inhibition of cell viability of the HK-2 cells by CCK-8 method. HK-2 cells treated with glibenclamide at a concentration of 45umol/L, gliclazide 1058umol/L, glimepiride 130 umol/L did not significantly affect cell viability. So, the above concentrations were used for our following experiments.

### Pro-apoptotic effect of glibenclamide on PTECs was alleviated, as well as an attenuated gliclazide protection, were seen with $K_{ATP}$ channel opening

To investigate the role of $K_{ATP}$ channels in SUs-induced PTECs injury, the HK-2 cells were treated with or without 100uM of the putative $K_{ATP}$ channel opener, DZ, for 24 h. Annexin-V binding and propidium iodide staining were used to detect apoptotic changes in HK-2 cells. As shown in Fig. 1, glibenclamide promoted the apoptosis of PTECs significantly ($P < 0.05$); the apoptosis rate (Q2 + Q4) in glimepiride-treated group was not different from the control group($P > 0.05$). However, the effect was opposite in gliclazide group, where the apoptosis rate was reduced ($P < 0.05$). What's more, the above effects of glibenclamide and gliclazide were alleviated by DZ. In contrast, exposure to glimepiride with or without DZ did not induce a significant change in the number of apoptotic cells.

Bcl-2 is a crucial inhibitor and Bax is the promoter of apoptosis. Our results of western blotting showed that Bcl-2 was downregulated significantly ($P < 0.01$) and Bax was upregulated ($P < 0.05$) in glibenclamide group compared with that of control group (Fig. 2). The expression of Bax was upregulated significantly in glimepiride group compared to control group ($P < 0.01$), even though there was no significant difference in Bcl-2 expression. However, the results were opposite in gliclazide group, the expression of Bcl-2 was upregulated and Bax was downregulated significantly (all $P < 0.01$). The effects of glibenclamide, glimepiride and gliclazide on apoptosis were restored or even reversed by DZ, a putative $K_{ATP}$ channel opener.

### The decreased autophagy-related protein and ratio of LC3-II/LC3-I were reversed by opening $K_{ATP}$ channel

Apoptosis and autophagy are two important cellular processes with complex and interacting protein networks.

The mechanisms linking autophagy and apoptosis are not fully defined, however, our previous study found that there was a negative correlation between apoptosis and autophagy in PTECs (Zhang et al. 2017). A high level of constitutive basal autophagy is observed in PTECs, which is proved an indispensable process in this part of kidney (Isaka et al. 2011; Weide & Huber, 2011). When autophagy is initiated, LC3 is processed from LC3-I to LC3-II. The increase of LC3-II and/or the ratio of LC3-II/LC3-I can be an indicator of the activation of autophagy to some degrees (Dancourt & Melia, 2014). As shown in Fig. 3, the expression of LC3-II and the ratio of LC3-II/LC3-I were increased in gliclazide and decreased in glibenclamide group significantly as compared with control ($P < 0.01$, $P < 0.01$). While their expressions did not show apparent difference in glimepiride group ($P > 0.05$). DZ upregulated the expressions of above two indicators more remarkable in glibenclamide than that in glimepiride group as compared with control group. These reversal changes were not found in gliclazide-treated HK-2 cells with or without DZ. The above results indicate that different SUs might have different effects on autophagy, and the changes of autophagy-related protein in glibenclamide can be reversed by opening the $K_{ATP}$ channel.

## Discussion

Increasing evidences suggest that apoptosis of tubular epithelial cells, especially PTECs, play an important role in the progression of DKD (Wakino et al. 2015; De Nicola et al. 2014; Singh et al. 2008). Sulfonylureas have been reported to accelerate apoptosis and dysfunction of pancreatic beta cells due to sustained enhancement of $Ca^{2+}$ influx and stimulated production of reactive oxygen species (ROS) (Efanova et al. 1998; Iwakura et al. 2000; Tsubouchi et al. 2005). Although SUs have long been utilized for their hypoglycemic properties in DKD patients, little evidence has been reported about their influences on the progression of DKD. The purpose of our study was to explore the effects and possible mechanisms of three widely prescribed SUs on the apoptosis of PTECs. The results showed that glibenclamide increased apoptosis of PTECs significantly, whereas the apoptosis of PTECs treated with gliclazide was reduced. Although glimepiride did not significantly increase the apoptosis rate of PTECs, the expression of proapoptotic protein Bax was increased in this group. Moreover, the increased apoptosis induced by glibenclamide, as well as the increase of Bax expression caused by glimepiride, could be alleviated or even restored obviously by $K_{ATP}$ channel opener, implying that closure of the $K_{ATP}$ channel might contribute to the apoptosis induced by specific SUs.

Why different SUs have different effects on apoptosis of PTECs? The $K_{ATP}$ channels are hetero-octameric complexs of pore-forming inwardly rectifier $K^{+}$ (Kir6) channel-forming subunits associated with regulatory SUR

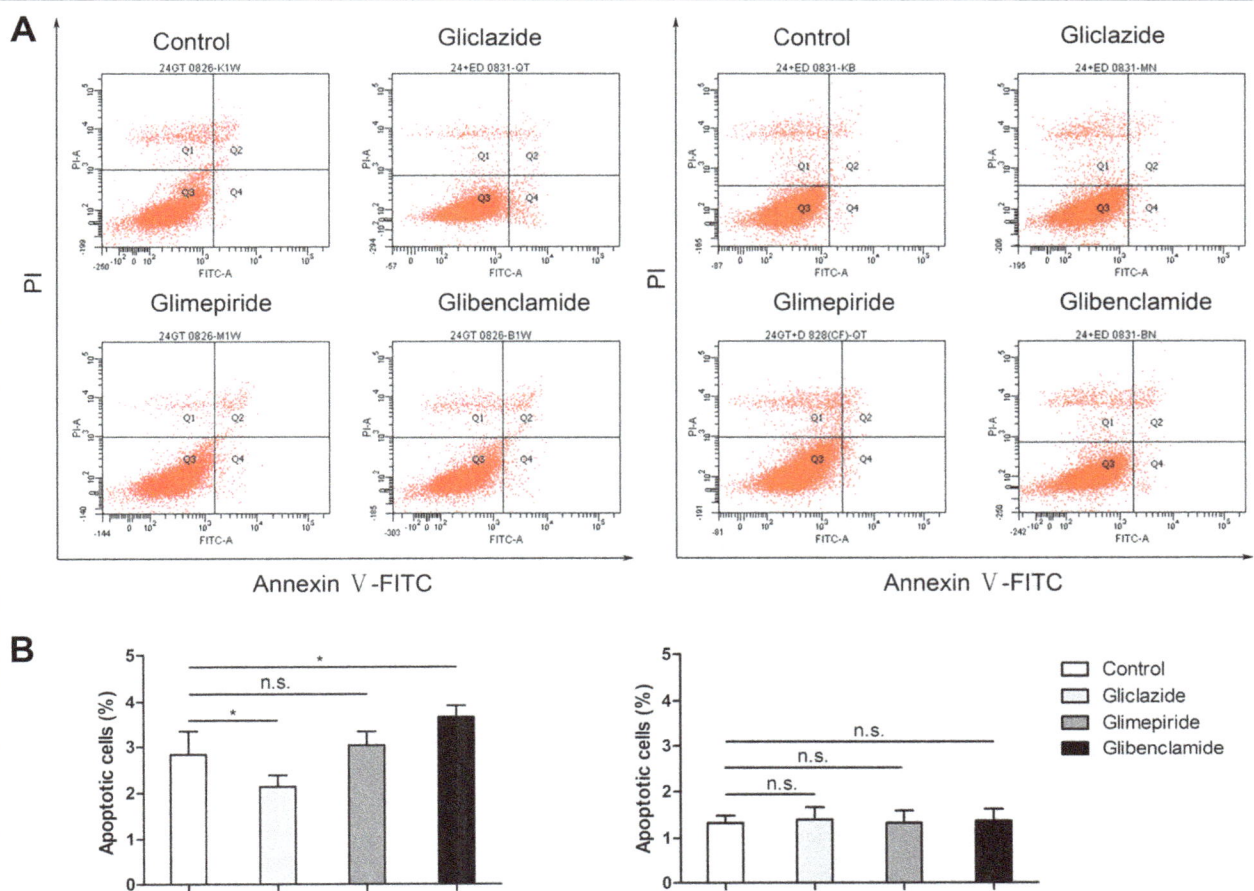

**Fig. 1** Effect of diazoxide on SUs-induced apoptosis was determined with Annexin V-FITC/PI staining by flow cytometry. **a** Flow cytometry results with Annexin V-FITC/PI staining. Cells were treated with SUs (left) and $K_{ATP}$ channel opener (right), DZ, as described above. After culture for 24 h, cells were harvested and then apoptosis was analyzed with an Annexin V-FITC Apoptosis Detection Kit by flow cytometry. Cells were classified as healthy cells (Annexin $V^-$, $PI^-$), early apoptotic cells (Annexin $V^+$, $PI^-$), late apoptotic cells (Annexin $V^+$, $PI^+$), and damaged cells (Annexin $V^-$, $PI^+$). **b** The ratio of apoptosis among different experiment groups. Apoptosis ratio was early apoptosis percentage plus late apoptosis percentage. The date were presented as the mean ± SD. Columns, mean of three independent experiments; bars, SD; * $p < 0.05$, ** $p < 0.01$, n.s. not significant

subunits (Inagaki et al. 1995). Two Kir6-encoding genes, KCNJ8 (Kir6.1) and KCNJ11 (Kir6.2), and 2 SUR genes, ABCC8 (SUR1) and ABCC9 (SUR2), encode mammalian $K_{ATP}$ subunits, but alternative RNA splicing can cause multiple SUR protein variants(e.g. SUR2A and SUR2B) that confer distinct physiological and pharmacological properties on the channel complex (Inagaki et al. 1996; Chutkow et al. 1996; Babenko et al. 2000). SUR endow the channel with sensitivity to SUs (Tucker et al. 1997). In addition to stimulating the insulin secretion by binding with SUR1 on the membrane of islet beta cell, SUs could also bound to its specific SURs in various other extrapancreatic tissues in the body, causing $K_{ATP}$ channel closure (Tsubouchi et al. 2005; Babenko et al. 2000; Liu et al. 2016). It has been estimated that cardiac and skeletal muscle channels contain Kir6.2 and SUR2A, and smooth muscle $K_{ATP}$ channel are formed by the coupling of SUR2B with either Kir6.2 or Kir6.1 (Liu et al. 2015). Either

glibenclamide or glimepiride could inhibit both Kir6.2/SUR1 and Kir6.2/SUR2A currents with high affinity, promoting closure of the $K_{ATP}$ channel and reducing ischemic preconditioning (Thompson et al. 2013). SUR2B is widely expressed in the kidney, particularly in proximal tubule, ascending limb, and the collecting duct, where it presumably mediates, in part, $K^+$ transport (Chutkow et al. 2002). Evidence suggests that the effect of SUs on these $K_{ATP}$ channels in different tissues varies. Considering the different effects of the three SUs on apoptosis in HK-2 cells, several possible mechanisms can be proposed.

First, conventional and modern SUs may display different sensitivity and specificity towards $K_{ATP}$ channels on PTECs. The binding of glibenclamide with $K_{ATP}$ channels is unselective and hardly reversible (Chutkow et al. 2001). Although the selectivity of glimepiride with $K_{ATP}$ channels is similar in SUR1 (in pancreas) and SUR2 (extrapancreatic tissues), but it dissociates quickly from

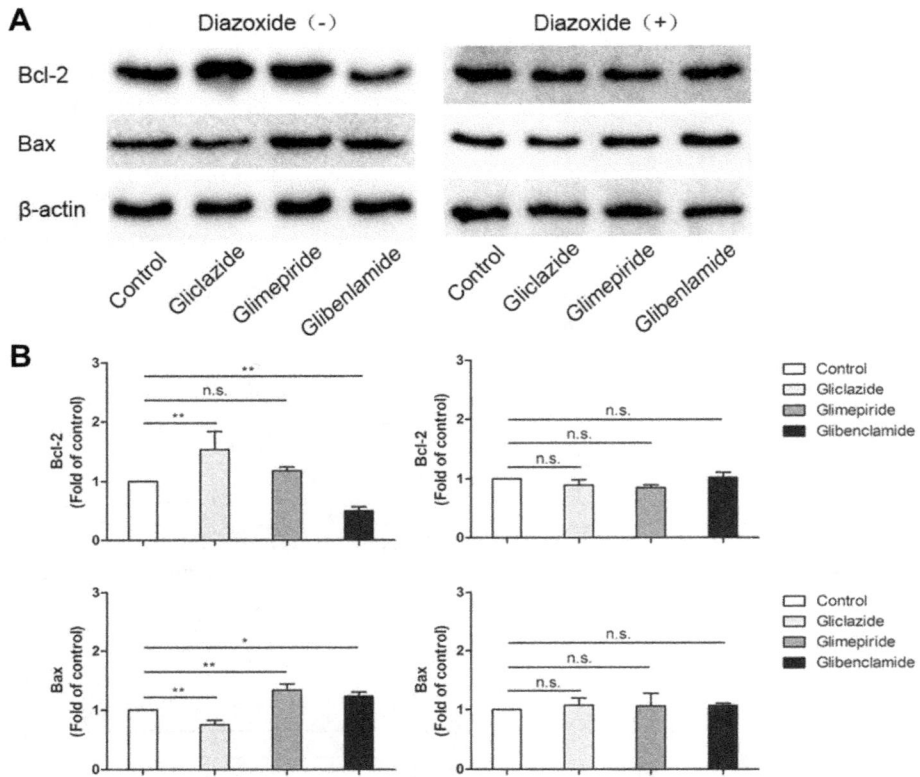

**Fig. 2** Bcl-2 and Bax expression in SUs and SUs + DZ groups. **a** Representative image of Western Blot of cells extracts. **b** Quantificaton of Western Blot results. Mean ± SD of three independent experiments *$P < 0.05$ versus control, ** $p < 0.01$, n.s. not significant

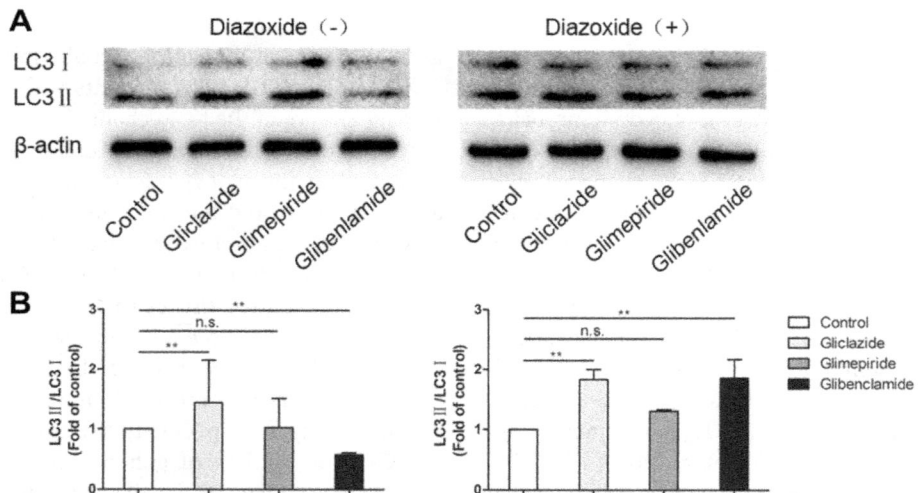

**Fig. 3** . Effect of SUs and SUs + DZ on expression of autophagy-related protein. LC3I and LC3II expression in SUs and SUs + DZ groups. **a** Western Blot analysis of cells extracts confirmed almost complete loss of LC3I to LC3II conversion after treated with DZ. **b** Quantificaton of Western Blot results. Mean ± SD of three independent experiments * $P < 0.05$ versus control, ** $p < 0.01$, n.s. not significant

the binding site and its blockage is reversible (Kakkar et al. 2006). On the other side, gliclazide shares with glibenclamide and glimepiride a sulphonylurea moiety but does not possess a carbox-amido-ethyl-phenyl group attached to the phenyl-sulphonyl group, which in part explains its specific interaction with the SUR1 and producing a reversible inhibition of $K_{ATP}$ channels (Ashcroft & Gribble, 2000). Such different binding selectivity and reversibility of these SUs may have produced different interactions in apoptosis of PTECs.

Second, several reports have shown that oxidative stress play an important role in the impairment of renal tubular function. Glibenclamide and glimepiride were reported to stimulate ROS production in the pancreatic beta cell line MIN6 (Tsubouchi et al. 2005). The increased ROS production is a causative mechanism for the apoptosis of β-cells induced by them. In contrast, gliclazide did not significantly stimulate ROS production. Beyond that, gliclazide, a modern SUs with a bicycle-octyl ring structure, scavenged ROS, inhibited NADPH oxidase and glomerular macrophage infiltration with suppression of ICAM-1, and prevented renal damage (Onozato et al. 2004). Similar effects might exist as the potentially protective mechanism of gliclazide that is different from other SUs.

Third, mechanisms other than $K_{ATP}$ channel are involved in PTEC apoptosis (Gribble et al. 1998). We could not exclude the possibility that these factors play a role in the process of apoptosis induced by specific SUs.

These evidences suggest that glibenclamide and glimepiride, especial the former, might promote the apoptosis of PTECs through closing the $K_{ATP}$ channel by binding to the SUR.

What might be the possible mechanisms of SUs induced apoptosis of PTECs by closing $K_{ATP}$ channel? It has been reported that SUs can induce apoptosis in β-cells or clonal β-cell lines under certain conditions, however, the mechanism is still unidentified (Beesley et al. 1999). Kim et al. (Kim et al. 2012) reported that SUs could induces apoptosis not only by elevated cytosolic $Ca^{2+}$ but also by dysregulation of $Ca^{2+}$ homeostasis through interfere with the endoplasmic reticulum stress (ERS). ERS is involved in a number of physiological and pathological processes, including diabetes. The ability of renal tubular cells to cope with ERS is essential for maintaining normal renal function (Ashcroft, 2006). Recent research suggests that ERS is a major factor in renal tubular cell apoptosis resulting from ischemic acute kidney injury (Sliwinska et al. 2012). Therefore, SUs' closure of $K_{ATP}$ channels, increased intracellular $Ca^{2+}$, which might have caused the ERS and triggered the apoptosis of PTECs. Apoptosis induction by specific SUs depends on different SUR isoform expression in different tissues. SUR2B was reported to express in PTECs, which may be regarded as the main target of SUs, responsible for mediating the process.

Autophagy is a highly conserved cytoprotective process, which allows cells to mitigate various types of cellular stress (Kim et al. 2012). Several groups have shown that autophagy plays a critical role in maintaining tubule homeostasis and integrity under conditions of stress (Inoue et al. 2010; Periyasamy-Thandavan et al. 2008; Yang et al. 2008; Jiang et al. 2010). More importantly, Shuya Liu et al. (Liu et al. 2012) found that proximal tubule cells depend more than any other tubule segment on basal autophagic activity. Our previous study also showed that impairment of autophagy play an important role in high glucose (HG)-induced apoptosis of PTECs. Whereas, the upregulation of autophagy in HK-2 cells could protect against HG-mediated apoptosis (Zhang et al. 2017). Here, our results suggested that impairment of autophagy induced by SUs might also contribute to the apoptosis of PTECs. In addition, our results are consistent with previous observations that autophagy protects PTECs from injury and apoptosis (Dong et al. 2015; Xu et al. 2016). Other research indicates that increased cytosolic $Ca^{2+}$ levels regulated by $K_{ATP}$ channels play a role in impairing autophagy, which is associated with neurodegenerative disorders (Hambrock et al. 2006). Altogether these studies brought an assumption that SUs could interfere with autophagy through their action on $K_{ATP}$ channels, which then play a part in SUs-induced apoptosis of PTECs.

Over the past decades, although several studies focused on the hypoglycemic effects of SUs on DKD treatment, few studies paid attention to the direct effect of SUs on kidney, especially their effects on the apoptosis of PTECs. Emerging evidences showed that $K_{ATP}$ channels are involved in regulating energy metabolism and maintaining the homeostasis in podocyte and renal tubular cells (Kim et al. 1999; Meijer & Codogno, 2008; Havasi & Dong, 2016). Our study finds that different SUs induce the apoptosis of proximal tubular epithelial cell differently. Glibenclamide and glimepiride, in particular the former may promote the apoptosis of PTECs; those effects may be reversed by DZ. Gliclazide, on the other hand, decreased the apoptosis of PTECs. Calcium overload induced by closure of $K_{ATP}$ channels might contribute to the impairment of autophagy and subsequent activation of apoptosis. Further precise mechanisms remain to be determined.

There are several limitations in this study, first of which being lack of a *SUR2* gene knockdown group. Second, the autophagy activity in tubular cells has not yet been elucidated in detail in this study. Third, only three common SUs included in our study, whether our findings could be generalized to other SUs need to be examined in further study.

## Conclusions

In summary, our study provides evidence for the first time that SUs, such as glibenclamide, could induce apoptosis in

PTECs through a $K_{ATP}$ channel-dependent manner and this effect could be reversed by DZ. Our data also indicated that different SUs induce apoptosis differently in PTECs. SUs should not be regarded as a homogeneous drug class in terms of their tissue specificity and their effects on extra-pancreatic cells. The clinical relevance of extra-pancreatic action of SUs is being widely discussed and remains controversial. Although it is still uncertain if SUs are harmful to renal cells, a more appropriate strategy for diabetes treatment would be to use drugs acting specifically on the β-cell $K_{ATP}$ channels.

## Abbreviations

DKD: Diabetic kidney disease; DMSO: Dimethyl sulfoxide; DZ: Diazoxide; ERS: Endoplasmic reticulum stress; HG: High glucose; $K_{ATP}$: Channel: ATP-dependent potassium channel; PTECs: Proximal tubular epithelial cells; ROS: Reactive oxygen species; SURs: Sulfonylurea receptors; SUs: Sulfonylureas; T2DM: Type 2 diabetes mellitus

## Funding

This study is supported by grants from the National Natural Science Foundation of China (81570742), Jinan Science & Technology Development Program, China (201602172), Shandong Provincial Natural Science Foundation, China (ZR2017LH025).

## Authors' contributions

LL and JD conceived and designed the study. XZ, XS and TX performed the experiments and interpreted the results. RZ assisted in conducting the experiments and analyzed the data. RZ, XZ wrote the manuscript. TX, CX and ZZ edited the figures in the manuscript. All authors read and approved the final version of the manuscript. LL and JD contributed equally to this work.

## Competing interests

The authors declare that they have no competing interests.

## Author details

[1]Department of Endocrinology, Shandong Provincial Qianfoshan Hospital, Shandong University, Jinan, Shandong, China. [2]Department of Endocrinology, Qilu Hospital of Shandong University, Jinan, Shandong, China. [3]Division of Endocrinology, Department of Internal Medicine, Shandong University of Traditional Chinese Medicine, Jinan, Shandong, China. [4]Department of Internal Medicine, Division of Endocrinology, Qilu Hospital of Shandong University, No. 107, Wenhuaxi Road, Jinan, Shandong, China. [5]Department of Internal Medicine, Division of Endocrinology, Shandong Provincial Qianfoshan Hospital, Shandong University, No. 16766, Jingshi Road, Jinan, Shandong, China.

## References

Ashcroft FM. K(ATP) channels and insulin secretion: a key role in health and disease. Biochem Soc Trans. 2006;34(Pt 2):243–6.

Ashcroft FM, Gribble FM. Tissue-specific effects of sulfonylureas: lessons from studies of cloned K(ATP) channels. J Diabetes Complicat. 2000;14(4):192–6.

Assad AR, Delou JM, Fonseca LM, Villela NR, Nascimento JH, Vercosa N, Lopes AG, Capella MA. The role of KATP channels on propofol preconditioning in a cellular model of renal ischemia-reperfusion. Anesth Analg. 2009;109(5):1486–92.

Babenko AP, Gonzalez G, Bryan J. Pharmaco-topology of sulfonylurea receptors. Separate domains of the regulatory subunits of K(ATP) channel isoforms are required for selective interaction with K(+) channel openers. J Biol Chem. 2000;275(2):717–20.

Barzilay JI, Lovato JF, Murray AM, Williamson J, Ismail-Beigi F, Karl D, Papademetriou V, Launer LJ. Albuminuria and cognitive decline in people with diabetes and normal renal function. Clin J Am Soc Nephrol. 2013;8(11):1907–14.

Beesley AH, Qureshi IZ, Giesberts AN, Parker AJ, White SJ. Expression of sulphonylurea receptor protein in mouse kidney. Pflugers Archiv. 1999;438(1):1–7.

Chutkow WA, Pu J, Wheeler MT, Wada T, Makielski JC, Burant CF, McNally EM. Episodic coronary artery vasospasm and hypertension develop in the absence of Sur2 K(ATP) channels. J Clin Invest. 2002;110(2):203–8.

Chutkow WA, Samuel V, Hansen PA, Pu J, Valdivia CR, Makielski JC, Burant CF. Disruption of Sur2-containing K(ATP) channels enhances insulin-stimulated glucose uptake in skeletal muscle. Proc Natl Acad Sci U S A. 2001;98(20):11760–4.

Chutkow WA, Simon MC, Le Beau MM, Burant CF. Cloning, tissue expression, and chromosomal localization of SUR2, the putative drug-binding subunit of cardiac, skeletal muscle, and vascular KATP channels. Diabetes. 1996;45(10):1439–45.

Dancourt J, Melia TJ. Lipidation of the autophagy proteins LC3 and GABARAP is a membrane-curvature dependent process. Autophagy. 2014;10(8):1470–1.

De Nicola L, Gabbai FB, Liberti ME, Sagliocca A, Conte G, Minutolo R. Sodium/glucose cotransporter 2 inhibitors and prevention of diabetic nephropathy: targeting the renal tubule in diabetes. Am J Kidney Dis. 2014;64(1):16–24.

Dong G, Liu Y, Zhang L, Huang S, Ding HF, Dong Z. mTOR contributes to ER stress and associated apoptosis in renal tubular cells. Am J Physiol Renal Physiol. 2015;308(3):F267–74.

Efanova IB, Zaitsev SV, Zhivotovsky B, Kohler M, Efendic S, Orrenius S, Berggren PO. Glucose and tolbutamide induce apoptosis in pancreatic beta-cells. A process dependent on intracellular Ca2+ concentration. J Biol Chem. 1998;273(50):33501–7.

Giannico G, Cortes P, Baccora MH, Hassett C, Taube DW, Yee J. Glibenclamide prevents increased extracellular matrix formation induced by high glucose concentration in mesangial cells. Am J of physiol Renal Physiol. 2007;292(1):F57–65.

Gribble FM, Reimann F. Sulphonylurea action revisited: the post-cloning era. Diabetologia. 2003;46(7):875–91.

Gribble FM, Tucker SJ, Seino S, Ashcroft FM. Tissue specificity of sulfonylureas: studies on cloned cardiac and beta-cell K(ATP) channels. Diabetes. 1998;47(9):1412–8.

Hambrock A, de Oliveira Franz CB, Hiller S, Osswald H. Glibenclamide-induced apoptosis is specifically enhanced by expression of the sulfonylurea receptor isoform SUR1 but not by expression of SUR2B or the mutant SUR1(M1289T). J Pharmacol Exp Ther. 2006;316(3):1031–7.

Havasi A, Dong Z. Autophagy and tubular cell death in the kidney. Semin Nephrol. 2016;36(3):174–88.

Ilatovskaya DV, Levchenko V, Lowing A, Shuyskiy LS, Palygin O, Staruschenko A. Podocyte injury in diabetic nephropathy: implications of angiotensin II-dependent activation of TRPC channels. Sci Rep. 2015;5:17637.

Inagaki N, Gonoi T, Clement JP, Wang CZ, Aguilar-Bryan L, Bryan J, Seino S. A family of sulfonylurea receptors determines the pharmacological properties of ATP-sensitive K+ channels. Neuron. 1996;16(5):1011–7.

Inagaki N, Gonoi T, JPt C, Namba N, Inazawa J, Gonzalez G, Aguilar-Bryan L, Seino S, Bryan J. Reconstitution of IKATP: an inward rectifier subunit plus the sulfonylurea receptor. Science. 1995;270(5239):1166–70.

Inoue K, Kuwana H, Shimamura Y, Ogata K, Taniguchi Y, Kagawa T, Horino T, Takao T, Morita T, Sasaki S, et al. Cisplatin-induced macroautophagy occurs prior to apoptosis in proximal tubules in vivo. Clin Exp Nephrol. 2010;14(2):112–22.

Isaka Y, Kimura T, Takabatake Y. The protective role of autophagy against aging and acute ischemic injury in kidney proximal tubular cells. Autophagy. 2011;7(9):1085–7.

Iwakura T, Fujimoto S, Kagimoto S, Inada A, Kubota A, Someya Y, Ihara Y, Yamada Y, Seino Y. Sustained enhancement of ca(2+) influx by glibenclamide induces apoptosis in RINm5F cells. Biochem Biophys Res Commun. 2000;271(2):422–8.

Jiang M, Liu K, Luo J, Dong Z. Autophagy is a renoprotective mechanism during in vitro hypoxia and in vivo ischemia-reperfusion injury. Am J Pathol. 2010;176(3):1181–92.

Kakkar R, Ye B, Stoller DA, Smelley M, Shi NQ, Galles K, Hadhazy M, Makielski JC, McNally EM. Spontaneous coronary vasospasm in KATP mutant mice arises from a smooth muscle-extrinsic process. Circ Res. 2006;98(5):682–9.

Kim JA, Kang YS, Lee SH, Lee EH, Yoo BH, Lee YS. Glibenclamide induces apoptosis through inhibition of cystic fibrosis transmembrane conductance regulator (CFTR) cl(–) channels and intracellular ca(2+) release in HepG2 human hepatoblastoma cells. Biochem Biophys Res Commun. 1999;261(3):682–8.

Kim JY, Lim DM, Park HS, Moon CI, Choi KJ, Lee SK, Baik HW, Park KY, Kim BJ. Exendin-4 protects against sulfonylurea-induced beta-cell apoptosis. J Pharmacol Sci. 2012;118(1):65–74.

Liu R, Wang H, Xu B, Chen W, Turlova E, Dong N, Sun CL, Lu Y, Fu H, Shi R, et al. Cerebrovascular safety of sulfonylureas: the role of KATP channels in neuroprotection and the risk of stroke in patients with type 2 diabetes. Diabetes. 2016;65(9):2795–809.

Liu S, Hartleben B, Kretz O, Wiech T, Igarashi P, Mizushima N, Walz G, Huber TB. Autophagy plays a critical role in kidney tubule maintenance, aging and ischemia-reperfusion injury. Autophagy. 2012;8(5):826–37.

Liu SY, Tian HM, Liao DQ, Chen YF, Gou ZP, Xie XY, Li XJ. The effect of gliquidone on KATP channels in pancreatic beta-cells, cardiomyocytes, and vascular smooth muscle cells. Diabetes Res Clin Pract. 2015;109(2):334–9.

Magri CJ, Fava S. Albuminuria and glomerular filtration rate in type 2 diabetes mellitus. Minerva urologica e nefrologica = The Italian journal of urology and nephrology. 2011;63(4):273–80.

Meijer AJ, Codogno P. Autophagy: a sweet process in diabetes. Cell Metab. 2008; 8(4):275–6.

Onozato ML, Tojo A, Goto A, Fujita T. Radical scavenging effect of gliclazide in diabetic rats fed with a high cholesterol diet. Kidney Int. 2004;65(3):951–60.

Periyasamy-Thandavan S, Jiang M, Wei Q, Smith R, Yin XM, Dong Z. Autophagy is cytoprotective during cisplatin injury of renal proximal tubular cells. Kidney Int. 2008;74(5):631–40.

Ryan MJ, Johnson G, Kirk J, Fuerstenberg SM, Zager RA, Torok-Storb B. HK-2: an immortalized proximal tubule epithelial cell line from normal adult human kidney. Kidney Int. 1994;45(1):48–57.

Shiraishi T, Tamura Y, Taniguchi K, Higaki M, Ueda S, Shima T, Nagura M, Nakagawa T, Johnson RJ, Uchida S. Combination of ACE inhibitor with nicorandil provides further protection in chronic kidney disease. Am J Physiol Renal Physiol. 2014;307(12):F1313–22.

Singh DK, Winocour P, Farrington K. Mechanisms of disease: the hypoxic tubular hypothesis of diabetic nephropathy. Nat Clin Pract Nephrol. 2008;4(4):216–26.

Sliwinska A, Rogalska A, Szwed M, Kasznicki J, Jozwiak Z, Drzewoski J. Gliclazide may have an antiapoptotic effect related to its antioxidant properties in human normal and cancer cells. Mol Biol Rep. 2012;39(5):5253–67.

Szamosfalvi B, Cortes P, Alviani R, Asano K, Riser BL, Zasuwa G, Yee J. Putative subunits of the rat mesangial KATP: a type 2B sulfonylurea receptor and an inwardly rectifying K+ channel. Kidney Int. 2002;61(5):1739 49.

Tahrani AA, Barnett AH, Bailey CJ. Pharmacology and therapeutic implications of current drugs for type 2 diabetes mellitus. Nat Rev Endocrinol. 2016;12(10): 566–92.

Thompson EM, Pishko GL, Muldoon LL, Neuwelt EA. Inhibition of SUR1 decreases the vascular permeability of cerebral metastases. Neoplasia. 2013;15(5):535–43.

Tojo A, Kinugasa S. Mechanisms of glomerular albumin filtration and tubular reabsorption. Int J Nephrol. 2012;2012:481520.

Tsubouchi H, Inoguchi T, Inuo M, Kakimoto M, Sonta T, Sonoda N, Sasaki S, Kobayashi K, Sumimoto H, Nawata H. Sulfonylurea as well as elevated glucose levels stimulate reactive oxygen species production in the pancreatic beta-cell line, MIN6-a role of NAD(P)H oxidase in beta-cells. Biochem Biophys Res Commun. 2005;326(1):60–5.

Tucker SJ, Gribble FM, Zhao C, Trapp S, Ashcroft FM. Truncation of Kir6.2 produces ATP-sensitive K+ channels in the absence of the sulphonylurea receptor. Nature. 1997;387(6629):179–83.

Wakino S, Hasegawa K, Itoh H. Sirtuin and metabolic kidney disease. Kidney Int. 2015;88(4):691–8.

Weide T, Huber TB. Implications of autophagy for glomerular aging and disease. Cell Tissue Res. 2011;343(3):467–73.

Xu Y, Guo M, Jiang W, Dong H, Han Y, An XF, Zhang J. Endoplasmic reticulum stress and its effects on renal tubular cells apoptosis in ischemic acute kidney injury. Ren Fail. 2016;38(5):831–7.

Yang C, Kaushal V, Shah SV, Kaushal GP. Autophagy is associated with apoptosis in cisplatin injury to renal proximal tubular epithelial cells. Am J Physiol Renal Physiol. 2008;294(4):F777–87.

Zhang XQ, Dong JJ, Cai T, Shen X, Zhou XJ, Liao L. High glucose induces apoptosis via upregulation of Bim expression in proximal tubule epithelial cells. Oncotarget. 2017;8(15):24119–29.

Zhang YJ, Zhang AQ, Zhao XX, Tian ZL, Yao L. Nicorandil protects against ischaemia-reperfusion injury in newborn rat kidney. Pharmacology. 2013; 92(5–6):245–56.

Zhou M, He HJ, Tanaka O, Suzuki R, Sekiguchi M, Yasuoka Y, Kawahara K, Itoh H, Abe H. Localization of the sulphonylurea receptor subunits, SUR2A and SUR2B, in rat renal tubular epithelium. Tohoku J Exp Med. 2008;214(3):247–56.

Zoja C, Zanchi C, Benigni A. Key pathways in renal disease progression of experimental diabetesNephrol Dial Transplant. 2015;30(Suppl 4):iv54–9.

# 10

# Effects of CREB1 gene silencing on cognitive dysfunction by mediating PKA-CREB signaling pathway in mice with vascular dementia

Xin-Rui Han[1,2†], Xin Wen[1,2†], Yong-Jian Wang[1,2†], Shan Wang[1,2], Min Shen[1,2], Zi-Feng Zhang[1,2], Shao-Hua Fan[1,2], Qun Shan[1,2], Liang Wang[1,2], Meng-Qiu Li[1,2], Bin Hu[1,2], Chun-Hui Sun[1,2], Dong-Mei Wu[1,2*], Jun Lu[1,2*] and Yuan-Lin Zheng[1,2*]

## Abstract

**Background:** As a form of dementia primarily affecting the elderly, vascular dementia (VD) is characterized by changes in the supply of blood to the brain, resulting in cognitive impairment. The aim of the present study was to explore the effects involved with cyclic adenosine monophosphate (cAMP) response element-binding (CREB)1 gene silencing on cognitive dysfunction through meditation of the protein kinase A (PKA)-CREB signaling pathway in mice with VD.

**Methods:** Both the Morris water maze test and the step down test were applied to assess the cognitive function of the mice with VD. Immunohistochemical and TUNEL staining techniques were employed to evaluate the positive expression rates of the protein CREB1 and Cleaved Caspase-3, as well as neuronal apoptosis among hippocampal tissues in a respective manner. Flow cytometry was applied to determine the proliferation index and apoptosis rate of the hippocampal cells among each group. Reverse transcription quantitative polymerase chain reaction and Western blot analysis methods were applied to detect the expressions of cAMP, PKA and CREB in hippocampal cells.

**Results:** Compared with the normal group, all the other groups exhibited impaired cognitive function, reduced cell numbers in the CAI area, positive expressions of CREB1 as well as positive optical density (OD) values. Furthermore, increased Cleaved Caspase-3 positive expression, OD value, proliferation index, apoptosis rate of hippocampal cells and neurons, were observed in the other groups when compared with the normal group, as well as lower expressions of cAMP, PKA and CREB1 and p-CREB1 (the shCREB1-1, H89 and shCREB1-1 + H89 groups < the VD group).

**Conclusion:** The key findings of the present study demonstrated that CREB1 gene silencing results in aggravated VD that occurs as a result of inhibiting the PKA-CREB signaling pathway, thus exasperating cognitive dysfunction.

**Keywords:** CREB1, PKA, CREB, Signaling pathway, Vascular dementia, Cognitive dysfunction

* Correspondence: wdm8610@jsnu.edu.cn; lu-jun75@163.com; ylzheng@jsnu.edu.cn
†Equal contributors
[1]Key Laboratory for Biotechnology on Medicinal Plants of Jiangsu Province, School of Life Science, Jiangsu Normal University, No. 101, Shanghai Road, Tongshan District, Xuzhou 221116, Jiangsu Province, People's Republic of China
Full list of author information is available at the end of the article

## Background

Representing the second leading cause of senile dementia behind that of Alzheimer's disease (AD), vascular dementia (VD) accounts for 17.6% of all cases of dementia in western countries, while studies have indicated this number to be even greater in the Eastern regions of the world, including in that of the Chinese and Japanese population's (Battistin & Cagnin, 2010). Cognitive dysfunction is widely thought to be the classical feature exhibited by patients suffering from dementia (McGirr et al., 2016). In generally terms, VD, can be understood as an acquired intellectual damage syndrome, characterized by various cerebral vascular diseases however, is predominately associated with ischemic cerebrovascular disease (You et al., 2017). Dementia including the subtype of VD, arises from impairments in cognitive function, motor function, functional domains and memory impairments (Lee, 2011; Li et al., 2015). At present, the precise pathogenesis of VD remains largely unclear (Gong et al., 2012). Therefore, it is necessary that the finer details of the molecular mechanism underlying the condition are elucidated, in order to identify more effective future treatment approaches.

As a 43 kDa protein and transcription factor, cyclic adenosine monophosphate (cAMP) responsive element-binding proteins (CREB) are members of the bZIP transcription factor superfamily (Ramakrishnan & Pace, 2011). In addition, by performing the downstream of various signals, CREB1 possesses gene expression regulatory abilities and plays an essential role in long-term memory formation, behavioral changes, immune function, metabolic function, as well as cell survival (Sadamoto et al., 2010). A previous study demonstrated that subjects with spatial memory impairment had lower hippocampal levels of CREB1 (Brightwell et al., 2004). CREB is a member of the family of leucine-zipper transcription factors, while CREB1 has been reported to promote cell signal transduction (Li et al., 2012). What's more, the phosphorylation of CREB1 has been highlighted due to its involvement in the synthesis of an array of proteins, of which play significant roles in neuronal functions, including that of protein kinase A (PKA) (Murphy Jr et al., 2013). PKA is the key mediator of the second messenger cAMP (Kleppe et al., 2011), and plays a positive role in the process of synaptic plasticity and long-term memory formation (Jarome et al., 2013). PKA is comprised of four sub-units: two regulatory sub-units and two catalytic sub-units, with the catalytic sub-units most commonly reported to bind to CREB as well as with the regulatory sub-units of cAMP (Hang et al., 2013). As an indispensable regulator of synaptic plasticity, the PKA/CREB signaling pathway plays a crucial role in the processes and functioning of learning and memory (Du et al., 2014). Studies have previously revealed that in the event that the PKA/CREB signaling pathway was to be inhibited, individuals would display learning and memory

deficits similar to that of patients suffering from AD (Chen et al., 2012). Based on the aforementioned literature, we are of the belief that CREB1 and the PKA/CREB signaling pathway are both involved in cognitive function, including that of the processes of memory formation and behavioral changes (Zheng et al., 2016; Cheng et al., 2015). Hence, the central objective of the present study was to elucidate the relationship of the CREB1 gene, the PKA-CREB signaling pathway and VD, in an attempt to form a basis in the search for a new treatment method for patients suffering from VD.

## Method
### Establishment of mouse model

A total of 80 male Kunming mice (aged 3-months), weighing approximately $34 \pm 2.5$ g (certificate number: 801032), were provided by the Animal Experiment Center of Hebei Medical University, and housed in controlled standard laboratory conditions ($21 \pm 2$ °C) for one week. The rats were granted free access to food and water, placed on a 12 h light-dark cycle, with relative humidity conditions of 40% ~ 70% and noise levels < 50 dB. Ten mice were then randomly selected as the normal group, while the other 70 mice were used in order to establish the VD mouse model (Higuchi et al., 2017). The VD mouse model was established based on the following procedure: bilateral carotid artery ischemia reperfusion combined with tail bleeding, anesthetized by means of intraperitoneal injection with 40 mg/kg 0.4% pentobarbital sodium solution, and immobilized on an operating table followed by routine sterilization, and routine disinfection. Through an anterior neck middle incision, the bilateral carotid arteries were bluntly dissected. Next, a No. 4 thread buckle was hooked to the artery, and a thread was tightened in order to stop bleeding for 20 min. Meanwhile, 1 cm of the tail was cut for bleeding (0.3 ml), and the bleeding was subsequently stopped by means of heat coagulation. The next day, the conditions were observed over a period of 30 min after reperfusion, and the skin was subsequently sutured. The local skin with an incision was injected with 2000 U gentamicin. After surgery, 2000 U penicillin was intramuscularly injected at regular intervals each day for 3 consecutive days. Changes in mice physical activity post model establishment were observed in order verify as to whether successful model establishment had been obtained (De Lucia et al., 2015). The mice in the VD group exhibited behavioral changes, such as sluggishness, reduced food intake, dry hair and slow response to external stimuli. All efforts were made to minimize animal suffering.

### Construction of CREB lentiviral vectors and grouping

RNA interference (RNAi) was applied to construct the shRNA lentiviral expression vector (pLenR-GPH vector) targeting CREB1 (shCREB1−1, shCREB1−2 and shCREB1−3) with the negative control (NC)-siRNA-CREB and positive control siRNA-glyceraldehyde-3-phosphate dehydrogenase (GAPDH). Based on the mRNA sequence of the NCBI nucleotide CREB1, two specific mouse CREB1 siRNA target sequences were designed. Double stranded DNA oligo comprised of interference sequences was synthesized, which were then directly connected to enzyme-digested carriers.

The mice were then assigned into 6 groups, namely: the normal, VD, NC, shCREB1 (shCREB1−1, shCREB1−2 and shCREB1−3 groups; each included 10 mice; the group exhibiting the best silence efficiency as per evaluation by means of reverse transcription quantitative polymerase chain reaction (RT-qPCR) was used for subsequent experiments), H89 (PKA-CREB signaling pathway inhibitor) and shCREB1 + H89 groups. Mice in the shCREB1 groups were injected with 20 μl of CREB1 siRNA lentiviral vectors at the caudal vein, while mice in the NC group were injected with 20 μl of unrelated sequence siRNA. An unrelated sequence of siRNA and CREB1 siRNA lentiviral vectors were encapsulated in the mixture of EntransterTM-invivo (Engreen Biosystem Co. Ltd., Beijing, China) with 10% glucose solution. Mice in the H89 group were intraperitoneal administered with 30 mg/kg 10 mol/L H89 (127243−85-0, Shanghai Peiyang Chemical Co. Ltd., Shanghai, China). The shCREB1 + H89 group were injected with CREB1 siRNA lentiviral vector, and then injected with H89. In order to ensure the identical equivalent injections were administered, all mice were injected in situ for every 72 h, with a total of three injections. After 15 d, one mouse in each of the shCREB1 groups was sacrificed by means of cervical dislocation, followed by peeling of the bilateral hippocampus. The shCREB1 group with the highest silencing efficiency was evaluated by RT-qPCR for later experiments.

### Detection of cognition function
On the 30th day, the cognition function of the mice was evaluated using the Morris water maze (MWM) test (Celik et al., 2016) and step-down test (Chi et al., 2017). In regard to the MWM test, a circular pool (130 cm in diameter and 50 cm in depth) was filled with water (19 °C−20 °C). According to the four cardinal points (at the four corners) marked in the wall, the pool was divided into four equal quadrants: the right lower, left lower, right upper and left upper. A platform was then placed in the right lower quadrant and submerged 1.5 cm below the surface of the water. (Battistin & Cagnin, 2010) The place navigation experiment was conducted according to the following: After training for 5 d, the mice were placed into the water facing the wall at the right lower, left lower, right upper and left upper quadrants successively, and the length of time required to find the

platform within 2 min was recorded. The time spent finding the platform was referred to as the latent time. If the mice found the platform within 2 min, the actual latent time was then recorded, if not, it would be aided in the form of gentle guidance to the platform and stationed for 10 s, and the latent time was then recorded as 2 min. (McGirr et al., 2016) The spatial probe experiment was performed according to the following: On the sixth day, the platform was removed, in order to allow the rats to find the platform based on their memory. The swimming time was set at 120 s, and the swimming track of each mouse was recorded during the preset time of 120 s. The number of times that the original platform was crossed and the residence time at the original platform quadrant were considered to be a reflection as to whether or not the mice had remembered the location of the original platform. Data acquisition and processing was completed using the MWM automatic image acquisition system. The WX-2 mouse electro-optical stimulation conditioned reflex platform (Institute of Materia Medica, Chinese Academy of Medical Sciences, Beijing, China) was used for the step-down test. A cuboid conditioning box was employed as the platform. The mice were placed toward the wall of the pool in a successive manner. A copper grid was placed on the bottom, and 36 V of alternating current was subsequently delivered to the device. A platform, 4.5 cm in diameter and height was placed on the front left corner of the conditioning box. After 5-d of feeding, the mice were placed in a conditioning box for adaption purposes for 3 min and followed by the prompt construction of an electric circuit. The time that the mice took to jump up onto the platform and steadied themselves 5 s after electric stimulation was recorded. The test was repeated 3 times for each mouse. The reaction time, latent time and number of errors were all kept record of.

### Hematoxylin and eosin (HE) staining for testing morphological changes
On the 15th d, the mice were sacrificed by means of cervical dislocation for further experiments. In each group, 4 mice were randomly selected and their brain tissues were immediately removed. The obtained brain tissues were then fixed with 4% paraformaldehyde for 24 h, dehydrated by 80%, 90%, 100% ethanol and N-butanol, and finally soaked and embedded in a wax box with 60 °C conditions. Next, 5 μm serial sections were made. After spread out and collected at 45 °C, the sections were baked for 1 h at 60 °C and dewaxed with xylene. The sections were then stained with routine HE (Beijing Solarbio Science & Technology Co. Ltd., Beijing, China), followed by dehydration with graded ethanol, cleaned with dimethylbenzene and mounted with neutral gum. Finally, the pathological changes of the hippocampal neurons in the mice were

observed under an optical microscope (XP-330, Shanghai Bing Yu Optical Instrument Co. Ltd., Shanghai, China).

## Immunohistochemical staining

Six brain tissues samples were randomly selected from each group. The streptavidin-biotin complex (SABC) method (Higuchi et al., 2017) was applied in order to evaluate the intercellular adhesion molecule-1 (ICAM-1) based on the instructions of the kit (BBSW042, Shenzhen Baoan Kang Biotechnology Co. Ltd., Shenzhen, China). The samples were then fixed with formaldehyde, embedded in paraffin, and made into 4 μm serial sections. The sections were then baked in an incubator at 60 °C for 1 h, conventionally dewaxed with xylene, dehydrated by graded ethanol and soaked in 3% $H_2O_2$ for 10 min. The sections were subsequently washed in distilled water, followed by antigen retrieval for 90 s at high pressure, and cooled at room temperature and washed with PBS. After the addition of 5% bovine serum albumin (BSA) blocking solution, the sections were incubated at 37 °C for 30 min. CREB1 rabbit anti-human (1: 100) (ab81289, Abcam Inc., Cambridge, MA, USA) was added to the sections, while Cleaved Caspase-3 (ab2302, Abcam Inc., Cambridge, MA, USA) as primary antibodies, and incubated at 4 °C overnight. The sections were then washed with PBS, added with biotin-labeled goat anti-rabbit antibody (HY90046, Shanghai Heng Yuan Biotechnology Co. Ltd., Shanghai, China) (1: 100 dilution) as second antibody, and incubated at 37 °C for 30 min. The sections were subsequently rinsed with PBS, followed by the addition of streptomycin avidin-peroxidase solution (Beijing Zhongshan Biotechnology Co. Ltd., Beijing, China), and incubated at 37 °C for 30 min. Afterward, the sections were washed with PBS, visualized with chromogen 3, 3-diaminobenzidine (DAB) (Beijing Bioss Biotechnology Co. Ltd., Beijing, China) at room temperature. The sections were then soaked in hematoxylin for 5 min, and washed with running water. After, the sections were rinsed in 1% hydrochloric acid alcohol for 4 s, allowing them to return to a blue color after 20 min of washing with running water. The criterion for judging CREB1 and Cleaved Caspase-3 positive cells was based on the observation of a brownish-yellow color exhibited by the positive cells. Using a low powered microscope, the same initially selected 5 random regions were selected, and the percentage of CREB1 and Cleaved Caspase-3 positive regions in each section was analyzed by Image J V1.8.0 software (National Institutes of Health, Bethesda, Maryland, USA). The positive expression rate = number of positive cells/total number of cells.

## Flow cytometry

The mice in each group sacrificed by means of decapitation, followed by stripping of the hippocampus, and fixing with 70% ethanol. Single cell suspension was prepared by mesh rubbing. The DNA staining of the apoptotic cells was performed based on the one step insertion method with iodide propidium. Expo32ADC was used to analyze the immunofluorescence data and calculate the percentage of apoptotic cells in a respective manner. Muticycle AV analysis software was applied for DNA cell cycle fitting analysis, as well as to calculate the percentage of cell distribution in each phase of the DNA histogram. The proliferation index (PI) was used to determine cell proliferation activity.

## TUNEL staining for neuronal apoptosis in hippocampal CA1 region

A total of 100 mg of hippocampal tissues were collected from each group, which were then subjected to a paraffin-embedded process, cut into sections, dewaxed and dehydrated. The sections were then cut into coronal sections according to the stereotactic atlases of the mouse brain (Wang et al., 2016a), and then fixed with 4% paraformaldehyde for 2 h. The sections were then incubated at 4 °C overnight in 20% sucrose phosphate buffer. The next day, 20 μm transverse sections of hippocampal tissue were made by – 22 °C cutting machine, followed by TUNEL staining of 10 sections of each mouse with TUNEL solution. The TUNEL Kit utilized was purchased from Boehringer Mannheim GmbH (24 Mannheim, Germany), and TUNEL staining was performed according to the instructions. The apoptotic neuronal cells were observed using a microscope, which were noted to have dark granules. In addition, 10 high power fields of vision (× 200) were selected from each group under the guidance of an optical microscope. The apoptotic nuclei and the number of cells were counted, were calculated and used to determine the apoptotic index (AI) (AI = the number of apoptotic neurons/total number of neurons) of the CA1 area in the hippocampus of each group. The procedure was repeated three time in order to obtain the mean value.

## RT-qPCR

A total of 30 mg hippocampal tissues were collected from each group, followed by the addition of 1 ml of Trizol reagent (Invitrogen, Carlsbad, CA, USA), and ground in an ice bath. Total RNA was extracted from the hippocampal tissues in accordance with the instructions of the Trizol reagents. The RNA purity and concentration were detected by means of ultraviolet spectrophotometry, and then samples with a purity of A260/A280 = 1.8–2.0 were subsequently adjusted to 1 ng/μl. Next, RNA was reverse transcribed into cDNA by PrimeScriptTM RT reagent Kit (Takara, RR047A, Beijing Think-Far Technology Co. Ltd., Beijing, China), and stored at – 80 °C for further use. The primers were designed and synthesized by Shanghai Sangon Biotech Company (Shanghai, China) (Table 1). SYBR Premix Ex TaqTM II (Takara, RR047A, Beijing Think far

**Table 1** The primer sequences of mRNA

| Gene | Amplification sequences of mRNA |
| --- | --- |
| cAMP | F: 5'-GCTAACCTCTACCGCCTCCT-3' |
|  | R: 5'-GGTCACTGTCCCCATACACC-3' |
| PKA | F: 5'-CAGGAAAGCGCTCCAGATAC-3' |
|  | R: 5'-AAGGGAAGGTTGGCGTTACT-3' |
| CREB | F: 5'-TACAGGATAGACTAGCCACTT-3' |
|  | R: 5'-AATATGTTTTCCTATCGGGGT-3' |
| β-actin | F: 5'-GGGCACAGTGTGGGTGAC-3' |
|  | R: 5'-CTGGCACCACACCTTCTAC-3' |

Notes: *cAMP* cyclic adenosine monophosphate, *PKA* protein kinase A, *CREB* cyclic adenosine monophosphate responsive element-binding; *mRNA* microRNA

Technology Co., Ltd., Beijing, China) was applied for RT-qPCR purposes. The reaction system was comprised of 5. 0 μl of SYBR Premix Ex Taq II, 0.4 μl of upstream and downstream primers (10 μmol/L) respectively, 1 μl of cDNA templates (50 ng), and the volume was then added to 10 μl by RNA enzyme-free water. The reaction conditions were as follows: pre-denaturation at 95 °C for 30 s; denaturation at 95 °C for 5 s, anneal at 58 °C for 30 s, and extension at 72 °C for 15 s, for 40 circles. The relative mRNA expressions were analyzed based on the $2^{-\Delta\Delta CT}$ method.

**Western blot analysis**

The bilateral cerebral hippocampi were dissected, added with protein lysate, and centrifuged at 12000 r/min for 20 min at 4 °C. An ultraviolet spectrophotometer (Shanghai Branch 752, Shanghai Daping Instrument Co. Ltd., Shanghai, China) was employed to determine the protein concentration, and then adjusted for Western blotting purposes. The extracted protein was added to the sample buffer and boiled at 95 °C for 10 min. The amount of protein per well was 30 μg. The samples were separated by 12% sodium dodecyl sulfatepolyacrylamide gel electrophoresis (SDS-PAGE) (Beijing Cellchip Biotechnology Co. Ltd., Beijing, China) at an electrophoresis voltage from 80 V to 120 V. The extracted proteins were electro transferred into 0.45 μm polyvinylidene difluoride (PVDF) membranes (Sigma Aldrich, St Louis, MO, USA). The membranes were then incubated in a blocking solution comprised of 5% nonfat dry milk, placed at room temperature and shaken for 2 h in a continuous manner. The membranes were then added with 50–100 μl rabbit anti-mouse primary antibody (1: 200, B103, Hangzhou Kitgen Biotechnology Co. Ltd., Hangzhou, China), and incubated at 4 °C overnight. The membranes were then added with 50–100 μl goat anti-rabbit secondary antibody (1: 200, cAMP, PKA, CREB and p-CREB) (SunShineBo, SN134, NanJing SunShine Biotechnology Co. Ltd., Nanjing, China), and shaken at room

temperature for 2 h. Finally, the reaction was visualized using enhanced chemiluminescence (ECL) kit (0164, Shanghai Shuojia Technology Co. Ltd., Shanghai, China), exposed and then developed (21475–466, VWR, Beijing NKO-GENE Biotechnology Co. Ltd., Beijing, China). Semi-quantitative analysis and photographic fixing were made using Image-Proplus (Media Cybernetics, Bethesda, Maryland, USA).

**Statistical analysis**

SPSS21.0 software (IBM, Armonk, NY, USA) was used for data analysis. Measurement data were presented as mean value ± standard deviation, while comparisons between groups were conducted using single factor analysis of variance. $p < 0.05$ was considered to be statistically significant.

## Results

### VD model is established successfully

The VD model was constructed by means of bilateral carotid artery ischemia reperfusion in combination with tail bleeding. There were distinct symptoms of nerve injury among all mice with bilateral common carotid artery ligation after operation. Compared with the normal group, the mice in the VD group exhibited notably reduced food intake, physical activity, sluggish action, dry hair and no response to external stimuli. These symptoms were noted to have improved after a period of time, while food intake and physical activity remained significantly reduced in comparison with the normal group.

### The shCREB1–1 group exhibits the optimal silence efficiency and is selected for the subsequent experiments

Three shRNA groups (shCREB1–1, shCREB1–2, shCREB1–3) targeting CREB1 were constructed in order to determine the one with the best silence efficiency for subsequent experimentation. RT-qPCR (Fig. 1) results demonstrated that compared with the NC group, the expression of CREB1 in three shRNA groups (shCREB1–1, shCREB1–2, shCREB1–3) targeting CREB1 was decreased ($p < 0.05$), however no significant difference was observed in relation to the expressions of CREB1 in the positive control group (siRNA-GAPDH) ($p > 0.05$). The shCREB1–1 group displayed significantly lower expressions of CREB1 and the optimal silence efficiency, compared with the shCREB1–2 and shCREB1–3 groups (all $p < 0.05$). Therefore, the shCREB1–1 group was selected for subsequent experimentation.

### Cognitive functions of mice injected with shCREB1–1 or/ and H89 are impaired

In order to observe the cognitive function of mice in each group, a platform test as well as the MWM test

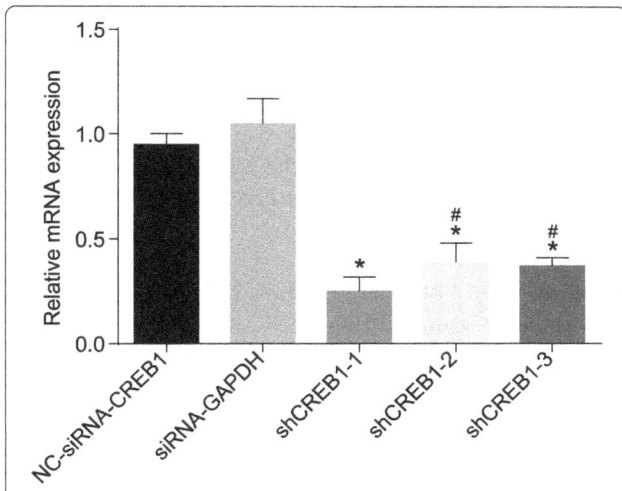

**Fig. 1** The shCREB1–1 group with best silence efficiency is selected for the subsequent experiments, Notes: $^*$, $p < 0.05$, compared with the NC-siRNA-CREB1 groups; #, $p < 0.05$, compared with the shCREB1–1 group; CREB1, cyclic adenosine monophosphate responsive element-binding protein 1; NC, negative control

was performed. The results of MWM test revealed that the latent time of mice in all groups decreased gradually during the five-day training period. Compared with the normal group, the latent time was significantly increased, while the number of times across the original platform as well as the time of residence in the original platform quadrant in other groups were reduced in all the other groups ($p < 0.05$); compared with the VD group, the latent time recorded was significantly increased, while the number of times recorded across the original platform and the time of residence at the original platform quadrant were reduced in the shCREB1–1, H89 and shCREB1–1 + H89 groups ($p < 0.05$) (Fig. 2a-b-c). The step-down test revealed that when compared with the normal group, there were significantly longer reaction times, notably shorter latent times and increased number of errors among the three groups (all $p < 0.05$). When compared with the VD group, the shCREB1–1, H89 and shCREB1–1 + H89 groups all had significant longer reaction times, notably shorter latent time and increased number of errors (all $p < 0.05$). There was no significant difference detected between the VD group and the NC group ($p > 0.05$) (Fig. 2d-e).

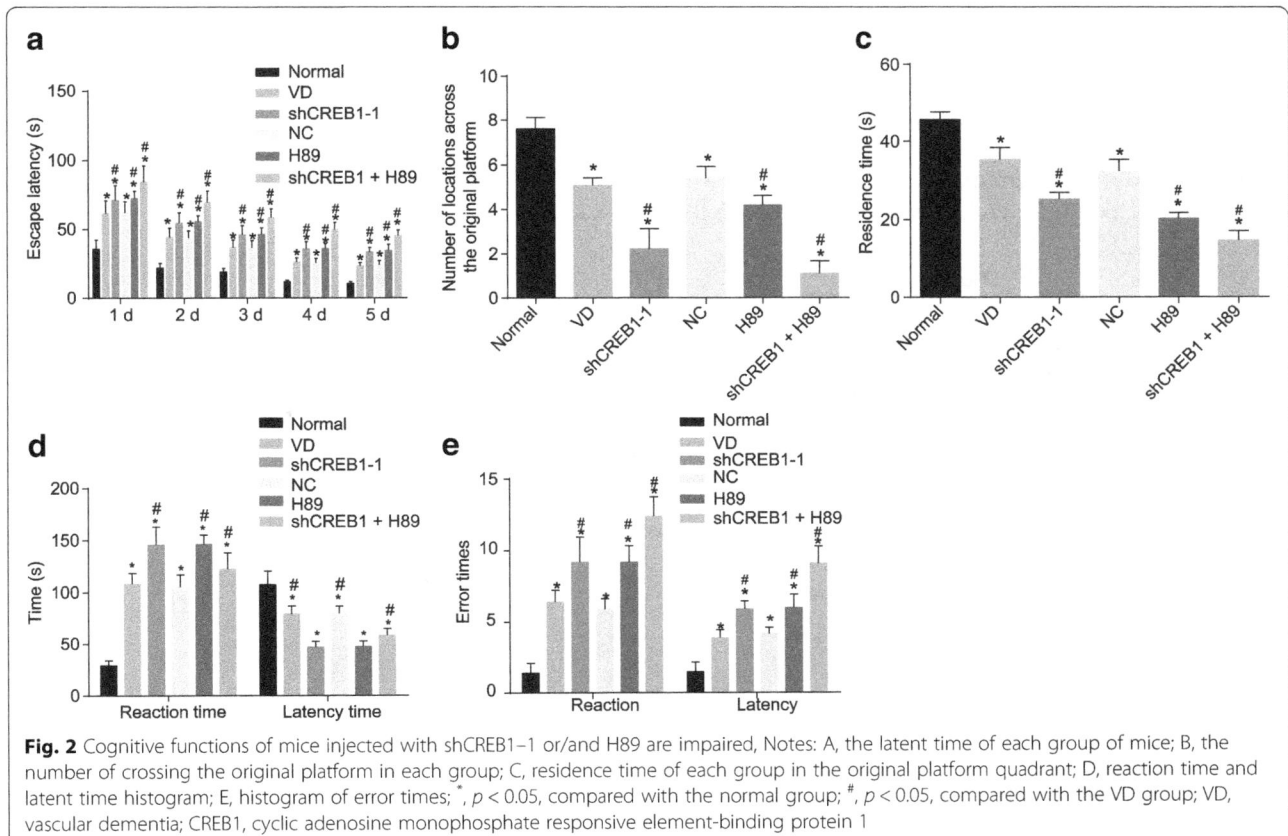

**Fig. 2** Cognitive functions of mice injected with shCREB1–1 or/and H89 are impaired, Notes: A, the latent time of each group of mice; B, the number of crossing the original platform in each group; C, residence time of each group in the original platform quadrant; D, reaction time and latent time histogram; E, histogram of error times; $^*$, $p < 0.05$, compared with the normal group; #, $p < 0.05$, compared with the VD group; VD, vascular dementia; CREB1, cyclic adenosine monophosphate responsive element-binding protein 1

## Pathological changes of hippocampal neurons among mice injected with shCREB1-1 and H89 exhibit the most significant changes

HE staining was conducted in order to explore the effects of shCREB1-1 or/and H89 on the pathological changes of the hippocampal neurons among the mice. The results of HE staining demonstrated that in the normal group, there were a number of pyramidal cells in the hippocampal CA1 area with compact and well-distributed arrangement, clear outline, neat border, large and round nucleus, distinct nucleolus, rich chromatin and limpid cytoplasm. Mice in the VD and NC groups had fewer pyramidal cells, with loose and disordered arrangements, with smaller, more deeply stained and pyknotic nucleus, in the hippocampal CA1 area. The nucleolus was faded with an intensely eosinophilic cytoplasm. Compared with the VD group, the shCREB1-1 group had fewer pyramidal cells, with a more distinct disarranged structure in the hippocampal CA1 area. The shCREB1-1 + H89 group recorded the most severe pathological changes of the hippocampal neurons (Fig. 3).

## Decreased positive expression rate of CREB1 and increased cleaved Caspase-3 in the hippocampal CA1 area of mice injected with shCREB1-1 or/and H89

Immunohistochemical staining was applied in order to elucidate the mechanism of shCREB1-1 or/and H89 on the positive expression rate of CREB1 and Cleaved Caspase-3 in the hippocampal CA1 area of mice. The immunohistochemical staining results illustrated in Fig. 4, revealed that CREB1 protein was expressed in cytoplasm, depicted by brown positive granules, while the cleaved caspase-3 positive cells presented brown granules. Compared with the normal group, all the other groups were determined to have a lower OD value of CREB1 protein

and higher OD value of Cleaved Caspase-3 protein in the hippocampal CA1 area (all $p < 0.05$) while comparisons with the VD group, the shCREB1-1, H89 and shCREB1-1 + H89 groups had significantly decreased average OD value of CREB1 protein and increased OD value of Cleaved Caspase-3 protein in the hippocampal CA1 area ($p < 0.05$). No significant difference was detected in the NC group.

## Increased PI and AI of hippocampal cells in mice injected with shCREB1-1 or/and H89

Flow cytometry was used to detect the PI and apoptotic rate of the hippocampal cells. Compared with the normal group, hippocampal cell PI and as well as the rate of apoptosis were significantly elevated in the VD group, the shCREB1-1 group, the NC group, the H89 group and the shCREB1-1 + H89 group ($p < 0.05$). Compared with the VD group, hippocampal cell PI and apoptotic rate in the shCREB1-1 group, the H89 group and the shCREB1-1 + H89 group were increased ($p < 0.05$); while no significant difference was detected in regard to PI and the rate of apoptosis of hippocampus in the NC group ($p > 0.05$) (Fig. 5).

## Increased neuronal apoptosis in hippocampal CA1 area of mice injected with shCREB1-1 or/and H89

TUNEL staining was applied in order to detect the AI of neurons in CA1 region in the hippocampus of mice. TUNEL staining (Fig. 6) results indicated that the apoptotic granules were brown in color. When compared with the normal group, all the other groups had significantly increased AI in the hippocampal CA1 area (all $p < 0.05$). The shCREB1-1, H89 and shCREB1-1 + H89 groups had significantly increased

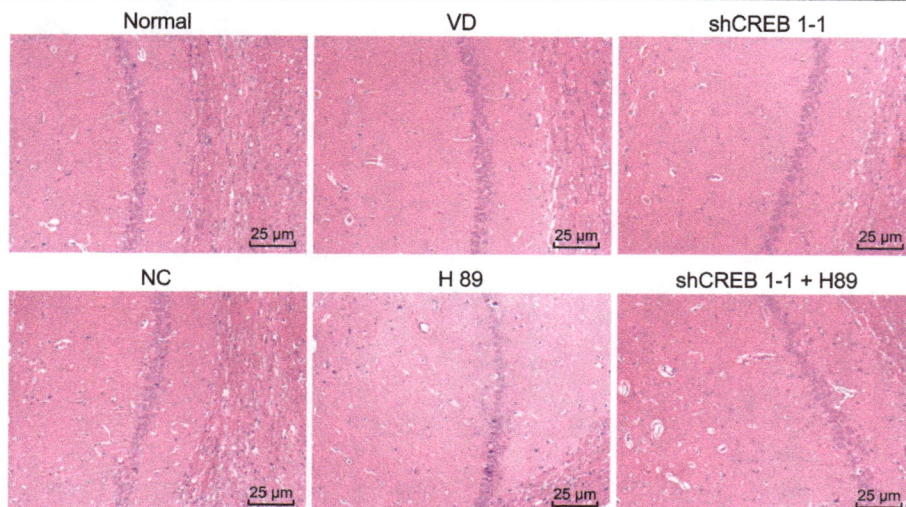

**Fig. 3** Pathological changes of hippocampal neurons of mice injected with shCREB1-1 and H89 are most serious, Note: CREB1, cyclic adenosine monophosphate responsive element-binding protein 1

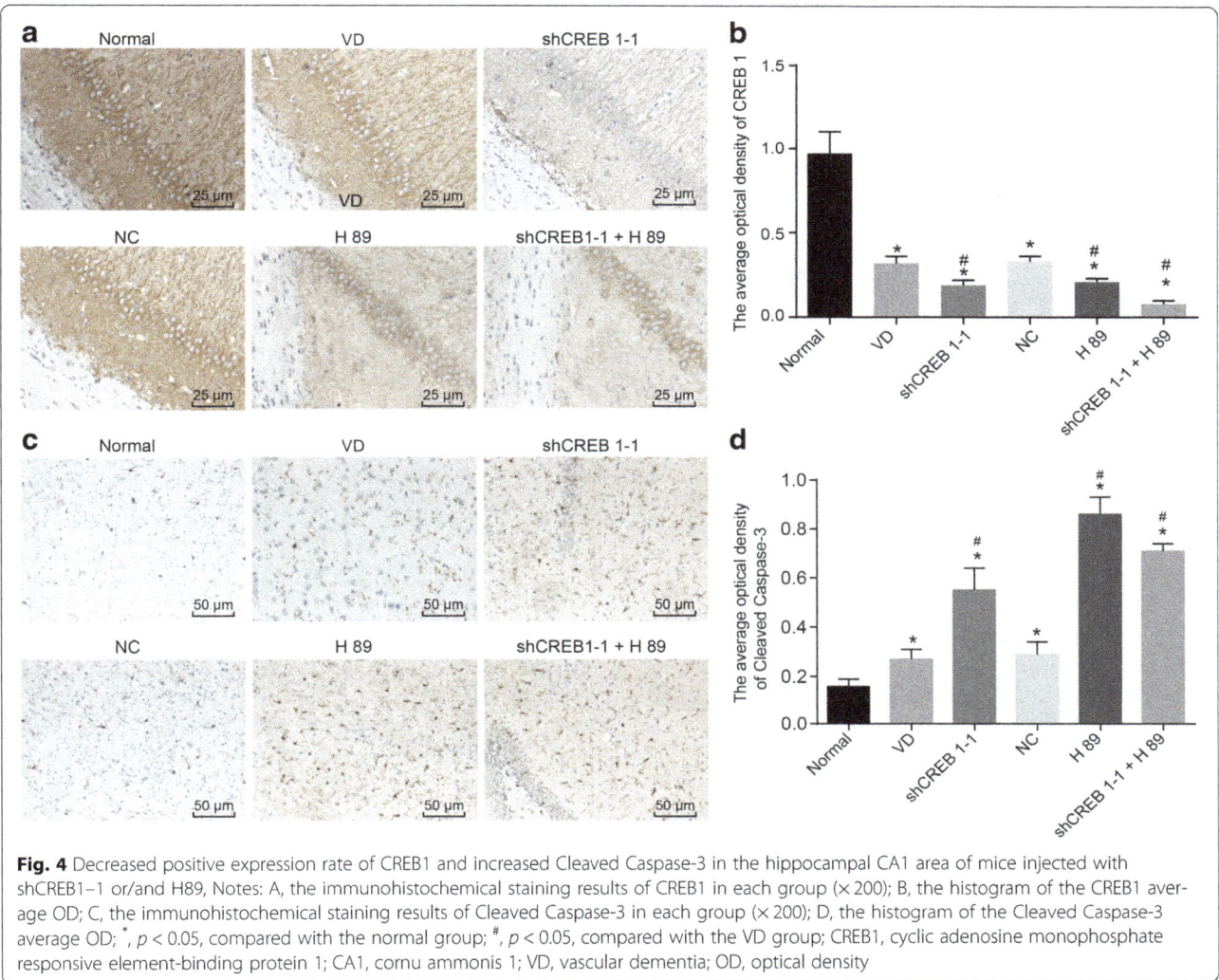

**Fig. 4** Decreased positive expression rate of CREB1 and increased Cleaved Caspase-3 in the hippocampal CA1 area of mice injected with shCREB1–1 or/and H89, Notes: A, the immunohistochemical staining results of CREB1 in each group (× 200); B, the histogram of the CREB1 average OD; C, the immunohistochemical staining results of Cleaved Caspase-3 in each group (× 200); D, the histogram of the Cleaved Caspase-3 average OD; *, $p < 0.05$, compared with the normal group; #, $p < 0.05$, compared with the VD group; CREB1, cyclic adenosine monophosphate responsive element-binding protein 1; CA1, cornu ammonis 1; VD, vascular dementia; OD, optical density

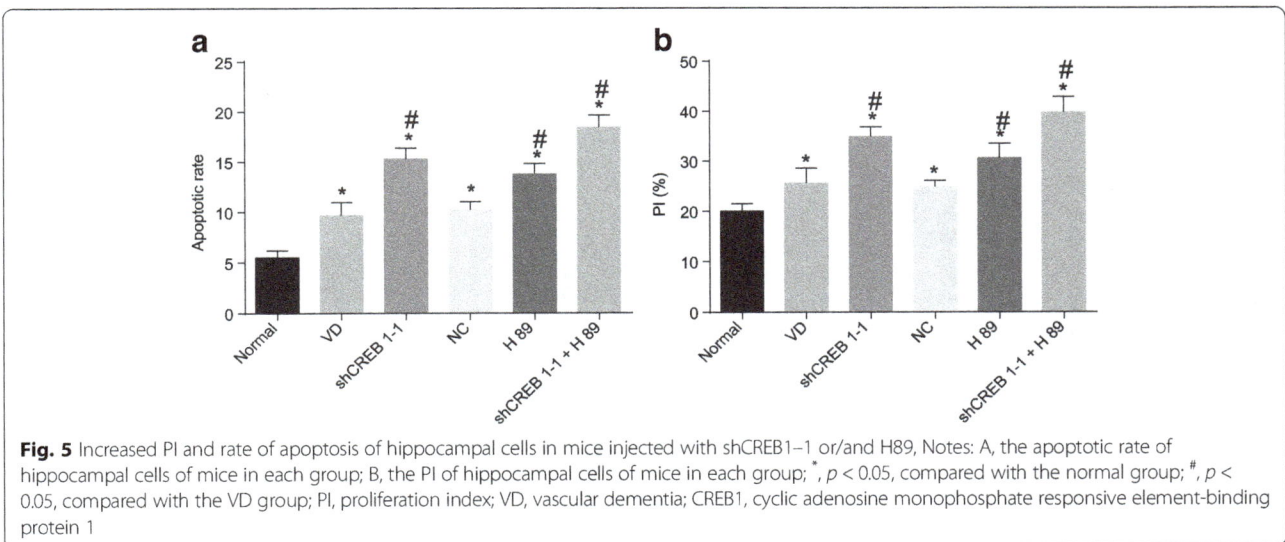

**Fig. 5** Increased PI and rate of apoptosis of hippocampal cells in mice injected with shCREB1–1 or/and H89, Notes: A, the apoptotic rate of hippocampal cells of mice in each group; B, the PI of hippocampal cells of mice in each group; *, $p < 0.05$, compared with the normal group; #, $p < 0.05$, compared with the VD group; PI, proliferation index; VD, vascular dementia; CREB1, cyclic adenosine monophosphate responsive element-binding protein 1

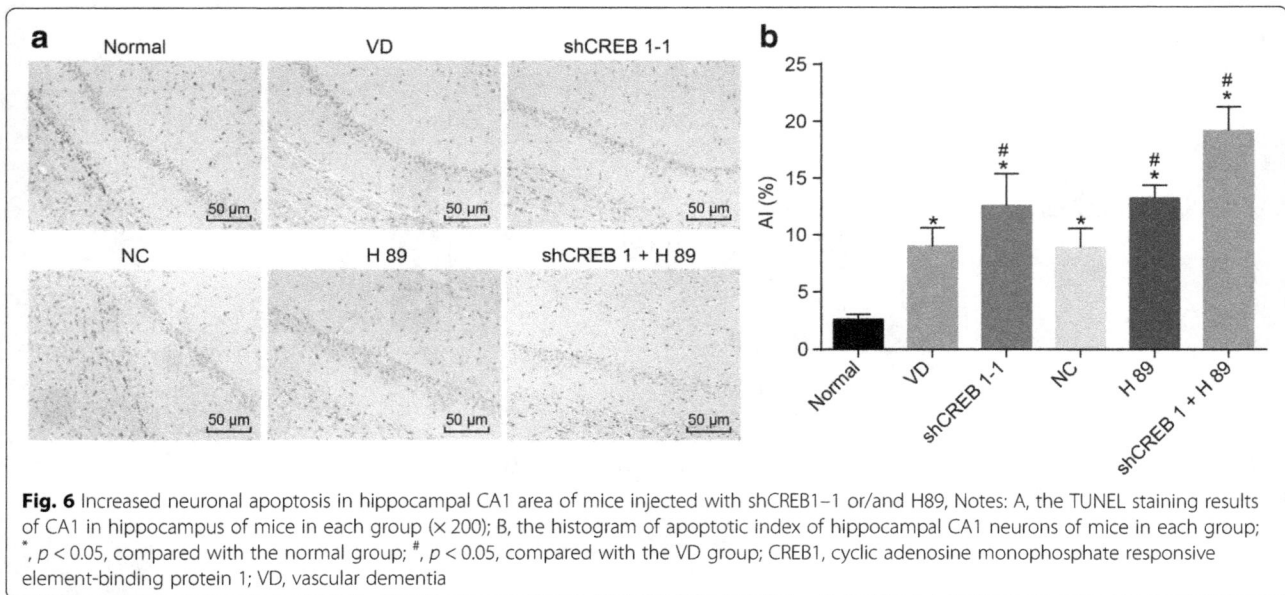

**Fig. 6** Increased neuronal apoptosis in hippocampal CA1 area of mice injected with shCREB1–1 or/and H89, Notes: A, the TUNEL staining results of CA1 in hippocampus of mice in each group (× 200); B, the histogram of apoptotic index of hippocampal CA1 neurons of mice in each group; *, $p < 0.05$, compared with the normal group; #, $p < 0.05$, compared with the VD group; CREB1, cyclic adenosine monophosphate responsive element-binding protein 1; VD, vascular dementia

AI in the hippocampal CA1 area when compared with the VD group ($p < 0.05$). There was no significant difference observed between the NC group and the VD group ($p > 0.05$).

### Decreased expression of cAMP, PKA, CREB1 and p-CREB1 in hippocampal tissues of mice with shCREB1–1 or/and H89

RT-qPCR and Western blot analysis were applied in order to identify the role of CREB1 gene silencing and PKA-CREB signaling pathway in the expression of cAMP, PKA, CREB1 and p-CREB1 in hippocampal tissues. The results (Fig. 7), of which revealed that, when compared with the normal group, all the other groups had decreased mRNA and protein expression of cAMP, PKA, CREB1 and p-CREB1 in hippocampal tissues (all

$p < 0.05$). The shCREB1–1, H89 and shCREB1–1 + H89 groups had significantly decreased mRNA and protein expressions of cAMP, PKA, CREB1 and p-CREB1 in hippocampal tissues when compared with the VD group ($p < 0.05$). No significant difference was detected between the NC group and the VD group (all $p > 0.05$).

### Discussion

Patients suffering from VD are widely known to manifest motor and cognitive impairments (Li et al., 2013). Studies have shown that when compared with the general population as well as patients with AD, patients with VD exhibit lower survival rates comparatively speaking (Bruandet et al., 2009). At present, there is a scarcity of effective drugs available to treat VD (Wang, 2014). Therefore, it is extremely urgent that novel treatments are developed to

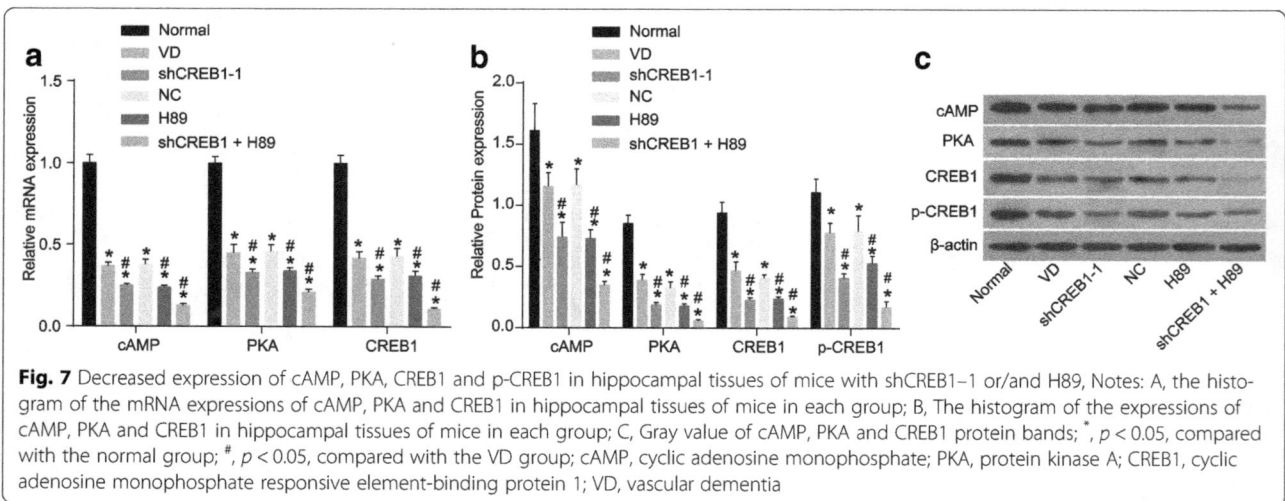

**Fig. 7** Decreased expression of cAMP, PKA, CREB1 and p-CREB1 in hippocampal tissues of mice with shCREB1–1 or/and H89, Notes: A, the histogram of the mRNA expressions of cAMP, PKA and CREB1 in hippocampal tissues of mice in each group; B, The histogram of the expressions of cAMP, PKA and CREB1 in hippocampal tissues of mice in each group; C, Gray value of cAMP, PKA and CREB1 protein bands; *, $p < 0.05$, compared with the normal group; #, $p < 0.05$, compared with the VD group; cAMP, cyclic adenosine monophosphate; PKA, protein kinase A; CREB1, cyclic adenosine monophosphate responsive element-binding protein 1; VD, vascular dementia

provide better outcomes for patients with VD. Previous literature has, stated that CREB was involved in cognitive function (Juhasz et al., 2011). Thus the present study, set out to investigate the CREB gene, which has the potential to provide new avenues in the treatment of VD. Our study mainly demonstrated that CREB1 gene silencing aggravated cognitive dysfunction through the suppression of the PKA-CREB signaling pathway in mice with VD.

A decreased expression of CREB1, declined cognitive function, decreased hippocampal cells, and higher apoptosis was detected among the mice with VD during our study. Previous studies have revealed that patients with cognitive dysfunction resulting from AD had significantly decreased expression of CREB1, which was observed in the findings of the current study (Nagakura et al., 2013). On the basis of the results of a previously conducted study, aged-impaired rats exhibited lower expressions CREB1 when compared with normal rats (Brightwell et al., 2004). In addition, a study recently conducted showed that the degeneration of hippocampal neurons could occur as a consequence of certain types of dementias, such as AD and VD (Zarow et al., 2005), with these dementias found to share an association with the apoptosis of neuronal cells (Guo et al., 2015).

Additionally, VD mice transfected with shCREB1−1 or H89 or both displayed elevated levels of cell apoptosis and decreased cell proliferation in mouse hippocampal CA1 region, as well as declined cognitive function. One study demonstrated that the degeneration of hippocampal neurons was observed among mice with disrupted CREB1 (Li et al., 2012), while a prior study highlighted the central role played by CREB1 in the development of neuronal cells in hippocampal CA1 region (Hebels et al., 2009). Evidence has been provided suggesting that increased CREB1 expression was accompanied by neuronal sprouting and increasing neurogenesis (Burcescu et al., 2005). Elisabetta Ciani et al. observed that downregulation of CREB was associated with the death of cerebellar granule neurons due to the effects of nitric oxide (Ciani et al., 2002). Importantly, studies have indicated that PKA not only activates pro-survival signals, but also acts to suppress pro-apoptotic signals induced by Rap1 (Saavedra et al., 2002). The PKA-CREB signaling pathway has also been previously emphasized upon due to its critical role in the process of memory acquisition (Vitolo et al., 2002). Interestingly, a previous study revealed that the PKA-CREB signaling pathway inhibitor could act to eliminate the beneficial effects of electroacupuncture on learning and memory (Zheng et al., 2016) , which was largely consistent with the results observed in the present study, in which silencing CREB1 or inhibiting the PKA-CREB signaling pathway was suggested to promote apoptosis, aggravate cognitive dysfunction and suppress hippocampal cell proliferation.

Furthermore, hippocampal cells transfected with shCREB1−1 or H89 or shCREB1−1 + H89 had descended expression levels of cAMP, PKA, CREB1 and p-CREB1, and increased expression of Cleaved Caspase-3. It has been suggested that CREB1 is the coding gene for CREB (Serretti et al., 2011). Evidence demonstrated that CREB, which plays a significant part in nerve system (Lonze & Ginty, 2002), can be activated through the phosphorylation of serine 133 by means of activating PKA (Gao et al., 2009). Signal transduction pathways converging on CREB and the subsequent modulation of the cAMP responsive genes transcription are widely accepted to be involved in therapeutic effect (Hellmann et al., 2012). Generally, cAMP is understood to be capable of activating PKA by binding the regulatory sub-units of PKA (Etique et al., 2007). A previous study indicated that cAMP activation could be influenced by CREB and PKA (Delghandi et al., 2005). Qian-Qian Li et al. demonstrated that rats with cognitive impairment exhibited lower expression of cAMP, PKA and CREB when compared with the normal group and the acupuncture group during their study (Li et al., 2015), which was in parallels with the findings of the our study. p-CREB1 is an important transcription factor which has been reported to be implicated in fibrogenesis (Wang et al., 2016b), while lower protein levels of p-CREB in the hippocampus have been linked with memory deficit (Min et al., 2012). Cleaved caspase-3 is well known as an executioner protease of apoptosis following brain ischemia, its expression has been predominantly correlated with cellular responses to stroke such as reactive astrogliosis and the infiltration of macrophages (Wagner et al., 2011). A recent study indicated that activated caspase-3 was also found in the plaques and blood vessels in VD brains (Day et al., 2015).

## Conclusion

Taken together, the present study provides encouraging evidence, illustrating that silencing of the CREB1 gene could act to exacerbate VD by inhibiting the activation of the PKA-CREB signaling pathway. Our study places emphasis on CREB1 gene and the PKA-CREB signaling pathway as a promising strategy for improved outcomes of patients with VD. Therefore, the identification of CREB1 and PKA-CREB signaling pathway may aid in facilitating the existing understanding of the mechanisms of VD, with potential of serving as a prognostic marker for the treatment of VD in the future. However, due to the limitations of sample size and fund, more detailed studies are needed to fully understand the specific mechanisms and to verify our conclusion and to explore the mechanism by which CREB1 mitigates VD in the future.

## Acknowledgements

We acknowledge and appreciate our colleagues for their valuable efforts and comments on this paper.


## Funding

This work was supported by the Priority Academic Program Development of Jiangsu Higher Education Institutions (PAPD); the 2016 "333 Project" Award of Jiangsu Province, the 2013 "Qinglan Project" of the Young and Middle-aged Academic Leader of Jiangsu College and University, the National Natural Science Foundation of China (grant number 81570531, 81571055, 81400902, 81271225, 81171012, 81672731 and 30950031), the Major Fundamental Research Program of the Natural Science Foundation of the Jiangsu Higher Education Institutions of China (13KJA180001), and grants from the Cultivate National Science Fund for Distinguished Young Scholars of Jiangsu Normal University.


## Authors' contributions

XRH, SW, ZFZ, CHS and DMW designed the study. XW, SHF, LW, MQL, JL and YLZ collated the data, designed and developed the database, carried out data analyses and produced the initial draft of the manuscript. YJW, MS, QS and BH contributed to drafting the manuscript. All authors contributed to the revision and approved the final submitted manuscript.


## Competing interests

The authors declare that they have no competing interests.


## Author details

[1]Key Laboratory for Biotechnology on Medicinal Plants of Jiangsu Province, School of Life Science, Jiangsu Normal University, No. 101, Shanghai Road, Tongshan District, Xuzhou 221116, Jiangsu Province, People's Republic of China. [2]College of Health Sciences, Jiangsu Normal University, No. 101, Shanghai Road, Tongshan District, Xuzhou 221116, Jiangsu Province, People's Republic of China.


## References

Battistin L, Cagnin A. Vascular cognitive disorder. A biological and clinical overview. Neurochem Res. 2010;35:1933–8.

Brightwell JJ, Gallagher M, Colombo PJ. Hippocampal CREB1 but not CREB2 is decreased in aged rats with spatial memory impairments. Neurobiol Learn Mem. 2004;81:19–26.

Bruandet A, et al. Alzheimer disease with cerebrovascular disease and vascular dementia: clinical features and course compared with Alzheimer disease. J Neurol Neurosurg Psychiatry. 2009;80:133–9.

Burcescu I, et al. Association study of CREB1 and childhood-onset mood disorders. Am J Med Genet B Neuropsychiatr Genet. 2005;137B:45–50.

Celik Y, et al. Is levetiracetam neuroprotective in neonatal rats with hypoxic ischemic brain injury? Bratisl Lek Listy. 2016;117:730–3.

Chen Y, et al. Alzheimer's beta-secretase (BACE1) regulates the cAMP/PKA/CREB pathway independently of beta-amyloid. J Neurosci. 2012;32:11390–5.

Cheng F, et al. Screening of the human Kinome identifies MSK1/2-CREB1 as an essential pathway mediating Kaposi's sarcoma-associated herpesvirus lytic replication during primary infection. J Virol. 2015;89:9262–80.

Chi CL, et al. Research on the role of GLP-2 in the central nervous system EPK signal transduction pathway of mice with vascular dementia. Eur Rev Med Pharmacol Sci. 2017;21:131–7.

Ciani E, et al. Nitric oxide protects neuroblastoma cells from apoptosis induced by serum deprivation through cAMP-response element-binding protein (CREB) activation. J Biol Chem. 2002;277:49896–902.

Day RJ, Mason MJ, Thomas C, Poon WW, Rohn TT. Caspase-cleaved tau co-localizes with early tangle markers in the human vascular dementia brain. PLoS One. 2015;10:e0132637.

De Lucia N, Grossi D, Trojano L. The genesis of graphic perseverations in Alzheimer's disease and vascular dementia. Clin Neuropsychol. 2015;29:924–37.

Delghandi MP, Johannessen M, Moens U. The cAMP signalling pathway activates CREB through PKA, p38 and MSK1 in NIH 3T3 cells. Cell Signal. 2005;17:1343–51.

Du H, et al. Cyclophilin D deficiency rescues Abeta-impaired PKA/CREB signaling and alleviates synaptic degeneration. Biochim Biophys Acta. 2014;1842:2517–27.

Etique N, et al. Ethanol-induced ligand-independent activation of ERalpha mediated by cyclic AMP/PKA signaling pathway: an in vitro study on MCF-7 breast cancer cells. Int J Oncol. 2007;31:1509–18.

Gao J, et al. Inactivation of CREB mediated gene transcription by HDAC8 bound protein phosphatase. Biochem Biophys Res Commun. 2009;379:1–5.

Gong X, et al. Down-regulation of IGF-1/IGF-1R in hippocampus of rats with vascular dementia. Neurosci Lett. 2012;513:20–4.

Guo HD, et al. Electroacupuncture suppressed neuronal apoptosis and improved cognitive impairment in the AD model rats possibly via downregulation of notch signaling pathway. Evid Based Complement Alternat Med. 2015;2015:393569.

Hang LH, et al. Involvement of spinal PKA/CREB signaling pathway in the development of bone cancer pain. Pharmacol Rep. 2013;65:710–6.

Hebels DG, et al. Molecular signatures of N-nitroso compounds in Caco-2 cells: implications for colon carcinogenesis. Toxicol Sci. 2009;108:290–300.

Hellmann J, et al. Repetitive magnetic stimulation of human-derived neuron-like cells activates cAMP-CREB pathway. Eur Arch Psychiatry Clin Neurosci. 2012; 262:87–91.

Higuchi T, et al. Flagellar filament structural protein induces Sjogren's syndrome-like sialadenitis in mice. Oral Dis. 2017;23:636–43.

Jarome TJ, et al. CaMKII, but not protein kinase a, regulates Rpt6 phosphorylation and proteasome activity during the formation of long-term memories. Front Behav Neurosci. 2013;7:115.

Juhasz G, et al. The CREB1-BDNF-NTRK2 pathway in depression: multiple gene-cognition-environment interactions. Biol Psychiatry. 2011;69:762–71.

Kleppe R, et al. The cAMP-dependent protein kinase pathway as therapeutic target: possibilities and pitfalls. Curr Top Med Chem. 2011;11:1393–405.

Lee AY. Vascular dementia. Chonnam Med J. 2011;47:66–71.

Li QQ, et al. Hippocampal cAMP/PKA/CREB is required for neuroprotective effect of acupuncture. Physiol Behav. 2015;139:482–90.

Li WZ, et al. Protective effect of bilobalide on learning and memory impairment in rats with vascular dementia. Mol Med Rep. 2013;8:935–41.

Li Y, et al. Integrated copy number and gene expression analysis detects a CREB1 association with Alzheimer's disease. Transl Psychiatry. 2012;2:e192.

Lonze BE, Ginty DD. Function and regulation of CREB family transcription factors in the nervous system. Neuron. 2002;35:605–23.

McGirr A, et al. Specific inhibition of phosphodiesterase-4B results in Anxiolysis and facilitates memory acquisition. Neuropsychopharmacology. 2016;41: 1080–92.

Min D, et al. Donepezil attenuates hippocampal neuronal damage and cognitive deficits after global cerebral ischemia in gerbils. Neurosci Lett. 2012;510:29–33.

Murphy GM Jr, et al. BDNF and CREB1 genetic variants interact to affect antidepressant treatment outcomes in geriatric depression. Pharmacogenet Genomics. 2013;23:301–13.

Nagakura A, et al. Characterization of cognitive deficits in a transgenic mouse model of Alzheimer's disease and effects of donepezil and memantine. Eur J Pharmacol. 2013;703:53–61.

Ramakrishnan V, Pace BS. Regulation of gamma-globin gene expression involves signaling through the p38 MAPK/CREB1 pathway. Blood Cells Mol Dis. 2011; 47:12–22.

Saavedra AP, et al. Role of cAMP, PKA and Rap1A in thyroid follicular cell survival. Oncogene. 2002;21:778–88.

Sadamoto H, et al. Learning-dependent gene expression of CREB1 isoforms in the molluscan brain. Front Behav Neurosci. 2010;4:25.

Serretti A, et al. A preliminary investigation of the influence of CREB1 gene on treatment resistance in major depression. J Affect Disord. 2011;128:56–63.

Vitolo OV, et al. Amyloid beta -peptide inhibition of the PKA/CREB pathway and long-term potentiation: reversibility by drugs that enhance cAMP signaling. Proc Natl Acad Sci U S A. 2002;99:13217–21.

Wagner DC, Riegelsberger UM, Michalk S, Hartig W, Kranz A, Boltze J. Cleaved caspase-3 expression after experimental stroke exhibits different phenotypes and is predominantly non-apoptotic. Brain Res. 2011;1381:237–42.

Wang H. Establishment of an animal model of vascular dementia. Exp Ther Med. 2014;8:1599–603.

Wang K, et al. Comparative study of voxel-based epileptic foci localization accuracy between statistical parametric mapping and three-dimensional stereotactic surface projection. Front Neurol. 2016a;7:164.

Wang P, Deng L, Zhuang C, Cheng C, Xu K. P-creb-1 promotes hepatic fibrosis through the transactivation of transforming growth factor-beta1 expression in rats. Int J Mol Med. 2016b;38:521–8.

You YN, et al. Assessing the quality of reports about randomized controlled trials of scalp acupuncture treatment for vascular dementia. Trials. 2017;18:205.

Zarow C, et al. Correlates of hippocampal neuron number in Alzheimer's disease and ischemic vascular dementia. Ann Neurol. 2005;57:896–903.

Zheng CX, et al. Electroacupuncture ameliorates learning and memory and improves synaptic plasticity via activation of the PKA/CREB signaling pathway in cerebral Hypoperfusion. Evid Based Complement Alternat Med. 2016;2016:7893710.

# Uncoupling of glycolysis from glucose oxidation accompanies the development of heart failure with preserved ejection fraction

Natasha Fillmore, Jody L. Levasseur, Arata Fukushima, Cory S. Wagg, Wei Wang, Jason R. B. Dyck and Gary D. Lopaschuk[*]

## Abstract

**Background:** Alterations in cardiac energy metabolism contribute to the development and severity of heart failure (HF). In severe HF, overall mitochondrial oxidative metabolism is significantly decreased resulting in a reduced energy reserve. However, despite the high prevalence of HF with preserved ejection fraction (HFpEF) in our society, it is not clear what changes in cardiac energy metabolism occur in HFpEF, and whether alterations in energy metabolism contribute to the development of contractile dysfunction.

**Methods:** We directly assessed overall energy metabolism during the development of HFpEF in Dahl salt-sensitive rats fed a high salt diet (HSD) for 3, 6 and 9 weeks.

**Results:** Over the course of 9 weeks, the HSD caused a progressive decrease in diastolic function (assessed by echocardiography assessment of E'/A'). This was accompanied by a progressive increase in cardiac glycolysis rates (assessed in isolated working hearts obtained at 3, 6, and 9 weeks of HSD). In contrast, the subsequent oxidation of pyruvate from glycolysis (glucose oxidation) was not altered, resulting in an uncoupling of glucose metabolism and a significant increase in proton production. Increased glucose transporter (GLUT)1 expression accompanied this elevation in glycolysis. Decreases in cardiac fatty acid oxidation and overall adenosine triphosphate (ATP) production rates were not observed in early HF, but both significantly decreased as HF progressed to HF with reduced EF (i.e. 9 weeks of HSD).

**Conclusions:** Overall, we show that increased glycolysis is the earliest energy metabolic change that occurs during HFpEF development. The resultant increased proton production from uncoupling of glycolysis and glucose oxidation may contribute to the development of HFpEF.

**Keywords:** Mitochondria, Fatty acid oxidation, Energy metabolism, Diastolic dysfunction, Cardiac hypertrophy

## Background

An abundance of evidence indicates that alterations in energy metabolism contribute to the severity of heart failure (Kato et al. 2010; Degens et al. 2006; Lei et al. 2004; Conway et al. 1991; Nascimben et al. 1995; Tian et al. 1996; Beer et al. 2002; Neubauer et al. 1999; Mori et al. 2013). This includes a decrease in overall cardiac mitochondrial oxidative metabolism as the severity of

heart failure increases (Conway et al. 1991; Nascimben et al. 1995; Tian et al. 1996; Beer et al. 2002; Neubauer et al. 1999; Lopaschuk et al. 2010). Improving cardiac efficiency, such as by either stimulating glucose oxidation or inhibiting fatty acid oxidation, can help to lessen the impact of this decrease in mitochondrial oxidative capacity, and can improve cardiac function in the failing heart (Kato et al. 2010; Masoud et al. 2014; Yamashita et al. 2009; Ussher et al. 2012; Stanley et al. 2005; Lopaschuk et al. 2003; Dyck et al. 2006; Dyck et al. 2004). However, there is not a consensus as to the importance of the specific energy metabolic changes to

---

[*] Correspondence: glopasch@ualberta.ca
Cardiovascular Research Centre, Mazankowski Alberta Heart Institute
University of Alberta, Edmonton, Canada

the development of heart failure. While it is generally believed that there is an increase in overall glucose metabolism in the failing heart, this may actually be specific to an increase in glucose uptake and glycolysis (Lei et al. 2004; Lopaschuk et al. 2010; Masoud et al. 2014). Whether mitochondrial oxidation of glucose, which supplies the majority of adenosine triphosphate (ATP) derived from glucose, is also increased in heart failure is debatable. In fact, myocardial glucose oxidation rates are decreased in mouse hearts subjected to cardiac hypertrophy and heart failure (Mori et al. 2013; Zhabyeyev et al. 2013; Zhang et al. 2013), and in pig hearts subjected to rapid-pacing induced heart failure (Schroeder et al. 2013).

The specific changes in glycolysis rates and glucose oxidation rates in heart failure are important because uncoupling of glycolysis and glucose oxidation has been shown to impair cardiac function. A selective increase in glycolysis relative to glucose oxidation uncouples glycolysis from glucose oxidation, which can result in the production of lactate and protons (Liu et al. 1996; Liu et al. 2002; Folmes et al. 2006). This rise in protons and drop in pH can reduce contractility of the adult heart by impairing troponin I sensitivity to calcium and inhibiting the slow calcium current (Chesnais et al. 1975; Vogel and Sperelakis 1977; Steenbergen et al. 1977; Schiaffino et al. 1993; Morimoto and Goto 2000). In addition, ATP is utilized to both remove these protons and maintain sodium and calcium homeostasis which decreases cardiac efficiency and contributes to the decrease in cardiac function (Lopaschuk et al. 2010).

Uncoupling of glycolysis and glucose oxidation may also contribute to the development of heart failure by increasing cardiac hypertrophy. Uncoupling of glycolysis and glucose oxidation is present in proliferative cells and is believed to be important in promoting cell growth. Otto Warburg first reported that cancer cells, which are characterized by high rates of proliferation, have high glycolysis rates even under aerobic conditions, a phenomenon called the "Warburg" effect (Vander Heiden et al. 2009; Warburg 1956). In addition, glycolysis is elevated in another form of cell growth, cardiac hypertrophy, which can lead to heart failure (Piao et al. 2010; Piao et al. 2013; Allard et al. 1994; Leong et al. 2002). A similar "Warburg" phenomena may also exist in the failing heart, which is frequently characterized by a relative rise in glycolysis and an overall decrease in mitochondrial oxidative metabolism (Lei et al. 2004; Conway et al. 1991; Nascimben et al. 1995; Tian et al. 1996; Beer et al. 2002; Neubauer et al. 1999; Lopaschuk et al. 2010; Zhang et al. 2013). This suggests that the coupling of glycolysis and glucose oxidation may be a promising target for the treatment of diseases characterized by abnormal cell growth. In fact, stimulation of glucose oxidation (by inhibition of pyruvate dehydrogenase kinase, PDK) has been

reported to be beneficial in multiple scenarios, including treatment of cancer, T-cells, cardiac hypertrophy, and heart failure (Kato et al. 2010; Liu et al. 1996; Bonnet et al. 2007; Gerriets et al. 2015).

While there is a substantial amount of evidence to indicate that heart failure with reduced ejection fraction (HFrEF) is commonly characterized by an overall decrease in oxidative metabolism and relative increase in glycolysis (which can result in increased uncoupling of glycolysis and glucose oxidation), there is a scarcity of research on metabolism in another common form of heart failure, heart failure with preserved ejection fraction (HFpEF). In this study we therefore examined mitochondrial oxidative metabolism and glycolysis during the development of HFpEF. This was examined using the Dahl salt-sensitive rat, a well characterized model of HFpEF (Horgan et al. 2014; Rapp and Dene 1985; Klotz et al. 2006), and cardiac energy metabolism was assessed after 3 weeks, 6 weeks, or 9 weeks on a high salt diet (HSD).

## Methods
### Animal protocol
Eight week old male Dahl salt-sensitive rats were either fed a standard low salt diet containing 0.3% NaCl (Research Diets, D10012G) or a high salt diet (HSD) (Research Diets, D11021901) containing 8% NaCl to induce HFpEF. Control rats were kept on the low salt diet while treatment groups were fed the HSD for 3, 6, or 9 weeks. Food and water were provided ad libitum. Rats were kept on a 12 h light:12 h dark cycle. All procedures on animals were approved by the University of Alberta Health Sciences Animal Welfare Committee and conformed to the Canadian Council on Animal Care guidelines (Canadian Council on Animal Care 2017).

### Echocardiography
In vivo cardiac function was assessed in rats anesthetized with 1–1.5% isoflurane using a Vevo 770 high resolution echocardiography imaging system (VisualSonics, Toronto) with a 30-MHz transducer (Zhong et al. 2010). Doppler and tissue doppler imaging were used to assess diastolic function: E'/A', E', E/A, E'/E, and isovolumetric relaxation time (IVRT). M-mode images were used to measure % Ejection fraction (%EF) and % Fractional shortening (%FS), to make left ventricle (LV) wall measurements [Interventricular septum end diastole (IVSd), LV internal diameter end diastole (LVIDd), LV posterior wall thickness end diastole (LVPWd), Interventricular septum end systole (IVSs), LV internal diameter end systole (LVIDs), LV posterior wall thickness end systole (LVPWs)], and to measure LV diameter and volume [left ventricular end diastolic diameter, left ventricular end systolic diameter, LV volume end diastole (LV Vol;d), LV volume end systole (LV Vol;s), and corrected LV mass].

## Isolated working heart perfusions

Rats were anesthetized with sodium pentobarbital (1 g/kg BW). Hearts were quickly excised from fully anesthetized rats, and were perfused in the working mode at a 11.5 mmHg left atrial preload and 80 mmHg aortic afterload, as previously described (Liu et al. 1996; Liu et al. 2002). Isolated working hearts were perfused with modified Krebs-Henseleit solution (118.5 mM NaCl, 25 mM NaHCO$_3$, 4.7 mM KCl, 1.2 mM MgSO$_4$, 1.2 mM KH$_2$PO$_4$, 2.5 mM CaCl$_2$) supplemented with 5 mM glucose, 0.5 mM lactate, and 0.8 mM palmitate bound to 3% fatty acid-free bovine serum albumin (BSA). To measure palmitate oxidation, glucose oxidation, glycolysis, and lactate oxidation [9,10-$^3$H] palmitate, [U-$^{14}$C] glucose, [5-$^3$H] glucose, or [U-$^{14}$C] lactate, respectively, were added to the Krebs-Henseleit solution. At 30 min of the 60 min perfusion, 100 μU/mL insulin was added to the Krebs-Henseleit solution. Glucose and lactate oxidation rates were assessed by measuring $^{14}$CO$_2$ production. Palmitate oxidation and glycolysis rates were assessed by measuring $^3$H$_2$O production. Proton production was determined by subtracting the glucose oxidation rate from the glycolysis rate and multiplying the result by 2 (Liu et al. 2002). Mechanical function was measured using a Powerlab acquisition system and a Transonic flow meter and probes were placed in the preload and afterload lines to measure cardiac output and aortic flow. Cardiac work (joules/min/g dry weight) was calculated by subtracting preload pressure from peak systolic pressure which was then multiplied by cardiac output and normalized against the heart dry weight. At the end of the aerobic perfusion protocol, hearts were immediately frozen in liquid N$_2$ and stored at − 80 °C (Barr and Lopaschuk 1997; Ussher et al. 2009).

## Western blot analysis

Standard western blot procedures were followed. Briefly, frozen ventricular tissue was homogenized for 30 s in buffer containing 50 mM Tris HCl, 1 mM EDTA, 10% glycerol, 0.02% Brij-35, 1 mM dithiothreitol (DTT), and protease and phosphatase inhibitors (Sigma). The homogenate was left on ice for 10 min and then centrifuged at 10,000 x g for 20 min. Protein concentration of supernatant was determined using a Bradford protein assay. SDS-polyacrylamide gel electrophoresis was used and protein was transferred onto a 0.45 μm nitrocellulose membrane. Membranes were blocked with 5% fat free milk for 1 h and probed with primary antibodies in 5% BSA overnight. Primary antibodies included pyruvate dehydrogenase (PDH; Cell Signaling 2784), phosphoSer293 PDH (Calbiochem AP1062), phosphoThr389 p70S6K (Cell Signaling 9206), p70S6K (Cell Signaling 9202), phosphoglycerate mutase 1 (PGAM1) (Cell Signaling 7534), hydroxyacyl coenzyme A dehydrogenase (HADH) (Abcam

ab93172), GLUT1 (Santa Cruz 1605), GLUT4 (Santa Cruz 1606), lactate dehydrogenase A (LDHA) (Santa Cruz 27,230), mitochondrial pyruvate carrier 1 (MPC1) (Cell Signaling 14,462), MPC2 (Cell Signaling 46,141), cytochrome c (Santa Cruz 8385) and hypoxia inducible factor (HIF)1α (Novus Biologicals 100–105)). Membranes were then washed 4 × 5 min in Tris-buffered saline tween, probed with secondary antibody, goat antirabbit (Santa Cruz 2054), goat antimouse (Santa Cruz 2055), or donkey antigoat (Jackson Immunoresearch 705,035,003), and again washed 4 × 5 min in Tris-buffered saline tween. Protein bands were then visualized with enhanced chemiluminescence (Perkin Elmer). Quantification was performed using Image J.

## Statistical analysis

Values are presented as mean ±SEM. One Way Analysis of Variance (ANOVA) with Bonferroni posthoc test was performed or Kruskal-Wallis test with Dunn's Multiple Comparison test was performed as appropriate using Prism software to determine statistical significance. Differences are considered significant if $p<0.05$. n size is indicated in the figure legends.

## Results

### Feeding a high salt diet (HSD) to Dahl salt-sensitive rats results in the progressive development of hypertrophy and diastolic dysfunction

When Dahl salt-sensitive rats were fed a HSD, a progressive decrease in diastolic function was observed over a 9 week period. In vivo echocardiography of the hearts showed a significant decrease in E'/A' (a measure of diastolic dysfunction) by 6 weeks following initiation of the HSD (Fig. 1a). In contrast, systolic function was largely preserved, with %EF decreasing slightly by 9 weeks (Fig. 1b), and %FS remaining unchanged (Table 1). This suggests that the rats developed HFpEF prior to developing heart failure with reduced ejection fraction (HFrEF). In isolated working hearts obtained from rats at each time period studied a progressive decrease in cardiac work was observed over the 9 week period (Fig. 1c), primarily due to a decrease in cardiac output (Table 2). This time frame for heart failure development agrees with other studies examining the development of heart failure in DSS rats fed a HSD (Rapp and Dene 1985; Klotz et al. 2006). The progressive development of diastolic dysfunction in the Dahl salt-sensitive rats following administration of the HSD was accompanied by an increase in LV mass (Fig. 1d), as well as an increase in IVSd and LVPWd (Fig. 1e, Table 1). At the same time the phosphorylation of p70S6k increased suggesting a stimulation of the mTOR pathway (which promotes cardiac hypertrophy) (Fig. 1f).

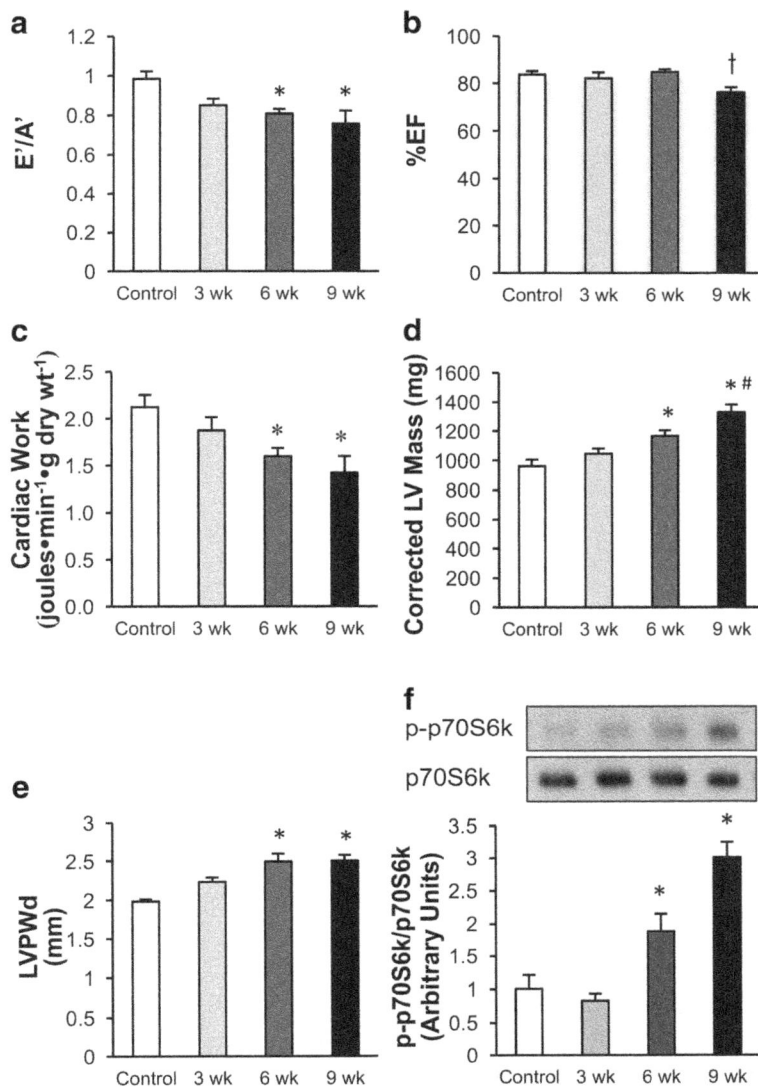

**Fig. 1** Time dependent effects of a high salt diet (HSD) on Dahl salt-sensitive rat cardiac function and hypertrophy. **a** Diastolic dysfunction was measured by E'/A'. **b** %EF was measured by echocardiography. **c** Cardiac work was measured during the isolated working heart perfusions. **d-e** Cardiac hypertrophy was measured by corrected LV mass and LVPWd using echocardiography. **f** Cardiac p-p70S6K/p70S6K protein expression was assessed in hearts obtained at each of the time periods studied. Measurements were made in Dahl salt-sensitive rats fed a low salt diet, 0.3% NaCl (Control) or a HSD, 8% NaCl, for 3, 6, or 9 weeks. n = 5–8 * $p < 0.05$ compared to Control. # $p < 0.05$ compared to 3 weeks. t $p < 0.05$ compared to 6 weeks. Values shown as mean ± SEM

## The development of diastolic dysfunction is accompanied by a decrease in cardiac mitochondrial oxidative metabolism in dahl salt-sensitive rats

Rates of overall energy metabolism were measured in isolated working hearts obtained at 3 weeks, 6 weeks, and 9 weeks of the HSD. A progressive decrease in fatty acid oxidation rates was observed following the HSD (Fig. 2a), although a significant decrease in fatty acid oxidation rates did not occur until 9 weeks of the HSD. In the presence of insulin, a similar time-dependent decrease in fatty acid oxidation was also observed (Table 3). In contrast, there was no change in glucose oxidation rates (Fig. 2b) or lactate oxidation rates (Fig. 2c) during the development of diastolic dysfunction, regardless of whether insulin was present (Table 3) or absent. The primary source of overall cardiac ATP production in all hearts originated from fatty acid oxidation (Fig. 2d). As a result, a decrease in overall cardiac ATP production rates were observed by 9 weeks of the HSD, which was primarily due to the observed decrease in fatty acid oxidation rates (Fig. 2d).

**Table 1** Effect of a high salt diet (HSD) on in vivo cardiac function in Dahl salt-sensitive rats

|  | Control | 3 weeks | 6 weeks | 9 weeks |
|---|---|---|---|---|
| EF (%) | 83.79 ±1.44 | 82.21 ±2.50 | 84.91 ±1.14 | 76.21 ±2.19$^{T}$ |
| FS (%) | 54.60 ±1.69 | 53.12 ±2.57 | 54.45 ±2.39 | 47.64 ±2.34 |
| LV Mass Corrected | 962.88 ±43.45 | 1045.85 ±36.11 | 1167.85 ±38.96$^{*}$ | 1328.94 ±52.37$^{*\#}$ |
| IVSd (mm) | 1.97 ±0.05 | 2.23 ±0.06$^{*}$ | 2.40 ±0.07$^{*}$ | 2.50 ±0.07$^{*\#}$ |
| LVIDd (mm) | 7.91 ±0.12 | 7.32 ±0.14$^{*}$ | 7.45 ±0.09 | 7.52 ±0.20 |
| LVPWd (mm) | 1.98 ±0.03 | 2.23 ±0.06 | 2.49 ±0.10$^{*}$ | 2.50 ±0.08$^{*}$ |
| IVSs (mm) | 3.40 ±0.05 | 3.67 ±0.10 | 3.68 ±0.09 | 3.68 ±0.15 |
| LVIDs (mm) | 3.87 ±0.18 | 3.46 ±0.23 | 3.40 ±0.09 | 4.25 ±0.08 |
| LVPWs (mm) | 3.45 ±0.12 | 3.68 ±0.11 | 3.77 ±0.08 | 3.65 ±0.13 |
| LV Vol;d | 335.75 ±10.95 | 283.11 ±12.35$^{*}$ | 294.62 ±7.78 | 301.74 ±17.16 |
| LV Vol;s | 51.99 ±6.28 | 45.76 ±6.96 | 47.51 ±3.37 | 81.30 ±3.62$^{*\#T}$ |
| E/E' | 19.04 ±2.18 | 20.49 ±1.95 | 18.82 ±1.22 | 18.29 ±1.51 |
| E/A | 1.60 ±0.11 | 1.64 ±0.07 | 1.33 ±0.15 | 1.40 ±0.20 |
| E'/A' | 0.98 ±0.04 | 0.85 ±0.03 | 0.81 ±0.02$^{*}$ | 0.76 ±0.07$^{*}$ |
| Tei Index | 0.65 ±0.03 | 0.72 ±0.04 | 0.78 ±0.05 | 0.76 ±0.05 |
| E' | 54.23 ±6.85 | 54.68 ±4.61 | 46.79 ±2.14 | 38.26 ±3.49 |
| IVRT (ms) | 24.32 ±0.60 | 22.68 ±0.68 | 27.97 ±1.76 | 28.13 ±1.63 |
| IVCT (ms) | 15.69 ±0.90 | 16.88 ±1.29 | 15.81 ±1.48 | 17.47 ±1.43 |
| HR (bpm) | 365.25 ±6.61 | 375.88 ±7.71 | 367.63 ±10.98 | 349.75 ±16.68 |
| L Kidney/TL (g/cm) | 0.31 ±0.01 | 0.34 ±0.01 | 0.34 ±0.01 | 0.38 ±0.03$^{*}$ |

In vivo cardiac function was measured via echocardiography in Dahl salt-sensitive rats fed a low salt diet, 0.3% NaCl (Control), or a high salt diet, 8% NaCl, for 3, 6, or 9 weeks. $n = 5–8$ * $p < 0.05$ compared to Control. * $p < 0.05$ compared to Control. $^{\#}$ $p < 0.05$ compared to 3 weeks. $^{T}$ $p < 0.05$ compared to 6 weeks. $n = 6–9$ Values shown as mean ±SEM % Ejection fraction (%EF); % Fractional shortening (%FS); left ventricle (LV); Interventricular septum end diastole (IVSd); LV internal diameter end diastole (LVIDd); LV posterior wall thickness end diastole (LVPWd); Interventricular septum end systole (IVSs); LV internal diameter end systole (LVIDs); LV posterior wall thickness end systole (LVPWs); LV volume end diastole (LV Vol;d); LV volume end systole (LV Vol;s); Isovolumetic relaxation time (IVRT); Isovolumetic contraction time (IVCT); Tibia length (TL); Heart rate (HR)

## Decreased glycolysis is an early energy metabolic change in hearts from Dahl salt-sensitive rats fed a HSD

The earliest energy metabolic change that occurred in Dahl-sensitive rats fed a HSD was an increase in glycolysis, which had already increased over 300% by 3 weeks of the HSD (Fig. 2e). This increase was also observed when insulin was present in the perfusate (Table 3), and prior to the onset of either HFpEF or HFrEF (Fig. 1). Since the increase in glycolysis during the development of diastolic dysfunction was not accompanied by an increase in glucose oxidation (Fig. 2b), an uncoupling of glycolysis from glucose oxidation occurred, resulting in a significant increase in proton production, even by 3 weeks of the HSD (Fig. 2f). This increased uncoupling of glycolysis and glucose oxidation and rise in proton production persisted in hearts perfused in the presence of insulin (Table 3). Since the uncoupling of glycolysis and glucose oxidation and elevation in proton

**Table 2** Effect of a high salt diet (HSD) on cardiac function ex vivo in Dahl salt-sensitive rats

|  | Control | 3 weeks | 6 weeks | 9 weeks |
|---|---|---|---|---|
| Heart rate (beats•min$^{-1}$) | 277.9 ±7.3 | 290.8 ±8.6 | 278.7 ±6.1 | 266.9 ±22.9 |
| Peak Systolic Pressure (mmHg) | 109.9 ±1.0 | 107.8 ±2.6 | 110.8 ±1.7 | 107.5 ±6.7 |
| Developed Pressure (mmHg) | 41.9 ±2.8 | 38.5 ±3.8 | 42.6 ±2.2 | 43.1 ±7.0 |
| Cardiac Output (ml•min$^{-1}$) | 50.4 ±2.2 | 45.7 ±1.9 | 41.6 ±2.2 | 38.5 ±3.1$^{*}$ |
| Coronary Flow (ml•min$^{-1}$) | 26.5 ±2.8 | 23.9 ±0.5 | 22.3 ±0.7 | 20.8 ±1.5 |
| Cardiac Work (joules•min$^{-1}$•g dry weight$^{-1}$) | 2.1 ±0.1 | 1.9 ±0.1 | 1.6 ±0.1$^{*}$ | 1.4 ±0.2$^{*}$ |

Cardiac function was measured in isolated working hearts from Dahl salt-sensitive rats fed a low salt diet, 0.3% NaCl (Control), or a high salt diet, 8% NaCl, for 3, 6, or 9 weeks. $n = 3–5$ * $p < 0.05$ compared to Control. Values shown as mean ±SEM

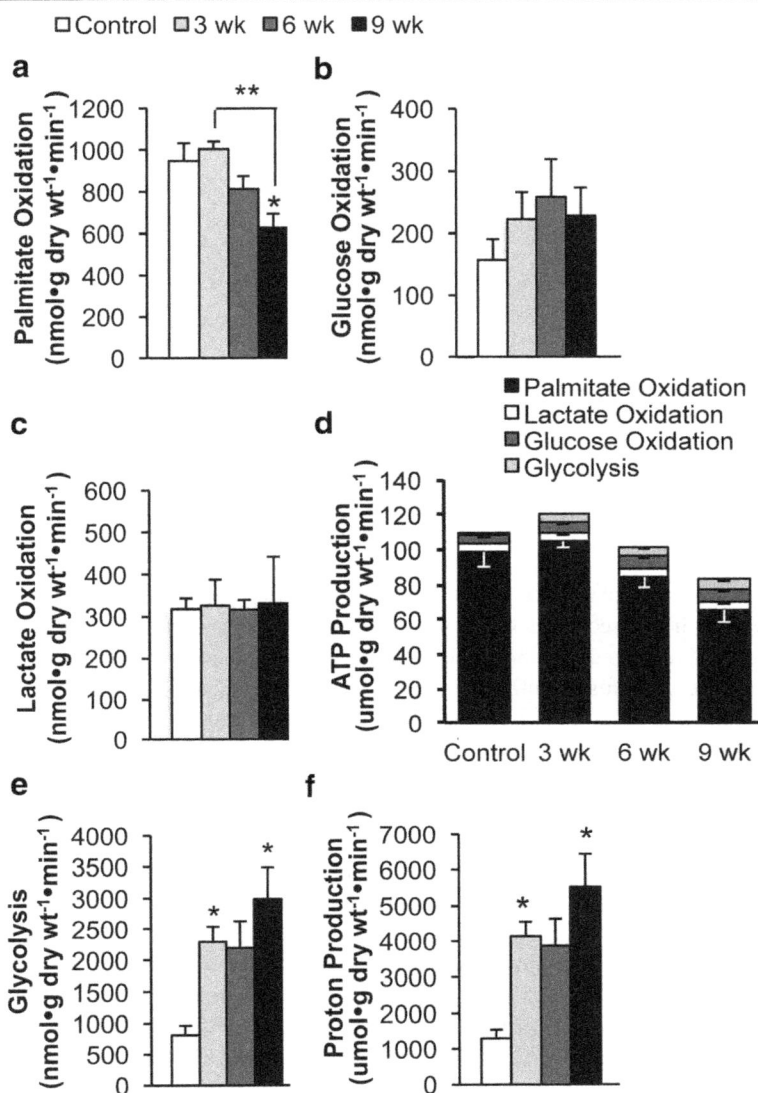

**Fig. 2** Time dependent effects of a high salt diet (HSD) on palmitate oxidation, glucose oxidation, glycolysis, and lactate oxidation in Dahl salt-sensitive rat hearts. **a** Palmitate oxidation, (**b**) Glucose oxidation, (**c**) Lactate oxidation, (**d**) ATP production, (**e**) Glycolysis, and (**f**) Proton production were measured in hearts from Dahl salt-sensitive rats fed a low salt diet, 0.3% NaCl (Control) or a HSD, 8% NaCl, for 3, 6, or 9 weeks. Energy metabolic rates were assessed in isolated working hearts. Proton production was calculated based on glycolysis and glucose oxidation rates. Contribution to ATP production was calculated from the metabolic rates assessed using the isolated working heart perfusion in Dahl salt-sensitive rats. $n = 3–5$ * $p < 0.05$ compared to Control. Values shown as mean ± SEM

production occurs early during the development of diastolic dysfunction, a possible causal link between the uncoupling of glycolysis and glucose oxidation and the development of HFpEF may exist.

Even though glycolysis rates in the hearts remained elevated as HFrEF developed (i.e. by 9 weeks of the HSD), the increase in ATP production originating from glycolysis did not compensate for the decrease in ATP production that occurred as a result of the decrease in fatty acid oxidation (Fig. 2d, Table 3).

**Increased GLUT1 expression may contribute to the increased uncoupling of glycolysis from glucose oxidation observed during the development of diastolic dysfunction**

Examination of the expression of various proteins involved in glucose metabolism indicated that a change in glucose transport may contribute to the rise in glycolysis seen during the development of diastolic dysfunction. A progressive increase in GLUT1 expression was seen in Dahl salt-sensitive rat hearts during the HSD (Fig. 3a

**Table 3** Effect of insulin (100 µU/ml) on cardiac metabolism in Dahl salt-sensitive rats fed a high salt diet (HSD)

|  | Control | 3 weeks | 6 weeks | 9 weeks |
|---|---|---|---|---|
| Glycolysis | 1231.3 ±234.8 | 2390.9 ±390.4 | 2090.6 ±647.2 | 2982.2 ±734.1 |
| Glucose Oxidation | 312.2 ±20.6 | 519.0 ±119.7 | 464.8 ±113.6 | 493.0 ±166.7 |
| Palmitate Oxidation | 983.5 ±47.5 | 931.0 ±38.2 | 796.9 ±43.8 | 616.3 ±56.9[*] |
| Lactate Oxidation | 377.0 ±46.2 | 426.5 ±95.0 | 339.6 ±62.4 | 275.0 ±113.7 |
| Proton Production | 1838.3 ±454.1 | 3743.8 ±558.6 | 3251.6 ±1073.8 | 4978.3 ±1197.6 |
| ATP Production |  |  |  |  |
| Glycolysis | 2.5 ±0.5 | 4.8 ±0.8 | 4.2 ±1.3 | 6.0 ±1.5 |
| Glucose Oxidation | 9.1 ±0.6 | 15.1 ±3.5 | 13.5 ±3.3 | 14.3 ±4.8 |
| Palmitate Oxidation | 102.3 ±4.9 | 96.8 ±4.0 | 82.9 ±4.6 | 64.1 ±5.9[*#] |
| Lactate Oxidation | 5.5 ±0.7 | 6.2 ±1.4 | 4.9 ±0.9 | 4.0 ±1.6 |
| Total | 115.6 ±3.3 | 122.8 ±6.2 | 106.4 ±10.2 | 88.3 ±11.0 |

Energy metabolic rates (nmol●g dry $wt^{-1}$●$min^{-1}$) were measured during the working heart perfusion. Contribution to ATP production (µmol●g dry $wt^{-1}$●$min^{-1}$) was calculated from the metabolic rates assessed via the isolated working heart perfusion in Dahl salt-sensitive rats. These results are from Dahl salt-sensitive rats fed a low salt diet, 0.3% NaCl (Control), or a high salt diet, 8% NaCl, for 3, 6, or 9 weeks. n = 3–5 * $p < 0.05$ compared to Control. # $p < 0.05$ compared to 3 weeks. Values shown as mean ±SEM

and b). Since GLUT1 mediates glucose uptake independent of insulin, it suggests that increased GLUT1 expression may be involved in the elevated glycolysis rates observed even when hearts were perfused without insulin (Fig. 2e). While PGAM1 and GLUT4 (the insulin-dependent glucose transporter) expression were not significantly altered during the development of diastolic dysfunction, LDHA was significantly increased after 3 weeks on the HSD (Fig. 3d). This isoform of LDH favors the conversion of pyruvate to lactate. This suggests that LDHA may contribute to the initial increase in uncoupling of glycolysis and glucose oxidation observed in response to the HSD. HIF1α, a transcription factor regulating glycolysis, was not altered by the HSD (Fig. 3e).

We also examined the expression of mitochondrial enzymes that might contribute to the changes in cardiac energy metabolism observed in response to the HSD. No significant changes were observed in PDH expression, the rate-limiting enzyme for glucose oxidation (Fig. 4a). While phosphorylation of PDH by PDH kinase decreases PDH activity, we observed no change in pPDH during the development of diastolic dysfunction (Fig. 4a and b). This lack of change in pPDH correlates with the lack of change in glucose oxidation rates during the development of diastolic dysfunction (Fig. 2b). We also looked at the expression of the mitochondrial pyruvate carrier. Interestingly, MPC1 expression was increased after 6 weeks on the HSD, but MPC2 expression was not significantly altered (Fig. 4c and d). In addition, cytochrome c protein expression was not significantly altered (Fig. 4f). Since acetylation has been shown to regulate mitochondrial oxidative metabolism we also assessed the effect of the HSD on overall acetylation. However, overall lysine acetylation was not significantly altered in hearts of Dahl salt-sensitive rats fed a HSD (Additional file 1).

## Discussion

Alterations in cardiac energy metabolism are thought to be an important contributor to the severity of heart failure. However, there is confusion as to what changes in cardiac energy metabolism occur in heart failure, although it is generally believed that in HFrEF fatty acid metabolism decreases while overall glucose metabolism increases (Kato et al. 2010; Ingwall 2007; Davila-Roman et al. 2002). In this study we directly determined for the first time that the earliest cardiac energy metabolic changes that occurs in HFpEF is a dramatic increase in glycolysis. This metabolic change occurs prior to the development of HFpEF. Of interest, is that this increase in glycolysis occurs without a parallel change in glucose oxidation, which results in increased uncoupling of glycolysis and glucose oxidation. This is notable as previously published research has shown that increasing this uncoupling of glycolysis and glucose oxidation can result in intracellular acidosis, which can impair cardiac function (Liu et al. 1996; Liu et al. 2002; Steenbergen et al. 1977). An increased uncoupling of glycolysis and glucose oxidation has also been reported in other more severe models of heart failure such as in rodent hearts subjected to coronary artery ligation (CAL) (Masoud et al. 2014). Further, in one study abdominal aortic banding induced changes in cardiac metabolite levels indicative of increased uncoupling of glycolysis and glucose oxidation due to elevated glycolysis (Seymour et al. 2015). Our data also confirms that fatty acid oxidation decreases in HFrEF. There is evidence indicating that a reduction in fatty acid oxidation may contribute to diastolic dysfunction. For example, it was recently reported that overexpressing Acetyl Coenzyme A Carboxylase both prevented diastolic dysfunction and reduced cardiac fatty acid oxidation in mice treated with Angiotensin II (Choi et al. 2016;

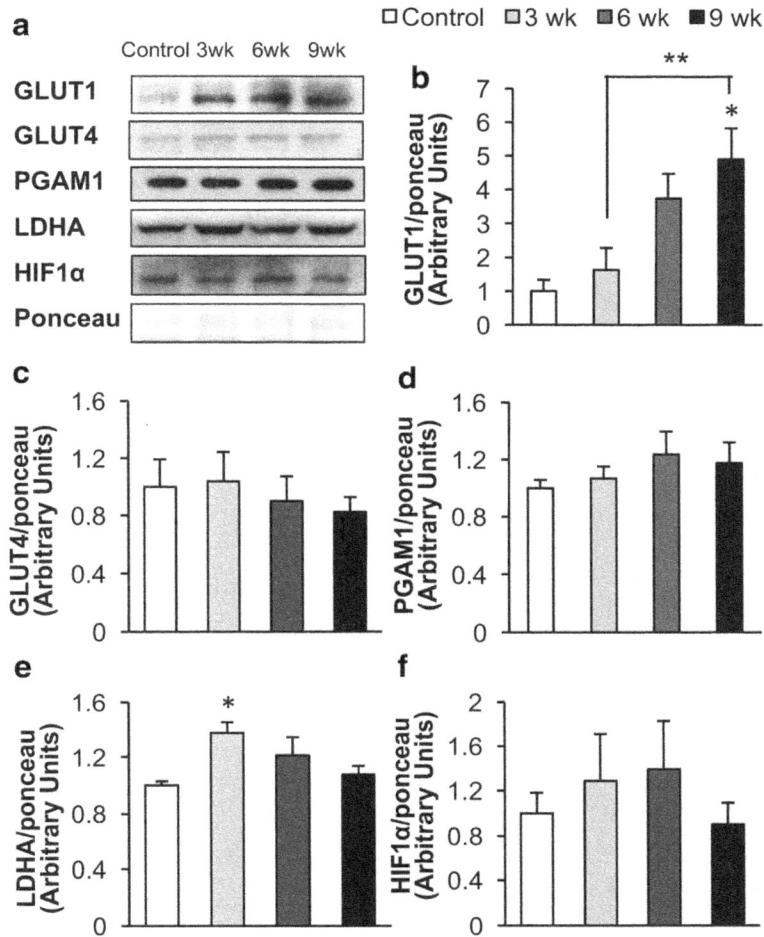

**Fig. 3** Effect of a high salt diet (HSD) on Dahl salt-sensitive rat heart glucose metabolic enzymes. **a** Representative western blots. **b** GLUT1, (**c**) GLUT4, (**d**) PGAM1, (**e**) LDHA expression, and (**f**) HIF1α protein expression was measured in hearts from Dahl salt-sensitive rats fed either a low salt diet, 0.3% NaCl (Control) or a HSD, 8% NaCl, for 3, 6, or 9 weeks. $n = 4$–9 * $p < 0.05$ compared to Control. ** $p < 0.05$ between compared groups. Values shown as mean ± SEM

Helge et al. 1996). However, of importance is that the decrease in fatty acid oxidation seen in the failing heart in our study did not precede the onset of diastolic dysfunction. As a result, it is unlikely that a decrease in fatty acid oxidation is contributing to the early development of diastolic dysfunction in heart failure.

While it is often cited that in heart failure the heart switches from fatty acid to glucose metabolism, our data suggests that it is more accurate to suggest that a decrease in overall cardiac mitochondrial oxidative metabolism occurs in HFrEF, accompanied by a relative increase in glycolysis. Despite glucose oxidation being the major source of glucose derived ATP production, glucose oxidation rates are not increased during the development of systolic dysfunction (Kato et al. 2010; Lopaschuk et al. 2010; Zhabyeyev et al. 2013; Zhang et al. 2013; Liu et al. 1996; Liu et al. 2002). In fact, in mouse models of HFrEF, we actually observed a decrease

in glucose oxidation rates (Zhabyeyev et al. 2013; Zhang et al. 2013).

There are several potential explanations for this rise in cardiac glycolysis in diastolic dysfunction. One possibility may be that the overall decrease in mitochondrial oxidative metabolism (which we have previously reported in hearts from HFpEF mice), results in a compensatory rise in glycolysis (Kato et al. 2010; Beer et al. 2002; Masoud et al. 2014; Zhang et al. 2013; Neubauer 2007). The decrease in cardiac ATP production after 9 weeks on a HSD appears to be solely due to a drop in fatty acid oxidation, as glucose and lactate oxidation remained unchanged. In an effort to determine what was responsible for this decrease in fatty acid oxidation we examined the expression of enzymes involved in fatty acid oxidation and mitochondrial oxidative metabolism. It has been previously reported that the cardiac expression of proteins involved in fatty acid oxidation and overall mitochondrial oxidative

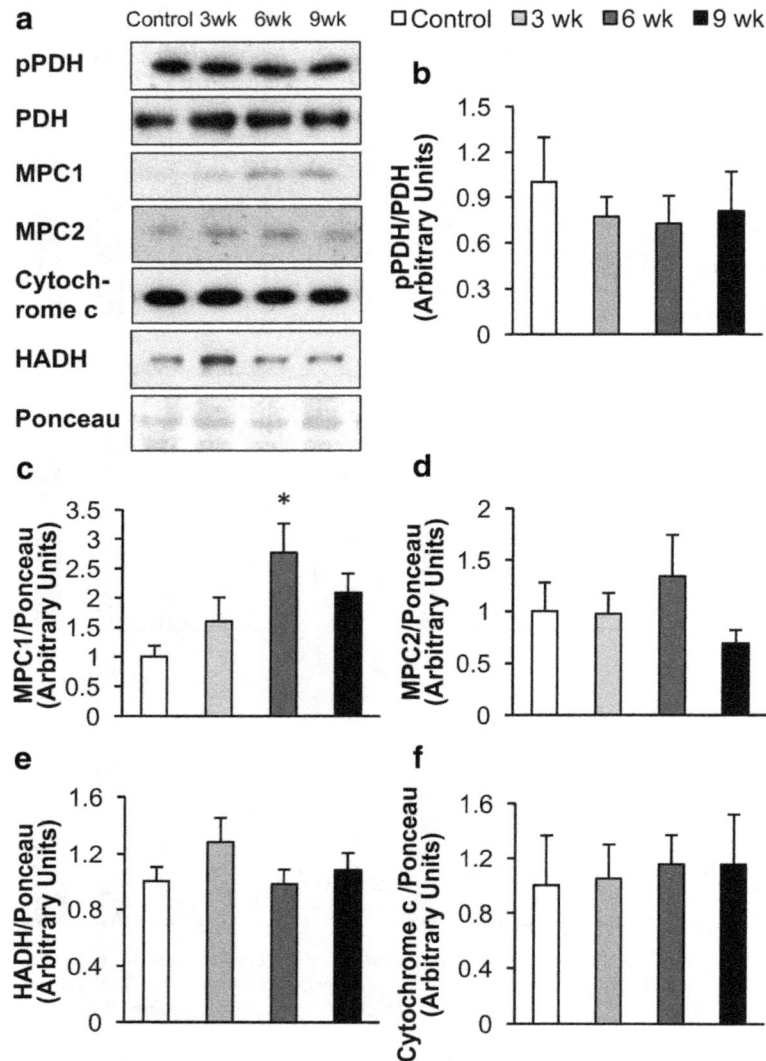

**Fig. 4** Effect of a high salt diet (HSD) on the cardiac expression of proteins involved in oxidative metabolism. **a** Representative western blots. **b** pPDH Ser293/PDH, (**c**) MPC1, (**d**) MPC2, (**e**) HADH, and (**f**) cytochrome c protein expression was measured in hearts from Dahl salt-sensitive rats fed a low salt diet, 0.3% NaCl (Control) or a HSD, 8% NaCl, for 3, 6, or 9 weeks. $n = 4$–9 * $p < 0.05$ compared to Control. Values shown as mean ± SEM

metabolism are decreased in severe heart failure (Zhang et al. 2013; Lai et al. 2014). However, we did not observe a change in the expression of ß-hydroxyacyl CoA dehydrogenase or cytochrome c in the heart (Fig. 4), enzymes involved in fatty acid oxidation and mitochondrial oxidative metabolism, respectively. Alternatively, the decrease in cardiac work may be lowering cardiac fatty acid oxidation rates. Cardiac fatty acid oxidation rates remained unchanged during the development of diastolic dysfunction when normalized against cardiac work (Control, 410.4 ±41.8; 3 weeks, 498.5 ±38; 6 weeks, 502.2 ±31.4; 9 weeks, 388.0 ±16.1 nmol•g dry wt$^{-1}$•min$^{-1}$) (Online Resource 1). While it is possible that a reduction in fatty acid

oxidation is causing the decrease in cardiac function, we speculate that the reduction in cardiac fatty acid oxidation is a consequence of reduced cardiac work.

Increased capacity for glycolysis or glucose transport may also be responsible for the rise in glycolysis during development of diastolic dysfunction and heart failure. Although we did not observe a change in the expression of the glycolytic enzyme PGAM1, we did find an increase in LDHA protein expression after 3 weeks on the HSD and a later rise in GLUT1 protein expression (Fig. 4). LDH isoforms that contain LDHA are more likely to convert pyruvate to lactate, as opposed to catalyzing the opposite reaction. Therefore, increased LDHA protein expression could be contributing to the early rise in glycolysis and increased uncoupling of glycolysis and glucose oxidation in response to the HSD.

Increased cardiac GLUT1 expression may also contribute to the rise in glycolysis. In support of this, glycolysis is elevated in hearts overexpressing GLUT1 and is decreased in hearts lacking GLUT1 (Liao et al. 2002; Pereira et al. 2014). However, studies that regulate GLUT1 expression report mixed results on the role of GLUT1 in the development of heart failure. While overexpression of GLUT1 has been reported to prevent pressure overload induced heart failure in mouse hearts, deletion of GLUT1 does not affect the rate of development of pressure overload induced heart failure. The GLUT1 knockout mouse has elevated fatty acid oxidation and reduced glucose oxidation, which would be expected to decrease cardiac efficiency and may explain why these hearts are not resistant pressure overload induced heart failure (Pereira et al. 2014). However, the results from these two studies do not preclude the possibility that a more acute up-regulation of GLUT1 expression could increase glycolysis and impair cardiac function.

Based on these results we hypothesize that stimulating glucose oxidation may be a promising strategy for treating and potentially preventing the development of HFpEF. As mentioned earlier, stimulating cardiac glucose oxidation is associated with an increase in cardiac efficiency and an improvement in cardiac function (Kato et al. 2010; Masoud et al. 2014; Yamashita et al. 2009; Ussher et al. 2012; Stanley et al. 2005; Lopaschuk et al. 2003; Dyck et al. 2006; Dyck et al. 2004). Stimulating cardiac glucose oxidation can also be beneficial in the context of obesity and diabetes, which can lead to heart failure (Ussher et al. 2009; Lewis et al. 2016; Nicholl et al. 1991). Furthermore, treatment of Dahl salt sensitive rats with dichloroacetate (DCA) decreases plasma lactate levels (an indirect indication of elevated glycolysis), and improves cardiac function (Kato et al. 2010). However, in this study intervention with DCA was at a later stage of heart failure development, which was also associated with changes in systolic function. In the future it will be important to determine if stimulating glucose oxidation with more potent PDK inhibitors can lessen or even prevent the development of HFpEF.

## Conclusions

This study directly characterized the changes in cardiac energy metabolism that occur in diastolic dysfunction. We demonstrate that the earliest cardiac metabolic change that occurs during the development of diastolic dysfunction is an increase in glycolysis, with no change in carbohydrate or fatty acid oxidation. The rise in glycolysis resulted in increased uncoupling of glycolysis and glucose oxidation and an increased proton production,

which occurs early during the development of diastolic dysfunction. Our findings combined with previous work suggest that the coupling of glycolysis and glucose oxidation is important in maintaining normal cardiac function and may contribute to the development of HFpEF. While these results suggest that decreasing the uncoupling of glycolysis and glucose oxidation may be a promising strategy for the treatment of heart failure, more work is needed to determine if therapeutically improving the coupling of glycolysis and glucose oxidation can treat HFpEF.

## Additional file

Additional file 1: Figure S1. Effect of a high salt diet (HSD) on overall protein acetylation. Total protein acetylation levels were measured in hearts from Dahl salt-sensitive rats fed a low salt diet, 0.3% NaCl (Control) or a HSD, 8% NaCl, for 3, 6, or 9 wk. $n = 6–9$ Values shown as mean ± SEM. (TIFF 3225 kb)

### Abbreviations
%EF: % Ejection fraction; %FS: % Fractional shortening; ANOVA: One Way Analysis of Variance; ATP: Adenosine triphosphate; Bpm: beats per minute; BSA: Bovine serum albumin; CAL: Coronary artery ligation; DCA: Dichloroacetate; DTT: Dithiothreitol; GLUT1: Glucose transporter 1; GLUT4: Glucose transporter 4; HADH: Hydroxyacyl coenzyme A dehydrogenase; HF: Heart failure; HFpEF: Heart failure with preserved ejection fraction; HFrEF: Heart failure with reduced ejection fraction; HIF1α: Hypoxia inducible factor 1α; HR: Heart rate; HSD: High salt diet; IVRT: Isovolumetric relaxation time; IVSd: Interventricular septum end diastole; IVSs: Interventricular septum end systole; LDHA: Lactate dehydrogenase A; LV Vol;d: Left ventricle volume end diastole; LV Vol;s: Left ventricle volume end systole; LV: Left ventricle; LVIDd: Left ventricle internal diameter end diastole; LVIDs: Left ventricle internal diameter end systole; LVPWd: Left ventricle posterior wall thickness end diastole; LVPWs: Left ventricle posterior wall thickness end systole; MPC1: Mitochondrial pyruvate carrier 1; MPC2: Mitochondrial pyruvate carrier 2; PDH: Pyruvate dehydrogenase; PGAM1: Phosphoglycerate mutase 1

### Acknowledgements
We thank the Cardiovascular Research Centre Core for assessment of in vivo cardiac function.

### Funding
This work was supported by an Alberta Innovates – Health Solutions Interdisciplinary Team Grant via Alberta Heart; and the Canadian Institutes of Health Research [to G.D.L. and to J.R.B.D]. G.D.L. is an Alberta Innovates – Health Solutions Scientist and N.F. holds an Alberta Innovates – Health Solutions studentship.

### Authors' contributions
NF designed the study, collected, analyzed and interpreted the data, and wrote the manuscript. JLL, AF, CSW, and WW collected, analyzed, and interpreted data for the study. JRBD revised the manuscript and contributed to the discussion. GDL designed the study, contributed to the discussion, and wrote the manuscript. The final manuscript was approved by all authors.

**Competing interests**
The authors declare that they have no competing interests.

**References**

Allard MF, Schonekess BO, Henning SL, English DR, Lopaschuk GD. Contribution of oxidative metabolism and glycolysis to ATP production in hypertrophied hearts. Am J Physiol Heart Circ Physiol. 1994;267:H742–H50.

Barr RL, Lopaschuk GD. Direct measurement of energy metabolism in the isolated working rat heart. J Pharmacol Toxicol Methods. 1997;38:11–7.

Beer M, Seyfarth T, Sandstede J, Landschutz W, Lipke C, Kostler H, et al. Absolute concentrations of high-energy phosphate metabolites in normal, hypertrophied, and failing human myocardium measured noninvasively with (31)P-SLOOP magnetic resonance spectroscopy. J Am Coll Cardiol. 2002;40:1267–74.

Bonnet S, Archer SL, Allalunis-Turner J, Haromy A, Beaulieu C, Thompson R, et al. A mitochondria-K+ channel axis is suppressed in cancer and its normalization promotes apoptosis and inhibits cancer growth. Cancer Cell. 2007;11:37–51.

Canadian Council on Animal Care. (2017) Guide to the care and use of experimental animals. 2nd. Ottawa, Ontario. [cited 2017 Sept 16]. Available from: http://www.ccac.ca/.

Chesnais JM, Coraboeuf E, Sauviat MP, Vassas JM. Sensitivity to H, li and mg ions of the slow inward sodium current in frog atrial fibres. J Mol Cell Cardiol. 1975;7:627–42.

Choi YS, de Mattos AB, Shao D, Li T, Nabben M, Kim M, et al. Preservation of myocardial fatty acid oxidation prevents diastolic dysfunction in mice subjected to angiotensin II infusion. J Mol Cell Cardiol. 2016;100:64–71.

Conway MA, Allis J, Ouwerkerk R, Niioka T, Rajagopalan B, Radda GK. Detection of low phosphocreatine to ATP ratio in failing hypertrophied human myocardium by 31P magnetic resonance spectroscopy. Lancet. 1991;338:973–6.

Davila-Roman VG, Vedala G, Herrero P, de las Fuentes L, Rogers JG, Kelly DP, et al. Altered myocardial fatty acid and glucose metabolism in idiopathic dilated cardiomyopathy. J Am Coll Cardiol. 2002;40:271–7.

Degens H, de Brouwer KF, Gilde AJ, Lindhout M, Willemsen PH, Janssen BJ, et al. Cardiac fatty acid metabolism is preserved in the compensated hypertrophic rat heart. Basic Res Cardiol. 2006;101:17–26.

Dyck JR, Cheng JF, Stanley WC, Barr R, Chandler MP, Brown S, et al. Malonyl coenzyme a decarboxylase inhibition protects the ischemic heart by inhibiting fatty acid oxidation and stimulating glucose oxidation. Circ Res. 2004;94:e78–84.

Dyck JR, Hopkins TA, Bonnet S, Michelakis ED, Young ME, Watanabe M, et al. Absence of malonyl coenzyme a decarboxylase in mice increases cardiac glucose oxidation and protects the heart from ischemic injury. Circulation. 2006;114:1721–8.

Folmes CD, Clanachan AS, Lopaschuk GD. Fatty acids attenuate insulin regulation of 5'-AMP-activated protein kinase and insulin cardioprotection after ischemia. Circ Res. 2006;99:61–8.

Gerriets VA, Kishton RJ, Nichols AG, Macintyre AN, Inoue M, Ilkayeva O, et al. Metabolic programming and PDHK1 control CD4+ T cell subsets and inflammation. J Clin Invest. 2015;125:194–207.

Helge JW, Richter EA, Kiens B. Interaction of training and diet on metabolism and endurance during exercise in man. J Physiol. 1996;492(Pt 1):293–306.

Horgan S, Watson C, Glezeva N, Baugh J. Murine models of diastolic dysfunction and heart failure with preserved ejection fraction. J Card Fail. 2014;20:984–95.

Ingwall JS. On substrate selection for ATP synthesis in the failing human myocardium. Am J Physiol Heart Circ Physiol. 2007;293:H3225–6.

Kato T, Niizuma S, Inuzuka Y, Kawashima T, Okuda J, Tamaki Y, et al. Analysis of metabolic remodeling in compensated left ventricular hypertrophy and heart failure. Circ Heart Fail. 2010;3:420–30.

Klotz S, Hay I, Zhang G, Maurer M, Wang J, Burkhoff D. Development of heart failure in chronic hypertensive dahl rats: focus on heart failure with preserved ejection fraction. Hypertension. 2006;47:901–11.

Lai L, Leone TC, Keller MP, Martin OJ, Broman AT, Nigro J, et al. Energy metabolic reprogramming in the hypertrophied and early stage failing heart: a multisystems approach. Circ Heart Fail. 2014;7:1022–31.

Lei B, Lionetti V, Young ME, Chandler MP, d'Agostino C, Kang E, et al. Paradoxical downregulation of the glucose oxidation pathway despite enhanced flux in severe heart failure. J Mol Cell Cardiol. 2004;36:567–76.

Leong HS, Grist M, Parsons H, Wambolt RB, Lopaschuk GD, Brownsey R, et al. Accelerated rates of glycolysis in the hypertrophied heart: are they a methodological artifact? Am J Physiol Endocrinol Metab. 2002;282:E1039–45.

Lewis AJ, Neubauer S, Tyler DJ, Rider OJ. Pyruvate dehydrogenase as a therapeutic target for obesity cardiomyopathy. Expert Opin Ther Targets. 2016;20:755–66.

Liao R, Jain M, Cui L, D'Agostino J, Aiello F, Luptak I, et al. Cardiac-specific overexpression of GLUT1 prevents the development of heart failure attributable to pressure overload in mice. Circulation. 2002;106:2125–31.

Liu B, Clanachan AS, Schulz R, Lopaschuk GD. Cardiac efficiency is improved after ischemia by altering both the source and fate of protons. Circ Res. 1996;79:940–8.

Liu Q, Docherty JC, Rendell JCT, Clanachan AS, Lopaschuk GD. High levels of fatty acids delay the recovery of intracellular pH and cardiac efficiency in post-ischemic hearts by inhibiting glucose oxidation. J Am Coll Cardiol. 2002;39: 718–25.

Lopaschuk GD, Barr R, Thomas PD, Dyck JR. Beneficial effects of trimetazidine in ex vivo working ischemic hearts are due to a stimulation of glucose oxidation secondary to inhibition of long-chain 3-ketoacyl coenzyme a thiolase. Circ Res. 2003;93:e33–7.

Lopaschuk GD, Ussher JR, Folmes CD, Jaswal JS, Stanley WC. Myocardial fatty acid metabolism in health and disease. Physiol Rev. 2010;90:207–58.

Masoud WG, Ussher JR, Wang W, Jaswal JS, Wagg CS, Dyck JR, et al. Failing mouse hearts utilize energy inefficiently and benefit from improved coupling of glycolysis and glucose oxidation. Cardiovasc Res. 2014;101:30–8.

Mori J, Alrob OA, Wagg CS, Harris RA, Lopaschuk GD, Oudit GY. ANG II causes insulin resistance and induces cardiac metabolic switch and inefficiency: a critical role of PDK4. Am J Physiol Heart Circ Physiol. 2013;304:H1103–13.

Morimoto S, Goto T. Role of troponin I isoform switching in determining the pH sensitivity of ca(2+) regulation in developing rabbit cardiac muscle. Biochem Biophys Res Commun. 2000;267:912–7.

Nascimben L, Friedrich J, Liao R, Pauletto P, Pessina AC, Ingwall JS. Enalapril treatment increases cardiac performance and energy reserve via the creatine kinase reaction in myocardium of Syrian myopathic hamsters with advanced heart failure. Circulation. 1995;91:1824–33.

Neubauer S. The failing heart–an engine out of fuel. N Engl J Med. 2007;356: 1140–51.

Neubauer S, Remkes H, Spindler M, Horn M, Wiesmann F, Prestle J, et al. Downregulation of the Na+-Creatine cotransporter in failing human myocardium and in experimental heart failure. Circulation. 1999;100:1847–50.

Nicholl TA, Lopaschuk GD, McNeill JH. Effects of free fatty acids and dichloroacetate on isolated working diabetic rat heart. Am J Phys. 1991;261: H1053–9.

Pereira RO, Wende AR, Olsen C, Soto J, Rawlings T, Zhu Y, et al. GLUT1 deficiency in cardiomyocytes does not accelerate the transition from compensated hypertrophy to heart failure. J Mol Cell Cardiol. 2014;72:95–103.

Piao L, Fang YH, Cadete VJ, Wietholt C, Urboniene D, Toth PT, et al. The inhibition of pyruvate dehydrogenase kinase improves impaired cardiac function and electrical remodeling in two models of right ventricular hypertrophy: resuscitating the hibernating right ventricle. J Mol Med. 2010;88:47–60.

Piao L, Sidhu VK, Fang YH, Ryan JJ, Parikh KS, Hong Z, et al. FOXO1-mediated upregulation of pyruvate dehydrogenase kinase-4 (PDK4) decreases glucose oxidation and impairs right ventricular function in pulmonary hypertension: therapeutic benefits of dichloroacetate. J Mol Med. 2013;91:333–46.

Rapp JP, Dene H. Development and characteristics of inbred strains of Dahl salt-sensitive and salt-resistant rats. Hypertension. 1985;7:340–9.

Schiaffino S, Gorza L, Ausoni S. Troponin isoform switching in the developing heart and its functional consequences. Trends Cardiovasc Med. 1993;3:12–7.

Schroeder MA, Lau AZ, Chen AP, Gu Y, Nagendran J, Barry J, et al. Hyperpolarized (13)C magnetic resonance reveals early- and late-onset changes to in vivo pyruvate metabolism in the failing heart. Eur J Heart Fail. 2013;15:130–40.

Seymour AM, Giles L, Ball V, Miller JJ, Clarke K, Carr CA, et al. In vivo assessment of cardiac metabolism and function in the abdominal aortic banding model of compensated cardiac hypertrophy. Cardiovasc Res. 2015;106:249–60.

Stanley WC, Morgan EE, Huang H, McElfresh TA, Sterk JP, Okere IC, et al. Malonyl-CoA decarboxylase inhibition suppresses fatty acid oxidation and reduces lactate production during demand-induced ischemia. Am J Physiol Heart Circ Physiol. 2005;289:H2304–9.

Steenbergen C, Deleeuw G, Rich T, Williamson JR. Effects of acidosis and ischemia on contractility and intracellular pH of rat heart. Circ Res. 1977;41:849–58.

Tian R, Nascimben L, Kaddurah-Daouk R, Ingwall JS. Depletion of energy reserve via the Creatine kinase reaction during the evolution of heart failure in Cardiomyopathic hamsters. J Mol Cell Cardiol. 1996;28:755–65.

Ussher JR, Koves TR, Jaswal JS, Zhang L, Ilkayeva O, Dyck JR, et al. Insulin-stimulated cardiac glucose oxidation is increased in high-fat diet-induced obese mice lacking malonyl CoA decarboxylase. Diabetes. 2009;58:1766–75.

Ussher JR, Wang W, Gandhi M, Keung W, Samokhvalov V, Oka T, et al. Stimulation of glucose oxidation protects against acute myocardial infarction and reperfusion injury. Cardiovasc Res. 2012;94:359–69.

Vander Heiden MG, Cantley LC, Thompson CB. Understanding the Warburg effect: the metabolic requirements of cell proliferation. Science. 2009;324:1029–33.

Vogel S, Sperelakis N. Blockade of myocardial slow inward current at low pH. Am J Phys. 1977;233:C99–103.

Warburg O. On the origin of cancer cells. Science. 1956;123:309–14.

Yamashita T, Honda M, Takatori H, Nishino R, Minato H, Takamura H, et al. Activation of lipogenic pathway correlates with cell proliferation and poor prognosis in hepatocellular carcinoma. J Hepatol. 2009;50:100–10.

Zhabyeyev P, Gandhi M, Mori J, Basu R, Kassiri Z, Clanachan A, et al. Pressure-overload-induced heart failure induces a selective reduction in glucose oxidation at physiological afterload. Cardiovasc Res. 2013;97:676–85.

Zhang L, Jaswal JS, Ussher JR, Sankaralingam S, Wagg C, Zaugg M, et al. Cardiac insulin-resistance and decreased mitochondrial energy production precede the development of systolic heart failure after pressure-overload hypertrophy. Circ Heart Fail. 2013;6:1039–48.

Zhong J, Basu R, Guo D, Chow FL, Byrns S, Schuster M, et al. Angiotensin-converting enzyme 2 suppresses pathological hypertrophy, myocardial fibrosis, and cardiac dysfunction. Circulation. 2010;122:717–28.

# 12

# Asymmetric expression of H19 and ADIPOQ in concave/convex paravertebral muscles is associated with severe adolescent idiopathic scoliosis

Heng Jiang[1†], Fu Yang[2,3†], Tao Lin[1†], Wei Shao[1], Yichen Meng[1], Jun Ma[1], Ce Wang[1], Rui Gao[1*] and Xuhui Zhou[1*] ⓘ

## Abstract

**Background:** Adolescent idiopathic scoliosis (AIS) is the most common paediatric spinal deformity. The etiology and pathology of AIS remain unexplained, and have been reported to involve a combination of genetic and epigenetic factors. Since paravertebral muscle imbalance plays an important role in the onset and progression of scoliosis, we aimed to investigate transcriptomic differences by RNA-seq and identify significantly differentially expressed transcripts in two sides of paravertebral muscle in AIS.

**Methods:** RNA-seq was performed on 5 pairs of paravertebral muscle from 5 AIS patients. Significantly differentially expressed transcripts were validated by quantitative reverse polymerase chain reaction. Gene expression difference was correlated to clinical characteristics.

**Results:** We demonstrated that ADIPOQ mRNA and H19 is significantly differentially expressed between two sides of paravertebral muscle, relatively specific in the context of AIS. Relatively low H19 and high ADIPOQ mRNA expression levels in concave-sided muscle are associated with larger spinal curve and earlier age at initiation. We identified miR-675-5p encoded by H19 as a mechanistic regulator of ADIPOQ expression in AIS. We demonstrated that significantly reduced CCCTC-binding factor (CCTF) occupancy in the imprinting control region (ICR) of the H19 gene in the concave-sided muscle contributes to down-regulated H19 expression.

**Conclusions:** RNA-seq revealed transcriptomic differences between two sides of paravertebral muscle in AIS patients. Our findings imply that transcriptomic differences caused by epigenetic factors in affected individuals may account for the structural and functional imbalance of paravertebral muscle, which can expand our etiologic understanding of this disease.

**Keywords:** Adolescent idiopathic scoliosis, Transcriptome, Paravertebral muscle, H19, ADIPOQ

## Background

Adolescent idiopathic scoliosis (AIS) is characterized by a three-dimensional deformity of the spine that occurs in the absence of underlying vertebral anomalies or obvious physiological defects (Altaf et al. 2013). The etiology and pathogenesis of AIS remain poorly explained, largely because of the genetic heterogeneity and lack of appropriate, tractable animal models (Boswell and Ciruna 2017). Genetic studies including traditional linkage analysis (Salehi et al. 2002), subsequent genome-wide association studies (Takahashi et al. 2011; Kou et al. 2013; Zhu et al. 2015; Sharma et al. 2011) and exome sequencing (Buchan et al. 2014; Haller et al. 2016) for AIS have identified more than 50 susceptible genetic variants, of which the function in AIS pathogenesis is yet undefined. On the other hand, numerous studies have suggested that some other factors, such as neuromuscular dysfunction (Wajchenberg et al. 2016; Grimes et al. 2016), and environment factors (Burwell et al. 2011) are associated with this disease.

---

* Correspondence: rgaospine@163.com; xhzhouspine@163.com
†Heng Jiang, Fu Yang and Tao Lin contributed equally to this work.
[1]Department of Orthopedics, Changzheng Hospital, Second Military Medical University, No.415 Fengyang Road, Shanghai, People's Republic of China
Full list of author information is available at the end of the article

The onset of scoliosis typically coincides with the adolescent growth spurt and the affected individuals are at a risk of increasing deformity until growth ceases. It has been reported that brace treatment significantly decreased the progression of high-risk curves, but still around 28% of AIS patients experienced exacerbation of scoliosis during or after bracing with undefined mechanism (Weinstein et al. 2013). Though several single nucleotide polymorphisms (SNPs) of certain genes such as neurotrophin-3 (Qiu et al. 2012; Ogura et al. 2017), and some parameters including the level of platelet calmodulin (Lowe et al. 2004) have been testified as predictors for spinal deformity progression in AIS, no method has been recommended for clinical use as diagnostic criteria (Noshchenko et al. 2015).

Functional and clinical assessments have correlated AIS with paravertebral muscle imbalance (Zapata et al. 2015; Wong 2015). Measurement of electromyography activity of the paravertebral muscles showed a higher amplitude of motor unit potentials on the convexity side (Stetkarova et al. 2016). In histological studies of multifidus muscles, increased proportion of type I fibers on the convex side and lower proportion of type I fibers on the concave side of the scoliotic curve have been reported (Stetkarova et al. 2016). Moreover, higher progression of AIS correlates significantly with the increased proportion of type I fibers on the convex side (Stetkarova et al. 2016). We have previously demonstrated that the muscle volumetric and fatty infiltration imbalance occur in all of the levels of the vertebrae involved in the major curve of AIS with larger muscle volume on the convex side and higher fatty infiltration rate in the concave side (Jiang et al. 2017). Some studies have uncovered asymmetric expression of melatonin receptor (Wong 2015) and transforming growth factor-beta signaling (Nowak et al. 2014) in bilateral paravertebral muscles of AIS. There are also some interesting findings that some AIS risk loci identified by genetic study located in regions near or within genes associated with muscle biogenesis (Sharma et al. 2015a). These evidences indicated that paravertebral muscle might play an important role in the initiation and progression of AIS. Nonetheless, the mechanism of the complex muscle tissue changes remains unclear. This study employed RNA-seq to evaluate whole transcriptomic changes in the concave- and convex-sided paravertebral muscle at the apex level of the main curve in patients with AIS. And our data identified differential expression of H19 and ADIPOQ mRNA between the two sides of paravertebral muscle in AIS patients. More importantly, lower expression of H19 and higher expression of ADIPOQ mRNA in concave-sided muscle correlate positively with curve severity and age at initiation.

## Methods

### Patients

The research project was approved by the ethics department of Shanghai Changzheng Hospital, Shanghai. We have consensus with all participants. All the procedures were done under the Declaration of Helsinki and relevant policies in China.

We collected 5 pairs of paravertebral muscle samples from 5 AIS patients during spinal surgery (mean age 14.20 ± 1.92 yrs.; female; $n = 5$) for RNA-seq. Paravertebral muscle samples were obtained from both sides of multifidus muscle of AIS patients at the apex level of the main curve. Muscle tissues were stored in liquid nitrogen immediately. To validate the differentially expressed transcripts identified by RNA-seq, 60 pairs of paravertebral muscle tissues were obtained from different patients with AIS during surgery. AIS was diagnosed and classified based on the Lenke classification. The clinical characteristics of the enrolled patients were summarized in Additional file 1: Table S1. Samples of patients with congenital scoliosis (CS) were collected from both sides of multifidus muscle at the apex level of the curve at surgery in 25 age-matched individuals during spinal surgery. CS patients enrolled in this study had major thoracic curves and similar magnitudes of curves compared with those of AIS patients ($54.48 ± 10.09$ vs. $59.32 ± 15.43$, $p = 0.09$, Additional file 1: Figure S1). And 16 age-matched patients undergoing spinal surgery for thoracic spinal fracture were enrolled as non-AIS group and the multifidus muscle samples were obtained at the upper level of the instrumented vertebra.

### Total RNA extraction and RNA-seq

Total RNA was isolated from fresh-frozen tissue samples and extracted using TRIzol reagent (Invitrogen, Carlsbad, CA, USA). Total RNA quality and quantity were determined using a Nanodrop 8000 UV-Vis spectrometer (Thermo Scientific Inc., Waltham, MA, USA). RNA-seq was performed using total RNA samples with a quantity greater than 10 µg and an RNA integrity number > 6.0. If the quantity of total RNA was less than 10 µg or the RNA integrity number was less than 6.0, another muscle sample was used for RNA isolation. Library construction for whole transcriptome sequencing was performed using the Truseq RNA sample preparation v2 kit (Illumina, San Diego, CA, USA) as described previously (Hong et al. 2017).

### Quantitative real-time polymerase chain reaction (qRT-PCR)

Total RNA was extracted and then reverse-transcribed into cDNA using the cDNA Reverse Transcription Kit from Applied Biosystems (Foster City, CA, USA). qRT-PCR was conducted using SYBR Green Master Mix on the ABI 7900HT fast real-time PCR System (Applied

Biosystems, Waltham, MA, USA). The following thermal settings were used: 95 °C for 10 min followed by 40 cycles of 95 °C for 15 s and 60 °C for 1 min. The primers used for H19, miR-675-5p, PCK1, FABP4, SCD, PLIN1, ADIPOQ, U6 (internal control for miRNAs), and 18 s (internal control for mRNAs and lncRNAs) are listed in Additional file 1: Table S2. The $\Delta\Delta$Ct method was used to calculate the relative expression level of mRNAs or miRNAs on both sides and fold change was presented related to convex side.

### Cell culture
Human skeletal muscle satellite cells (HSkMSC) were obtained from ZhongQiaoXinZhou Biotech Co. (Shanghai, China) and cultured at sub-confluent density in growth medium consisting of Ham's F-10 supplemented with 20% fetal bovine serum (FBS) and 1% antibiotics (PeSt). All cell-based in vitro experiments were repeated in triplicate. To initiate differentiation into myotubes, Ham's F-10/20% FBS was removed from cells and Dulbecco's modified Eagle's medium (DMEM) containing 1% PeSt/4% FBS was added for 48 h. After this, medium was changed to DMEM containing 1% PeSt/2% FBS. Differential medium was changed every 3 days, and cells were harvested at the indicated times. The HEK293T cells were obtained from Cellbank (SIBS, Shanghai, China) and cultured in DMEM with 10% FBS and 1% antibiotics.

### RNA oligoribonucleotides and transient transfection
A chemically-modified double-stranded miR-675-5p mimic and the corresponding miRNA mimic control (mimic NC) were obtained from RiboBio Co. (Guangzhou, China). Inhibitor of miR-675-5p and the corresponding inhibitor control (inhibitor NC) were from RiboBio Co. (Guangzhou, China). The sequences are listed in Additional file 1: Table S2. Cells at 70–80% confluence were transfected with miRNA mimics, or inhibitors using Lipofectamine 2000 (Invitrogen, Carlsbad, CA, USA) according to the manufacturer's instructions as described previously (Dey et al. 2014).

### Dual luciferase reporter assay
The 3′-untranslated region (3′UTR) of ADIPOQ was amplified with 5′-GCCTCCTGAATTTATTATTGTTC-3′ and 5′-GTT CGG TGT GGT AGA CCG A-3′, and subcloned in psiCheck-2 (Promega, Madison, WI, USA). As specificity control, the seed sequence GGCTC of miR-675-5p target sites on the 3′UTR of ADIPOQ was replaced by GGGGG using site-directed mutagenesis. HEK293T cells grown in 48-well plates were transfected with 100 nM miR-675 mimic or control, 40 ng luciferase reporter, and 4 ng pRL-TK, plasmid expressing Renilla luciferase (Promega) using Lipofectamine 2000 (Invitrogen). The Renilla/firefly luciferase activities were measured 24 h after transfection using the Dual Luciferase Reporter Assay System (Promega). All luciferase values were normalized to those of Renilla luciferase and expressed as fold-induction relative to the basal activity.

### Western blotting
Cells were harvested, washed with PBS, and lysed in RIPA buffer. Proteins were separated by 12% sodium dodecyl sulfate–polyacrylamide gel electrophoresis and transferred to polyvinylidene fluoride membranes. Primary antibodies against ADIPOQ (Abcam, Cambridge, UK) and beta-actin (Cell Signaling Technology,Bevereverly, MA, USA) were diluted 1:1,000. The intensities of the bands obtained by Western blotting analysis were quantified using ImageJ software (http://rsb.info.nih.gov/ij/). The background was subtracted, and the signal of each target band was normalized to that of the beta-actin band.

### Chromatin immunoprecipitation (ChIP) assay
ChIP assays were performed using the SimpleChIP Plus Enzymatic Chromatin IP kit (Cell Signaling Technology) according to the manufacturer's instructions. When harvesting tissue, unwanted material such as fat and necrotic material was removed. Then the tissue was cross-linked with 1.5% formaldehyde for 20 min. Nuclei preparation and chromatin digestion was performed by micrococcal nuclease. Chromatin was sonicated on ice to generate chromatin fragments of 150–900 bp. Antibodies against CTCF (Cell Signaling Technology) or negative control rabbit IgG (Cell Signaling Technology) were used in chromatin immunoprecipitation. Then chromatin was eluted from antibody/protein G magnetic beads and reverse cross-linked. Input control DNA or immunoprecipitated DNA was quantified by standard PCR method, using SimpleChIP Human H19/IGF2 ICR Primers (Cell Signaling Technology). The following thermal settings were used: 95 °C for 5 min followed by 34 cycles of 95 °C for 30s, 62 °C for 30s and 72 °C for 30s, then 72 °C for 5 min. PCR product was analyzed by 10% polyacrylamide gel electrophoresis and the signal of each target band was quantified using ImageJ software mentioned above.

### Statistical analysis
Statistical analyses were performed using SPSS version 16.0 (SPSS, Chicago, IL, USA). All data are expressed as mean ± standard deviation (SD). Differences between groups were analyzed using Student's t-test. In cases of multiple-group testing, one-way analysis of variance was conducted. Pearson correlation test was used to analyze the correlation between the expression difference of genes and the clinical parameters. A two-tailed value of $p < 0.05$ was considered statistically significant.

## Results

### Transcriptomic alterations in the concave and convex side of paravertebral muscle of AIS patients

RNA-seq was performed for 5 pairs of paravertebral muscle tissues from 5 AIS patients. Differentially expressed genes (DEG) analysis using the R-based DESeq package identified a total of 40 genes differentially expressed between the convex and concave side of paravertebral muscles. The gene expression profiles of the sample were visualized and compared using the heat maps (Fig. 1a). DEGs (showed in Additional file 1: Table S3) in two sides of paravertebral muscles of AIS patients clustered together and there were 16 genes higher expressed in the convex side relative to the concave side.

To understand the biological meaning of DEGs, KEGG enrichment analysis of DEGs were conducted. The prominently over-represented pathways included those for peroxisome proliferator-activated receptor (PPAR) signaling pathway (fold enrichment = 31.5; $p = 3.01E-07$; FDR = 1.38E-05), glycolysis/gluconeogenesis (fold enrichment = 20.3; $p = 3.75E-04$; FDR = 6.84E-03), adipocytokine signaling pathway (fold enrichment = 19.2; $p = 4.46E-04$; FDR = 6.84E-03), pyruvate metabolism (fold enrichment = 21.8; $p = 3.62E-03$; FDR = 4.17E-02) and vascular smooth muscle contraction (fold enrichment = 7.6; $p = 2.77E-02$; FDR = 2.54E-01) (Fig. 1b). It is interesting to note that several genes related with PPAR signaling pathway, such as PCK1, FABP4, SCD, PLIN1, ADIPOQ, MSTN, showed a higher expression in the concave side of the paravertebral muscles, since PPAR signaling pathway plays a major regulatory role in postnatal myogenesis and muscle fiber type (Wang et al. 2004; Chandrashekar et al. 2015).

### Significantly differentially expressed transcripts between two sides of paravertebral muscle of AIS patients

To test the quality of RNA-seq, we screened for the expression of 5 PPAR signaling pathway related genes (FABP4, SCD, PLIN1, ADIPOQ, MSTN, the expression of PCK1 was not quantified as its expression level was too low to be detected by qPCR) using qPCR in a series of 10 pairs of muscle samples from AIS patients. In addition, H19, a long noncoding RNA functioning in skeletal muscle differentiation and regeneration (Dey et al. 2014), which showed a differential expression in RNA-seq results, was also included. At first, we investigated the expression of specific markers of adipocytes (PPARγ, C/EBPα) and myocytes (Myog, MHC) to ensure a similar muscle tissue rate biopsy in each side (Additional file 1: Figure S2). The mRNA of ADIPOQ, FABP4, and MSTN genes showed significantly higher expressions ($p < 0.001$, 0.027, 0.004, respectively), while H19 showed significantly lower expression in concave-sided muscle tissue ($p = 0.023$) (Fig. 2a) when compared to convex-side.

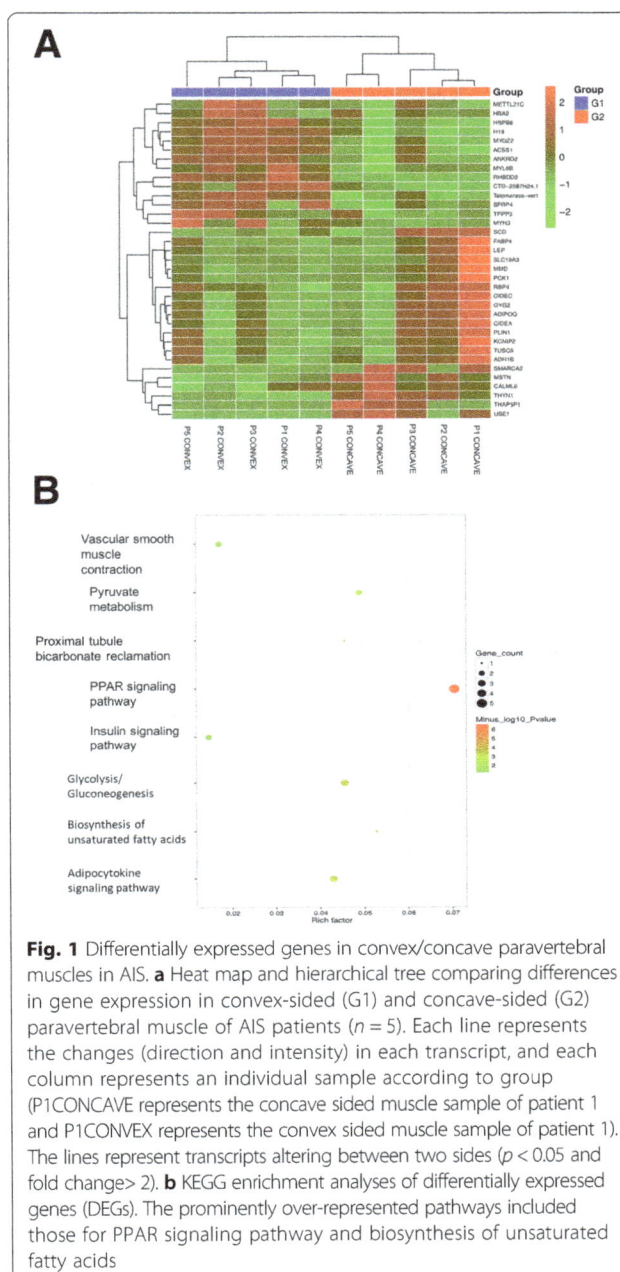

Fig. 1 Differentially expressed genes in convex/concave paravertebral muscles in AIS. **a** Heat map and hierarchical tree comparing differences in gene expression in convex-sided (G1) and concave-sided (G2) paravertebral muscle of AIS patients ($n = 5$). Each line represents the changes (direction and intensity) in each transcript, and each column represents an individual sample according to group (P1CONCAVE represents the concave sided muscle sample of patient 1 and P1CONVEX represents the convex sided muscle sample of patient 1). The lines represent transcripts altering between two sides ($p < 0.05$ and fold change> 2). **b** KEGG enrichment analyses of differentially expressed genes (DEGs). The prominently over-represented pathways included those for PPAR signaling pathway and biosynthesis of unsaturated fatty acids

Since the expression of ADIPOQ mRNA and H19 showed the most significant difference and recent studies have uncovered that they both play fundamental roles in regulation of muscle metabolic and contractile function (Dey et al. 2014; Iwabu et al. 2010), we measured ADIPOQ mRNA and H19 expressions in a second AIS cohort of 50 pairs of muscle tissues to validate the differential expression. Both genes showed significantly differential expression (ADIPOQ, $p < 0.001$; H19, $p = 0.040$) in two sides of the paravertebral muscles (Fig. 2b).

To verify whether the mRNA of ADIPOQ and H19 are also dysregulated in patients with congenital scoliosis

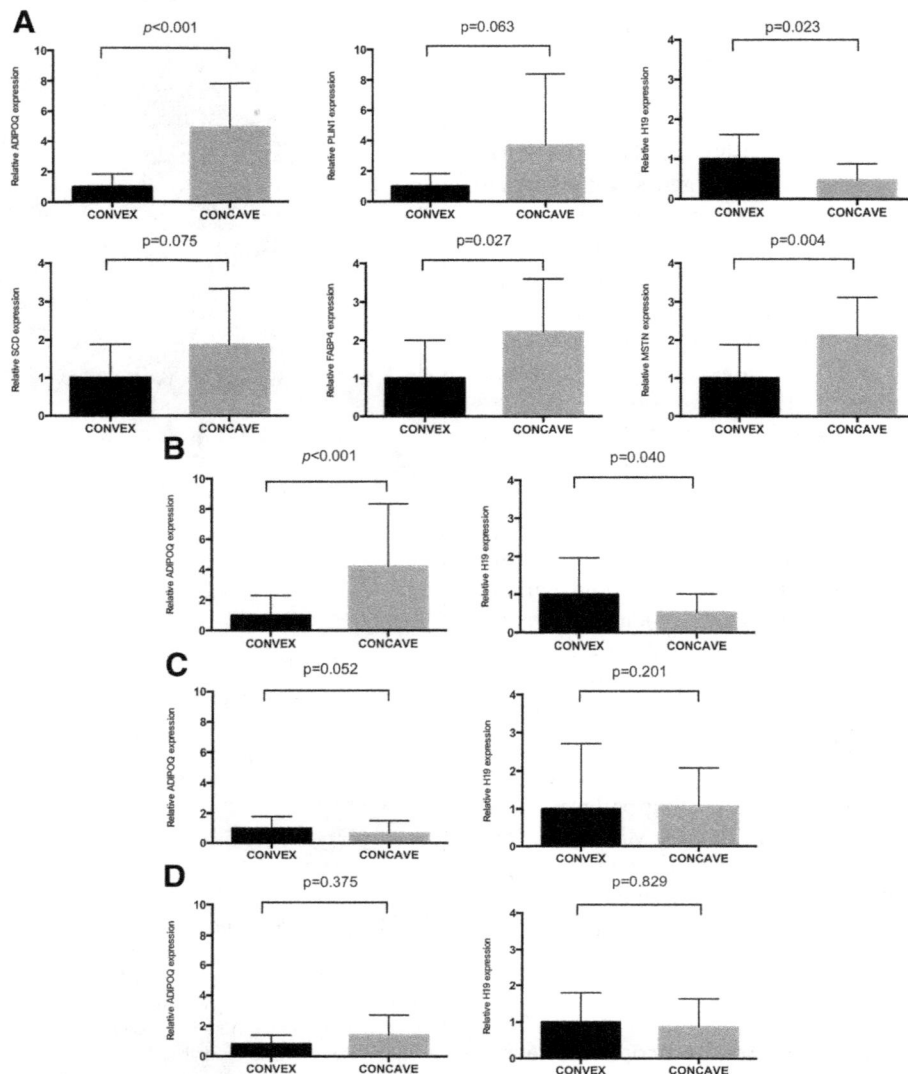

**Fig. 2** H19 and ADIPOQ mRNA is significantly differentially expressed between two sides of paravertebral muscle of AIS patients. Paravertebral muscles were obtained during the fusion surgery. Tissue samples were processed for assessment of expression of mRNA of PPAR signaling pathway related genes (SCD, FABP4, ADIPOQ, PLIN1, MSTN) and H19, as described in Materials and Methods. For (**a**) AIS patients (n = 10), the mRNA of ADIPOQ, FABP4, MSTN genes and H19 showed significantly differential expression in concave/convex muscle tissues. For (**b**) AIS patients (n = 50), ADIPOQ mRNA and H19 are still significantly differentially expressed between two sides of muscle tissues. For (**c**) age-matched CS group (n = 25), ADIPOQ mRNA or H19 expression showed no significant difference between convex and concave sided muscle tissue. For (**d**) age-matched non-AIS group (n = 16), ADIPOQ mRNA or H19 expression showed no significant difference between right and left sided muscle tissue. Results are expressed as mean ± SEM, and the relative expression of the studied genes are represented as fold change related to the convex side

(CS), we assessed ADIPOQ mRNA and H19 expression in 25 paired muscle samples of CS. Neither ADIPOQ mRNA nor H19 expression showed significant differences between convex and concave sided muscle tissue (p = 0.052 and 0.201, respectively) (Fig. 2c).

To further ascertain whether this differential expression was specifically present in AIS patients, we analyzed ADIPOQ mRNA and H19 expression in muscle tissues obtained from a series of 16 age-matched patients undergoing spinal surgery for thoracic spinal

fracture. Neither ADIPOQ mRNA nor H19 expression showed significant differences between right and left sided muscle tissue (p = 0.375 and 0.829 respectively) (Fig. 2d).

**ADIPOQ and H19 expression in patients with AIS is associated with curve severity and age at initiation**

Then we were interested in comparing features of clinical characteristics, such as the magnitude of spinal curve, age at menarche, body mass index and age at initiation, between different samples with different ADIPOQ and H19 expression patterns. We classified the enrolled 60 AIS patients studied in Fig. 2 as group A and group B. In group A, the expression level of H19 was lower and ADIPOQ mRNA higher in concave-sided muscle tissues compared with the corresponding convex side (low H19/high ADIPOQ). And the remained patients were included in group B. Patients in group A showed a larger magnitude of spinal curve ($p = 0.031$) and earlier age at initiation ($p = 0.032$) compared with that of group B. And patients in group A tend to have a decreased BMI, but the difference is not significant ($p = 0.056$) (Fig. 3).

We also performed correlation analysis to identify whether gene expression difference between two sides of paravertebral muscles was related to these clinical parameters. The relative expression difference of H19 (concave-convex) was significantly correlated with Cobb's angle ($r = 0.638$, $p < 0.001$) and age at initiation ($r = -0.295$, $p = 0.011$) (Fig. 4a-c), and the relative expression difference of ADPOQ mRNA (concave-convex) was also significantly correlated with spinal curve ($r = -0.4926$, $p < 0.001$) and age at initiation ($r = 0.230$, $p = 0.039$) (Fig. 4b, c). The expression difference of H19 or ADIPOQ mRNA

showed no significant correlation with patients' age at menarche or BMI (Additional file 1: Figure S3).

### H19 regulated the expression of ADIPOQ by miR-675-5p

H19 is a long non-coding RNA of which transcription persists only in skeletal muscle in adult, and functions as a primary miRNA precursor for microRNA-675 (miR-675) which generates two mature miRNAs, namely miR-675-5p and miR-675-3p (Lewis et al. 2016). MiR-675-5p and miR-675-3p mediate the regulatory function of H19 in skeletal muscle differentiation (Dey et al. 2014). So, we quantified expression of miR-675-5p and miR-675-3p using qRT-PCR in AIS patients and identified that both of two miRNA showed significantly higher expressions in convex-sided muscle tissue (Fig. 5a, Additional file 1: Figure S4A). Moreover, we demonstrated that the expression levels of miR-675-5p and miR-675-3p in muscle tissue were positively correlated with that of H19 ($r = 0.701$, $p < 0.001$; $r = 0.689$, $p < 0.001$, respectively) (Fig. 5b, Additional file 1: Figure S4B).

The miRNA machinery is a regulator of gene expression and we assumed that this kind of epigenetic regulation was involved in the imbalanced ADIPOQ expression as the expression difference of ADIPOQ

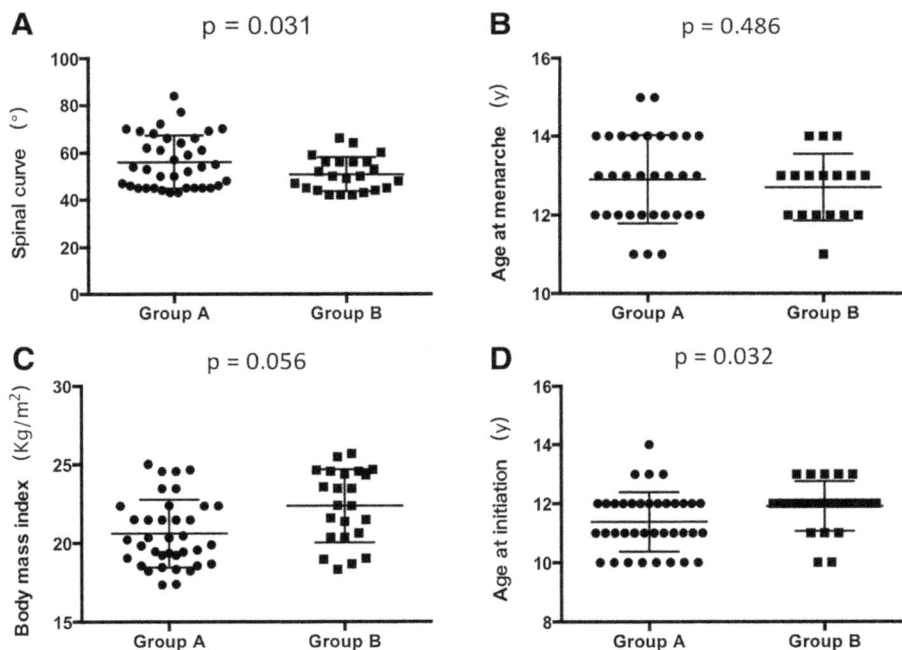

**Fig. 3** ADIPOQ mRNA and H19 expression pattern in paravertebral muscles of AIS patients is associated with curve severity and age at initiation. Patients with lower H19 and higher ADIPOQ mRNA expression levels in concave-sided muscles were included in Group A ($n = 37$), and the remained patients were included in group B ($n = 23$). For (**a**), Patients in Group A showed a bigger spinal curve ($p = 0.031$) compared with patients in Group B. For (**b**), Group A and Group B showed no difference in age at menarche ($p = 0.486$). For (**c**), Patients in Group A tended to have a declined body mass index (BMI) ($p = 0.056$). For (D), Patients in Group A ($n = 37$) showed an earlier age at initiation ($p = 0.032$) compared with patients in Group B ($n = 23$). Results are expressed as mean ± SEM

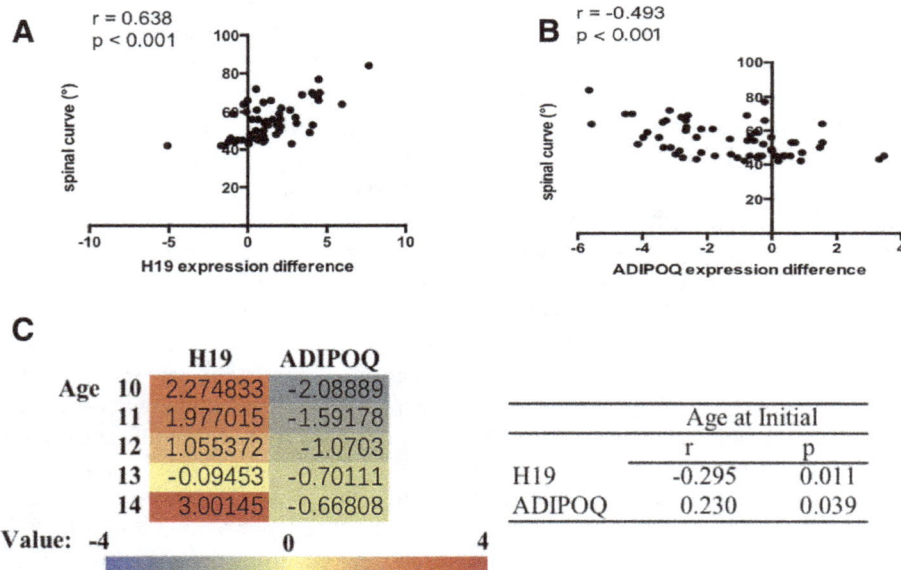

**Fig. 4** Expression difference of H19 and ADIPOQ mRNA in paravertebral muscles of AIS patients is associated with curve severity and age at initiation. The relative expression difference of studied genes was calculated as the relative expression level of one gene in concave sided muscle minus that in convex sided. For (**a**), correlation analysis identified that the relative expression difference of H19 in AIS patients ($n = 60$) was positively correlated with the magnitude of spinal curve. For (**b**), the relative expression difference of ADIPOQ mRNA in AIS patients ($n = 60$) was negatively correlated with the magnitude of spinal curve. For (**c**), Heat map showed significant correlation of the expression difference of H19 and ADIPOQ mRNA in AIS patients ($n = 60$) with age at initiation of AIS

mRNA represented an opposite direction compared with H19. We performed bioinformatics algorithms using RNA22 software scanning for miRNAs potentially targeting ADIPOQ mRNA (Miranda et al. 2006). The transcript of ADIPOQ was found to contain several putative miR-675-5p-binding sites but not miR-675-3p (Additional file 1: Table S4). Among these, miR-675-5p possessed the maximum likelihood of binding to the 3'UTR of ADIPOQ (3403–3428 nt) ($\Delta G = -17.70$Kcal/mol). Thus, we chose this target site and subcoloned the 3'UTR of ADIPOQ mRNA in the Renillaluciferase expression cassette (Luc-3'UTR) of a luciferase reporter construct. The ectopic overexpression of miR-675-5p significantly ($p < 0.0001$) inhibited luciferase activity in the ADIPOQ construct, while mutation of the miR-675-5p-binding site abolished the inhibitory effect of miR-675-5p on ADIPOQ reporter activity (Fig. 5c). Then we assessed the expression of ADIPOQ in HSMCs overexpressing miR-675-5p. Compared with the negative control, miR-675-5p substantially reduced the protein levels of ADIPOQ during HSMC differentiation (Fig. 5d). In a reciprocal experiment, we inhibited the endogenous miR-675-5p using antisense inhibitor and observed increased levels of ADIPOQ (Fig. 5e). These data demonstrate that miR-675-5p can silence ADIPOQ expression, which is also reflected in vivo where a significant ($r = -0.615$, $p < 0.001$, Fig. 5f) inverse correlation of

ADIPOQ mRNA and miR-675-5p expression in muscle samples studied in Fig. 2.

### H19 expression was regulated by CTCF occupancy in the H19 imprinting control region (ICR)

H19 is an imprinted gene, which is abundantly expressed maternally in embryonic tissues but is strongly repressed after birth (Dey et al. 2014; Keniry et al. 2012; Gabory et al. 2010). The H19- insulin like growth factor (IGF2) gene locus contains differentially methylated regions that control parent-of-origin expression. It is reported that epigenetic-related dysregulation of H19 may play complex roles in different disorders, including stenotic aortic valves disease (Hadji et al. 2016). Thus, we profiled both sides of paravertebral muscles for the level of CpG methylation in the promoter region of H19 ($\sim -900$ bp from the transcription start site) and found no differences between two sides (Additional file 1: Figure S6).

The CTCF protein binding to the ICR of the H19 gene promotes enhancer function at the H19 prompter, which is another important mechanism controlling H19 expression (Ideraabdullah et al. 2011; Phillips and Corces 2009). To determine the differences of the CTCF-binding status at the H19 ICR, we analyzed the levels of CTCF occupancy in this region ($\sim -4$ k bp from the transcription start site) in both sides of paravertebral muscles using CHIP assay. The occupancy of CTCF

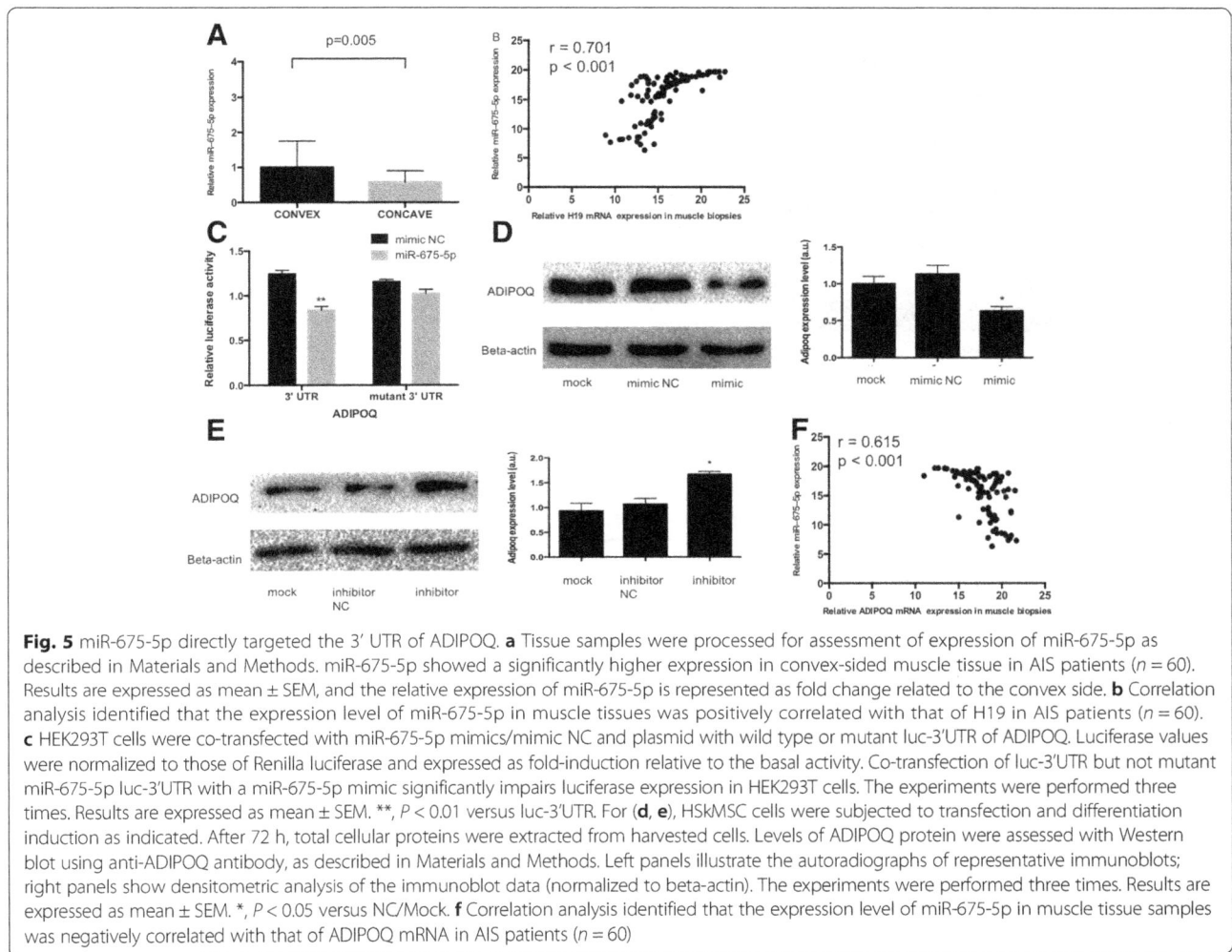

**Fig. 5** miR-675-5p directly targeted the 3' UTR of ADIPOQ. **a** Tissue samples were processed for assessment of expression of miR-675-5p as described in Materials and Methods. miR-675-5p showed a significantly higher expression in convex-sided muscle tissue in AIS patients (n = 60). Results are expressed as mean ± SEM, and the relative expression of miR-675-5p is represented as fold change related to the convex side. **b** Correlation analysis identified that the expression level of miR-675-5p in muscle tissues was positively correlated with that of H19 in AIS patients (n = 60). **c** HEK293T cells were co-transfected with miR-675-5p mimics/mimic NC and plasmid with wild type or mutant luc-3'UTR of ADIPOQ. Luciferase values were normalized to those of Renilla luciferase and expressed as fold-induction relative to the basal activity. Co-transfection of luc-3'UTR but not mutant miR-675-5p luc-3'UTR with a miR-675-5p mimic significantly impairs luciferase expression in HEK293T cells. The experiments were performed three times. Results are expressed as mean ± SEM. **, $P < 0.01$ versus luc-3'UTR. For (**d**, **e**), HSkMSC cells were subjected to transfection and differentiation induction as indicated. After 72 h, total cellular proteins were extracted from harvested cells. Levels of ADIPOQ protein were assessed with Western blot using anti-ADIPOQ antibody, as described in Materials and Methods. Left panels illustrate the autoradiographs of representative immunoblots; right panels show densitometric analysis of the immunoblot data (normalized to beta-actin). The experiments were performed three times. Results are expressed as mean ± SEM. *, $P < 0.05$ versus NC/Mock. **f** Correlation analysis identified that the expression level of miR-675-5p in muscle tissue samples was negatively correlated with that of ADIPOQ mRNA in AIS patients (n = 60)

protein in the H19 ICR significantly decreased in the concave-sided muscle tissue (Fig. 6).

## Discussion

AIS is a common and unexplained spinal deformity in children and poses an increasing burden on global health. The phenotypic heterogeneity of AIS patients makes it difficult to form any efficient strategy to prevent this disease or its progression (Altaf et al. 2013). One of the biggest challenges in etiologic research of AIS is that the affected individuals present no obvious structural deficiencies or pathologic changes in the vertebral column and associated soft tissues, expect the curvation of the spine (Weinstein and Dolan 2015). So numerous theories have been put forward to define the disease mechanisms, including genetic predisposition (Gorman et al. 2012), neuromuscular dysfunction (Wajchenberg et al. 2016), and environment factors (Burwell et al. 2011). The fact that scoliosis is frequently seen as a part of the phenotypic spectrum of heritable

syndromes, in particular, disorders of neuromuscular development, also serves as a reminder of the importance of the muscle imbalance in AIS pathogenesis (Hresko 2013). By studying the differentially expressed transcripts between two sides of paravertebral muscle of AIS patients, we aimed to identify drivers or key molecules for AIS-associated paravertebral muscle changes.

Here, we demonstrate that H19 shows a higher expression in convex-sided muscle and ADIPOQ higher expression in concave side. H19 is a paternally-imprinted gene that does not encode a protein, but rather a 2.3-Kb ncRNA (Borensztein et al. 2013). It is reported that H19 can promote skeletal muscle differentiation and regeneration (Dey et al. 2014), and regulate glucose metabolism in muscle cells as well (Gao et al. 2014). Adiponectin (ApN) encoded by ADIPOQ gene, is a circulating hormone and it has been demonstrated that during skeletal muscle differentiation, myotubes represent an autocrine system for ApN production (Fiaschi et al. 2009). In addition, low ADIPOQ expression associates with

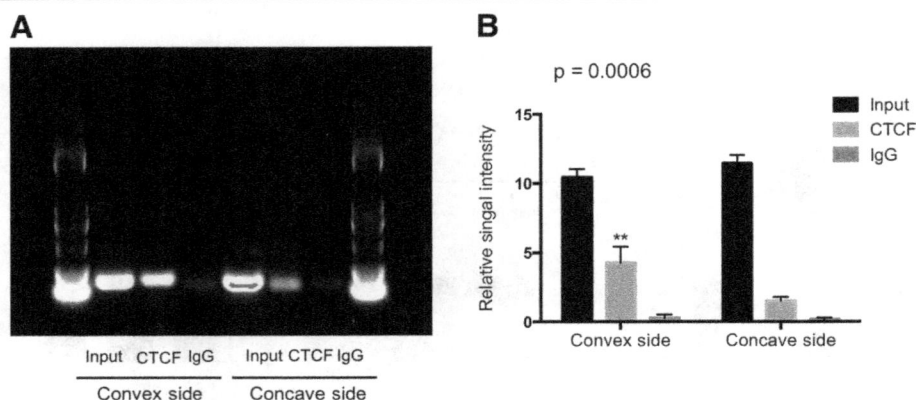

**Fig. 6** H19 expression was regulated by CTCF occupancy in the H19 imprinting control region. **a, b** Paravertebral muscles were harvested from AIS patients during the fusion surgery. The tissues were subjected to Nuclei preparation and chromatin digestion, and the CTCF-binding status at the H19 ICR were assessed with CHIP assay, as described in Materials and Methods. **a** represent electrophoretogram of PCR product by 10% polyacrylamide gel electrophoresis. **b** CTCF occupancy in the H19 ICR showed significantly reduced occupancy in the concave-sided muscle tissue samples. The experiments were performed three times. Results are expressed as mean ± SEM. $n = 4$ in each group. **, $P < 0.01$ versus concave side

degenerative muscle disease, such as Duchenne muscular dystrophy (Abou-Samra et al. 2015). Here, we demonstrate for the first time that H19 and ADIPOQ expressions are inconsistent in two sides of the paravertebral muscle in AIS patients.

Our data demonstrate that lower H19 levels and higher ADIPOQ levels in concave-sided muscle tissues significantly correlate with larger spinal curve and earlier age at initiation. Moreover, our data demonstrate that the relative differential expression of H19 and ADIPOQ (concave-convex) significantly correlate with spinal curve and age at initiation. But we didn't find asymmetric expression of H19 or ADIPOQ between two sides of paravertebral muscles of age-matched CS patients or non-scoliotic controls. Taken together, the evidence suggests that an asymmetric expression of H19 and ADIPOQ is a relatively specific event in AIS disease progression.

In this study, we identified imbalanced-expressed H19 regulatory mechanism that induces ADIPOQ differential expression in two sides of paravertebral muscles in AIS. We demonstrate that ADIPOQ mRNA is targeted by miR-675-5p, a miRNA encoded by H19. Consistent with this, the expression levels of miR-675-5p in muscle tissues positively correlate with that of H19 and negatively correlate with that of ADIPOQ. H19-derived miR-675-5p has been reported to directly target DNA replication initiation factor Cdc6 to promote skeletal muscle differentiation (Dey et al. 2014) and inhibit adipocyte differentiation of mesenchymal stem cells through down-regulating HDACs (Huang et al. 2016). Our data demonstrate that ADIPOQ is a novel target gene of miR-675-5p.

Muscle derived ApN has been reported to participate in the activation of autophagy, which is required for muscle differentiation (Gamberi et al. 2016). In skeletal muscle, ApN exerts its metabolic effects through

adiponectin receptor1 (AdipoR1) (Delaigle et al. 2004). ApN has been suggested as a main effector in the regulation of muscle lipid metabolism by stimulating fatty-acid oxidation (Yamauchi et al. 2002). Thus dysregulated ADIPOQ expression may contribute to the fatty infiltration imbalance of paravertebral muscle in AIS (Additional file 1: Figure S7) (Jiang et al. 2017). ApN has also been reported to modulate oxidative stress-induced mitophagy and alleviate skeletal muscle inflammation through miR-711 (Boursereau et al. 2017). In consideration of oxidative stress and local inflammation have been associated with muscle dysfunction (Acharyya et al. 2007; Powers et al. 2012), the lower ADIPOQ levels in the convex-sided muscle may contribute to the paravertebral muscle weakness in convex side (Martinez-Llorens et al. 2010). On the other hand, ApN has been reported to increase mitochondria and oxidative myofiber in skeletal muscle through activation of CaMKK, AMPK, SIRT1, which were correlated with increased type I myofiber, insulin resistance and exercise endurance and supported the view of stronger muscle contraction of concave-sided paravertebral muscle in AIS (Iwabu et al. 2010; Abou-Samra et al. 2015). The existence of an increased proportion of type I fibers on the convex-sided paravertebral muscles in AIS suggests the existence of additional regulatory mechanisms of myofiber identity and muscle performance.

Epigenetic mechanisms, including DNA methylation and transcription regulator CTCF have been reported to be involved in the regulation of H19 expression (32). Loss of CTCF binding, regional CpG methylation and spread of heterochromatin have been shown in different disorders such as myotonic dystrophy caused by expanded CTG repeats (Cho et al. 2005). We evaluated in both sides of paravertebral muscles the level of CTCF occupancy in

ICR and found reduced CTCF occupancy in the concave side. On the other hand, CpG methylation level in the promoter region of H19 showed no significant difference. These data thus suggest that CTCF occupancy changes in ICR of H19 might contribute to dysregulation of its expression in AIS. However, the mechanism of altered CTCF occupancy in two sides of muscle tissue in AIS remains unknown. There is increasing evidence that several environmental factors, such as dietary factors and sports, can reshape the epigenome and cause transcriptional changes in different tissues including skeletal muscle (Jacobsen et al. 2012; Feil and Fraga 2012). In one study, a 3-month exercise training was shown to induce modifications in DNA methylation that were associated to gene expression changes concordant with muscle functional and structural remodeling (Lindholm et al. 2014). Interestingly, some environmental factors have been reported to be involved in the etiopathogenesis and phenotypic expression of AIS (Burwell et al. 2011; Grivas et al. 2006; McMaster 2011). It has been reported that AIS to be positively associated with classical ballet training (Watanabe et al. 2017) and negatively associated with skating and horse riding classes (McMaster et al. 2015). Hence, further work is necessary to examine whether and how these factors alter CTCF occupancy of ICR of H19, particularly in the context of AIS.

The mRNA of MSTN gene showed significantly higher expressions in concave-sided muscle tissue in the first cohort ($n = 10$). But the difference was not significant in the second cohort ($n = 50$, Additional file 1: Figure S5). Myostatin, encoded by MSTN, is predominantly expressed in skeletal muscles and is a potent negative regulator of muscle growth and development (Rodriguez et al. 2014). It has been demonstrated that the muscle volumetric imbalance occur in all of the levels of the vertebrae involved in the major curve of AIS with larger muscle volume on the convex side (Jiang et al. 2017). Myostatin inactivation can induce skeletal muscle hypertrophy, while its overexpression or systemic administration causes muscle atrophy (Rodriguez et al. 2014; Sharma et al. 2015b). In our study, no difference expression of MSTN in AIS patients suggests the existence of additional regulatory mechanisms of muscle mass. In addition, KEGG enrichment analysis of DEGs showed genes involved in pathways of glycolysis/gluconeogenesis, adipocytokine signaling pathway, pyruvate metabolism and vascular smooth muscle contraction may be associated with the imbalance of paravertebral muscle in AIS patients. It is worthwhile to note that MYH3 expression showed imbalance in RNA-seq. MYH3 encodes embryonic myosin and its mutations contribute to spondylocarpotarsal synostosis (SCT), which is a skeletal disorder characterized by fused vertebrae (including scoliosis and lordosis) and fused carpal and tarsal joints

(Cameron-Christie et al. 2018). And it is reported that MYH3 SCT mutations may influence the mechanics of contractility in muscle fibers between the neural arches and lead to SCT (Zieba et al. 2017). Whether the asymmetric expression of MYH3 in convex/concave paravertebral muscles is involved in the etiology of AIS should be further validated.

## Conclusion

We provide evidence that H19 and ADIPOQ are expressed inconsistently in paravertebral muscles, and more importantly, lower H19 levels and higher ADIPOQ levels in concave-sided muscle tissues positively correlate with spinal curve and age at initiation. These data suggest an important role of H19 and ADIPOQ in the onset or progression of scoliosis. Our results imply AIS may be a disease of genetically predisposed individuals with some environmental stress, which influence the epigenome and transcriptional changes in paravertebral muscles, overwhelm the stability of the spine and result in scoliosis, which can expand our etiologic understanding of this disease.

## Additional file

**Additional file 1: Table S1.** Clinical characteristics of enrolled AIS patients. **Table S2.** Sequence of RNA and DNA Oligonucleotides. **Table S3.** Differentially expressed genes (DEG) from RNA-seq. **Table S4.** The miR-675-5p potential target sites in ADIPOQ transcript according to the RNA22 software. **Figure S1.** Representative radiographic data of the CS patients enrolled in this study. **Figure S2.** Similar muscle tissue rate biopsy in each side of AIS patients. **Figure S3.** Expression difference of H19 or ADIPOQ mRNA in paravertebral muscles of AIS patients is not associated with age at menarche and BMI. **Figure S4.** The relative expression of miR-675-3p in concave/convex sided paravertebral muscles and the correlation of the expression level between miR-675-3p and miR-675-5p. **Figure S5.** The relative expression of MSTN mRNA in a larger AIS cohort. **Figure S6.** CpG methylation in the promoter region of H19 showed no difference between two sides of AIS patients. **Figure S7.** Fatty infiltration imbalance of deep paravertebral muscles in AIS patients. (DOCX 4564 kb)

### Abbreviations
AIS: Adolescent idiopathic scoliosis; CCTF: CCCTC-binding factor; CS: Congenital scoliosis; DEG: Differentially expressed genes; ICR: Imprinting control region; SNPs: Single nucleotide polymorphisms

### Funding
This study was supported by grants from the National Natural Science Foundation of China (81772305).

### Authors' contributions
HJ analyzed and interpreted the RNA-seq data and was a major contributor in writing the manuscript. FY analyzed the RNA-seq data, performed cell culture and differentiation, and was a major contributor in writing the manuscript. TL collected the muscle tissue, performed the qRT-PCR the transplant, and was a major contributor in writing the manuscript. WS analyzed the clinical

information of the patients and modified the manuscript. YCM performed cell transfection and collected the clinical information of the patients enrolled. JM performed luciferase reporter assay and analyzed the RNA-seq data. CW performed western blotting assay and analyzed the clinical information of the patients. RG performed the ChIP assay, modified the manuscript and guided the revision of the manuscript. XHZ collected the muscle tissue and modified the manuscript. All authors read and approved the final manuscript.

## Competing interests

The authors declare that they have no competing interests.

## Author details

[1]Department of Orthopedics, Changzheng Hospital, Second Military Medical University, No.415 Fengyang Road, Shanghai, People's Republic of China. [2]Department of Medical Genetics, Second Military Medical University, Shanghai, People's Republic of China. [3]Shanghai Key Laboratory of Cell Engineering (14DZ2272300), Shanghai, People's Republic of China.

## References

Abou-Samra M, Lecompte S, Schakman O, Noel L, Many MC, Gailly P, et al. Involvement of adiponectin in the pathogenesis of dystrophinopathy. Skelet Muscle. 2015;5:25.

Acharyya S, Villalta SA, Bakkar N, Bupha-Intr T, Janssen PM, Carathers M, et al. Interplay of IKK/NF-kappaB signaling in macrophages and myofibers promotes muscle degeneration in Duchenne muscular dystrophy. J Clin Invest. 2007;117(4):889–901.

Altaf F, Gibson A, Dannawi Z, Noordeen H. Adolescent idiopathic scoliosis. BMJ. 2013;346:f2508.

Borensztein M, Monnier P, Court F, Louault Y, Ripoche MA, Tiret L, et al. Myod and H19-Igf2 locus interactions are required for diaphragm formation in the mouse. Development. 2013;140(6):1231–9.

Boswell CW, Ciruna B. Understanding idiopathic scoliosis: a new zebrafish School of Thought. Trends Genet. 2017;33(3):183–96.

Boursereau R, Abou-Samra M, Lecompte S, Noel L, Brichard SM. New targets to alleviate skeletal muscle inflammation: role of microRNAs regulated by adiponectin. Sci Rep. 2017;7:43437.

Buchan JG, Alvarado DM, Haller GE, Cruchaga C, Harms MB, Zhang T, et al. Rare variants in FBN1 and FBN2 are associated with severe adolescent idiopathic scoliosis. Hum Mol Genet. 2014;23(19):5271–82.

Burwell RG, Dangerfield PH, Moulton A, Grivas TB. Adolescent idiopathic scoliosis (AIS), environment, exposome and epigenetics: a molecular perspective of postnatal normal spinal growth and the etiopathogenesis of AIS with consideration of a network approach and possible implications for medical therapy. Scoliosis. 2011;6(1):26.

Cameron-Christie SR, Wells CF, Simon M, Wessels M, Tang CZN, Wei W, et al. Recessive Spondylocarpotarsal synostosis syndrome due to compound heterozygosity for variants in MYH3. Am J Hum Genet. 2018;102(6):1115–25.

Chandrashekar P, Manickam R, Ge X, Bonala S, McFarlane C, Sharma M, et al. Inactivation of PPARbeta/delta adversely affects satellite cells and reduces postnatal myogenesis. Am J Physiol Endocrinol Metab. 2015;309(2):E122–31.

Cho DH, Thienes CP, Mahoney SE, Analau E, Filippova GN, Tapscott SJ. Antisense transcription and heterochromatin at the DM1 CTG repeats are constrained by CTCF. Mol Cell. 2005;20(3):483–9.

Delaigle AM, Jonas JC, Bauche IB, Cornu O, Brichard SM. Induction of adiponectin in skeletal muscle by inflammatory cytokines: in vivo and in vitro studies. Endocrinology. 2004;145(12):5589–97.

Dey BK, Pfeifer K, Dutta A. The H19 long noncoding RNA gives rise to microRNAs miR-675-3p and miR-675-5p to promote skeletal muscle differentiation and regeneration. Genes Dev. 2014;28(5):491–501.

Feil R, Fraga MF. Epigenetics and the environment: emerging patterns and implications. Nat Rev Genet. 2012;13(2):97–109.

Fiaschi T, Cirelli D, Comito G, Gelmini S, Ramponi G, Serio M, et al. Globular adiponectin induces differentiation and fusion of skeletal muscle cells. Cell Res. 2009;19(5):584–97.

Gabory A, Jammes H, Dandolo L. The H19 locus: role of an imprinted non-coding RNA in growth and development. BioEssays. 2010;32(6):473–80.

Gamberi T, Modesti A, Magherini F, D'Souza DM, Hawke T, Fiaschi T. Activation of autophagy by globular adiponectin is required for muscle differentiation. Biochim Biophys Acta. 2016;1863(4):694–702.

Gao Y, Wu F, Zhou J, Yan L, Jurczak MJ, Lee HY, et al. The H19/let-7 double-negative feedback loop contributes to glucose metabolism in muscle cells. Nucleic Acids Res. 2014;42(22):13799–811.

Gorman KF, Julien C, Moreau A. The genetic epidemiology of idiopathic scoliosis. European spine journal : official publication of the European Spine Society, the European Spinal Deformity Society, and the European Section of the Cervical Spine Research Society. 2012;21(10):1905–19.

Grimes DT, Boswell CW, Morante NF, Henkelman RM, Burdine RD, Ciruna B. Zebrafish models of idiopathic scoliosis link cerebrospinal fluid flow defects to spine curvature. Science. 2016;352(6291):1341–4.

Grivas TB, Vasiliadis E, Mouzakis V, Mihas C, Koufopoulos G. Association between adolescent idiopathic scoliosis prevalence and age at menarche in different geographic latitudes. Scoliosis. 2006;1:9.

Hadji F, Boulanger MC, Guay SP, Gaudreault N, Amellah S, Mkannez G, et al. Altered DNA methylation of long noncoding RNA H19 in calcific aortic valve disease promotes mineralization by silencing NOTCH1. Circulation. 2016; 134(23):1848–62.

Haller G, Alvarado D, McCall K, Yang P, Cruchaga C, Harms M, et al. A polygenic burden of rare variants across extracellular matrix genes among individuals with adolescent idiopathic scoliosis. Hum Mol Genet. 2016;25(1):202–9.

Hong SN, Joung JG, Bae JS, Lee CS, Koo JS, Park SJ, et al. RNA-seq reveals transcriptomic differences in inflamed and noninflamed intestinal mucosa of Crohn's disease patients compared with Normal mucosa of healthy controls. Inflamm Bowel Dis. 2017;23(7):1098–108.

Hresko MT. Clinical practice. Idiopathic scoliosis in adolescents. N Engl J Med. 2013;368(9):834–41.

Huang Y, Zheng Y, Jin C, Li X, Jia L, Li W. Long non-coding RNA H19 inhibits adipocyte differentiation of bone marrow mesenchymal stem cells through epigenetic modulation of histone deacetylases. Sci Rep. 2016;6:28897.

Ideraabdullah FY, Abramowitz LK, Thorvaldsen JL, Krapp C, Wen SC, Engel N, et al. Novel cis-regulatory function in ICR-mediated imprinted repression of H19. Dev Biol. 2011;355(2):349–57.

Iwabu M, Yamauchi T, Okada-Iwabu M, Sato K, Nakagawa T, Funata M, et al. Adiponectin and AdipoR1 regulate PGC-1alpha and mitochondria by ca(2+) and AMPK/SIRT1. Nature. 2010;464(7293):1313–9.

Jacobsen SC, Brons C, Bork-Jensen J, Ribel-Madsen R, Yang B, Lara E, et al. Effects of short-term high-fat overfeeding on genome-wide DNA methylation in the skeletal muscle of healthy young men. Diabetologia. 2012;55(12):3341–9.

Jiang J, Meng Y, Jin X, Zhang C, Zhao J, Wang C, et al. Volumetric and fatty infiltration imbalance of deep paravertebral muscles in adolescent idiopathic scoliosis. Med Sci Monit. 2017;23:2089–95.

Keniry A, Oxley D, Monnier P, Kyba M, Dandolo L, Smits G, et al. The H19 lincRNA is a developmental reservoir of miR-675 that suppresses growth and Igf1r. Nat Cell Biol. 2012;14(7):659–65.

Kou I, Takahashi Y, Johnson TA, Takahashi A, Guo L, Dai J, et al. Genetic variants in GPR126 are associated with adolescent idiopathic scoliosis. Nat Genet. 2013;45(6):676–9.

Lewis A, Lee JY, Donaldson AV, Natanek SA, Vaidyanathan S, Man WD, et al. Increased expression of H19/miR-675 is associated with a low fat-free mass index in patients with COPD. J Cachexia Sarcopenia Muscle. 2016;7(3):330–44.

Lindholm ME, Marabita F, Gomez-Cabrero D, Rundqvist H, Ekstrom TJ, Tegner J, et al. An integrative analysis reveals coordinated reprogramming of the epigenome and the transcriptome in human skeletal muscle after training. Epigenetics. 2014;9(12):1557–69.

Lowe TG, Burwell RG, Dangerfield PH. Platelet calmodulin levels in adolescent idiopathic scoliosis (AIS): can they predict curve progression and severity? Summary of an electronic focus group debate of the IBSE. Eur Spine J. 2004; 13(3):257–65.

Martinez-Llorens J, Ramirez M, Colomina MJ, Bago J, Molina A, Caceres E, et al. Muscle dysfunction and exercise limitation in adolescent idiopathic scoliosis. Eur Respir J. 2010;36(2):393–400.

McMaster ME. Heated indoor swimming pools, infants, and the pathogenesis of adolescent idiopathic scoliosis: a neurogenic hypothesis. Environ Health : a global access science source. 2011;10:86.

McMaster ME, Lee AJ, Burwell RG. Physical activities of patients with adolescent idiopathic scoliosis (AIS): preliminary longitudinal case-control study historical evaluation of possible risk factors. Scoliosis. 2015;10:6.

Miranda KC, Huynh T, Tay Y, Ang YS, Tam WL, Thomson AM, et al. A pattern-based method for the identification of MicroRNA binding sites and their corresponding heteroduplexes. Cell. 2006;126(6):1203–17.

Noshchenko A, Hoffecker L, Lindley EM, Burger EL, Cain CM, Patel VV, et al. Predictors of spine deformity progression in adolescent idiopathic scoliosis: a systematic review with meta-analysis. World J Orthop. 2015;6(7):537–58.

Nowak R, Kwiecien M, Tkacz M, Mazurek U. Transforming growth factor-beta (TGF- beta) signaling in paravertebral muscles in juvenile and adolescent idiopathic scoliosis. Biomed Res Int. 2014;2014:594287.

Ogura Y, Kou I, Takahashi Y, Takeda K, Minami S, Kawakami N, et al. A functional variant in MIR4300HG, the host gene of microRNA MIR4300 is associated with progression of adolescent idiopathic scoliosis. Hum Mol Genet. 2017; 26(20):4086–92.

Phillips JE, Corces VG. CTCF: master weaver of the genome. Cell. 2009;137(7): 1194–211.

Powers SK, Smuder AJ, Judge AR. Oxidative stress and disuse muscle atrophy: cause or consequence? Current opinion in clinical nutrition and metabolic care. 2012;15(3):240–5.

Qiu Y, Mao SH, Qian BP, Jiang J, Qiu XS, Zhao Q, et al. A promoter polymorphism of neurotrophin 3 gene is associated with curve severity and bracing effectiveness in adolescent idiopathic scoliosis. Spine (Phila Pa 1976). 2012; 37(2):127–33.

Rodriguez J, Vernus B, Chelh I, Cassar-Malek I, Gabillard JC, Hadj Sassi A, et al. Myostatin and the skeletal muscle atrophy and hypertrophy signaling pathways. Cell Mol Life Sci. 2014;71(22):4361–71.

Salehi LB, Mangino M, De Serio S, De Cicco D, Capon F, Semprini S, et al. Assignment of a locus for autosomal dominant idiopathic scoliosis (IS) to human chromosome 17p11. Hum Genet. 2002;111(4–5):401–4.

Sharma M, McFarlane C, Kambadur R, Kukreti H, Bonala S, Srinivasan S. Myostatin: expanding horizons. IUBMB Life. 2015b;67(8):589–600.

Sharma S, Gao X, Londono D, Devroy SE, Mauldin KN, Frankel JT, et al. Genome-wide association studies of adolescent idiopathic scoliosis suggest candidate susceptibility genes. Hum Mol Genet. 2011;20(7):1456–66.

Sharma S, Londono D, Eckalbar WL, Gao X, Zhang D, Mauldin K, et al. A PAX1 enhancer locus is associated with susceptibility to idiopathic scoliosis in females. Nat Commun. 2015a;6:6452.

Stetkarova I, Zamecnik J, Bocek V, Vasko P, Brabec K, Krbec M. Electrophysiological and histological changes of paraspinal muscles in adolescent idiopathic scoliosis. Eur Spine J : official publication of the European Spine Society, the European Spinal Deformity Society, and the European Section of the Cervical Spine Research Society. 2016;25(10):3146–53.

Takahashi Y, Kou I, Takahashi A, Johnson TA, Kono K, Kawakami N, et al. A genome-wide association study identifies common variants near LBX1 associated with adolescent idiopathic scoliosis. Nat Genet. 2011;43(12):1237–40.

Wajchenberg M, Astur N, Kanas M, Martins DE. Adolescent idiopathic scoliosis: current concepts on neurological and muscular etiologies. Scoliosis Spinal Disord. 2016;11:4.

Wang YX, Zhang CL, Yu RT, Cho HK, Nelson MC, Bayuga-Ocampo CR, et al. Regulation of muscle fiber type and running endurance by PPARdelta. PLoS Biol. 2004;2(10):e294.

Watanabe K, Michikawa T, Yonezawa I, Takaso M, Minami S, Soshi S, et al. Physical activities and lifestyle factors related to adolescent idiopathic scoliosis. J Bone Joint Surg Am. 2017;99(4):284–94.

Weinstein SL, Dolan LA. The evidence base for the prognosis and treatment of adolescent idiopathic scoliosis: the 2015 Orthopaedic Research and Education Foundation clinical research award. J Bone Joint Surg Am. 2015; 97(22):1899–903.

Weinstein SL, Dolan LA, Wright JG, Dobbs MB. Effects of bracing in adolescents with idiopathic scoliosis. N Engl J Med. 2013;369(16):1512–21.

Wong C. Mechanism of right thoracic adolescent idiopathic scoliosis at risk for progression; a unifying pathway of development by normal growth and imbalance. Scoliosis. 2015;10:2.

Yamauchi T, Kamon J, Minokoshi Y, Ito Y, Waki H, Uchida S, et al. Adiponectin stimulates glucose utilization and fatty-acid oxidation by activating AMP-activated protein kinase. Nat Med. 2002;8(11):1288–95.

Zapata KA, Wang-Price SS, Sucato DJ, Dempsey-Robertson M. Ultrasonographic measurements of paraspinal muscle thickness in adolescent idiopathic scoliosis: a comparison and reliability study. Pediatr Phys Ther : the official publication of the Section on Pediatrics of the American Physical Therapy Association. 2015;27(2):119 25.

Zhu Z, Tang NL, Xu L, Qin X, Mao S, Song Y, et al. Genome-wide association study identifies new susceptibility loci for adolescent idiopathic scoliosis in Chinese girls. Nat Commun. 2015;6:8355.

Zieba J, Zhang W, Chong JX, Forlenza KN, Martin JH, Heard K, et al. A postnatal role for embryonic myosin revealed by MYH3 mutations that alter TGFβ signaling and cause autosomal dominant spondylocarpotarsal synostosis. Sci Rep. 2017;7(1):41803.

# 13

# Exploring the biological functional mechanism of the HMGB1/TLR4/MD-2 complex by surface plasmon resonance

Mingzhu He[1*] ⓘ, Marco E. Bianchi[2], Tom R. Coleman[1], Kevin J. Tracey[3] and Yousef Al-Abed[1*]

## Abstract

**Background:** High Mobility Group Box 1 (HMGB1) was first identified as a nonhistone chromatin-binding protein that functions as a pro-inflammatory cytokine and a Damage-Associated Molecular Pattern molecule when released from necrotic cells or activated leukocytes. HMGB1 consists of two structurally similar HMG boxes that comprise the pro-inflammatory (B-box) and the anti-inflammatory (A-box) domains. Paradoxically, the A-box also contains the epitope for the well-characterized anti-HMGB1 monoclonal antibody "2G7", which also potently inhibits HMGB1-mediated inflammation in a wide variety of in vivo models. The molecular mechanisms through which the A-box domain inhibits the inflammatory activity of HMGB1 and 2G7 exerts anti-inflammatory activity after binding the A-box domain have been a mystery. Recently, we demonstrated that: 1) the TLR4/MD-2 receptor is required for HMGB1-mediated cytokine production and 2) the HMGB1–TLR4/MD-2 interaction is controlled by the redox state of HMGB1 isoforms.

**Methods:** We investigated the interactions of HMGB1 isoforms (redox state) or HMGB1 fragments (A- and B-box) with TLR4/MD-2 complex using Surface Plasmon Resonance (SPR) studies.

**Results:** Our results demonstrate that: 1) intact HMGB1 binds to TLR4 via the A-box domain with high affinity but an appreciable dissociation rate; 2) intact HMGB1 binds to MD-2 via the B-box domain with low affinity but a very slow dissociation rate; and 3) HMGB1 A-box domain alone binds to TLR4 more stably than the intact protein and thereby antagonizes HMGB1 by blocking HMGB1 from interacting with the TLR4/MD-2 complex.

**Conclusions:** These findings not only suggest a model whereby HMGB1 interacts with TLR4/MD-2 in a two-stage process but also explain how the A-box domain and 2G7 inhibit HMGB1.

**Keywords:** HMGB1, TLR4/MD-2 complex, Surface plasmon resonance (SPR), Antagonist, TLR4-signaling

## Background

As its name implies, High Mobility Group Box 1 (HMGB1) is a small protein that migrates rapidly on SDS-PAGE gels and was first identified as a nonhistone chromatin-binding protein that has important biological activities in human health and diseases (Kang et al. 2014; Andersson and Tracey 2011; VanPatten and Alabed 2017). HMGB1 resides in the nucleus of most eukaryotic cells, where it functions as a transcriptional regulator facilitating the binding of several regulatory protein complexes to DNA (Wang et al. 2007; Stros 2010). Upon cellular activation, injury or death, HMGB1 translocates to the cytoplasm, where it can activate autophagy by interacting with beclin-1 (Kang et al. 2010), and to the extracellular medium, where it acts as a prototypic Damage Associated Molecular Pattern (DAMP) molecule. This DAMP has cytokine, chemokine, and growth factor activities, orchestrating the inflammatory and immune responses (Bianchi et al. 2017). When extracellular HMGB1 is released passively from damaged necrotic cells or actively from immune and/or stressed cells, it promotes inflammatory responses by binding to key pattern recognition receptors such as the Receptor for Advanced Glycation Endproducts (RAGE) and Toll-like

* Correspondence: mhe@northwell.edu; yalabed@northwell.edu
[1]Center for Molecular Innovation, The Feinstein Institute for Medical Research, 350 Community Drive, Manhasset, New York 11030, USA
Full list of author information is available at the end of the article

Receptors (TLRs) (Schmidt et al. 2000). Upon binding to its receptors, HMGB1 induces nuclear translocation of nuclear factor-κB (NF-κB), leading to secretion of pro-inflammatory cytokines including tumor necrosis factor-α (TNF-α), interleukin-6 (IL-6), and interleukin-1β (IL-1β) (Wu et al. 2016).

HMGB1 is highly conserved among various species, with 99% identity between human, rat and bovine protein sequences (Sessa and Bianchi 2007). Structurally, HMGB1 consists of a single 215-amino acid polypeptide organized into two DNA-binding domains linked by a short basic hinge, and an acidic C-terminal tail (Stros 2010) (Fig. 1). Each of the DNA binding, L-shaped HMG-box domains, termed A-box and B-box, is approximately 80 amino acids long and about 43% identical to the other (Read et al. 1993; Weir et al. 1993). The C-terminal tail consists of 30 acidic residues (aspartates and glutamates) (Weir et al. 1993). HMGB1 has three conserved, redox sensitive cysteines (Fig. 1). Two of the cysteine residues are located in A-box: Cys23 and Cys45. These residues can rapidly form an intramolecular disulfide bond, and the redox reaction is reversible (Sahu et al. 2008). The formation of the disulfide bond in the A-box induces significant structural change in the loop, particularly, the flipping of Phe38 ring which is the key residue interacting with cisplatinated DNA (Wang et al. 2013). The third cysteine residue, Cys106, remains in its reduced state in B-box (Yang et al. 2013a). The oxidative state of the three cysteines determines the receptor preference of extracellular HMGB1 (Yang et al. 2013a).

HMGB1-TLR4 signaling has been strongly implicated in the pathogenesis of sterile injury (Maroso et al. 2010; Yang et al. 2013b). TLR4-deficient animals are significantly protected from tissue injury during hepatic ischemia. TLR4, a pivotal receptor for activation of innate immunity, including cytokine release and tissue damage, is required for HMGB1-dependent activation of macrophage TNF release, whereas RAGE and TLR2 are dispensable. TLR4 activity and interaction with its ligands depend on a molecular collaboration with the extracellular adaptor protein Myeloid Differentiation factor 2 (MD-2) (Miyake 2004; Visintin et al. 2006). Surface plasmon resonance (SPR) studies indicate that HMGB1 binds specifically to TLR4/MD-2, and that this binding

requires cysteine 106 (Yang et al. 2010). Recently, we demonstrated that MD-2 binds specifically to the disulfide isoform of HMGB1 and not to the other isoforms (Yang et al. 2015a).

Structure–function analyses demonstrated that exogenous B-box recapitulates the cytokine activity of full length HMGB1 and stimulates TNF- release from macrophages. TNF-stimulating activity localizes to 20 amino acids within B-box (B1-B20, HMGB1 amino acids 89 to 108) (Li et al. 2003). In contrast, despite a 40% sequence identity with B-box, A-box not only possesses no TNF-stimulating activity but also acts as an antagonist of HMGB1, and can compete with HMGB1 for binding sites on the surface of activated macrophages and suppresses HMGB1-induced pro-inflammatory cytokines release (Yang et al. 2004). Recombinant A-box was found protective in established preclinical inflammatory disease models (Andersson and Tracey 2011; Venereau et al. 2016), including mouse models of sepsis (Yang et al. 2004; Suda et al. 2006), lung injury induced by LPS, hepatitis, severe acute pancreatitis, ischemia-reperfusion injury in the heart, cerebral ischemia, and epilepsy (Maroso et al. 2010; Andrassy et al. 2008; Muhammad et al. 2008; Yuan et al. 2009). The specific mechanism of how A-box antagonizes HMGB1 remains unknown. Adding to this mystery is the fact that the A-box contains the epitope of the anti-HMGB1 monoclonal antibody, 2G7. How 2G7 inhibits HMGB1 activity through binding to the A-box remains unknown.

As it has long been known that A-box acts as a potent HMGB1 antagonist in many experimental models, we sought to address the underlying molecular mechanism using surface plasmon resonance (SPR). We found that A-box binds to TLR4 with a comparable equilibrium dissociation constant ($K_D$) to HMGB1, but with a 10-fold slower dissociation rate than that of HMGB1. We propose that A-box antagonizes HMGB1 by blocking HMGB1-TLR4 binding sites, thus preventing HMGB1/TLR4/MD-2 complex formation.

## Methods
### Reagents
Human TLR4/MD-2 complex, human MD-2, TLR4 were obtained from R&D Systems.

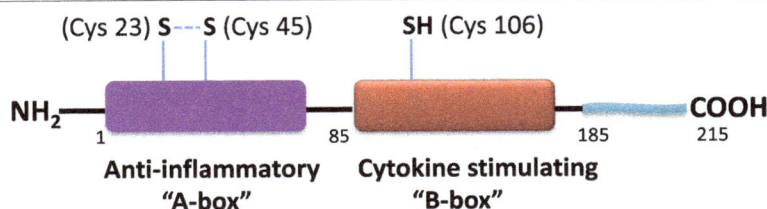
**Fig. 1** HMGB1 is composed of two box domains that individually have unique biological functions

Recombinant HMGB1 was expressed in *E. coli* and purified to homogeneity as described previously (Wang et al. 1999; Li et al. 2004). DTT reduced HMGB1 was prepared as previously described (Yang et al. 2012). The non-oxidizable HMGB1 3S mutant, where serines replace cysteines, was provided by HMGBiotech (Milan, Italy). Recombinant GST-A-box, GST-B-box and GST protein were expressed in *E. coli* and purified to homogeneity as previously described (Li et al. 2003; Yang et al. 2004; Li et al. 2004). Recombinant A-box without GST tag was also provided by HMGBiotech (Milan, Italy). A-box with or without GST tag showed comparable binding activity in our SPR assay (Additional file 1: Figure S4), both types of A-box were utilized in this study. Typically, LPS content in the protein preparations was less than 1 pg LPS/μg protein.

### Surface plasmon resonance analysis

Biacore T200 (GE Healthcare, USA) was used for real-time binding interaction studies. Binding reactions were done in HBS-EP buffer from BIAcore, containing 10 mM hepes, 150 mM NaCl, 3 mM EDTA and 0.05% surfactant p20, pH 7.4. At least 3 independent experiments were performed.

### TLR4/MD-2 or TLR4 and redox forms of HMGB1 binding analyses

A slow, high-level immobilization of TLR4/MD-2 or rhTLR4 protein was obtained on a CM5 series chip (GE Healthcare). The TLR4/MD-2 complex was diluted to a concentration of 20 μg/mL in 10 mM Acetate buffer (pH 4.5). A 1:1 mixture of N-hydroxysuccinimide and N-ethyl-N-(dimethyaminopropyl)carbodiimide was used to activate 2 flow-cells of the CM5 chip. One flow-cell was used as a reference and thus immediately blocked upon activation with 1 M ethanolamine (pH = 8.5). The sample flow-cell was injected with the diluted TLR4/MD-2 at a flow rate of 10 μL/min. The TLR4/MD-2 injection was stopped when the surface plasmon resonance reached ~ 1200 RU. For TLR4/MD-2 and HMGB1 isoform kinetics assays, HMGB1 isoforms were sequentially injected at a flow rate of 30 μL/min for 60s at 25 °C; the dissociation time was set for 1 min. The concentrations were 31.25, 62.5, 125, 250, 500, 1000 nM for disulfide and reduced HMGB1; 310, 625, 1250, 2500, 5000 nM for 3S mutant HMGB1. The rhTLR4 protein was diluted to a concentration of 20 μg/mL in 10 mM Acetate buffer (pH 5.0) and was immobilized on the CM5 chip according to the same amine coupling method described above. The TLR4 injection was stopped when the surface plasmon resonance reached ~ 800 RU. For TLR4 and HMGB1 isoform kinetics assays, HMGB1 isoforms were sequentially injected at a flow rate of 30 μL/min for 60s at 25 °C, the dissociation time

was set for 1–2 min. The concentrations were 31.25, 62.5, 125, 250, 500, 1000 nM for disulfide and reduced HMGB1; 250, 500, 1000, 2000, 4000, 8000 nM for 3S mutant HMGB1. The equilibrium dissociation constant ($K_D$) for individual analytes was obtained to evaluate the binding affinity by using the BIAEvaluation 2.0 software (GE Healthcare) supposing a 1:1 binding ratio.

### TLR4/MD-2 and GST-A-box or GST-B-box binding analyses

TLR4/MD-2 protein was immobilized onto a CM5 series chip (GE Healthcare) by amine coupling chemistry. GST protein alone was used as negative control (Additional file 1: Figures S2-S3). GST-A-box or GST-B-box were sequentially injected over immobilized TLR4/MD-2 (1100 RU) at a flow rate of 30 μL/min for 60s at 25 °C; the dissociation time was set for 1 min. The concentrations were 150, 310, 625, 1250, 2500, 5000 nM for GST-A-box and GST-B-box. The association and dissociation phases of GST-A-box were separately fitted to a 1:1 L binding model provided in the BIAevaluation 2.0 software. Binding affinity of GST-B-box was determined by global fitting of data to a steady-state affinity model in the BIAEvaluation 2.0.

### TLR4 and GST-A-box or GST-B-box binding analyses

TLR4 protein was immobilized onto a CM5 series chip (GE Healthcare) by amine coupling chemistry. GST-A-box was sequentially injected over the immobilized TLR4 (800 RU) at a flow rate of 30 μL/min for 60s at 25 °C; the dissociation time was set for 2 min. The concentrations were 310, 625, 1250, 2500, 5000, 10,000 nM. The equilibrium dissociation constant ($K_D$) was obtained by using the BIAEvaluation 2.0 software (GE Healthcare) supposing a 1:1 binding ratio. 1 μM and 5 μM GST-B-box was injected over the immobilized TLR4 at a flow rate of 30 μL/min for 60s at 25 °C, however there has no observed binding activity. GST protein alone was used as negative control; no binding was observed (Additional file 1: Figures S2-S3).

### MD-2 and GST-A-box or GST-B-box binding analyses

GST-A-box or B-box protein was immobilized onto a CM5 series chip (GE Healthcare) by amine coupling chemistry. MD-2 was sequentially injected over the immobilized GST-A-box (750 RU) or GST-B-box (1000 RU) at a flow rate of 30 μL/min for 60s at 25 °C; the dissociation time was set for 1 min. The concentrations were 17, 31.25, 62.5, 125, 250, 500 nM. Apparent equilibrium dissociation constants ($K_D$) were determined by global fitting of data to a steady-state affinity model in the BIAEvaluation 2.0 software. Binding affinity and kinetics data of HMGB1 isoforms and segments to TLR4/MD-2 receptors are listed in Additional file 1: Tables S1-2S. Data shown in this report are representative of three independent experiments.

## Biacore analysis of complex formation among TLR4/MD-2, TLR4, A-box and HMGB1

The assay was performed using the HBS-EP buffer from BIAcore as described above. HMGB1 (100 nM) was injected on a TLR4/MD-2 complex sensor chip surface followed by HBS buffer or HMGB1 (100 nM) or TLR4/MD-2 (100 nM) or mixture of two proteins (1:1 M ratio) using the dual injection command. In competition experiments, A-box (10 μM) was injected on a TLR4 sensor chip surface followed by 2-fold dilutions of HMGB1 (2.5–5 μg/ml) using the dual injection command. In separate experiments, HMGB1 (500 nM) was injected on a TLR4 sensor chip surface, followed by A-box using the dual injection command (Additional file 1: Figure S5).

## Results

### The TLR4/MD-2 complex is sensitive to the oxidative state of HMGB1, while TLR4 is not

Recent studies emphasize that the redox states of the three conserved cysteine residues within HMGB1 regulate its receptor-binding ability and subsequent biological outcome including its pro-inflammatory activity (Yang et al. 2013a). In 2015, we demonstrated that MD-2 binds specifically to the cytokine-inducing disulfide isoform of HMGB1, whereas fully reduced or sulfonyl HMGB1 had 1000-fold lower binding affinity for MD-2

(Yang et al. 2015b). To further clarify the underlying molecular mechanisms, we examined whether the TLR4/MD-2 complex or TLR4 alone could discriminate various HMGB1 isoforms. We tested reduced HMGB1 and the non-oxidizable HMGB1 3S mutant, generated by replacing all three cysteines with serines. To begin, the TLR4/MD-2 complex was coated on the CM5 sensor chip, and then probed with each of the three HMGB1 isoforms (Fig. 2a-c). Consistent with previous findings (Yang et al. 2012), the disulfide HMGB1 isoform binds to TLR4/MD-2 in a concentration-dependent manner, with relatively high affinity, an apparent equilibrium dissociation constant ($K_D$) of $0.42 \pm 0.01$ μM (Fig. 2a). In contrast, DTT-reduced HMGB1 and the non-oxidizable 3S mutant bind TLR4/MD-2 complex with $\sim$ 10-fold lower affinity (apparent $K_D = 3.93 \pm 0.01$ and $3.02 \pm 0.02$ μM, respectively, Fig. 2b & c). These results are consistent with the finding that reduced HMGB1 and 3S do not induce cytokine expression in macrophages (Yang et al. 2013a; Venereau et al. 2012). The sensorgrams also demonstrate that the disulfide HMGB1 has a 10-fold faster association rate (ka = $2.86 \pm 0.03 \times 10^5$ M$^{-1}$ s$^{-1}$, Additional file 1: Table S2) relative to the other isoforms.

Previously, we reported that HMGB1 was incapable of directly binding to TLR4 in the absence of MD-2 (Yang

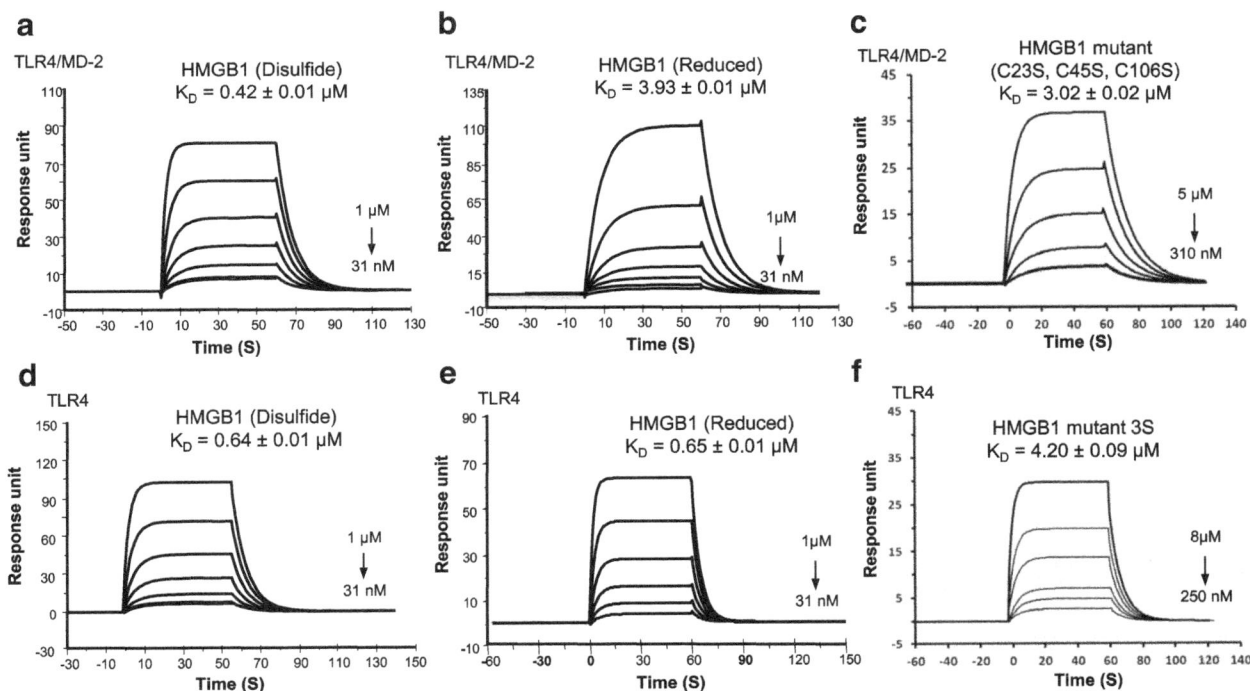

**Fig. 2** SPR analyses of redox forms of HMGB1 binding to TLR4/MD-2 complex or TLR4. **a-c** TLR4/MD-2 complex was coated on the CM5 chip; disulfide HMGB1 binds to complex with a $K_D$ of $0.42 \pm 0.01$ μM; reduced HMGB1 binds with a $K_D$ of $3.93 \pm 0.01$ μM; HMGB1 3S mutant binds with a $K_D$ of $3.02 \pm 0.02$ μM. **d-f** TLR4 was coated on the chip; HMGB1 binds to TLR4 with a $K_D$ of $0.64 \pm 0.01$ μM; reduced HMGB1 binds with a $K_D$ of $0.65 \pm 0.01$ μM; HMGB1 3S mutant binds with a $K_D$ of $4.20 \pm 0.09$ μM. Data are representative of three repeats

et al. 2015a). In this study, we revisited this observation and refined the experimental conditions (immobilization levels and/or switching ligand and analyte) for this binding assay. Using these optimized conditions we found that disulfide HMGB1 does bind to TLR4 (coated on the sensor chip) in a concentration-dependent manner with an apparent $K_D$ of $0.64 \pm 0.01$ μM (Fig. 2d). Next, the other isoforms of HMGB1 were injected onto the TLR4 sensor chip to investigate which redox state of HMGB1 was most conducive to binding (Fig. 2e-f). Reduced HMGB1 bound to TLR4 with a comparable equilibrium dissociation constant $K_D = 0.65 \pm 0.01$ μM (Fig. 2e), indicating that a disulfide bond between C23 and C45 has a negligible influence on the binding to TLR4. However, the sensorgrams demonstrated a 2-fold slower dissociation rate (kd = $0.128 \pm 0.002$ s$^{-1}$, Additional file 1: Table S2) for disulfide HMGB1 compared with reduced HMGB1, indicating that the complex with TLR4 is more stable once formed. We also found that 3S, where C23, C45 and C106 are mutated to serines, binds to TLR4 with a weaker affinity (apparent $K_D = 4.20 \pm 0.09$ μM) (Fig. 2f), suggesting that three cysteine residues within HMGB1 are essential for binding to TLR4.

## A-box binds to TLR4/MD-2 complex and major binding sites are located on TLR4

As mentioned above, A-box has been widely used as an HMGB1 antagonist in many inflammatory disease models. Exogenous A-box has been reported to antagonize full-length HMGB1 by competitively binding to RAGE (Zhang et al. 2008); it was also described to interact with CXCL12 and thus competes with the HMGB1 for signaling via CXCR4 (Schiraldi et al. 2012). In the present study, we investigated the A-box–Toll-like receptor 4 (TLR4) interaction using SPR. TLR4/MD-2, TLR4 or MD-2 were individually immobilized on the CM5 sensor chip; recombinant GST-A-box was

passed through the chips to analyze the binding activity. We observed that GST-A-box had a high affinity to TLR4 with apparent $K_D$ of $0.59 \pm 0.01$ μM, compared to the TLR4/MD-2 ($K_D = 1.21 \pm 0.02$ μM) (Fig. 3a-b). In addition, the sensorgrams showed that GST-A-box interacted with TLR4/MD-2 and TLR4 in comparable association, but different dissociation rate constants (Additional file 1: Tables S1-S2). For example, GST-A-box associated to TLR4/MD-2 at a rate of $3.08 \pm 0.85 \times 10^4$ M$^{-1}$ s$^{-1}$ and dissociated at $0.037 \pm 0.01$ s$^{-1}$; while associated to TLR4 at $2.20 \pm 0.02 \times 10^4$ M$^{-1}$ s$^{-1}$ and dissociated at a 3-fold slower rate of $0.013 \pm 0.01$ s$^{-1}$. On the contrary, only weak binding activity was observed on the MD-2 immobilized chip (Additional file 1: Figure S1). Therefore, we asked whether GST-A-box binds to MD-2 in the reverse orientation. We immobilized GST-A-box on the CM5 chip; MD-2 was injected as analyte. The sensorgram showed that MD-2 had a weak association rate with GST-A-box and the affinity of GST-A-box binding to MD-2 ($K_D = 3.25 \pm 0.17$ μM) was much lower than binding to TLR4 or TLR4/MD-2 (Fig. 3c, Additional file 1: Tables S1-S2). Taken together, these results confirmed that A-box alone binds to the TLR4/MD-2 complex and major binding site(s) are likely located on TLR4.

## B-box binds to MD-2 but not TLR4

To evaluate the binding of B-box to the TLR4/MD-2 complex in detail, SPR analyses were performed. Akin to previous reports (Yang et al. 2010), the GST-B-box binds to TLR4/MD-2 in a concentration-dependent manner, with an apparent equilibrium dissociation constant $K_D$ of $5.78 \pm 0.22$ μM (Fig. 4a), 6-fold weaker than GST-A-box (Fig. 3a). The sensorgram showed that GST-B-box has a fast association to TLR4/MD-2 complex and is quickly dissociated by washing, suggesting that the

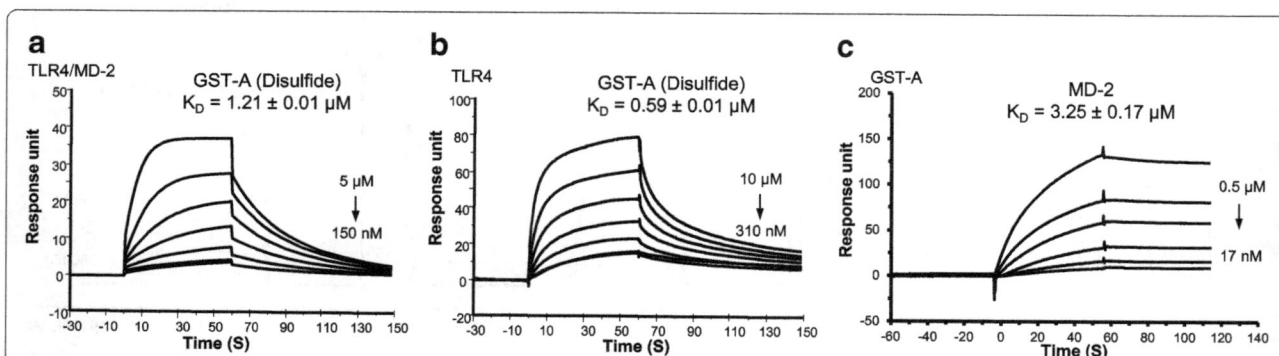

Fig. 3 SPR analyses of GST-A-box binding to TLR4/MD-2, TLR4 and MD-2. a TLR4/MD-2 complex was coated on the CM5 chip, GST-A-box binds to complex with a $K_D$ of $1.21 \pm 0.02$ μM. b TLR4 was coated on the chip, GST-A-box binds to TLR4 with a $K_D$ of $0.59 \pm 0.01$ μM. c GST-A-box was coated on the CM5 chips, MD-2 was used as analyte, MD-2 binds to GST-A-box with a $K_D$ of $3.25 \pm 0.17$ μM. GST tag was used as negative control. Data are representative of three repeats

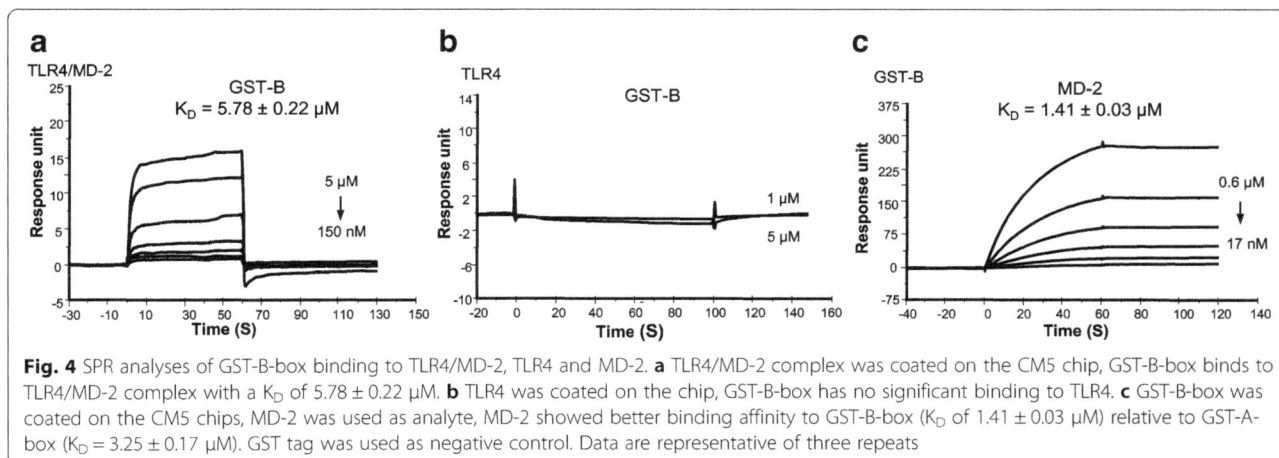

**Fig. 4** SPR analyses of GST-B-box binding to TLR4/MD-2, TLR4 and MD-2. **a** TLR4/MD-2 complex was coated on the CM5 chip, GST-B-box binds to TLR4/MD-2 complex with a $K_D$ of 5.78 ± 0.22 µM. **b** TLR4 was coated on the chip, GST-B-box has no significant binding to TLR4. **c** GST-B-box was coated on the CM5 chips, MD-2 was used as analyte, MD-2 showed better binding affinity to GST-B-box ($K_D$ of 1.41 ± 0.03 µM) relative to GST-A-box ($K_D$ = 3.25 ± 0.17 µM). GST tag was used as negative control. Data are representative of three repeats

complex between GST-B-box and TLR4/MD-2 is not remarkably stable. Surprisingly, when GST-B-box was applied to immobilized TLR4, no significant binding was observed (Fig. 4b), and this lack of interaction was confirmed in the reverse orientation experiment (not shown). When GST-B-box was injected over immobilized MD-2, no binding activity was found (Additional file 1: Figure S1); in contrast, MD-2 showed a concentration-dependent binding to immobilized GST-B-box with a $K_D$ of 1.41 ± 0.03 µM (Fig. 4c). The extremely slow off-rate indicated that the complex between GST-B-box and MD-2, once formed, was much more stable than the complex formed by GST-A-box. These data indicate that B-box alone binds to MD-2, but not to TLR4, suggesting that the binding of B-box to the TLR4/MD-2 complex occurs via the MD-2 subunit.

## Plausible mechanism of HMGB1-TLR4 signaling and the role of A-box as antagonist

Binding of HMGB1 to TLR4 has been shown to activate the MyD88 signaling pathway, thus resulting in the release of pro-inflammatory cytokines (Ugrinova and Pasheva 2017). It is unknown whether HMGB1 recognition by the TLR4/MD-2 complex shares similarities with other prototypical activators of TLR4 signaling, such as lipopolysaccharide (LPS). In the last decade, the crystal structures of the LPS receptors and accessory proteins have been characterized. Recently, Kim and coworkers reconstituted the entire cascade of LPS transfer to TLR4/MD-2 in a total internal reflection fluorescence (TIRF) microscope in a single-molecule analysis, reveling that a single LPS molecule bound to CD14 is transferred to TLR4/MD-2 in a TLR4-dependent manner (Kim and Kim 2017). Upon binding of LPS to a hydrophobic pocket in MD-2, two LPS-bound TLR4/MD-2 complexes form an M-shaped dimer, followed by activation of the signaling pathway (Kim and Kim 2017).

We hypothesized that HMGB1 may act in a manner similar to LPS, binding to TLR4/MD-2 complex and then inducing the dimerization of HMGB1/TLR4/MD-2 complexes, which brings together the cytosolic toll/interleukin-1 receptor (TIR) domains of TLR4 to recruit downstream adaptor molecules. To examine the details of the binding of HMGB1 to the TLR4/MD-2 complex, we immobilized one ligand on a Biacore CM5 sensor chip and used a sequential dual-injection method where the second analyte is injected after the first analyte with zero dissociation time. If a two-step increase in the bound mass is observed, we infer that the second analyte can bind to the complex of the ligand and first analyte; conversely, a decrease or unchanged signal after the second injection suggests that the first and second analytes compete for binding to the ligand, and then a ternary complex is not formed.

HMGB1 (100 nM) was applied to the TLR4/MD-2 sensor chip surface and reached a steady state signal of ~30 RU (Fig. 5a). When blank control (HBS buffer) was injected as second analyte, the binding signal was decreased due to the dissociation of bound HMGB1. When a second injection of TLR4/MD-2 (100 nM) was made, no additional binding was observed. When HMGB1 (100 nM) was injected as second analyte, the binding signal was unchanged. Instead, when a mixture of HMGB1 and TLR4/MD-2 (1:1 M ratio) was injected, we observed a significant increase of the binding signal immediately after injection. These data suggest that HMGB1 induces dimerization between TLR4/MD-2 complexes, which could be the key step in the HMGB1-TLR4 signaling pathway. We next considered whether, as an HMGB1 antagonist, A-box exerts its role through interference with the formation of the HMGB1/TLR4/MD-2 complex. We immobilized TLR4 on the CM5 sensor chip and injected 10 µM A-box to reach a steady state binding of ~ 150 RU; after adding HMGB1 as second analyte, no

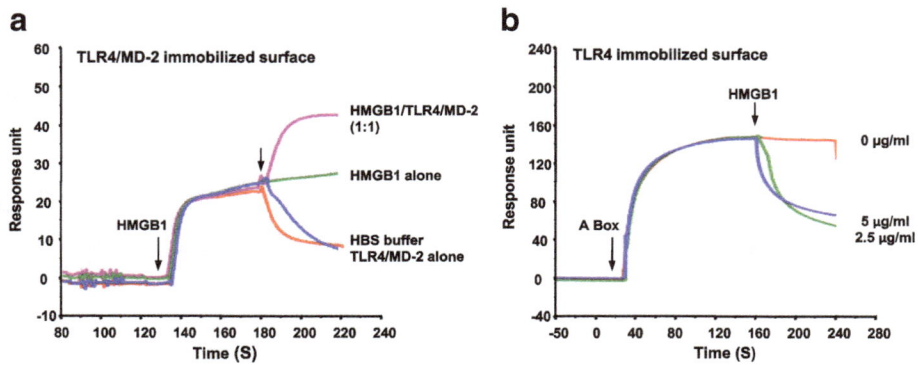

**Fig. 5** Ternary complex formation among TLR4/MD-2, TLR4, A-box and HMGB1. **a** Biacore sensorgram showing molecular interactions, after injecting HMGB1 (100 nM) followed immediately by HBS buffer, HMGB1 (100 nM) or TLR4/MD-2 (100 nM) or mixture of the latter (100 nM each) onto a TLR4/MD-2 sensor chip surface. **b** Injecting A-box (10 μM), followed immediately by A-box (0 μg/ml of HMGB1) or HMGB1 (2.5 and 5 μg/ml) onto a TLR4 sensor chip surface

complex with HMGB1 was seen (Fig. 5b). Similarly, we observed a decrease of the binding signal when we injected HMGB1 followed by A-box (data not shown, Additional file 1: Figure S5). These data demonstrated that A-box directly competes with HMGB1 for binding to TLR4.

## Discussion

We propose the mechanism of HMGB1-induced TLR4 signaling outlined in Scheme 1. Real-time SPR studies showed that: 1) the binding of HMGB1 to TLR4/MD-2 complex is mostly contributed by the A-box domain whose major binding site(s) are located on TLR4; 2) B-

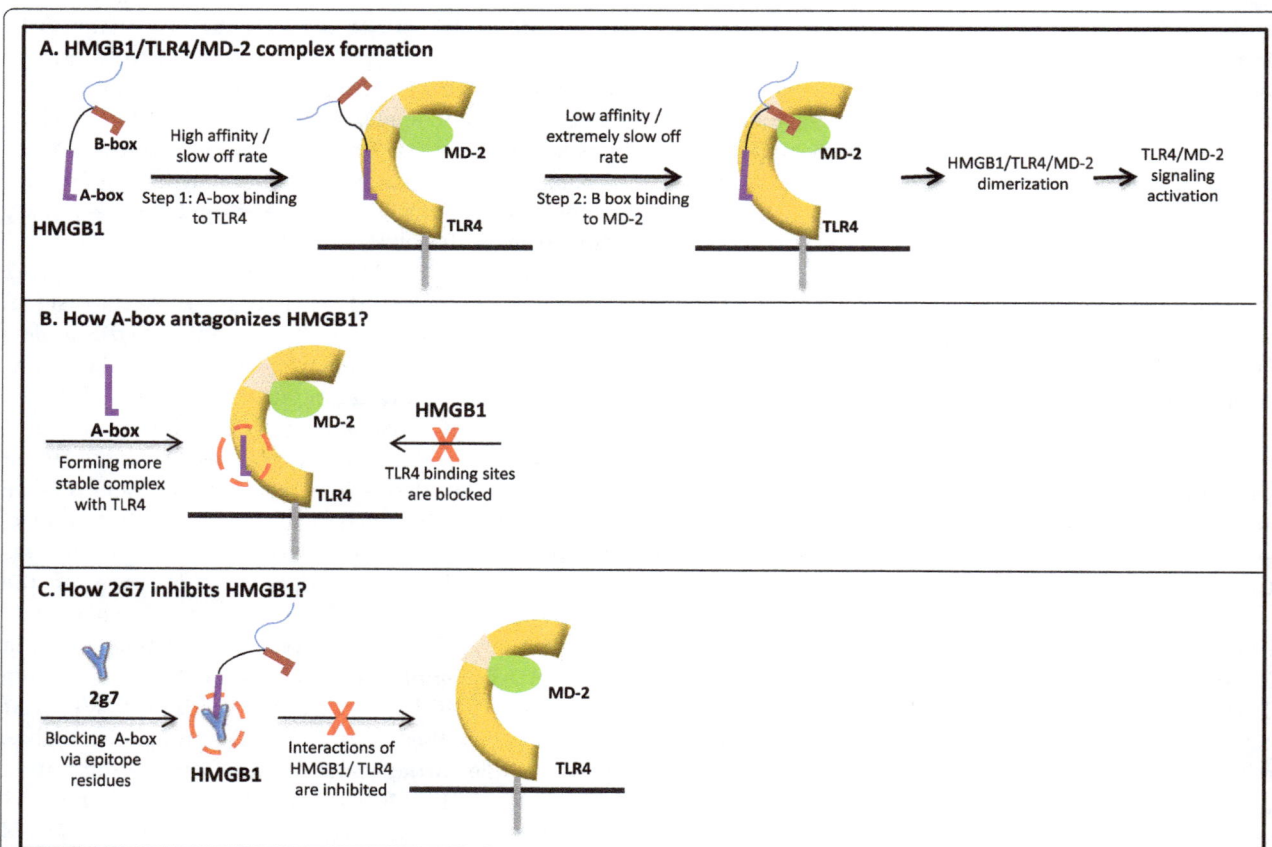

**Scheme 1** Proposed mechanism of HMGB1-TLR4 interaction and role of anti-HMGB1 antibody (2G7)

box binds to MD-2; and 3) the HMGB1/TLR4/MD-2 complex can dimerize with another HMGB1/TLR4/MD-2 complex. Our results suggest that HMGB1/TLR4/MD-2 interaction is initiated by HMGB1-TLR4 binding via the A-box domain (high affinity and slow off-rate, Scheme 1a) and, once in close proximity, the HMGB1 B-box domain binds to MD-2 (low affinity but extremely slow off-rate, Scheme 1a). In addition, SPR studies also suggest that A-box functions as an HMGB1 antagonist by blocking the first step of HMGB1 binding to TLR4 (Scheme 1b). A-box and HMGB1 bind to TLR4 with comparable equilibrium dissociation constants ($K_D$), but with quite different dissociation rates (Additional file 1: Table S2), indicating that the complex formed between A-box and TLR4 is more stable than that formed by HMGB1. As hypothesized in the Scheme 1b, when A-box and HMGB1 are present, A-box occupies and blocks HMGB1/TLR4 binding sites, preventing downstream full-length HMGB1/TLR4/MD-2 interactions, thus inhibiting TLR4/MD-2 signal activation.

Previously, SPR studies reported by Yang et al. (Yang et al. 2010) showed that anti-HMGB1 monoclonal antibody (mAb) 2G7 also inhibited the binding of HMGB1 to TLR4/MD-2. This antibody has been extensively used by researchers to block HMGB1 activity both in vitro and in vivo (Venereau et al. 2016; Ugrinova and Pasheva 2017). The epitope in HMGB1 that binds to 2G7 has been identified within amino acids 53–63 of the A-box subunit (Qin et al. 2006). However, the molecular mechanisms whereby binding of 2G7 to A-box has anti-inflammatory activity remained elusive. Based upon the finding of A-box as an HMGB1 antagonist, we speculate that mAb 2G7 would share similar mechanism to inhibit HMGB1 activity (Scheme 1c) by blocking HMGB1-TLR4 interactions.

## Conclusions

In summary, SPR studies showed that HMGB1 and its fragments (A-box and B-box) individually interact with the TLR4/MD-2 receptor with different binding and kinetic parameters. Our study also reveals that HMGB1 likely activates TLR4 signaling through inducing TLR4/MD-2 dimerization. The HMGB1 recognition cascade can be disrupted by the antagonistic A-box fragment due to its higher binding affinity to TLR4 or by blocking A-box with anti-HMGB1 mAb 2G7. Ongoing studies further detailing HMGB1/TLR4/MD-2 interactions will facilitate the design and development of therapeutics to inhibit HMGB1-mediated inflammation.

## Additional file

**Additional file 1: Table S1.** Binding affinity of HMGB1 isoforms and segments. **Table S2.** Kinetics data of HMGB1 isoforms and segments. **Figure S1.** SPR analyses of GST-A-box and GST-B box binding to MD-2.

**Figure S2.** SPR analyses of GST-A-box binding to TLR4/MD-2, TLR4. **Figure S3.** SPR analyses of GST-B-box binding to TLR4/MD-2, TLR4. **Figure S4.** SPR analyses of GST-A-box and A-box binding to TLR4/MD-2, TLR4. **Figure S5.** Ternary complex formation among TLR4, A-box and HMGB1. (DOCX 241 kb)

## Abbreviations
DAMP: Damage Associated Molecular Pattern; DNA: Deoxyribonucleic acid; HMGB1: High Mobility Group Box 1; IL-1β: Interleukin-1β; IL-6: Interleukin-6; $K_D$: Equilibrium dissociation constant; LPS: Lipopolysaccharide; MD-2: MYELOID Differentiation factor 2; NF-kB: Nuclear factor-κB; RAGE: Receptor for Advanced Glycation Endproducts; SDS-PAGE: Sodium dodecyl sulfate –polyacrylamide gel electrophoresis; SPR: Surface plasmon resonance; TIR: Toll/interleukin-1 receptor; TIRF: Total internal reflection fluorescence; TLRs: Toll-like Receptors (TLRs); TNF-α: Tumor necrosis factor

## Acknowledgments
We acknowledge Dr. Sonya VanPatten with help in manuscript editing.

## Funding
This work was supported by funding from the Feinstein Institute for Medical Research and National Institutes of Health (NIH) Grant S10 RR033072–01 to Y.A-A, and by Associazione Italiana Ricerca sul Cancro (AIRC) Grant IG 18623 to M.E.B.

## Authors' contributions
Conception and design of experiments, and development of assays: MH, KJT, YAA. Acquisition of data, and/or analysis and interpretation of data: MH, MEB, YAA. Drafting the manuscript: MH, MEB, TRC, YAA. Revising the manuscript: MH, MEB, TRC, KJT, YAA. Final approval prior to submission: MH, MEB, TRC, KJT, YAA.

## Competing interests
YAA is on patents related to HMGB1 antagonists, and MEB on patents related to the HMGB1 3S mutant.

## Author details
[1]Center for Molecular Innovation, The Feinstein Institute for Medical Research, 350 Community Drive, Manhasset, New York 11030, USA. [2]Chromatin Dynamics Unit, Division of Genetics and Cell Biology, San Raffaele University and San Raffaele Scientific Institute IRCCS, Via Olgettina 58, 20132 Milan, Italy. [3]Center for Biomedical Science, and Center for Bioelectronic Medicine, The Feinstein Institute for Medical Research, 350 Community Drive, Manhasset, New York 11030, USA.

## References
Andersson U, Tracey KJ. HMGB1 is a therapeutic target for sterile inflammation and infection. Annu Rev Immunol. 2011;29:139–62.
Andrassy M, et al. High-mobility group Box-1 in ischemia-reperfusion injury of the heart. Circulation. 2008;117:3216–26.
Bianchi ME, et al. High-mobility group box 1 protein orchestrates responses to tissue damage via inflammation, innate and adaptive immunity, and tissue repair. Immunol Rev. 2017;280:74–82.
Kang R, Livesey KM, Zeh HJ, Lotze MT, Tang D. HMGB1: a novel Beclin 1-binding protein active in autophagy. Autophagy. 2010;6:1209–11.
Kang R, et al. HMGB1 in health and disease. Mol Asp Med. 2014;40:1–116.
Kim SJ, Kim HM. Dynamic lipopolysaccharide transfer cascade to TLR4/MD2 complex via LBP and CD14. BMB Rep. 2017;50:55–7.

Li J, et al. Structural basis for the proinflammatory cytokine activity of high mobility group box 1. Mol. Med (Manhasset, NY, U. S.). 2003;9:37–45.

Li J, et al. Recombinant HMGB1 with cytokine-stimulating activity. J Immunol Methods. 2004;289:211–23.

Maroso M, et al. Toll-like receptor 4 and high-mobility group box-1 are involved in ictogenesis and can be targeted to reduce seizures. Nat Med (N Y, NY, U S). 2010;16: 413–9.

Miyake K. Endotoxin recognition molecules, toll-like receptor 4-MD-2. Semin Immunol. 2004;16:11–6.

Muhammad S, et al. The HMGB1 receptor RAGE mediates ischemic brain damage. J Neurosci. 2008;28:12023–31.

Qin S, et al. Role of HMGB1 in apoptosis-mediated sepsis lethality. J Exp Med. 2006;203:1637–42.

Read CM, Cary PD, Crane-Robinson C, Driscoll PC, Norman DG. Solution structure of a DNA-binding domain from HMG1. Nucleic Acids Res. 1993;21:3427–36.

Sahu D, Debnath P, Takayama Y, Iwahara J. Redox properties of the A-domain of the HMGB1 protein. FEBS Lett. 2008;582:3973–8.

Schiraldi M, et al. HMGB1 promotes recruitment of inflammatory cells to damaged tissues by forming a complex with CXCL12 and signaling via CXCR4. J Exp Med. 2012;209:551–63.

Schmidt AM, Yan SD, Yan SF, Stern DM. The biology of the receptor for advanced glycation end products and its ligands. Biochim Biophys Acta, Mol Cell Res. 2000;1498:99–111.

Sessa L, Bianchi ME. The evolution of high mobility group box (HMGB) chromatin proteins in multicellular animals. Gene. 2007;387:133–40.

Stros M. HMGB proteins: interactions with DNA and chromatin, Biochim. Biophys. Acta, gene Regul. Mech. 2010;1799:101–13.

Suda K, et al. Anti-high-mobility group box chromosomal protein 1 antibodies improve survival of rats with sepsis. World J Surg. 2006;30:1755–62.

Ugrinova I, Pasheva E. HMGB1 protein: a therapeutic target inside and outside the cell. Adv Protein Chem Struct Biol. 2017;107:37–76.

VanPatten S, Alabed Y. (2017) High mobility group Box-1 (HMGb1) - current wisdom, and advancement as a potential drug target. J Med Chem. https://pubs.acs.org/doi/10.1021/acs.jmedchem.7b01136

Venereau E, et al. Mutually exclusive redox forms of HMGB1 promote cell recruitment or proinflammatory cytokine release. J Exp Med. 2012;209:1519–28.

Venereau E, et al. HMGB1 as biomarker and drug target. Pharmacol Res. 2016;111:534–44.

Visintin A, Iliev DB, Monks BG, Halmen KA, Golenbock DT. MD-2. Immunobiology. 2006;211:437–47.

Wang H, et al. HMG-1 as a late mediator of endotoxin lethality in mice. Science (Washington, D C). 1999;285:248–51.

Wang J, et al. Redox-sensitive structural change in the A-domain of HMGB1 and its implication for the binding to cisplatin modified DNA. Biochem Biophys Res Commun. 2013;441:701–6.

Wang Q, Zeng M, Wang W, Tang J. The HMGB1 acidic tail regulates HMGB1 DNA binding specificity by a unique mechanism. Biochem Biophys Res Commun. 2007;360:14–9.

Weir HM, et al. Structure of the HMG box motif in the B-domain of HMG1. EMBO J. 1993;12:1311–9.

Wu H, et al. High mobility group Box-1: a missing link between diabetes and its complications. Mediat Inflamm. 2016;2016:3896147.

Yang H, Antoine DJ, Andersson U, Tracey KJ. The many faces of HMGB1: molecular structure-functional activity in inflammation, apoptosis, and chemotaxis. J Leukoc Biol. 2013a;93:865–73.

Yang H, et al. Reversing established sepsis with antagonists of endogenous high-mobility group box 1. Proc Natl Acad Sci U S A. 2004;101:296–301.

Yang H, et al. A critical cysteine is required for HMGB1 binding to toll-like receptor 4 and activation of macrophage cytokine release. Proc Natl Acad Sci U S A. 2010;107:11942–7.

Yang H, et al. Redox modification of cysteine residues regulates the cytokine activity of high mobility group box-1 (HMGB1). Mol Med (Manhasset, NY, U S). 2012;18:250–9.

Yang H, et al. MD-2 is required for disulfide HMGB1-dependent TLR4 signaling. J Exp Med. 2015a;212:5–14.

Yang H, et al. Aspirin delays mesothelioma growth by inhibiting HMGB1-mediated tumor progression. Cell Death Dis. 2015b;6:e1786.

Yang Z, et al. TLR4 as receptor for HMGB1-mediated acute lung injury after liver ischemia/reperfusion injury. Lab Investig. 2013b;93:792–800.

Yuan H, et al. Protective effect of HMGB1 a box on organ injury of acute pancreatitis in mice. Pancreas (Hagerstown, MD, U S). 2009;38:143–8.

Zhang C-L, Shu M-G, Qi H-W, Li L-W. Inhibition of tumor angiogenesis by HMGB1 a box peptide. Med Hypotheses. 2008;70:343–5.

# 14

# The role of KIBRA in reconstructive episodic memory

Armin Zlomuzica[1][*][†], Friederike Preusser[1][†], Susanna Roberts[2], Marcella L. Woud[1], Kathryn J. Lester[2,3], Ekrem Dere[4,5], Thalia C. Eley[2] and Jürgen Margraf[1]

## Abstract

**Background:** In order to retrieve episodic past events, the missing information needs to be reconstructed using information stored in semantic memory. Failures in these reconstructive processes are expressed as false memories. KIBRA single nucleotide polymorphism (rs17070145) has been linked to episodic memory performance as well as an increased risk of Alzheimer's disease and post-traumatic stress disorder (PTSD).

**Methods:** Here, the role of KIBRA rs17070145 polymorphism (male and female CC vs. CT/TT carriers) in reconstructive episodic memory in the Deese-Roediger-McDermott (DRM) paradigm was investigated in $N = 219$ healthy individuals.

**Results:** Female participants outperformed males in the free recall condition. Furthermore, a trend towards a *gender x genotype interaction* was found for false recognition rates. Female CT/TT carriers exhibited a lower proportion of false recognition rates for associated critical lures as compared to male CT/TT. Additionally, an association between KIBRA rs17070145 genotype, familiarity and recollection based recognition performance was found. In trials with correct recognition of listed items CT/TT carriers showed more "remember", but fewer "know" responses as compared to CC carriers.

**Discussion and conclusion:** Our findings suggest that the T-allele of KIBRA rs17070145 supports recollection based episodic memory retrieval and contributes to memory accuracy in a gender dependent manner. Findings are discussed in the context of the specific contribution of KIBRA related SNPs to reconstructive episodic memory and its implications for cognitive and emotional symptoms in dementia and PTSD.

**Keywords:** KIBRA, WWC1 gene, Episodic memory, False memories, Alzheimer's disease

## Background

Episodic memory refers to the ability to recollect personal experiences and specific events in terms of contextual details, specific perceptions, emotions, and thoughts (Tulving, 2002). Genetic variability seems to play a prominent role in the inter-individual variation in episodic memory performance (Volk et al., 2006). However, the relevant genes, gene clusters and their molecular pathways remain to be determined.

Recently, a genome-wide association study identified KIBRA as a potential candidate gene that is associated with the encoding and retrieval of episodic memories (Papassotiropoulos & de Quervain, 2011). KIBRA is abundantly expressed in brain regions such as the prefrontal cortex and hippocampus that are at the core of episodic memory formation and retrieval (Papassotiropoulos et al., 2006). In the hippocampus, the KIBRA gene is expressed in neurons. The KIBRA protein interacts with synaptopodin (Duning et al., 2008) and PKCζ (Büther et al., 2004), which are both involved in synaptic plasticity. An important role of KIBRA in development of brain architecture (Yoshihama et al., 2009; Johannsen et al., 2008) has also been confirmed. Genetic deletion of KIBRA in mice leads to impairments in hippocampal long-term potentiation as well as compromised memory performance (Makuch et al., 2011). At the behavioral level, a considerable number of studies confirmed an association between a single nucleotide polymorphism (SNP) of the KIBRA gene (rs17070145) and episodic memory performance, with T-allele carriers (CT/TT) of the SNP showing a superior performance relative to non-carriers (CC) (summarized in Milnik et al., 2012).

* Correspondence: armin.zlomuzica@rub.de
†Equal contributors
[1]Mental Health Research and Treatment Center, Ruhr-Universität Bochum, 150, 44780 Bochum, Germany
Full list of author information is available at the end of the article

However, findings regarding KIBRA and memory functions are inconclusive and depend on whether young or older adults are being examined and whether participants are healthy or suffer from neurological or neurodegenerative diseases (Nacmias et al., 2008; Need et al., 2008; Boraxbekk et al., 2015; Rodriguez-Rodriguez et al., 2009; Schaper et al., 2008); Vassos et al., 2010 summarized in Schwab et al., 2014. Imaging studies suggest that the genetic variation in KIBRA rs17070145 is also related to differences in patterns of brain activation during episodic retrieval, particularly in the hippocampal/medial temporal lobe region (Papassotiropoulos et al., 2006; Kauppi et al., 2011).

Since our capacity to recollect complex personal events is limited, episodic memories often contain only a selection or fragments of the original event information. With regard to retrieval, such fragmentary information has to be complemented with semantic information in order to reconstruct the original event as precise as possible (Pause et al., 2013; Loftus, 2005; Breeden et al., 2016). Errors during the reconstruction process of past events are expressed as false memories, i.e., subjects often tend to recall false information or recognize items incorrectly simply because they are semantically or visually related to correct information or items that were actually presented.

The DRM task was developed as in attempt to design a simple and fast task to induce and measure false memories under laboratory conditions (Deese, 1959; Roediger & McDermott, 1995). The DRM experimental procedure (see Pardilla-Delgado, 2017) can be easily applied (without further adaptations necessary) to children, adults, aged individuals, as well as to amnesic, neurological and psychiatric patients. To date, the DRM paradigm is considered *as a* gold standard for the investigation of psychological and biological factors underlying reconstructive processes (Gallo, 2010). In the DRM task, participants are first instructed to memorize lists of semantically related words (e.g., "dark", "night", etc.). Each of the words presented during the learning phase is highly associative of a word belonging to the gist or theme of the respective word list (referred to as the critical lure word: "black"). The critical lure representing the gist or theme of the lists of semantically related words, however, is not being presented. During the subsequent test phase, subjects often tend to recall and/or recognize both the unpresented critical lure word (false memories) and words presented during the initial learning phase (accurate memories). The reliability of the DRM task in creating false memories is well documented and reflected by its predominant use in false memory research.

Determining individual differences with respect to susceptibility to produce false memories in the DRM paradigm has a long tradition in the field (Deese, 1959; Roediger & McDermott, 1995). A number of decisive factors, including increased dissociative and delusional tendency (Laws & Bhatt, 2005; Winograd et al., 1998), high schizotypy (Saunders et al., 2012), and specific autobiographic memory retrieval style (Dewhurst et al., 2018), have been identified that predict high false recognition rates in healthy subjects. Contrarily, the contribution of genetic factors to individual differences in reconstructive episodic memories has been largely neglected (but see Zhu et al., 2013). Recently, Zhu et al., 2013 demonstrated that the 5-Hydroxytryptamine Receptor 2 (HTR2A) gene is significantly associated with the capacity to retrieve true, but not false memories during recognition in the DRM task.

So far research on the association between KIBRA rs17070145 and episodic memory has neglected the reconstructive nature of episodic memory functions. Both, the storage and retrieval of veridical and false episodic memories (as studied in the DRM paradigm) are supposed to be subserved by distinct brain regions, i.e. anterior and posterior regions of the medial temporal lobe, dentate gyrus and CA subregions of the hippocampus (Schacter et al., 1996; Schacter & Slotnick, 2004; Ramirez et al., 2013). Since KIBRA is abundantly expressed in the CA1 region of the hippocampus as well as the dentate gyrus (Papassotiropoulos et al., 2006; Yoshihama et al., 2009; Johannsen et al., 2008), suggesting a possible involvement of KIBRA in processes related to reconstructive episodic memory, we asked whether KIBRA related genotype effects exist for reconstructive episodic memory and whether these can be observed during recall and recognition memory performance in the DRM task.

The precise role of the hippocampus and its adjacent areas in recollection and familiarity-based recognition memory is still a matter of debate. Results from numerous neuropsychological, neuroimaging and neurophysiological studies implicate that the hippocampus and posterior parahippocampal cortex selectively support recollection-based recognition, whereas other regions (e.g. the rhinal cortex) mediate familiarity-based recognition (Ranganath et al., 2004; Suchan et al., 2008). Notably, there is preliminary evidence from imaging studies that KIBRA is associated with structural differences in areas which are selectively involved in recollection and familiarity-based recognition memory (Palombo et al., 2013). To explore the possibility that qualitative aspects of recognition performance might be differentially affected by KIBRA polymorphism, the remember/know judgment procedure was employed in our study.

Considerable evidence suggests that episodic memory performance differs between genders, with women showing superior retrieval in dependence of the learning material, i.e. verbal, spatial or autobiographical information (Andreano & Cahill, 2009; Herlitz et al., 1997). Furthermore, the association between KIBRA rs17070145 polymorphism and cognitive functions is more pronounced in healthy female subjects as compared to males or mixed samples (Wersching et al., 2011). We thus included gender as an additional important factor to determine the association between KIBRA and reconstructive episodic memory.

## Methods

### Participants

A total of $N = 219$ healthy students with no history of psychiatric disease and/or current psychoactive medication were tested. Twelve participants were excluded from analysis because they could not be genotyped ($n = 5$) or had incomplete test data ($n = 7$). Each participant was instructed to refrain from eating food and drinking beverages (except for water) 1 h prior to the experiment. Subjects received either financial allowance (10euro/h) or course credits for participation. All participants provided written informed consent. The study was approved by the local ethics committee of the University of Bochum and was carried out in accordance with the principles outlined by the Declaration of Helsinki.

### Experimental procedure

Participants were tested in the DRM paradigm according to a slightly modified procedure by Roediger & McDermott, 1995. Briefly, all subjects were instructed to memorize word lists for a subsequent memory test. The learning material comprised 8 word lists which were derived from Stadler et al., 1999 word list inventory and translated to German. Each word list consisted of 15 words which were semantically related to a specific theme word, which was not presented during the learning phase itself (e.g. "cold" was a theme word and was not presented, but instead its highly associative words "hot", "snow", "warm" etc. were presented).

Words of each list were presented both as auditory (via earphones by a pre-recorded female voice) and visual stimuli on the computer screen. Words of a list were presented with an inter-word delay of 750 ms, whereas word lists as a whole were presented with a delay of 10 s. The order of word presentation was chosen according to the associative strength with the theme word (from the associatively strongest word to the weakest one). After the learning phase, each participant completed an unrelated distraction task for approximately 15 min to prevent rehearsal. Subsequently, each participant was asked to recall as many words as possible from the initial learning phase and to write down these words on a sheet of paper. Participants were granted 4 min to recall and write down the words. After another distraction task, participants completed the recognition test.

During the recognition test, words that had been presented at serial positions 1, 5 and 10 of each word list during the initial learning phase ("listed items") as well as unrelated distractor words ("distractor items", i.e. words not presented during encoding and unrelated to listed items) and semantically-associated theme words ("critical lures", i.e. words not presented during encoding but highly related to listed items) were presented individually on a sheet of paper. Participants were asked to rate each word as old or new (i.e. according as to whether the word had been presented during the learning phase or not) as well as to categorize the words judged as "old" according to the Remember/Know/Guess procedure (Seamon et al., 2002).

### Questionnaires

In order to control for the impact of depressive symptoms, trait anxiety and stress sensitivity on the retrieval of accurate and false memories, each participant completed specifically selected items from the Depression Anxiety Stress Scales (DASS; Lovibond & Lovibond, 1995) prior to the encoding phase.

### Genotyping

DNA samples were collected using OG-100 Oragene saliva collection kits (DNA Genotek, Ontario, Canada). DNA extraction and genotyping were performed using established procedures according to the manufacturers protocol. The KIBRA rs17070145 polymorphism was genotyped by LGC Genomics (Hoddesdon, UK) using KASP technology with validated arrays. Five participants could not be genotyped, giving a genotyping success rate of 97.7%.

### Statistical procedures

Statistical procedures were conducted with the software package SPSS statistics Version 22 (IBM; Armonk, NY, USA: IBM Corp.). All analyses were performed using the dominant model of inheritance (CC vs. CT/TT). With respect to free recall, the proportion of listed items and critical lure items were entered as within-subjects factors while Genotype (CC vs. CT/TT) and Gender were entered as between-subjects factor in a mixed-design ANOVA. Measures of recognition memory (hit rates (=listed items classified as "old"; false memory rates (=critical lures classified as "old"; and false alarm rates (=distractor items classified as "old") were corrected prior to analyses according to the procedure by Snodgrass & Corwin, 1988. Genotype and gender differences in these recognition memory scores were assessed using mixed ANOVAs and a series of univariate analyses. Remember/Know/Guess Judgments were analyzed by a series of 2 (Genotype) × 2 (Gender) × 3 (Item-type; critical lures, distractors, listed items) mixed ANOVAs.

Bonferroni-correction for multiple testing was applied where indicated and simple effects analyses were conducted following a significant interaction or main effect. Where appropriate, degrees of freedom were corrected by Greenhouse-Geiser estimates of sphericity. $P$-values $< 0.05$ were considered to be significant.

## Results

For the KIBRA polymorphism, 97 subjects were homozygous for the C allele, 26 for the T allele, while 84 subjects were heterozygous for the C/T alleles. The distribution of allele frequencies (C = 67.15%, T = 32.85%) and the hereby observed genotypes were in Hardy-Weinberg equilibrium, $P = 0.2486$.

As displayed in Table 1, CC and CT/TT carriers were comparable with respect to age, gender distribution and their scores on any of the subscales of the DASS, all P ≥ 0.291.

### Free recall condition

As indicated by a significant main effect for item-type, $F(1, 203) = 131.287$, $P < 0.001$, subjects recalled a greater proportion of listed items [0.34 ± 0.01 (mean ± SE)] than critical lures (0.15 ± 0.01). Furthermore, we found an item-type x gender interaction, $F(1, 203) = 5.033$, $P = 0.026$, with female participants (0.36 ± 0.01) recalling a greater proportion of listed items than males (0.31 ± 0.01), $P = 0.003$.

No other main or interaction effects attained statistical significance, all P ≥ 0.215. With respect to the total number of words recalled, females (M = 46.76, SD = 1.31) again outperformed males (M = 41.33, SD = 1.45), $F(1, 203) = 7.780$, $P = 0.006$, while no effects for genotype were evident (main effect and interaction, all P ≥ 0.243). In addition, genotypes and genders were comparable in the number of distractors being recalled (main or interaction effects, all P ≥ 0.05).

### Recognition memory

Discriminability scores for hit rates, false memory rates, and false alarm rates in male and female CC and CT/TT carriers are summarized in Table 2. A mixed ANOVA

**Table 1** Demographic characteristics of the different genotypes

| Variable | CC (n = 97) | CT/TT (n = 110) | P - value |
|---|---|---|---|
| | M (SD) | M (SD) | |
| Age (years) | 24.47 (4.87) | 25.34 (6.59) | 0.291 |
| Gender % female) | 53.6% | 56.4% | 0.398 |
| DASS | | | |
| Depression | 2.38 (2.53) | 2.82 (3.45) | 0.306 |
| Anxiety | 2.76 (2.97) | 2.51 (2.52) | 0.507 |
| Stress | 6.07 (3.99) | 6.46 (4.43) | 0.507 |

*DASS* Depression Anxiety Stress Scales

**Table 2** Hit rates, false memory rates and false alarm rates

| | | Hits | False memories | False alarms |
|---|---|---|---|---|
| | | M ± SE | M ± SE | M ± SE |
| CC | Male | .82 ± .02 | .62 ± .04 | .13 ± .01 |
| | Female | .83 ± .01 | .64 ± .03 | .13 ± .02 |
| | Total | .82 ± .01 | .63 ± .02 | .13 ± .01 |
| CT/TT | Male | .83 ± .01 | .66 ± .03 | .14 ± .02 |
| | Female | .83 ± .01 | .56 ± .03 | .11 ± .01 |
| | Total | .83 ± .01 | .60 ± .02 | .12 ± .01 |
| Total | Male | .83 ± .01 | .64 ± .02 | .13 ± .01 |
| | Female | .83 ± .01 | .60 ± .02 | .12 ± .01 |

with type of recognition (hit rates, false memories, false alarms) as within-subjects factor as well as genotype and gender as between-subjects factor revealed a significant main effect for type of recognition, F (1.553, 315.258) = 1156.324, $P < .001$ (Greenhouse-Geiser: ε = 0.776), and a significant gender x genotype interaction, F (1, 203) = 4.050, $P = 0.045$, as well as a trend towards a three-way interaction, F(1.553, 315.258) = 2.409, $P = 0.105$ (Greenhouse-Geiser: ε = 0.776). Interestingly, a series of univariate analyses showed that carriers of the T-allele did not differ from CC homozygotes in their hit rates, F (1, 203) = 0.152, $P = 0.697$, and false alarm rates, F (1, 203) = 0.004, $P = 0.948$, with these patterns not being subjected to gender differences (genotype x gender interaction, all P ≥ 0.328). However, the interaction between gender and genotype emerged for false memory rates, F (1,203) = 4.140, $P = 0.043$, while the main effects themselves were non-significant, all P ≥ 0.190. As shown in Fig. 1, there was a modulation of gender-specific effects by rs17070145 genotype, with females being less prone to false memories than males within the group of T-allele carriers ($P = 0.016$). Furthermore, there was a tendency for female carriers of the T-allele to have a lower proportion of false memories than their counterparts of the CC group ($P = 0.052$). After correcting for repeated testing of the different recognition indices (hit rates, false memories, and false alarms), the gender x genotype interaction for false memory rates did not remain significant ($P_{corr} = .129$).

### Remember / know / guess judgments
#### Listed items

A significant main effect for response-type, F(1.301, 264.149, = 300.352, $P < 0.001$ (Greenhouse-Geiser: ε = 0.651), and a significant response-type x genotype interaction, F (1.301, 264.149) = 4.891, $P = 0.019$; Greenhouse-Geiser: ε = 0.651) were found. As displayed in Fig. 2a, carriers of the T-allele exhibited a significantly greater proportion of "remember" judgments as compared to CC carriers (P = 0.016), while the opposite was

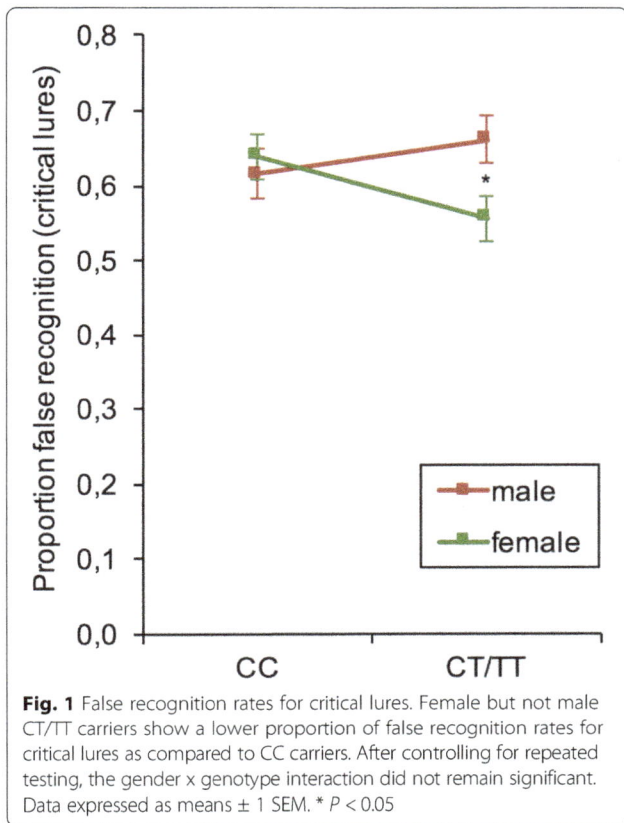

**Fig. 1** False recognition rates for critical lures. Female but not male CT/TT carriers show a lower proportion of false recognition rates for critical lures as compared to CC carriers. After controlling for repeated testing, the gender x genotype interaction did not remain significant. Data expressed as means ± 1 SEM. * P < 0.05

true for "know" judgments (P = 0.037). In addition, gender differences (interaction response-type x gender, F (1.301, 246.149) = 3.927, P = 0.038; Greenhouse-Geiser: ε = 0.651) were observed for the readout response types. Analysis of simple effects revealed that females had a significantly lower proportion of know responses (P = 0.023) and a tendency towards more remember responses (P = 0.061) than males.

### Critical lures
As indicated by a significant main effect for response-type F(1.925, 390.749) = 9.789, P < 0.001 (Greenhouse Geiser: ε = 0.962), critical lures were more frequently judged to be remembered than either guessed or known (Fig. 2b). No other effects attained statistical significance, all P ≥ 0.162.

### Distractor items
Only the main effect for response-type, F(1.780, 361.408) = 29.982, P < 0.001 (Greenhouse-Geiser: ε = 0.890), attained statistical significance (all other effects, P ≥ 0.05), with distractors being most frequently subjected to guess judgments (Fig. 2c).

### Discussion
In the present study, we examined the contribution of KIBRA polymorphism in the reconstruction of past episodes as measured by the DRM paradigm. In the free recall condition, we found that female participants outperformed males in terms of total number of items correctly retrieved. This effect is consistent with previous findings on gender differences in episodic memory performance by showing that women show superior performance relative to men, especially on verbal memory tasks (Herlitz & Rehnman, 2008). The explanation for the observed sex differences in episodic memory is still a matter of debate (Herlitz & Rehnman, 2008). Interestingly, accuracy in the correct recognition condition of listed items was not significantly different between males and females or CC and CT/TT carriers of the KIBRA rs17070145 polymorphism. In contrast, we found a significant *gender x genotype interaction* for false recognition rates of critical lures. In particular, female CT/TT carriers exhibited a lower proportion of false recognition

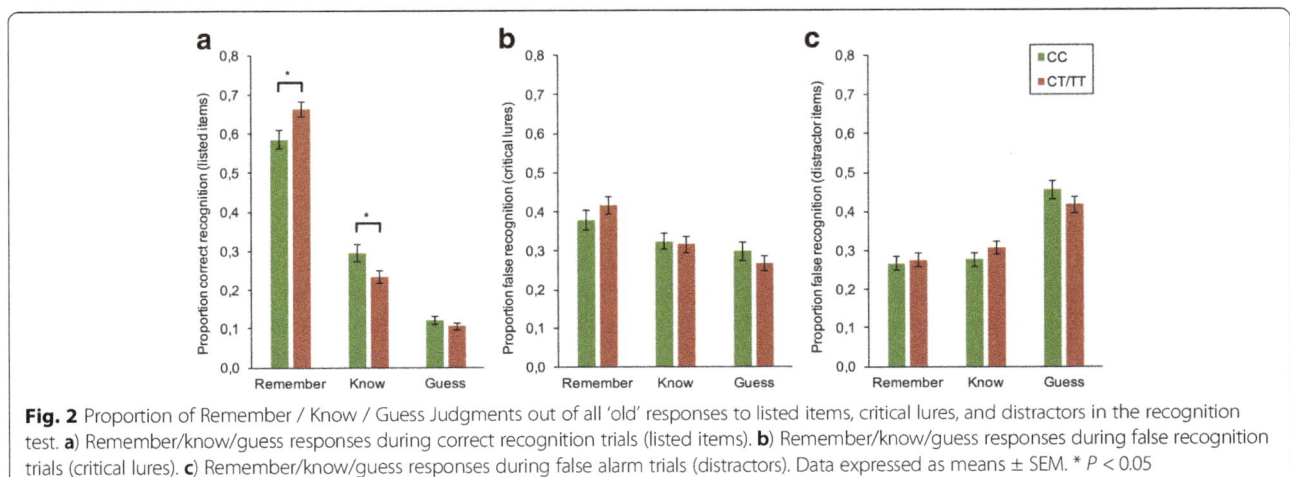

**Fig. 2** Proportion of Remember / Know / Guess Judgments out of all 'old' responses to listed items, critical lures, and distractors in the recognition test. **a)** Remember/know/guess responses during correct recognition trials (listed items). **b)** Remember/know/guess responses during false recognition trials (critical lures). **c)** Remember/know/guess responses during false alarm trials (distractors). Data expressed as means ± SEM. * P < 0.05

rates as compared to male CT/TT carriers and a tendency to be less prone to false recognition of critical lures than female CC carriers. This effect however, did not remain significant after correcting for repeated testing. Thus, our preliminary results tentatively support previous findings on the association between KIBRA polymorphism, gender and cognitive functions (Wersching et al., 2011), but (perhaps due to relatively small sample sizes) failed to reach statistical significance. Results regarding the principal role of KIBRA polymorphism on memory functions are rather inconclusive (summarized in Schwab et al., 2014). In healthy subjects, the T-allele of the KIBRA rs17070145 seem to be associated with significantly better (Schaper et al., 2008; Vassos et al., 2010; Kauppi et al., 2011; Almeida et al., 2008; Preuschhof et al., 2010), slightly better (Witte et al., 2016) or unchanged (Need et al., 2008) declarative memory performance relative to non-carriers of the T-allele. These inconsistencies might be due to methodological differences, i.e. the use of different tasks for the measurement of episodic memory functions. Similar to our results, Wersching et al., 2011 used a neuropsychological test battery and failed to find main effects of the KIBRA rs17070145 genotype on immediate and delayed memory performance. Instead, a significant interaction between gender and rs17070145 genotype was observed for working memory performance (for example in the Digit span test). Furthermore, the same study also reports that gender determines the effect of rs17070145 on executive functioning. Thus, it is possible that our findings regarding false recognition performance are related to an interaction between gender and rs17070145 genotype that modulates working memory and executive functions. Interestingly, working memory capacity seems to be closely related to the susceptibility to false memories (Leding, 2012) and false recognition rates can be significantly reduced by improving executive control functions (McCabe & Smith, 2002). Similarly, Zhang et al., 2009 proposed that the KIBRA rs17070145 T-allele could differentially modulate hippocampal functions such as long-term memory and those functions related to the prefrontal cortex (i.e, working memory capacity). Thus, the putative explanation behind the interactive effects of KIBRA genotype and gender on false recognition performance might be the differential effect of KIBRA in processes related to working memory, executive functions and long-term memory, all of which contribute to differences in the susceptibility to produce false memories. From the methodological perspective, our results thus argue for considerations of gender (Wersching et al., 2011) and task specific demands (Zhang et al., 2009) as important variables in the interpretation of results related to the association of KIBRA and complex cognitive functions such as reconstructive episodic memory.

Another important finding of this study was the association of KIBRA and confidence ratings during recognition memory. While there were no genotype differences in overall recognition performance, the T-allele of the KIBRA rs17070145 polymorphism was associated with differences in qualitative aspects of recognition memory. In particular, in trials with correct recognition of listed items, participants showed significantly more "remember" responses as compared to "know" and "guess" responses. Likewise, "know" responses were significantly higher than "guess" responses during the correct recognition of listed items. Most importantly however, a significant response-type x genotype interaction was evident, indicating that, CT/TT carriers showed more "remember", but fewer "know" responses as compared to CC carriers during the correct recognition of listed items. One explanation for these findings might be that the T-allele of the KIBRA rs17070145 polymorphism supports recollection-based episodic memory retrieval. According to dual process models of recognition memory, recollection refers to the conscious retrieval of items plus the contextual details encountered during the encoding phase. In contrast, the mere knowing that the item was on the list without remembering the contextual details refers to familiarity-based retrieval processes. Tulving, 1985 proposed that the semantic and episodic memory systems are operating on these two retrieval processes to a different degree. Furthermore, the identified brain structures subserving these different recognition memory processes do not necessarily overlap (Eldridge et al., 2000; Aggleton et al., 2005; Yonelinas et al., 2002). Studies using the remember/know procedure have shown that an intact hippocampus is most probably required for recollection (Aggleton et al., 2005) whereas hippocampal recruitment during familiarity-based retrieval is not obligatory (Ranganath et al., 2004; Suchan et al., 2008). KIBRA is abundantly expressed in the hippocampus. Female T-allele carriers show larger hippocampal volumes relative to non-T-allele carriers (Palombo et al., 2013), an effect which was recently replicated in older healthy adults (Witte et al., 2016). Such structural differences observed in T-carriers and non-carriers of KIBRA rs17070145 might represent an underlying mechanism for the herein observed differences in retrieval characteristics. Indeed, recollection memory can be predicted on the basis of hippocampal longitudinal volume ratios (Poppenk & Moscovitch, 2011). Of course, this conclusion is rather speculative, considering the limited data at hand, especially since we did not perform structural functional magnetic resonance imaging to support this conclusion.

Another compelling but speculative explanation of the behavioral effects observed in the present study could be a genotype-related difference in brain activation patterns.

Using a face-profession paired associative learning task (which is intended to measure episodic memory), Papassotiropoulos et al., 2006 found a significantly higher brain activation in the hippocampus and parahippocampal gyrus of CC homozygotes relative to T-carriers during the retrieval but not encoding phase. In a similar task applied to a sample of elderly non-demented subjects, Kauppi et al., 2011 also found differences in hippocampal activation between CC homozygotes and T-allele carriers during retrieval. However, in contrast to the findings obtained by Papassotiropoulos et al., 2006, both a lower activation of medial temporal lobe regions as well as a slower response time was reported in CC homozygous (Kauppi et al., 2011). Hence, it can be concluded that KIBRA rs17070145 genotype-related differences in brain activation patterns exist which do not necessarily lead to equivalent genotype-related differences in episodic memory performance (Papassotiropoulos et al., 2006; Kauppi et al., 2011). Diminished hippocampal functioning in CC homozygous carriers (Papassotiropoulos et al., 2006; Kauppi et al., 2011) corroborate our results, implicating a beneficial effect of KIBRA T-allele in episodic memory mainly due to a qualitatively different retrieval process (i.e. recollection based retrieval) and thus more efficient hippocampal recruitment during recognition performance. Thus, it would be valuable to implement remember/know judgements in future imaging studies to get more insight into the functional link between KIBRA, hippocampal structure and functionality and episodic memory processing.

The following limitations of this study need to be considered. First, the sample size was relatively small for genetic association studies and the herewith associated limited statistical power might explain why we only found a trend towards a gender x genotype interaction for false recognition rates. Interestingly, studies with much smaller sample sizes report similar trends towards an effect (Witte et al., 2016) or even significant effects (Nacmias et al., 2008; Schaper et al., 2008) of KIBRA polymorphism on cognitive functions. In contrast to previous studies, our DRM task is relatively difficult to implement, laborious and more time-consuming. When taking the latter into account, our sample size is substantially larger relative to other genetic association studies employing the DRM procedure (see (Montag et al., 2014). Nevertheless, future studies with larger samples would be beneficial to derive definite conclusions regarding the role of gender and KIBRA genotype on reconstructive memory in the DRM task.

Furthermore, it is conceivable that other genetic factors might play a role in the relationship between KIBRA polymorphism, gender and reconstructive memory. For example, it was repeatedly shown that another gene, CLSTN2 (calsyntenin 2) interacts with KIBRA to modulate episodic memory performance in healthy individuals (Papassotiropoulos et al., 2006; Preuschhof et al., 2010) and depressed elderly subjects (Pantzar et al., 2014). Similar to KIBRA, CLSTN2 is expressed in memory-related brain regions such as the hippocampus (Papassotiropoulos et al., 2006; Hintsch et al., 2002), suggesting a possible involvement in processes related to episodic memory storage and retrieval. Also, we did not employ any structural and/or functional neuroimaging measures, thus any conclusion about underlying neuronal mechanisms mediating the herein observed behavioral effect remain speculative. Such additional measures, however, would be helpful, especially with regard to possible changes in medial temporal lobe/hippocampal activations which go along with our finding of genotype-related differences in familiarity and recollection-based retrieval. Given that the participants in our study were healthy young students the clinical implication of our findings and any extrapolation of the findings are not possible. Nevertheless, there are some important clinical implications that can be derived from this study. It has been shown that non-carriers of the KIBRA rs17070145 T-allele exhibit an increased risk of late-onset Alzheimer's disease (Corneveaux et al., 2010) which might be related to lower glucose metabolism in brain regions involved in the processing of episodic memories. Similarly, a possible association between KIBRA and the risk of developing strong traumatic memories in survivors of mass conflict (Wilker et al., 2013) has been demonstrated by array-based SNP genotyping. Individuals suffering from PTSD and Alzheimer's disease show distinct neuropsychological profiles with specific alterations in different aspects of episodic memory functioning. Thus, it could be predicted that the KIBRA (rs17070145) T-allele might have a protective role in both Alzheimer's disease and PTSD.

## Conclusion

The present study extends previous findings on the possible role of KIBRA on cognitive functions. We add new data showing a trend towards an interactive effect of KIBRA rs17070145 genotype and gender on reconstructive episodic memory, in particular regarding the susceptibility to produce false memories in healthy young adults. Furthermore, we demonstrated an association of KIBRA rs17070145 polymorphism and differences in qualitative aspects of recognition memory, suggesting a beneficial role of the T-allele in supporting recollection-based retrieval processes. We conclude that examining the contribution of genetic variations in KIBRA related SNPs to such systematic alterations in episodic memory functioning might be helpful to counteract the occurrence of cognitive and emotional symptoms in dementia and PTSD (Schneider et al., 2010) and lead to the development of novel therapeutic interventions.

## Funding

This study was funded by a research grant to JM by the Alexander von Humboldt Foundation (http://www.humboldt-foundation.de/web/start.html) and a research grant to AZ by the Deutsche Forschungsgemeinschaft (ZL 59/2–1). This work was also partly supported by grants from the UK MRC; G0901874/1 (TCE) and MR/J011762/1 (TCE & KJL). This study presents independent research partly funded by the NIHR. The views expressed are those of the author(s) and not necessarily those of the NHS, the NIHR or the Department of Health. The funders had no role in study design, data collection and analysis, decision to publish, or preparation of the manuscript.

## Authors' contributions

AZ designed the study. AZ and FP analyzed and interpreted the data and wrote the manuscript. SR, KJL and TCE conducted genotyping analysis. MLW, ED and JM discussed the results and implications and commented on the manuscript at all stages. All authors read and approved the final manuscript.

## Competing interests

The authors declare that they have no competing interests.

## Author details

[1]Mental Health Research and Treatment Center, Ruhr-Universität Bochum, 150, 44780 Bochum, Germany. [2]Institute of Psychiatry, Psychology and Neuroscience, MRC Social, Genetic and Developmental Psychiatry Centre, King's College London, London, UK. [3]School of Psychology, University of Sussex, Brighton, UK. Teaching and Research Unit, Life Sciences (UFR927), University Pierre and Marie Curie, Paris, France. Clinical Neuroscience, Max Planck Institute of Experimental Medicine, Göttingen, Germany.

## References

Aggleton JP, et al. Sparing of the familiarity component of recognition memory in a patient with hippocampal pathology. Neuropsychologia. 2005;43:1810–23.

Almeida OP, et al. KIBRA genetic polymorphism influences episodic memory in later life, but does not increase the risk of mild cognitive impairment. J Cell Mol Med. 2008;12:1672–6.

Andreano JM, Cahill L. Sex influences on the neurobiology of learning and memory. Learn Mem. 2009;16:248–66.

Boraxbekk CJ, et al. Investigating the influence of KIBRA and CLSTN2 genetic polymorphisms on cross-sectional and longitudinal measures of memory performance and hippocampal volume in older individuals. Neuropsychologia. 2015;78:10–7.

Breeden P, Dere D, Zlomuzica A, Dere E. The mental time travel continuum: on the architecture, capacity, versatility and extension of the mental bridge into the past and future. Rev Neurosci. 2016;27:421–34.

Büther K, Plaas C, Barnekow A, Kremerskothen J. KIBRA is a novel substrate for protein kinase Cζ. Biochem Biophys Res Commun. 2004;317:703–7.

Corneveaux JJ, et al. Evidence for an association between KIBRA and late-onset Alzheimer's disease. Neurobiol Aging. 2010;31:901–9.

Deese J. On the prediction of occurrence of particular verbal intrusions in immediate recall. J Exp Psychol. 1959;58:17–22.

Dewhurst SA, Anderson RJ, Berry DM, Garner SR. (2018) Individual differences in susceptibility to false memories: the effect of memory specificity. Q J Exp Psychol, in press. http://journals.sagepub.com/doi/full/10.1080/17470218.2017.1345961

Duning K, et al. KIBRA modulates directional migration of podocytes. J Am Soc Nephrol. 2008;19:1891–903.

Eldridge LL, Knowlton BJ, Furmanski CS, Bookheimer SY, Engel SA. Remembering episodes: a selective role for the hippocampus during retrieval. Nat Neurosci. 2000;3:1149–52.

Gallo DA. False memories and fantastic beliefs: 15 years of the DRM illusion. Mem Cogn. 2010;38:833–48.

Herlitz A, Nilsson LG, Backman L. Gender differences in episodic memory. Mem Cogn. 1997;25:801–11.

Herlitz A, Rehnman J. Sex differences in episodic memory. Curr Dir Psychol Sci. 2008;17:52–6.

Hintsch G, et al. The calsyntenins–a family of postsynaptic membrane proteins with distinct neuronal expression patterns. Mol Cell Neurosci. 2002;21:393–409.

Johannsen S, Duning K, Pavenstadt H, Kremerskothen J, Boeckers TM. Temporal-spatial expression and novel biochemical properties of the memory-related protein KIBRA. Neuroscience. 2008;155:1165–73.

Kauppi K, Nilsson LG, Adolfsson R, Eriksson E, Nyberg L. KIBRA polymorphism is related to enhanced memory and elevated hippocampal processing. J Neurosci. 2011;31:14218–22.

Laws KR, Bhatt R. False memories and delusional ideation in normal healthy subjects. Pers Individ Dif. 2005;39:775–81.

Leding JK. Working memory predicts the rejection of false memories. Memory. 2012;20:217–23.

Loftus EF. Planting misinformation in the human mind: a 30-year investigation of the malleability of memory. Learn Mem. 2005;12:361–6.

Lovibond SH, Lovibond PF. Manual for the depression anxiety stress scales. Sydney: Psychology Foundation; 1995.

Makuch L, et al. Regulation of AMPA receptor function by the human memory associated gene KIBRA. Neuron. 2011;71:1022–9.

McCabe DP, Smith AD. The effect of warnings on false memories in young and older adults. Mem Cogn. 2002;30:1065–77.

Milnik A, et al. Association of KIBRA with episodic and working memory: a meta-analysis. Am J Med Genet B Neuropsychiatr Genet. 2012;159B:958–69.

Montag C, et al. The role of the BDNF Val66Met polymorphism in individual differences in long-term memory capacity. J Mol Neurosci. 2014;54:796–802.

Nacmias B, et al. KIBRA gene variants are associated with episodic memory performance in subjective memory complaints. Neurosci Lett. 2008;436:145–7.

Need AC, et al. Failure to replicate effect of Kibra on human memory in two large cohorts of European origin. Am J Med Genet B Neuropsychiatr Genet. 2008;147B:667–8.

Palombo DJ, et al. KIBRA polymorphism is associated with individual differences in hippocampal subregions: evidence from anatomical segmentation using high-resolution MRI. J Neurosci. 2013;33:13088–93.

Pantzar A, et al. Interactive effects of KIBRA and CLSTN2 polymorphisms on episodic memory in old-age unipolar depression. Neuropsychologia. 2014;62:137–42.

Papassotiropoulos A, de Quervain DJF. Genetics of human episodic memory: dealing with complexity. Trends Cogn Sci. 2011;15:381–7.

Papassotiropoulos A, et al. Common KIBRA alleles are associated with human memory performance. Science. 2006;314:475–8.

Pardilla-Delgado E, Payne JD. (2017) The Deese-Roediger-McDermott (DRM) Task: A Simple Cognitive Paradigm to Investigate False Memories in the Laboratory. J Vis Exp. (119), e54793.

Pause BM, et al. Perspectives on episodic-like and episodic memory. Front Behav Neurosci. 2013;7:33.

Poppenk J, Moscovitch M. A hippocampal marker of recollection memory ability among healthy young adults: contributions of posterior and anterior segments. Neuron. 2011;72:931–7.

Preuschhof C, et al. KIBRA and CLSTN2 polymorphisms exert interactive effects on human episodic memory. Neuropsychologia. 2010;48:402–8.

Ramirez S, et al. Creating a false memory in the hippocampus. Science. 2013;341:387–91.

Ranganath C, et al. Dissociable correlates of recollection and familiarity within the medial temporal lobes. Neuropsychologia. 2004;42:2–13.

Rodriguez-Rodriguez E, et al. Age-dependent association of KIBRA genetic variation and Alzheimer's disease risk. Neurobiol Aging. 2009;30:322–4.

Roediger H, McDermott K. Creating false memories: remembering words not presented in lists. J Exp Psychol Learn Mem Cogn. 1995;21:803–14.

Saunders J, Randell J, Reed P. Recall of false memories in individuals scoring high in schizotypy: memory distortions are scale specific. J Behav Ther Exp Psychiatry. 2012;43:711–5.

Schacter DL, Slotnick SD. The cognitive neuroscience of memory distortion. Neuron. 2004;44:149–60.

Schacter DL, et al. Neuroanatomical correlates of veridical and illusory recognition memory: evidence from positron emission tomography. Neuron. 1996;17:267–74.

Schaper K, Kolsch H, Popp J, Wagner M, Jessen F. KIBRA gene variants are associated with episodic memory in healthy elderly. Neurobiol Aging. 2008; 29:1123–5.

Schneider A, et al. KIBRA: a new gateway to learning and memory? Front Aging Neurosci. 2010;2:4.

Schwab LC, Luo V, Clarke CL, Nathan PJ. Effects of the KIBRA single nucleotide polymorphism on synaptic plasticity and memory: a review of the literature. Curr Neuropharmacol. 2014;12:281–8.

Seamon JG, et al. Are false memories more difficult to forget than accurate memories? The effect of retention interval on recall and recognition. Mem Cogn. 2002;30:1054–64.

Snodgrass JG, Corwin J. Pragmatics of measuring recognition memory: applications to dementia and amnesia. J Exp Psychol Gen. 1988;117:34–50.

Stadler MA, Roediger HL 3rd, McDermott KB. Norms for word lists that create false memories. Mem Cogn. 1999;27:494–500.

Suchan B, Gayk AE, Schmid G, Köster O, Daum I. Hippocampal involvement in recollection but not familiarity across time: a prospective study. Hippocampus. 2008;18:92–8.

Tulving E. Memory and consciousness. Can Psychol. 1985;26:1–12.

Tulving E. Episodic memory: from mind to brain. Annu Rev Psychol. 2002;53:1–25.

Vassos E, et al. Evidence of association of KIBRA genotype with episodic memory in families of psychotic patients and controls. J Psychiatr Res. 2010;44:795–8.

Volk HE, McDermott KB, Roediger HL, Todd RD. Genetic influences on free and cued recall in long-term memory tasks. Twin Res Hum Genet. 2006;9:623–31.

Wersching H, et al. Impact of common KIBRA allele on human cognitive functions. Neuropsychopharmacology. 2011;36:1296–304.

Wilker S, et al. The role of memory-related gene WWC1 (KIBRA) in lifetime posttraumatic stress disorder: evidence from two independent samples from African conflict regions. Biol Psychiatry. 2013;74:664–71.

Winograd E, Peluso JP, Glover TA. Individual differences in susceptibility to memory illusions. Appl Cogn Psychol. 1998;12:S5–S27.

Witte AV, Kobe T, Kerti L, Rujescu D, Floel A. Impact of KIBRA polymorphism on memory function and the hippocampus in older adults. Neuropsychopharmacology. 2016;41:781–90.

Yonelinas AP, et al. Effects of extensive temporal lobe damage or mild hypoxia on recollection and familiarity. Nat Neurosci. 2002;5:1236–41.

Yoshihama Y, Hirai T, Ohtsuka T, Chida K. KIBRA Colocalizes with protein kinase Mzeta (PKM zeta) in the mouse hippocampus. Biosci Biotechnol Biochem. 2009;73:147–51.

Zhang H, Kranzler HR, Poling J, Gruen JR, Gelernter J. Cognitive flexibility is associated with KIBRA variant and modulated by recent tobacco use. Neuropsychopharmacology. 2009;34:2508–16.

Zhu B, et al. True but not false memories are associated with the HTR2A gene. Neurobiol Learn Mem. 2013;106:204–9.

# 15

# Adenosine A$_{2A}$ receptor antagonists act at the hyperoxic phase to confer protection against retinopathy

Rong Zhou[1,2†], Shuya Zhang[1,2†], Xuejiao Gu[1,2], Yuanyuan Ge[1,2], Dingjuan Zhong[1,2], Yuling Zhou[1,2], Lingyun Tang[1,2], Xiao-Ling Liu[1,2*] and Jiang-Fan Chen[1,2*]

## Abstract

**Background:** Retinopathy of prematurity (ROP) remains a major cause of childhood blindness and current laser photocoagulation and anti-VEGF antibody treatments are associated with reduced peripheral vision and possible delayed development of retinal vasculatures and neurons. In this study, we advanced the translational potential of adenosine A$_{2A}$ receptor (A$_{2A}$R) antagonists as a novel therapeutic strategy for selectively controlling pathological retinal neovascularization in oxygen-induced retinopathy (OIR) model of ROP.

**Methods:** Developing C57BL/6 mice were exposed to 75% oxygen from postnatal (P) day 7 to P12 and to room air from P12 to P17 and treated with KW6002 or vehicle at different postnatal developmental stages. Retinal vascularization was examined by whole-mount fluorescence and cross-sectional hematoxylin-eosin staining. Cellular proliferation, astrocyte and microglial activation, and tip cell function were investigated by isolectin staining and immunohistochemistry. Apoptosis was analyzed by TUNEL assay. The effects of oxygen exposure and KW6002 treatment were analyzed by two-way ANOVA or Kruskal-Wallis test or independent Student's t-test or Mann-Whitney U test.

**Results:** The A$_{2A}$R antagonist KW6002 (P7-P17) did not affect normal postnatal development of retinal vasculature, but selectively reduced avascular areas and neovascularization, with the reduced cellular apoptosis and proliferation, and enhanced astrocyte and tip cell functions in OIR. Importantly, contrary to our prediction that A$_{2A}$R antagonists were most effective at the hypoxic phase with aberrantly increased adenosine-A$_{2A}$R signaling, we discovered that the A$_{2A}$R antagonist KW6002 mainly acted at the hyperoxic phase to confer protection against OIR as KW6002 treatment at P7-P12 (but not P12-P17) conferred protection against OIR; this protection was observed as early as P9 with reduced avascular areas and reduced cellular apoptosis and reversal of eNOS mRNA down-regulation in retina of OIR.

**Conclusions:** As ROP being a biphasic disease, our identification of the hyperoxic phase as the effective window, together with selective and robust protection against pathological (but not physiological) angiogenesis, elevates A$_{2A}$R antagonists as a novel therapeutic strategy for ROP treatment.

**Keywords:** Retinopathy of prematurity, Oxygen-induced retinopathy, Adenosine A$_{2A}$ receptor, KW6002

* Correspondence: lxl@mail.eye.ac.cn; chenjf555@gmail.com
†Rong Zhou and Shuya Zhang contributed equally to this work.
[1]Institute of Molecular Medicine, School of Optometry and Ophthalmology and Eye Hospital, Wenzhou Medical University, 270 Xueyuan Road, Wenzhou 325027, Zhejiang, China
Full list of author information is available at the end of the article

## Background

Retinopathy of prematurity (ROP) remains a major cause of childhood blindness in many parts of the world (Chen et al. 2008; Gilbert 2008; Dhaliwal et al. 2009; Husain et al. 2013; Smith et al. 2013; Hellstrom et al. 2013; Hartnett 2015). As this disease of premature infants is believed to be largely driven by hypoxia-induced factor-1α (HIF-1α) signaling pathway and vascular endothelial growth factor (VEGF) levels in retina (Penn et al. 2008; Cavallaro et al. 2014; Campochiaro 2015), with characteristic hypoxia-induced pathological angiogenesis (Cavallaro et al. 2014; Fleck and McIntosh 2008; Hartnett and Penn 2012), current study of therapeutic development for ROP has largely focused on anti-VEGF therapy. Anti-VEGF antibody has been shown successful in a clinical trial to reduce the recurrence rate in stage III of ROP infants (Mintz-Hittner et al. 2011). However, intraocular injections of anti-VEGF antibody are invasive and repeated injection is associated with the risk of endophthalmitis. Importantly, as VEGF being an important cellular survival factor, the anti-VEGF treatment has been associated with serious concerns about the unintended effects of anti-VEGF agents on delayed development of retinal vasculatures and neurons, and on brain development of preterm infants (Nishijima et al. 2007; Saint-Geniez et al. 2008). Thus, alternative and less-invasive ROP therapeutic strategies with targets other than VEGF are critically needed to improve the ROP management and the quality of life for a growing number of premature infants.

We propose that drugs targeting adenosine (particularly $A_{2A}$) receptor signaling offer therapeutic advantage by selectively controlling pathological angiogenesis with minimal effect on normal retinal and brain development (for a review see Chen et al. 2017). The validity of $A_{2A}R$ signaling as a promising and novel therapeutic target is supported by rapid (minutes) local increase of adenosine level associated with upregulation of enzymes responsible for generating and maintaining adenosine concentration and delayed (~ 24 h) upregulation of $A_{2A}R$ in oxygen-induced retinopathy (OIR) model of ROP (Elsherbiny et al. 2013; Lutty and McLeod 2003; Liu et al. 2017), diabetic retina of rat with proliferative retinopathy (Vindeirinho et al. 2013) and other pathological conditions (Chen et al. 2013; Frick et al. 2009; Schingnitz et al. 2010; Linden 2011). Aberrantly increased adenosine-$A_{2A}R$ signaling thus represents a *local* "find-me" signal and renders a unique "purinergic chemotaxis" for a *local* resolution to pathological conditions (Chen et al. 2013). Moreover, the variants of human $A_{2A}R$ gene are associated with reduced risk of developing diabetic retinopathy in a prospective study (Charles et al. 2011). In support for this proposal, our recent studies with genetic knockout of $A_{2A}Rs$ or $A_1Rs$ suggested that in OIR, the most frequently used model for ocular pathological angiogenesis, genetic inactivation of $A_{2A}R$ or $A_1R$ did not influence normal postnatal development of retinal vasculature, but selectively attenuated pathological angiogenesis (Liu et al. 2010; Zhang et al. 2015), whereas $A_1R$ activity differentially modulated hyperoxia-induced vaso-obliteration and hypoxia-induced revascularization (Zhang et al. 2015). This proposal is further substantiated by a recent large prospective phase III clinical study "Caffeine Therapy for Apnea of Prematurity" showing severe ROP (as a secondary outcome in a two-year follow-up observation) was less common in infants assigned to chronic caffeine (a non-selective adenosine receptor antagonist) treatment compared with the control (Schmidt et al. 2007), and by pharmacological studies revealing that chronic caffeine treatment selectively attenuates retinal vasculopathy in OIR model (Zhang et al. 2017; Aranda et al. 2016). Thus, $A_{2A}R$ antagonism may represent novel and promising pharmacological strategy to control retinal pathological angiogenesis in ROP with distinct advantage over other anti-VEGF antibody strategies, which may be necessary not only for pathological angiogenesis, but also for normal retinal vascularization and brain development (LeBlanc et al. 2013).

However, the effectiveness and selectivity of $A_{2A}R$ antagonist-mediated protection against pathological angiogenesis (without affecting normal retinal vascularization) in ROP models have not been tested directly. In this study, the $A_{2A}R$ antagonist KW6002, a drug already in clinical phase III trials for Parkinson's disease treatment with noted safety profile for aging population (Chen et al. 2013), was used to demonstrate the efficacy and selectivity of $A_{2A}R$ antagonist control of ROP without affecting normal retinal vascular development. Importantly, contrary to our prediction that $A_{2A}R$ antagonists are most effective at the hypoxic phase with aberrantly increased adenosine-$A_{2A}R$ signaling, we discovered that the $A_{2A}R$ antagonist KW6002 mainly acted at the hyperoxic phase to confer protection against OIR. As ROP being a biphasic disease, targeting the initial vaso-obliteration stage offers therapeutic advantage to preserve developing retinal vascular function and prevent progression to the proliferative phase of ROP. Thus, our identification of the hyperoxic phase as the effective therapeutic window, together with selective and robust protection against pathological (but not physiological) angiogenesis and possible cellular mechanisms (i.e. neuronal cell death and endothelial nitric oxide synthase (eNOS) activity), elevates $A_{2A}R$ antagonists as a novel therapeutic strategy for treatment of ROP.

## Methods

### Mouse model of oxygen-induced retinopathy (OIR)

C57BL/6 J mice from the Animal Laboratory of Wenzhou Medical University (Wenzhou, China) were used in this study. The OIR model described previously by Smith and colleagues was adopted (Liu et al. 2010; Smith et al. 1994).

Briefly, seven-days old C57BL/6 J mice kept with the foster/nursing mothers were exposed to 75% oxygen for 5 days [from postnatal day 7(P7) to P12 (with P0 being the day for pup delivery)] to induce vaso-obliteration. At P12, the mice were returned to room air (21% oxygen) to induce retinal neovascularizaion, which was maximal at P17. Age-matched mice kept in room air throughout postnatal development (P0-P17) served as "Room-air Controls". The foster mothers were rotated between the mice exposed to hyperoxia and the mice kept in room air every 8 h.

All procedures with animals in this study were performed in accordance with the Association for Research in Vision and Ophthalmology (ARVO) Statement for the Use of Animals in Ophthalmic and Vision Research and were approved by the Institutional Animal Care and Use Committee of Wenzhou Medical University.

## KW6002 treatment
KW6002 was prepared freshly in 15% DMSO, 15% castrol oil and 70% phosphate buffer saline (PBS), as we described previously (Chen et al. 2001). For each drug treatment, littermates from the same breeding were randomly divided into the drug treatment and control groups. For each treatment condition, at least 2–3 litters were used for the experiment. KW6002 was administered by intraperitoneal injection (i.p.) at dose of 10 mg/kg at different postnatal developmental stages (P7 or P12) and for different period (P7-P17, P7-P12,P12-P17 or P7-P9) every other day or every day. The mice received vehicle in the same volume and with the same intervals served as the control group.

## Fluorescence immunostaining of whole-mount retinas
Fluorescence staining of whole-mounted retinas was performed as previously described (Connor et al. 2009). Mice were euthanized at P12 and P17 and eyes were enucleated and fixed with 4% paraformaldehyde for 1 h. The corneas were removed with scissors along the limbus, and then intact retinas were dissected. Retinas were blocked and permeabilized in PBS containing 0.5% Triton-X-100 overnight at 4 °C. Then retinas were incubated with 10 μg/ml isolectin B4 (Molecular Probes, Life Technologies, Carlsbad, CA, USA)overnight at 4 °C. Retinas were then incubated with anti-glial fibrillary acidic protein (GFAP) mouse monoclonal antibody (1:500, Sigma-Aldrich, St. Louis, MO, USA) for 12 h at 4 °C, followed by incubation with fluorescence-conjugated secondary antibodies (1:500, Invitrogen, Life Technologies, Carlsbad, CA,USA) for 2 h, and then whole-mounted. Retinas were washed with PBS and mounted on microscope slides in mounting medium. Retinas were examined by Laser Scanning Microscope (Zeiss 510; Carl Zeiss). Areas of vaso-obliteration and vitreoretinal neovascular tufts were quantified by using Adobe Photoshop CS 5 software. Eight non-overlapping and randomly selected microscopic fields per retina

were imaged by confocal scanning laser microscopy (LSM 710; Carl Zeiss, Oberkochen, Germany) to assess the formation of endothelial tip cells;four non-overlapping and randomly selected microscopic fields in the avascular area per retina were imaged by confocal scanning laser microscopy to assess astrocyte function.

To assess normal postnatal development of retinal angiogenesis, C57BL/6 J mice littermates received vehicle (breeding in room air) were sacrificed and the eyes were harvested at P17, respectively. Whole-mount retinas were stained with isolectin B4. Eight non-overlapping and randomly selected microscopic fields per retina and whole-mounted retina were assessed for morphology and distribution of retinal vessels at P17. Vessels in the three layers (superficial, intermediate and deep) were skeletonized (Kornfield and Newman 2014), and the total vessel length in each microscopic field was calculated using Image-Pro Plus software. Vessel density was quantified as the ratio of the total vessel length to microscopic field.

## Neovascular quantification
Quantification of neovascularization was performed according to the procedure described previously (Liu et al. 2010; Smith et al. 1994). The extent of neo-vascularization was evaluated by counting the number of neovascular nuclei, which were defined as the nuclei of cells extended beyond the inner limiting membrane of the retina into the vitreous body. In this study, eyes of 10 mice from each group were examined and analyzed. For each eye, 20 retinal sections (excluding the optic nerve) were evaluated. All neovascular nuclei were counted under 400× magnifications with hematoxylin and eosin–stained retinal sections by an investigator who was blind to the specific group assignment.

## Semi-quantification of astrocyte in retinal Vaso-obliteration areas
After OIR exposure, mouse retinas were harvested on P17 to assess the astrocyte. GFAP staining of whole-mounted retinas were examined by fluorescence microscopy. The extent of astrocyte persistence in the obliterated zones were scored by the blind observer using the semi-quantitation method on a 1–6 scale as described previously (Dorrell et al. 2010; Liang et al. 2012). As indicated in Fig. 3e, the score of 1–2 indicated retinas with a large number of astrocytes in the vascular obliterated areas which formed a nearly normal astrocytic template. The score of 3–4 indicated retinas with substantial numbers of astrocytes remaining in the vascular obliterated areas (fewer than normal), but failed to form normal astrocytic template. The score of 5–6 indicated there were very few astrocytes in the vascular obliterated zone.

### Terminal deoxynucleotidyl transferase biotin-dUTP nick end labelling (TUNEL) assay

Retinal cell apoptosis was evaluated at P12 or P17. TUNEL staining was performed with the Roche In Situ Cell Death Detection kit (Roche Diagnostic, Basel, Switzerland) following the manufacturer's instructions. Ten-micrometer–thick cryostat sections with optic nerve head were permeabilized and antigen retrieval was performed by 0.1% sodium citrate buffer solution with 0.5% Triton X-100 for 5 min. After washing 3 times, the sections were incubated in TUNEL reaction solutions for 1 h in 37 °C, then washed and stained for another 5 min using DAPI (1:2000; Beyotime Biotechnology). TUNEL-positive cells were evaluated in three sections crossing the optic nerve per retina under fluorescent microscopy (Zeiss 510; Carl Zeiss).

### Immunohistochemistry

Mouse eyes were dissected and embedded in paraffin at P17 of OIR. For anti–proliferating cell nuclear antigen (PCNA) staining, after being deparaffinized and heated in 10 mM sodium citrate for antigen repairing, 3 retinal paraffin sections were blocked and permeabilized, then incubated with PCNA rabbit polyclonal antibody (1:200; Santa Cruz Biotechnology, SantaCruz, CA, USA). Fluorescence-conjugated secondary Abs (1:500; Thermo Fisher Scientific) were applied to detect positive signals.

For microglial activation by immunostaining with anti-Iba-1 antibody at P12/P17 of OIR, mouse eyes were dissected and embedded in optimum cutting temperature compound. Three cryostat sections with optic nerve head per retina were blocked and permeabilized, then incubated with the anti-Iba-1 rabbit polyclonal antibody (1:100; Wako, Osaka, Japan) overnight at 4 °C. Fluorescence-conjugated second antibodies (1:500; Invitrogen, Life Technologies) were applied for detecting the positive signal.

### Quantitative real-time reverse transcription PCR

The mRNA level of $A_1R$, $A_{2A}R$, VEGFA, and eNOS in retina harvested at P12 was done by the quantitative real-time polymerase chain reaction (qPCR) procedure as we have described previously (Zhang et al. 2017) using the following forward and reverse primers: $A_{2A}R$: forward,5'-CCGAATTCCACTCCGGTACA-3'; reverse, 5'-CAGTTGTTCCAGCCCAGCAT-3'; $A_1R$: forward, 5'-ATCCCTCTCCGGTACAAGACAGT-3'; reverse, 5'-ACTCAGGTTGTTCCAGCCAAAC-3'; VEGFA: forward, 5'-GAAAGGGTCAAAAACGAAAGC-3'; reverse, 5'-CGCTCTGAACAAGGCTCAC-3'; eNOS: forward, 5'-TGTGACCCTCACCGCTACAA-3'; reverse, 5'-GCACAATCCAGGCCCAATC-3'. GAPDH: forward, 5'- AGGTCGGTGTGAACGGATTTG-3'; reverse, 5'-TGTAGACCATGTAGTTGA GGTCA-3'.

### Statistical analysis

The data were presented as the mean ± standard error (SE). The effect of KW6002 versus vehicle was analyzed by independent Student's t-test or Mann-Whitney $U$ test. The effects of multiple factors were analyzed by two-way ANOVA followed by Bonferroni *post-hoc* test or Kruskal-Wallis test. These statistical analyses were performed with commercial analytical software (SPSS 25.0) with $p$ value < 0.05 being considered as statistically significant.

## Results

### Repeated KW6002 treatment did not affect normal postnatal development of retinal vasculature

To address whether KW6002 affects normal retinal vasculature during postnatal development, we analyzed development of the retinal vascular networks at P17 of C57BL/6 mice after repeated treatment with KW6002 (from P7 to P17, 10 mg/kg, i.p. every other day, Fig. 1a), by fluorescent staining of whole-mounted retinas under room air conditions (Fig. 1b). After exposure to room air from P0 to P21, the mice displayed normal development of the retinal vasculature, the superficial layer reaching near completion at P12. Both the superficial and the deep vascular layers from the optic disc to the periphery were well developed at P12-P17, and the intermediate layer was almost finished at P21. KW6002 treatment did not affect retinal vasculature in the superficial, intermediate and deep vascular plexus, as revealed by isolectin B4 analysis in whole-mounts retina scanned with laser scanning microscope (Fig. 1c). No avascular areas were detected at P17 in mice treated either with vehicle or KW6002 (Fig. 1b), indicating that the superficial retinal vasculature grew with similar rates and indistinguishable patterns of the vessels distribution between mice treated with vehicle or KW6002. Furthermore, morphology, distribution and density of three retinal vessels layers (superficial, intermediate and deep) were indistinguishable between mice treated with the vehicle and KW6002 when analyzed by confocal scanning laser microscopy at P17 (Fig. 1C). These analyses demonstrated that repeated KW6002 treatment did not affect normal postnatal development of retinal vasculature in mice.

### KW6002 treatment selectively and effectively reduced retinal avascular area and pathological angiogenesis at P17 in OIR

We first evaluated the effect of repeated KW6002 treatment for 10 days (from P7 to P17, 10 mg/kg, i.p. every other day, Fig. 2a) on vaso-obliteration and neovascularization by analyzing the avascular area and neovascular area with isolectin B4 staining in whole-mounted retina (Fig. 2b). Repeated treatment with KW6002 largely prevented hypoxia-induced retinopathy. Quantitative analysis

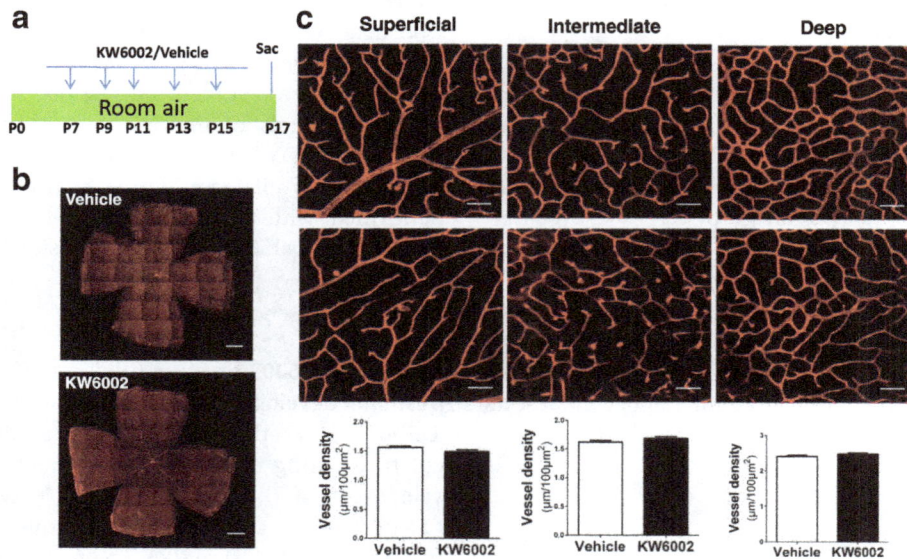

**Fig. 1** KW6002 treatment did not affect normal postnatal development of retinal vasculature. **a** Schematic of the experimental design: KW6002 was administered by intraperitoneal injection at volume of 10 mg/kg from P7 to P15 every other day. Mice were euthanized at P17.(Sac:Sacrifice). **b** Mouse whole-mount retinas from KW6002- and vehicle-treated mice were harvested and immune-stained with isolectin B4. The retinal vasculature morphologies were indistinguishable between KW6002- or vehicle-treated pups at P17 in room-air. Scale bar: 500 μm. **c** The retinal vasculatures of the superficial, intermediate and deep vascular layers were examined at P17 by isolectin B4 staining of whole-mount retinas. The distributions of three retinal vascular layers were displayed in distinct confocal planes. Vessel density was quantified as the ratio of the total vessel length to microscopic field. The vessel densities of the superficial, intermediate and deep plexuses were indistinguishable between KW6002-treated and vehicle-treated pups. Scale bar: 50 μm

demonstrated that KW6002 treatment reduced avascular area by 74.2% ($P < 0.001$) and neovascular area by 55.0% ($P < 0.001$) compared to the vehicle-treated mice (Fig. 2c). Independent and quantitative analysis of neovascular nuclei numbers in cross sections demonstrated that KW6002 treatment for 10 days markedly reduced pathological angiogenesis with reduced neovascular nuclei in retina of OIR ($46.85 \pm 4.53$) compared to vehicle-treated mice ($23.03 \pm 2.105$) ($P < 0.001$, Fig. 2d, e). These studies demonstrated that repeated KW6002 treatment protects against oxygen-induced vaso-obliteration and pathological angiogenesis.

**KW6002-induced protection against OIR was associated with increased astrocyte and endothelial tip cell functions and decreased cellular proliferation and apoptosis at P17**

We further investigated the cellular basis underlying the KW6002 effects on pathological angiogenesis by analyzing function of astrocytes and endothelial tip cells in retina of mice treated with KW6002 or vehicle at P17 stage of OIR. Consistent with the previous study (Weidemann et al. 2010), GFAP-positive cells with normal morphology were mainly detected in the peripheral vascular areas while GFAP-positive cells with abnormal morphology were detected in the avascular area of retina by immunofluorescence staining. Using the semi-quantitative method described by Dorrell et al. (Dorrell et al. 2010), we estimated

GFAP expression in the avascular area. Analysis showed that OIR markedly reduced GFAP-positive cells, as expected, but KW6002 partially reversed this reduction of astrocyte function in retina compared to the vehicle-treated retina (Fig. 3e). Quantitative analysis revealed that the number of endothelial tip cells in retina was significantly increased by KW6002 treatment compared to the vehicle group (Fig. 3a). Because pathologic angiogenesis is characterized by proliferation of endothelial cells in the hypoxic phase, we analyzed expression of PCNA, a marker for cellular proliferation, at P17 of OIR (Fig. 3b). KW6002 treatment decreased the number of PCNA-positive cells in the retina. TUNEL assay showed that most TUNEL-positive signals were found within the outer nuclear layer, in which mainly photoreceptor cells were distributed (Fig. 3c). Quantitative analysis showed that KW6002 treatment decreased TUNEL-positive signals in retinas compared with vehicle group. Collectively, KW6002 treatment enhanced function of astrocyte and endothelial tip cells and reduced cellular proliferation and apoptosis to confer protection against oxygen-induced pathological angiogenesis in retina at P17 of OIR. Microglial activation in retinas was assessed by Iba-1 immunohistochemistry antibody at P17. OIR increased microglial activation in retina but KW6002 did not have a major effect on microglial activation in retina at P17 (Fig. 3d).

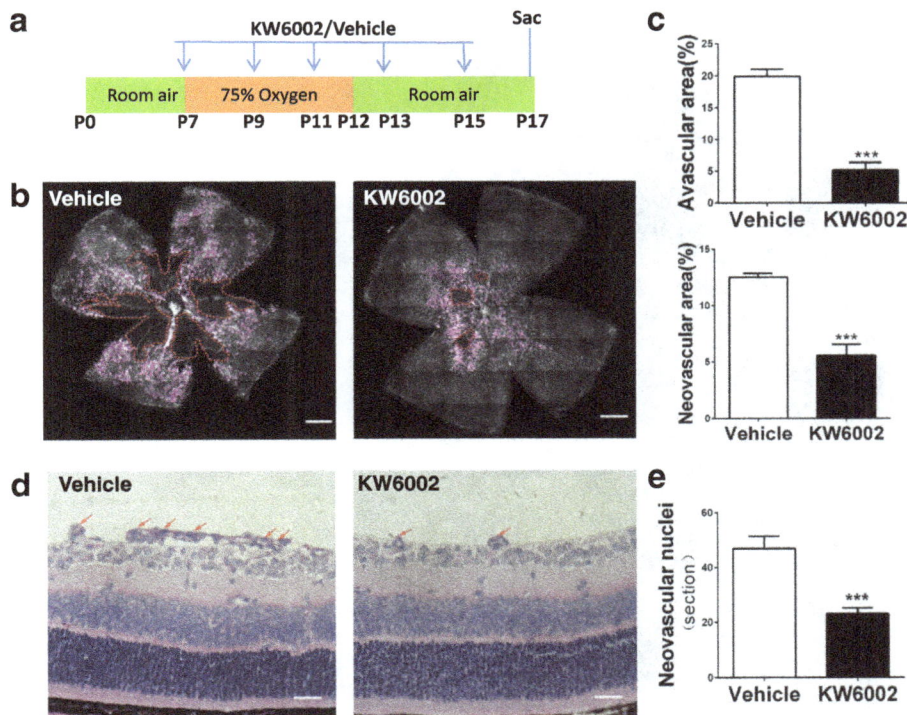

**Fig. 2** KW6002 treatment attenuated retinal avascular area and pathological angiogenesis at P17 in OIR. **a** Schematic of the experimental design: KW6002 was administered by intraperitoneal injection at volume of 10 mg/kg from P7 to P15 every other day. OIR mice were euthanized at P17. **b** Following the OIR, retinal vasculatures from KW6002- and vehicle-treated mice were visualized by whole-mount isolectin B4 at P17. Avascular areas are indicated by red dotted line. Neovascularization tufts are indicated by purple line. Scale bar: 500 μm. **c** Quantitative analysis of avascular areas by isolectin B4 and the neovascular tufts area showed that KW6002 treatment reduced avascular areas(Student's t-test) and neovascular tufts area(Mann-Whitney $U$ test)compared to the vehicle-treated pups. ***$P < 0.001$, $n = 11$–13/group. **d** Representative H-E staining images showing the neovascular nuclei numbers (red arrow) on the vitreal side of the inner limiting membrane. Scale bar: 20 μm. **e** Quantitative histochemical analysis showed that KW6002 treatment (P7–17) reduced neovascular nuclei numbers as compared to the vehicle-treated pups. ***$P < 0.001$, Student's t-test, $n = 11$–13 /group

### KW6002 treatment at P7–12 (but not P12–17) was required to confer protection against OIR

To define the effective therapeutic window, we treated the mice with KW6002 in three different treatment regimens (i.e. P7-P12, P12-P17 and P7-P17, Fig. 4d, d, f). KW6002 treatment at P7–12 ($8.25 \pm 0.85\%$) or 7–17 ($5.07 \pm 0.82\%$) was effective in reducing avascular area by 49.9% ($p < 0.001$) and 74.5% ($p < 0.001$), respectively, comparing to the vehicle-treated control (Fig. 4a, b, c, d). In addition, quantitative analysis confirmed that KW6002 treatment at P7–12 ($8.29 \pm 0.62\%$) or 7–17 ($4.76 \pm 0.76\%$) was effective in neovascularization tufts towards the vitreous body by 17.6% ($p < 0.05$) and 63.44% ($p < 0.001$), respectively, comparing to the vehicle-treated control (Fig. 4a, b, c, d). By contrast, repeated KW6002 treatment at P12–17 was not effective in reducing vaso-obliteration or neovascularization (Fig. 4 e, f). Thus, the administration of KW6002 at P7–12 (i.e. the hyperoxic phase) is required to confer protection against OIR, whereas the injection of KW6002 at P12–17 (i.e. the hypoxic phase) is not sufficient to confer the protection.

### KW6002 treatment reduced hyperoxia-induced retinal vascular regression at P9 and 12 and cellular apoptosis at P12

Next, we further examined the protective effect of KW6002 treatment at the hyperoxic phase by analyzing hyperoxia-induced avascular area at P9 and P12 in whole-mounted retinas with isolectin B4 staining (Fig. 5a,c). Analysis revealed that KW6002 treatment reduced avascular areas in the central retina at P9 and P12. Quantitative analysis of retinal vaso-obliteration demonstrated that KW6002 treatment reduced avascular areas by 27.0% at P9 and 27.5% at P12, respectively, compared to the vehicle-treated mice (Fig. 5d, d).

Consistent with our previously (Zhang et al. 2015) and other studies (Duan et al. 2011; Ludewig et al. 2014; Narayanan et al. 2014), hyperoxia induced TUNEL-positive signals mainly within the inner nuclear layer (mainly neurons such as amacrine cells and bipolar cells) of the avascular area of OIR, in both KW6002- and vehicle-treated groups (Fig. 5e). Quantitative analysis showed that TUNEL-positive cells were

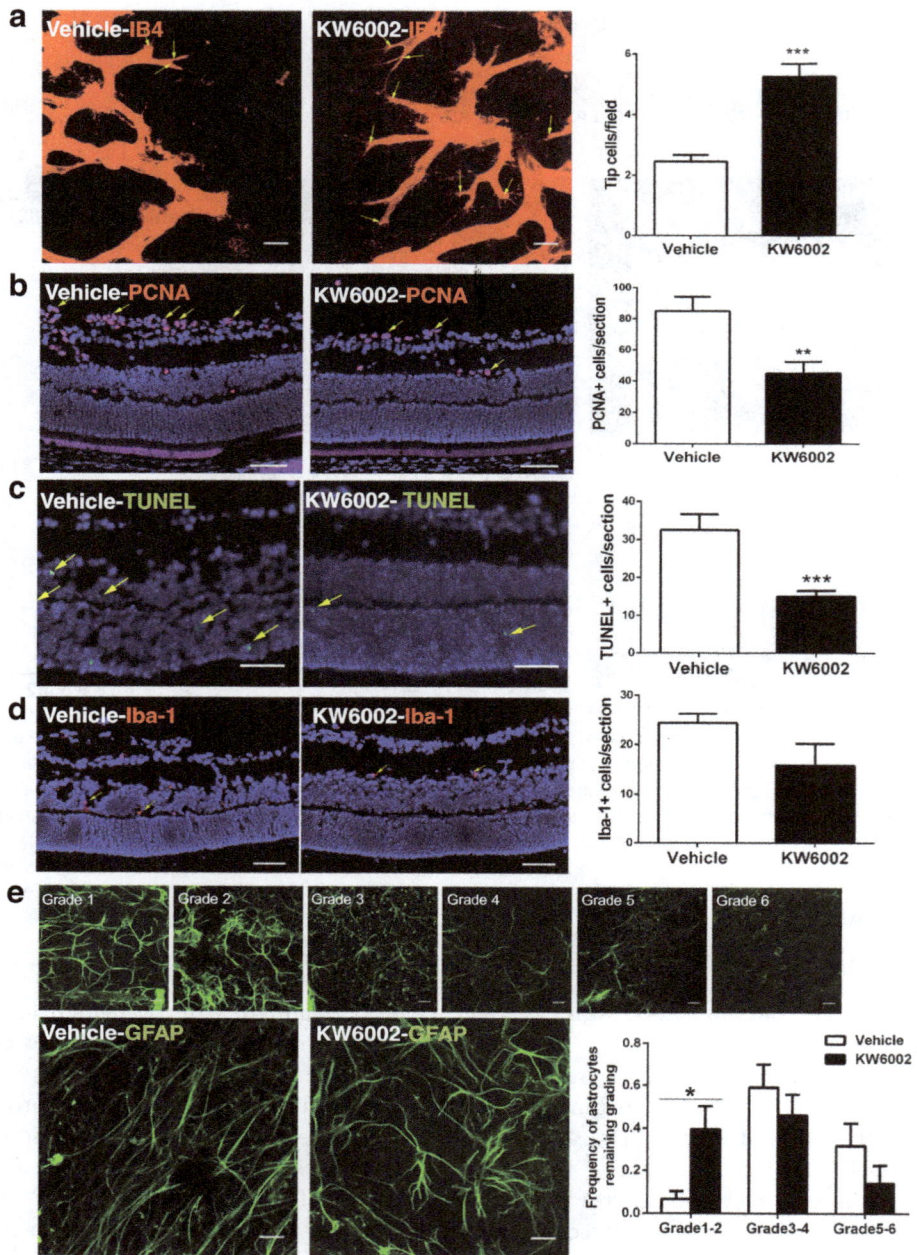

**Fig. 3** In OIR, the effect of KW6002 treatment on cellular proliferation, tip cell, astrocytes and microglial numbers, and apoptosis in retina at P17. **a** Endothelial tip cells in retina at P17 of OIR were stained with isolectin B4 (red). Scale bar: 20 μm. Quantitative analysis shows that KW6002 treatment increased tip cell number compared to the vehicle-treated pups (***$p < 0.001$, Student's t-test, $n = 11$–13/group). **b** Cell proliferation in retina was assessed by immunohistochemistry of PCNA at P17 of OIR. PCNA$^+$ cells (yellow arrow) were quantified. (**$p < 0.01$, Student's t-test, $n = 8$/group). Scale bar: 50 μm. **c** Apoptotic cells in retina were analyzed by TUNEL (green) staining and individual cells were visualized by DAPI (blue) staining at P17 of OIR. Retinal TUNEL-positive cells (yellow arrow) were quantified and analyzed. KW6002 treatment reduced cellular apoptosis in (**$p < 0.01$, Mann-Whitney U test, $n = 8$–9/group). Scale bar: 50 μm. **d** Microglial activation in retinas was assessed by immunofluorescence staining of Iba-1 at P17 of OIR. Retinal Iba-1-positive cells (yellow arrow) were quantified and analyzed. ($p > 0.01$, Student's t-test, $n = 8$/group). Scale bar: 50 μm. **e** Representative images show GFAP-positive cells in the avascular areas by anti-GFAP (green) staining at P17 of OIR. Scale bar: 20 μm. GFAP staining in the avascular area was graded on a scale from 1 to 6 as described in the Methods section. The grades of astrocytes from each treatment group were analyzed at P17 of OIR. KW6002 treatment enhanced GFAP staining (with the reduced grade) (*$p < 0.05$, Mann-Whitney U test, $n = 9$–12/group), Scale bar: 20 μm

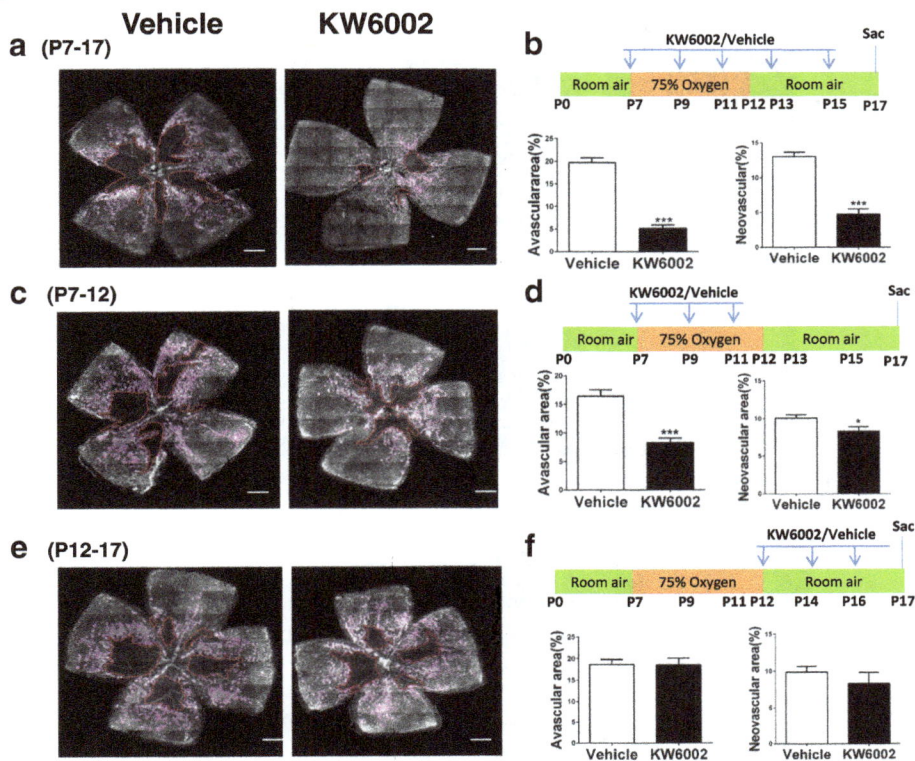

**Fig. 4** Effective therapeutic windows for KW6002 to confer protection against OIR. **a, c, e** Pups were treated with KW6002 (10 mg/kg) in different developmental stages (P7–17, P7–12, and P12–17) and retinal vasculatures were analyzed by whole-mount isolectin B4 staining at P17 of OIR. Avascular areas are shown by red dotted line. Neovascularization tufts are indicated by purple line. Scale bar: 500 µm. **b, d, f** Schematic of the experimental design: KW6002 was administered by intraperitoneal injection at volume of 10 mg/kg at different postnatal developmental stages (P7 or P12) and for different period (P7-P17, P7-P12 or P12-P17) every other day. OIR mice were euthanized at P17. **b, d, f** Avascular area (%) was quantified as a percentage of the whole retinal surface ($n = 7$–9/group). The neovascularization tufts area (%) was quantified as a percentage of whole retinal area ($n = 7$–9/group). ***$p < 0.001$, *$p < 0.05$, Student's t-test or Mann-Whitney $U$ test, $n = 7$–9/group

lower in mice treated with KW6002 than in mice treated with vehicle at P12 (Fig. 5f). These results confirmed that cellular apoptosis pattern after KW6002 treatment in OIR paralleled with the results of the avascular area, suggesting that KW6002 may reduce avascular areas partly by reducing hyperoxia-induced neuronal apoptosis in retina. We have performed analysis for microglial activation in retinas, and found that KW6002 treatment did not affect microglial activation at P12 (Fig. 5g, h).

**KW6002 treatment reversed hyperoxia-induced reduction of the mRNAs for A$_{2A}$R and eNOS at P12**

We further explored the possible mechanism underlying the A$_{2A}$R-mediated protection at the hyperoxic phase and found that in agreement with the early finding (Taomoto et al. 2000) A$_{2A}$R mRNA was reduced by hyperoxic exposure at P12 ($n = 6$, $p < 0.01$, Fig. 6b). This reduction of the A$_{2A}$R mRNA was reversed by KW6002 treatment. By contrast, A$_1$R mRNA in retina of OIR harvested at P12 was affected by neither to hyperoxia

or KW6002 treatment ($n = 6$, $p > 0.05$, Fig. 6a). Moreover, as eNOS and VEGF play important role for in the vaso-obliterative phase of ROP (Hartnett et al. 2008), we also examined the expression of eNOS and VEGF at P12 in eye exposed to hyperoxia and after KW6002 treatment (P7–12). Consistent with the previous study (Wang et al. 2013; Abdelsaid et al. 2014), both VEGF mRNA and eNOS mRNA levels were reduced after exposure to hyperoxia compared to the room air condition ($n = 6$, $p < 0.01$) (Fig. 6c, d). Importantly, KW6002 treatment reversed the reduction of eNOS but not VEGF mRNA in eye, suggesting the possible involvement of eNOS in A$_{2A}$R modulation of OIR (independent of VEGF) at the hyperoxia phase.

## Discussion

### A$_{2A}$R antagonists act at the hyperoxic phase to confer its protection against OIR

Current research efforts (such as anti-VEGF and other strategies) have largely focused on the hypoxic phase for proliferative angiogenesis is a key feature of ROP, driven

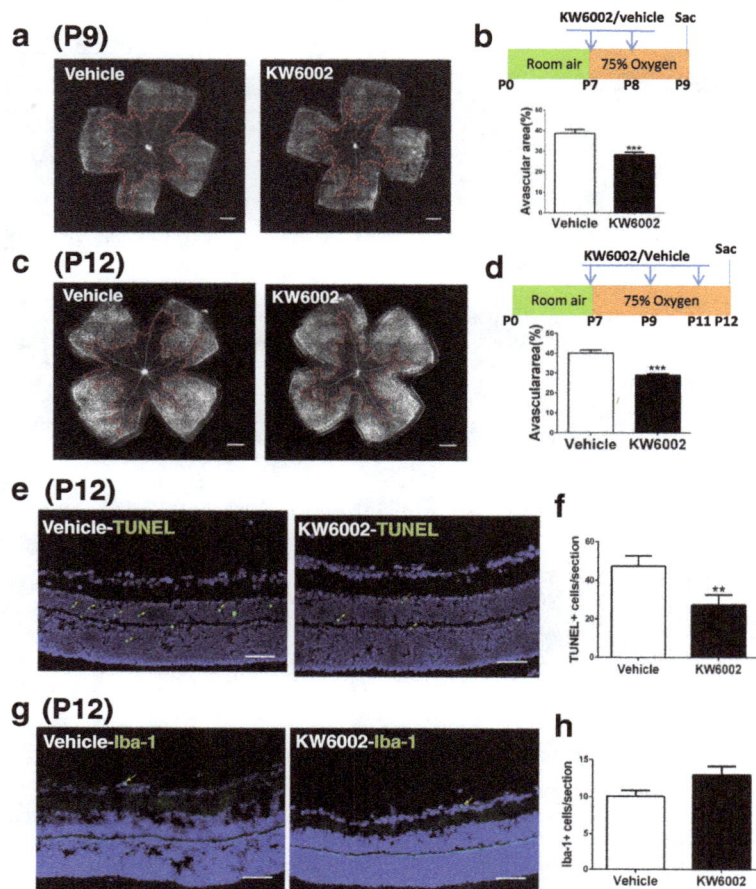

**Fig. 5** KW6002 treatment reduced hyperoxia-induced retinal vascular regression at P9 and P12 and cellular apoptosis at P12, does not affect the activation of microglia. Whole-mount retinas (**a**, **c**) or retinal cross-section (**e**, **g**) from the vehicle-OIR and KW6002 groups were harvested on P9 (**a**) or P12 (**c**, **e**, **g**) and examined by immunostaining with isolectin B4, or histological analysis by TUNEL or Iba-1. Representative images show the avascular areas (indicated by red dotted line) at P9 (**a**) and P12 (**c**) (Scale bar: 500 μm) and TUNEL$^+$ cells (indicated by yellow arrow) (**e**) or Iba-1$^+$ cells (indicated by yellow arrow) (**g**) in retinal sections at P12 (Scale bar: 50 μm). Areas of vaso-obliteration (**b**, **d**) and TUNEL$^+$ cells (**f**) or Iba-1+ cells (**h**) were quantified and analyzed **$P < 0.01$, ***$P < 0.001$, Student's t-test or Mann-Whitney $U$ testn = 8 /group

largely by HIF-1α signaling and VEGF pathway. Because hypoxia is associated with huge surge of adenosine signaling as result of increased expression of CD73/CD39 and $A_{2A}R$ mRNA and of hypoxia-induced inhibition of ADK and ENT (the enzyme responsible for adenosine degradation), $A_{2A}R$ antagonists are expected to act mainly at the hypoxic phase to blunt hypoxia-induced pathological angiogenesis. To our surprise, KW6002 treatment at P12–17 was in fact ineffective, whereas KW6002 treatment at P7–12 was effective in protecting against OIR. KW6002 treatment just at P7–8 was sufficient to confer protection against the damage to the developing retinal vessels (as indicated by reduced avascular area). Lack of protective effect of KW6002 upon administration at P12–17 may be interpreted as follows: direct, acute effect of KW6002 at the hypoxic phase alone is not sufficient and the *combined* effect of KW6002 at both phases is needed to confer its protection against OIR. The reduced pathological angiogenesis

by $A_{2A}R$ KO at P17 could be attributed to the action at the hyperoxic phase (in addition to the hypoxic phase) as the $A_{2A}R$ KO conceives at the early embryonic stage and throughout life. The finding of the required treatment of KW6002 at P7–12 is consistent with the protection against OIR by caffeine observed at P12 (Zhang et al. 2017), and with the finding of the importance of the hyperoxic phase in $A_1R$-mediated modulation of OIR (Zhang et al. 2015). Developmental factors may also contribute to the selective effect of $A_{2A}R$ antagonists at the hyperoxic phase. Retinal vasculature development at postnatal day 7 might be particularly sensitive to pharmacological interference, since from P7 onward the superficial capillaries start sprouting vertically in the retina to form, firstly, the deep, then the intermediated vascular plexus in the vitreous body of C57BL/6 mice (Smith et al. 1994; Stahl et al. 2010). In addition, KW6002 concentration may be higher at P7-P12 than P12-P17 following the same dose regime because of

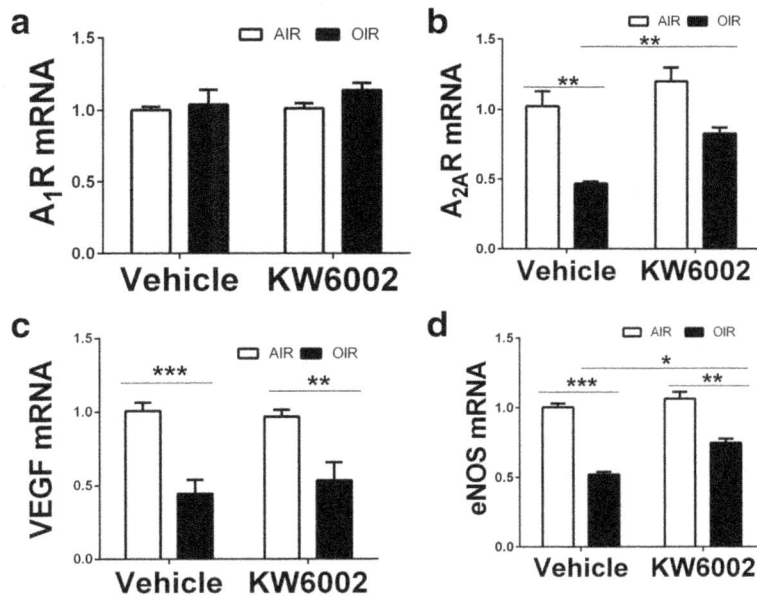

**Fig. 6** KW6002 treatment reversed hyperoxia-induced reduction of the mRNAs for $A_{2A}R$ and eNOS at P12. Retina of OIR and room air was dissected and harvested at P12 in retina after KW6002 or vehicle treatment (P7–12) and $A_{2A}R$ and $A_1R$ mRNAs as well as the mRNAs for VEGF and eNOS were determined by qPCR analysis. Compared to the room air group, $A_1R$ was affected by neither to hyperoxia or KW6002 treatment (**a**) whereas the mRNAs for $A_{2A}R$, VEGF and eNOS were reduced by hyperoxic exposure. KW6002 treatment reversed the reduction of $A_{2A}R$ mRNA and eNOS by hyperoxia (**b, c, d**). $n = 6$/group *$p < 0.05$, **$p < 0.01$, ***$p < 0.001$, two-way ANOVA followed by Bonferroni post-hoc test or Kruskal-Wallis test $n = 6$/group

different metabolism of drugs during postnatal development, as evidenced by caffeine treatment at different postnatal stages producing different steady-state levels of caffeine in human and rodents (Parsons and Neims 1981; Pearlman et al. 1989).

Intriguingly, despite clear vaso-obliteration at the retina center, the hyperoxic phase is associated with lack of "hypoxia" in the retina by in vivo labelling of hypoxic tissues/cells with nitroimidazole EF5 (Smith et al. 2012) and with the reduced expression of ecto-5′ nucleotidase (CD73) and $A_{2A}R$ (Lutty and McLeod 2003) and, presumably, adenosine level. Yet, the hyperoxic phase (P7–12 in OIR) is most critical to confer protection against OIR by KW6002, caffeine (Zhang et al. 2017) and $A_1R$ KO (Zhang et al. 2015). Where did adenosine level come from at the hyperoxic phase? This may be due to the fact that adenosine production is intrinsically linked to energy metabolism and biosynthetic processes (Chen et al. 2013), generating basal levels of adenosine intracellularly and extracellularly through effective bidirectional ENT activity. Consequently, there is always a finite amount of extracellular adenosine that is likely sufficient to activate the $A_{2A}R$ (with $K_d$ value at 1–10 nM) (Chen et al. 2013). Thus, despite low but nonetheless sufficient concentration of adenosine, KW6002 treatment primarily acts at the early stage of ROP to confer its protection.

The biphasic disease of ROP suggests that hyperoxic damage to developing retinal vasculatures is the primary and root cause of pathological angiogenesis in ROP despite the fact that pathological angiogenesis, the hallmark of ROP pathology, is most evident at the hypoxic phase of ROP (Sapieha et al. 2010). Thus, therapeutic strategies targeting the initial obliteration at the hyperoxia phase can preserve retinal endothelial and neuronal functions and to prevent progression to the proliferative phase of the disease. Our demonstration of the effective therapeutic window (i.e. P7–12) of KW6002 treatment argues that KW6002 treatment is more effective when administered during the early stage of ROP (i.e. when premature infants receive oxygen support) to prevent the devastating latter stage (the hypoxic phase) of the disease. Currently, caffeine treatment for sleep apnea of prematurity is used during the first 10 days after birth in preterm infants subjected to oxygen treatment (Schoen et al. 2014). $A_{2A}R$ antagonists and caffeine may be developed as *prophylactic* measures for ROP by targeting the hyperoxic and hypoxic phases to achieve maximal therapeutic benefits.

### $A_{2A}R$ antagonists protect against OIR by acting at the distinct mechanisms at the hyperoxic and hypoxic phases

The mechanisms underlying $A_{2A}R$ antagonist-induced protection at the hyperoxic phase are not clear.

Hyperoxia-induced reactive oxygen species (ROS) can promote apoptosis in ganglia cells and developing endothelial cells, and can inhibit endothelial cells proliferation and migration, leading to vaso-obliteration (Aiello et al. 1994; Alon et al. 1995). Accordingly, attenuation of the hyperoxia-induced avascular area by the $A_{2A}R$ antagonist is associated with the reduced neuronal apoptosis in the inner nuclear layer of the retina (i.e. TUNEL-positive cells). This is consistent with the previous finding that $A_{2A}R$ antagonists and $A_{2A}R$ KO exert protection against OIR (Liu et al. 2010) and seizure susceptibility (Georgiev et al. 1993) in neonates. In keep with this, caffeine treatment during the first 7 days after birth affected neonates sensitivity to ischemic brain injury (Bona et al. 1995), reduced white matter injury by preventing early differentiation of oligodendrocytes (Rivkees and Wendler 2011) and reduced the effects of NMDA on seizure susceptibility in neonates (Georgiev et al. 1993). As the $A_{2A}R$ activation can increase Nox2-dependent generation of ROS in some cell types (Ribe et al. 2008; Thakur et al. 2010), $A_{2A}R$ antagonists may attenuate cellular apoptosis in the inner ganglion cells by reducing ROS production by hyperoxic exposure. Furthermore, hyperoxic exposure has been shown to impair endothelium function (Garcia-Quintans et al. 2016) with depletion of the eNOS cofactor (6R)-5,6,7,8-tetrahydrobiopterin (BH4) (Edgar et al. 2015). Our observations that KW6002 treatment reversed the reduction of hyperoxia-induced of eNOS mRNA at P12 suggests that $A_{2A}R$ antagonists may specifically modulate hyperoxia-induced apoptosis and damage to developing retinal vessels through eNOS-ROS pathway. However, the interplay of the $A_{2A}R$ activity and eNOS in OIR are complex because eNOS can have both beneficial (via vasodilation) (Dimmeler et al. 1999) and detrimental (via production of ROS) (Brooks et al. 2001; Edgar et al. 2012) effects on retinal vascular (Edgar et al. 2012) development and because $A_{2A}R$ activation can either enhance (Carlstrom et al. 2011) or suppress (Dai et al. 2010; Lin et al. 2007) NOS activity depending on cellular type or local environment (e.g. glutamate). On the other hand, KW6002 reduced avascular areas and promoted revascularization by enhancing the functions of astrocytes and endothelial tip cells at the hypoxic phase at P17. Furthermore, a recent study with endothelial cell-specific A2AR knockout elegantly shows that A2AR control pathological neovascularization in the OIR mice by transcriptional modulation of glycolytic enzymes, via ERK- and Akt-dependent translational activation of HIF-1α protein, to promote glycolysis in endothelial cells and endothelial cell proliferation (Liu et al. 2017).

In this regard, we noted that both $A_{2A}R$ antagonist (Fig. 5c, d) and $A_1R$ KO (Zhang et al. 2015) reduced the oxygen-induced avascular areas at P12. Thus, adenosine acting at $A_{2A}R$ and $A_1R$ corporately controls oxygen-induced damage to developing retinal vasculature at the hyperoxic phase. This is in striking contrast to the fact that $A_{2A}Rs$ and $A_1Rs$ exert opposite control on angiogenesis at the hypoxic phase in OIR, as indicated by reduced avascular areas in $A_{2A}R$-KO mice (Liu et al. 2010) and increased avascular areas in $A_1R$-KO mice (Zhang et al. 2015). The different interactions between $A_{2A}R$ and $A_1R$ at the hyperoxia versus hypoxic phases likely reflect fundamentally different mechanisms of adenosine signaling action at these two phases. It would be critical to determine the retinal adenosine level at the hypoxic phase and to dissect out the specific mechanism of the $A_1R$ and $A_{2A}R$ interactions at P12 versus P17.

### Distinct features of $A_{2A}R$ antagonists versus anti-VEGF and caffeine therapeutic strategy in ROP

The present study also revealed additional features of $A_{2A}R$ antagonists in control of pathological angiogenesis with translational implications for ROP. At first, in contrast to anti-VEGF and other therapeutic strategies, $A_{2A}R$ antagonism selectively attenuated retinal pathological vaso-obliteration and neovascularization in OIR, but did not affect postnatal retinal vascularization (with normal morphology, density and distribution of retinal vessels), a feature shared by other adenosine-based manipulations including caffeine treatment (Zhang et al. 2017) and $A_{2A}R$ KO (Liu et al. 2010) and $A_1R$ KO (Zhang et al. 2015). However, the lingering concerns on the possible specific effect of the caffeine on embryonic development (Ma et al. 2014; Back et al. 2006) and possible postnatal development and maturation of cortical GABAergic neurons at the microstructural level after perinatal exposure to the caffeine (Favrais et al. 2014) should be taken into consideration carefully. This treatment confers distinct advantages over the currently testing anti-VEGF antibody treatment in ROP. This selectivity has been attributed to the aberrantly enhanced adenosine signaling (Lutty and McLeod 2003), which amplifies $A_{2A}R$ antagonist effect. However, our demonstration of the primary action of $A_{2A}R$ antagonists at the hyperoxic phase (with presumably relatively low adenosine signaling) suggests that additional mechanisms may be critical for preferential control of retinal vascularization by $A_{2A}R$ signaling at the hyperoxic phase. At second, protective effect of the $A_{2A}R$ antagonist against OIR ($\approx75\%$ avascular area by KW6002 at P17) is stronger/more robust than caffeine treatment (35%) and other experimental manipulations of adenosine signaling, including $A_{2A}R$ KO (~ 60%). The robust protection conferred by the $A_{2A}R$ antagonist may be attributed to the unique feature of $A_{2A}R$ antagonists targeting primarily at the hyperoxic phase. As such, $A_{2A}R$ antagonists are more effective at the hyperoxic phase (i.e. the early stage of ROP), whereas anti-VEGF treatment is more effective at the hypoxic phase (i.e. later stage of ROP, such as ROP stage II-III).

## Conclusion

Our identification of the hyperoxic phase as the effective window, together with selective and robust protection against pathological (but not physiological) angiogenesis, provide the preclinical evidence for translating $A_{2A}R$ antagonists as a novel therapeutic strategy for ROP treatment.

### Abbreviations
A2AR: Adenosine A2A receptor; eNOS: Endothelial nitric oxide synthase; HIF-1α: Hypoxia-induced factor-1α; OIR: Oxygen-induced retinopathy; ROP: Retinopathy of prematurity; VEGF: Vascular endothelial growth factor

### Acknowledgments
The authors thank Dr. Sergii Vakal (Wenzhou Medical University) for editing and proof-reading of the manuscript. This study was sponsored by the National Natural Science Foundation of China (Grants 81630040 to J.-F.C., 81600753 to S.Z., and 81100672 to R.Z.), the Start-up Fund from Wenzhou Medical University (Grants 89211010 and 89212012 to J.-F.C.), the Zhejiang Provincial Special Funds (Grant 604161241 to J.-F.C.), Key Laboratory of Vision Science, Ministry of Health, China (Grant 601041241 to J.-F.C.), the Central Government Special Fund for Local Universities' Development (Grant 474091314 to J.-F.C.), Zhejiang Provincial Natural Science Foundation Grant (Grant LY12H12007 to X.-LL; Grant LY17H120006 to R.Z.) and Public welfare science and technology plan project of Wenzhou city (Grant Y20160059 to R.Z.).

### Funding
This study was sponsored by the National Natural Science Foundation of China (Grants 81630040 to J.-F.C., 81600753 to S.Z., and 81100672 to R.Z.), the Start-up Fund from Wenzhou Medical University (Grants 89211010 and 89212012 to J.-F.C.), the Zhejiang Provincial Special Funds (Grant 604161241 to J.-F.C.), Key Laboratory of Vision Science, Ministry of Health, China (Grant 601041241 to J.-F.C.), the Central Government Special Fund for Local Universities' Development (Grant 474091314 to J.-F.C.), Zhejiang Provincial Natural Science Foundation Grant (Grant LY12H12007 to X.-LL; Grant LY17H120006 to R.Z.) and Public welfare science and technology plan project of Wenzhou city (Grant Y20160059 to R.Z.).

### Authors' contributions
RZ, SZ, X-LL and J-FC designed the experiment, analyzed the data and wrote the paper; RZ, SZ, XG, YG, DZ, YZ and LT performed the experiments, collected and analyzed the data. All authors read and approved the final manuscript.

### Competing interests
The authors declare that they have no competing interests as defined by Molecular Medicine, or other interests that might be perceived to influence the results and discussion reported in this paper.

### Author details
[1]Institute of Molecular Medicine, School of Optometry and Ophthalmology and Eye Hospital, Wenzhou Medical University, 270 Xueyuan Road, Wenzhou 325027, Zhejiang, China. [2]State Key Laboratory Cultivation Base and Key Laboratory of Vision Science, Ministry of Health, China and Zhejiang Provincial Key Laboratory of Ophthalmology and Optometry, Wenzhou Zhejiang, China.

## References
Abdelsaid MA, Matragoon S, Ergul A, El-Remessy AB. Deletion of Thioredoxin interacting protein (TXNIP) augments Hyperoxia-induced Vaso-obliteration in a mouse model of oxygen induced-retinopathy. PLoS One. 2014;9

Aiello LP, et al. Vascular endothelial growth factor in ocular fluid of patients with diabetic retinopathy and other retinal disorders. N Engl J Med. 1994;331:1480–7.

Alon T, et al. Vascular endothelial growth factor acts as a survival factor for newly formed retinal vessels and has implications for retinopathy of prematurity. Nat Med. 1995;1:1024–8.

Aranda JV, et al. Pharmacologic synergism of ocular ketorolac and systemic caffeine citrate in rat oxygen-induced retinopathy. Pediatr Res. 2016;80: 554–65.

Back SA, et al. Protective effects of caffeine on chronic hypoxia-induced perinatal white matter injury. Ann Neurol. 2006;60:696–705.

Bona E, Aden U, Fredholm BB, Hagberg H. The effect of long term caffeine treatment on hypoxic-ischemic brain damage in the neonate. Pediatr Res. 1995;38:312–8.

Brooks SE, et al. Reduced severity of oxygen-induced retinopathy in eNOS-deficient mice. Invest Ophthalmol Vis Sci. 2001;42:222–8.

Campochiaro PA. Molecular pathogenesis of retinal and choroidal vascular diseases. Prog Retin Eye Res. 2015;49:67–81.

Carlstrom M, Wilcox CS, Welch WJ. Adenosine a(2A) receptor activation attenuates tubuloglomerular feedback responses by stimulation of endothelial nitric oxide synthase. Am J Physiol-Renal. 2011;300:F457–64.

Cavallaro G, et al. The pathophysiology of retinopathy of prematurity: an update of previous and recent knowledge. Acta Ophthalmol. 2014;92:2–20.

Charles BA, et al. Variants of the adenosine a(2A) receptor gene are protective against proliferative diabetic retinopathy in patients with type 1 diabetes. Ophthalmic Res. 2011;46:1–8.

Chen JF, Eltzschig HK, Fredholm BB. Adenosine receptors as drug targets--what are the challenges? Nat Rev Drug Discov. 2013;12:265–86.

Chen JF, et al. Neuroprotection by caffeine and a(2A) adenosine receptor inactivation in a model of Parkinson's disease. J Neurosci. 2001;21 art. no.-RC143

Chen JF, et al. Adenosine receptors and caffeine in retinopathy of prematurity. Mol Asp Med. 2017;55:118–25.

Chen Y, et al. Risk factors for retinopathy of prematurity in six neonatal intensive care units in Beijing, China. Br J Ophthalmol. 2008;92:326–30.

Connor KM, et al. Quantification of oxygen-induced retinopathy in the mouse: a model of vessel loss, vessel regrowth and pathological angiogenesis. Nat Protoc. 2009;4:1565–73.

Dai SS, et al. Local glutamate level dictates adenosine a(2A) receptor regulation of Neuroinflammation and traumatic brain injury. J Neurosci. 2010;30:5802–10.

Dhaliwal C, Wright E, Graham C, McIntosh N, Fleck BW. Wide-field digital retinal imaging versus binocular indirect ophthalmoscopy for retinopathy of prematurity screening: a two-observer prospective, randomised comparison. Br J Ophthalmol. 2009;93:355–9.

Dimmeler S, Hermann C, Galle J, Zeiher AM. Upregulation of superoxide dismutase and nitric oxide synthase mediates the apoptosis-suppressive effects of shear stress on endothelial cells. Arterioscl Throm Vas. 1999;19:656–64.

Dorrell MI, et al. Maintaining retinal astrocytes normalizes revascularization and prevents vascular pathology associated with oxygen-induced retinopathy. Glia. 2010;58:43–54.

Duan LJ, Takeda K, Fong GH. Prolyl hydroxylase domain protein 2 (PHD2) mediates oxygen-induced retinopathy in neonatal mice. Am J Pathol. 2011; 178:1881–90.

Edgar K, Gardiner TA, van Haperen R, de Crom R, McDonald DM. eNOS overexpression exacerbates vascular closure in the Obliterative phase of OIR and increases Angiogenic drive in the subsequent proliferative stage. Invest Ophthalmol Vis Sci. 2012;53:6833–50.

Edgar KS, Matesanz N, Gardiner TA, Katusic ZS, McDonald DM. Hyperoxia depletes (6R)-5,6,7,8-tetrahydrobiopterin levels in the neonatal retina Implications for Nitric Oxide Synthase Function in Retinopathy. Am J Pathol. 2015;185:1769–82.

Elsherbiny NM, et al. Potential roles of adenosine deaminase-2 in diabetic retinopathy. Biochem Biophys Res Commun. 2013;436:355–61.

Favrais G, et al. Impact of common treatments given in the perinatal period on the developing brain. Neonatology. 2014;106:163–72.

Fleck BW, McIntosh N. Pathogenesis of retinopathy of prematurity and possible preventive strategies. Early Hum Dev. 2008;84:83–8.

Frick JS, et al. Contribution of adenosine A2B receptors to inflammatory parameters of experimental colitis. J Immunol. 2009;182:4957–64.

Garcia-Quintans N, et al. Oxidative stress induces loss of pericyte coverage and vascular instability in PGC-1 alpha-deficient mice. Angiogenesis. 2016;19:217–28.

Georgiev V, Johansson B, Fredholm BB. Long-term caffeine treatment leads to a decreased susceptibility to NMDA-induced clonic seizures in mice without changes in adenosine A1 receptor number. Brain Res. 1993;612:271–7.

Gilbert C. Retinopathy of prematurity: a global perspective of the epidemics, population of babies at risk and implications for control. Early Hum Dev. 2008;84:77–82.

Hartnett ME. Pathophysiology and mechanisms of severe retinopathy of prematurity. Ophthalmology. 2015;122:200–10.

Hartnett ME, Penn JS. Mechanisms and Management of Retinopathy of prematurity. N Engl J Med. 2012;367:2515–26.

Hartnett ME, et al. Neutralizing VEGF decreases tortuosity and alters endothelial cell division orientation in arterioles and veins in a rat model of ROP: relevance to plus disease. Invest Ophthalmol Vis Sci. 2008;49:3107–14.

Hellstrom A, Smith LEH, Dammann O. Retinopathy of prematurity. Lancet. 2013; 382:1445–57.

Husain SM, et al. Relationships between maternal ethnicity, gestational age, birth weight, weight gain, and severe retinopathy of prematurity. J Pediatr. 2013; 163:67–72.

Kornfield TE, Newman EA. Regulation of blood flow in the retinal trilaminar vascular network. J Neurosci. 2014;34:11504–13.

LeBlanc KH, Maidment NT, Ostlund SB. Repeated cocaine exposure facilitates the expression of incentive motivation and induces habitual control in rats. PLoS One. 2013;8:e61355.

Liang X, et al. TMP prevents retinal neovascularization and imparts neuroprotection in an oxygen-induced retinopathy model. Invest Ophthalmol Vis Sci. 2012;53:2157–69.

Lin CL, et al. Attenuation of experimental subarachnoid hemorrhage-induced cerebral vasospasm by the adenosine a(2A) receptor agonist CGS 21680. J Neurosurg. 2007;106:436–41.

Linden J. Regulation of leukocyte function by adenosine receptors. Adv Pharmacol. 2011;61:95–114.

Liu XL, et al. Genetic inactivation of the adenosine A2A receptor attenuates pathologic but not developmental angiogenesis in the mouse retina. Invest Ophthalmol Vis Sci. 2010;51:6625–32.

Liu ZP, et al. Endothelial adenosine A2a receptor-mediated glycolysis is essential for pathological retinal angiogenesis. Nat Commun. 2017;8

Ludewig P, et al. CEACAM1 confers resistance toward oxygen-induced vessel damage in a mouse model of retinopathy of prematurity. Invest Ophthalmol Vis Sci. 2014;55:7950–60.

Lutty GA, McLeod DS. Retinal vascular development and oxygen-induced retinopathy: a role for adenosine. Prog Retin Eye Res. 2003;22:95–111.

Ma ZL, et al. Excess caffeine exposure impairs eye development during chick embryogenesis. J Cell Mol Med. 2014;

Mintz-Hittner HA, Kennedy KA, Chuang AZ. Efficacy of intravitreal bevacizumab for stage 3+ retinopathy of prematurity. N Engl J Med. 2011;364:603–15.

Narayanan SP, et al. Arginase 2 deficiency reduces hyperoxia-mediated retinal neurodegeneration through the regulation of polyamine metabolism. Cell Death Dis. 2014;5

Nishijima K, et al. Vascular endothelial growth factor-a is a survival factor for retinal neurons and a critical neuroprotectant during the adaptive response to ischemic injury. Am J Pathol. 2007;171:53–67.

Parsons WD, Neims AH. Prolonged half-life of caffeine in healthy tem newborn infants. J Pediatr. 1981;98:640–1.

Pearlman SA, Duran C, Wood MA, Maisels MJ, Berlin CM Jr. Caffeine pharmacokinetics in preterm infants older than 2 weeks. Dev Pharmacol Ther. 1989;12:65–9.

Penn JS, et al. Vascular endothelial growth factor in eye disease. Prog Retin Eye Res. 2008;27:331–71.

Ribe D, et al. Adenosine a(2A) receptor signaling regulation of cardiac NADPH oxidase activity. Free Radic Biol Med. 2008;44:1433–42.

Rivkees SA, Wendler CC. Adverse and protective influences of adenosine on the newborn and embryo: implications for preterm white matter injury and embryo protection. Pediatr Res. 2011;69:271–8.

Saint-Geniez M, et al. Endogenous VEGF is required for visual function: evidence for a survival role on muller cells and photoreceptors. PLoS One. 2008;3:e3554.

Sapieha P, et al. Retinopathy of prematurity: understanding ischemic retinal vasculopathies at an extreme of life. J Clin Invest. 2010;120:3022–32.

Schingnitz U, et al. Signaling through the A2B adenosine receptor dampens endotoxin-induced acute lung injury. J Immunol. 2010;184:5271–9.

Schmidt B, et al. Long-term effects of caffeine therapy for apnea of prematurity. N Engl J Med. 2007;357:1893–902.

Schoen K, Yu T, Stockmann C, Spigarelli MG, Sherwin CM. Use of methylxanthine therapies for the treatment and prevention of apnea of prematurity. Paediatric Drugs. 2014;16:169–77.

Smith KS, Virkud A, Deisseroth K, Graybiel AM. Reversible online control of habitual behavior by optogenetic perturbation of medial prefrontal cortex. Proc Natl Acad Sci U S A. 2012;109:18932–7.

Smith LE, Hard AL, Hellstrom A. The Biology of Retinopathy of Prematurity How Knowledge of Pathogenesis Guides Treatment. Clin Perinatol. 2013;40:201–+.

Smith LE, et al. Oxygen-induced retinopathy in the mouse. Invest Ophthalmol Vis Sci. 1994;35:101–11.

Stahl A, et al. The mouse retina as an angiogenesis model. Invest Ophthalmol Vis Sci. 2010;51:2813–2826.

Taomoto M, McLeod DS, Merges C, Lutty GA. Localization of adenosine A2a receptor in retinal development and oxygen-induced retinopathy. Invest Ophthalmol Vis Sci. 2000;41:230–43.

Thakur S, Du JJ, Hourani S, Ledent C, Li JM. Inactivation of adenosine a(2A) receptor attenuates basal and angiotensin II-induced ROS production by Nox2 in endothelial cells. J Biol Chem. 2010;285:40104–13.

Vindeirinho J, Costa GN, Correia MB, Cavadas C, Santos PF. Effect of diabetes/hyperglycemia on the rat retinal Adenosinergic system. PLoS One. 2013;8

Wang XM, et al. (2013) LRG1 promotes angiogenesis by modulating endothelial TGF-beta signalling. Nature vol 499, pg 306.

Weidemann A, et al. Astrocyte hypoxic response is essential for pathological but not developmental angiogenesis of the retina. Glia. 2010;58:1177–85.

Zhang S, et al. Adenosine A1 receptors selectively modulate oxygen-induced retinopathy at the Hyperoxic and hypoxic phases by distinct cellular mechanisms. Invest Ophthalmol Vis Sci. 2015;56:8108–19.

Zhang SY, et al. Caffeine preferentially protects against oxygen-induced retinopathy. FASEB J. 2017;31:3334–48.

# 16

# Stachydrine protects eNOS uncoupling and ameliorates endothelial dysfunction induced by homocysteine

Xinya Xie[1], Zihui Zhang[1], Xinfeng Wang[1], Zhenyu Luo[1], Baochang Lai[1], Lei Xiao[1*] and Nanping Wang[2*]

**Abstract**

**Background:** Hyperhomocysteinemia (HHcy) is an independent risk factor for cardiovascular diseases (CVDs). Stachydrine (STA) is an active component in Chinese motherwort *Leonurus heterophyllus* sweet, which has been widely used for gynecological and cardiovascular disorders. This study is aimed to examine the effects of STA on homocysteine (Hcy)-induced endothelial dysfunction.

**Methods:** The effects of STA on vascular relaxation in rat thoracic aortas (TA), mesenteric arteries (MA) and renal arteries (RA) were measured by using Multi Myograph System. The levels of nitric oxide (NO), tetrahydrobiopterin (BH4) and guanosine 3', 5' cyclic monophosphate (cGMP) were determined. Endothelial nitric oxide synthase (eNOS) dimers and monomers were assayed by using Western blotting. GTP cyclohydrolase 1 (GTPCH1) and dihydrofolate reductase (DHFR) expressions were measured by using quantitative reverse transcriptase-PCR (qRT-PCR) and Western blotting.

**Results:** STA effectively blocked Hcy-induced impairment of endothelium-dependent vasorelaxation in rat TA, MA and RA. STA-elicited arterial relaxations were reduced by NOS inhibitor NG-nitro-L-arginine methyl ester (L-NAME) or the NO-sensitive guanylyl cyclase inhibitor 1H- [1, 2, 4] Oxadiazolo[4,3-a]quinoxalin-1-one (ODQ), but not by inducible iNOS inhibitor 1400 W nor the nonselective COX inhibitor indomethacin. Hcy caused eNOS uncoupling and decreases in NO, cGMP and BH4, which were attenuated by STA. Moreover, STA prevented decreases of GTPCH1 and DHFR levels in Hcy-treated BAECs.

**Conclusion:** We demonstrated that STA effectively reversed the Hcy-induced endothelial dysfunction and prevented eNOS uncoupling by increasing the expression of GTPCH1 and DHFR. These results revealed a novel mechanism by which STA exerts its beneficial vascular effects.

**Keywords:** Stachydrine, GTPCH1, DHFR, eNOS uncoupling, Vasorelaxation

## Background

Stachydrine (STA) is a major constituent of Chinese motherwort *Leonurus heterophyllus* sweet, which has been used in traditional medicine to promote blood circulation and dispel blood stasis (Yin et al., 2010). STA is also highly present in *L. japonicus*, *L. cardiaca* fruits, *Leonotis leonurus* (Kuchta et al., 2013) as well as in citrus fruits (Servillo et al., 2013). Several studies have shown that STA has protective effects on vascular endothelial cells (ECs).

STA protected endothelial against the injury induced by anoxia-reoxygenation (Yin et al., 2010). STA effectively reduced lipopolysaccharide (LPS)-induced endothelial inflammatory response via the inhibition of interleukin (IL-10) and thromboxane B 2 (TXB$_2$) secretion (Hu et al., 2015; Hu et al., 2012). STA inhibited the deleterious effect of high glucose on ECs and acted through the modulation of SIRT1 pathway (Servillo et al., 2013). However, little is known about STA on vascular relaxation, a common feature of endothelial function.

Hyperhomocysteinemia (HHcy) is an independent risk factor for various cardiovascular diseases (CVDs) (Karolczak et al., 2013; Baggott & Tamura, 2015).

* Correspondence: xiaolei0122@xjtu.edu.cn; nanpingwang2003@yahoo.com
[1]Cardiovascular Research Center, School of Basic Medical Sciences, Xi'an Jiaotong University, Xi'an 710061, China
[2]The Advanced Institute for Medical Sciences, Dalian Medical University, Dalian 116044, China

Homocysteine (Hcy) exerts its adverse effect on endothelial function by increasing oxidative stress and inhibiting the activity of endothelial nitric oxide synthase (eNOS) and decreasing nitric oxide (NO) production (Cheng et al., 2015). A critical determinant of eNOS activity is its cofactor tetrahydrobiopterin (BH4). BH4 can be formed either by a de novo biosynthetic pathway using the rate-limiting enzyme GTP-cyclohydrolase I (GTPCH1) or a salvage pathway from sepiapterin, which is dependent on dihydrofolate reductase (DHFR) (Hussein et al., 2015; Haruki et al., 2016). An inadequate level of BH4 makes eNOS no longer coupled to L-arginine oxidation (eNOS uncoupling) and results in the production of reactive oxygen species (ROS) rather than NO, thereby leading to vascular endothelial dysfunction (Takimoto et al., 2005).

In this study, we investigated the effects of STA on the Hcy-induced endothelial dysfunction and with the emphasis on its role in eNOS uncoupling and the underlying mechanism.

## Methods

### Reagents

STA was obtained from Cayman Chemical (Ann Arbor, MI, USA). Dimethyl sulfoxide (DMSO), 3-[4,5-dimethyl-thiazol-2-yl]-2,5-diphenyl-tetrazolium bromide (MTT), acetylcholine (ACh), indomethacin, NG-nitro-L-arginine methyl ester (L-NAME), 1H- (Yin et al., 2010; Kuchta et al., 2013; Hu et al., 2015) Oxadiazolo[4,3-a]quinoxalin-1-one (ODQ), 1400 W, Hcy, angiotensin II (Ang II), palmitic acid (PA) and rabbit polyclonal antibody to GTPCH1 were purchased from Sigma-Aldrich (St. Louis, MO, USA). The antibody against eNOS was purchased from Cell Signaling Technology (Danvers, MA, USA). Mouse monoclonal antibodies to DHFR and β-actin, HRP-conjugated anti-rabbit and anti-mouse IgG polyclonal antibodies were procured from Santa Cruz Biotechnology (Santa Cruz, CA, USA). ELISA kit for cGMP was obtained from R&D Systems Inc. (R&D Systems, MN, USA). BH4 ELISA kit was from MyBioSource Inc. (San Diego, CA, USA). Dulbecco's modified Eagle medium (DMEM), fetal bovine serum (FBS) and 4-amino-5-methylamino-2′, 7′-difluorofluorescein (DAF-FM) diacetate were obtained from Invitrogen (Carlsbad, CA, USA).

### Animals

Male Sprague-Dawley rats (8 weeks, 250–300 g) were obtained from the Experimental Animal Center of Xi'an Jiaotong University. Rats were housed in a specific pathogen-free environment under a 12 h/12 h light/dark cycle. Rats were killed with the inhalation of carbon dioxide. After death was ensured with cervical dislocation, the vessels were collected for later analysis.

### Cell culture and treatment

Bovine aorta endothelial cells (BAECs) were prepared as previously described (Wejksza et al., 2004)) and maintained in DMEM with 10% FBS, penicillin (100 U·ml$^{-1}$) and streptomycin (100 U·ml$^{-1}$). BAECs were treated with STA (0–10 μM) for 24 h or pre-treated with STA for 12 h following treatment with Hcy (500 μM) for another 12 h. BAECs within seven passages were used.

### Determination of cell viability

Cell viability was evaluated by the MTT assay. BAECs were seeded in 96-well plates and cultured until 80% confluence. Then, cells were treated with the indicated concentrations of STA for 24 h before incubation with 5 mg·ml$^{-1}$ MTT at 37 °C in 5% $CO_2$ atmosphere for 4 h. Next, the culture medium was removed and the formazan formed in the reaction was dissolved in 150 μl DMSO. The metabolized MTT was measured by using a spectrophotometer at 490 nm, and calculated by OD (test)/OD (control) × 100%.

### Nitric oxide (NO) assay

The levels of NO in the culture supernatants were assayed with the use of the Griess Reagent Nitrite Measurement Kit (Cell Signaling) to detect nitrite, a stable and nonvolatile breakdown product of NO. Briefly, 100 μl of supernatant was mixed with 100 μl of Griess reagent in a 96-well plate. Nitrite concentration was determined by detecting spectrophotometric absorbance at 550 nm and plotted against respective concentration in a standard curve (0–100 μM) derived from the nitrite standards. Culture media from cell-free wells was used as blank control. Intracellular NO concentrations were measured by using DAF-FM diacetate (4-Amino-5-Methyla-mino-2′,7′-Difluorofluorescein Diacetate). Briefly, BAECs seeded on glass coverslips and treated with different stimuli. By the end of treatment, the cells were incubated with DMEM containing 5 μM DAF-FM for 30 min in the dark at 37 °C and then washed with PBS. Images were obtained using the fluorescence microscopy. NO production was evaluated by measuring fluorescence intensity.

### Measurement of BH4

BH4 levels the cell lysates were measured by using a competitive ELISA kit. Briefly, ELISA plates pre-coated with a BH4-specific monoclonal antibody were used to incubate with the samples and test standards along with fixed amount of biotin-labelled BH4. Excess sample and reagents were washed off, and avidin conjugated to HRP was added to each well and incubated again. The 3,3′,5,5′-Tetramethylbenzidine (TMB) liquid substrate was then added to each well followed by incubation for 10 min. The enzyme substrate reaction was terminated and the product was measured spectrophotometrically at 450 nm. The concentration of BH4 in each sample was then calculated by comparing the optical density to a standard curve (Almudever et al., 2013).

## Measurement of cGMP levels in rat arterial rings

Rat aortic rings were incubated at 37 °C in 12-well culture plates containing Krebs solution gassed with 95% $O_2$ and 5% $CO_2$. Tissue lysates were prepared by homogenization with a Polytron homogenizer and centrifugation at 12,000×g for 20 min. The levels of cGMP were measured using an enzyme immunoassay kit in accordance to the instructions of the manufacturer.

## Measurement of vasorelaxation

Rat thoracic aortas (TA), mesenteric arteries (MA) and renal arteries (RA) were harvested and immediately transferred into oxygenated ice-cold Krebs solution containing NaCl (119 mM), KCl (4.7 mM), $NaHCO_3$ (25 mM), $CaCl_2$ (2.5 mM), $MgCl_2$ (1 mM), $KH_2PO_4$ (1.2 mM) and D-glucose (11 mM). In some experiments, the endothelial layer was denuded using 0.1% Triton X-100. After cleaned perivascular tissues, the arteries were cut into several rings (each in 2 mm length). Then the rings were suspended between two stainless steel hooks in a 5 mL organ bath filled with Krebs solution oxygenated with 95% $O_2$–5% $CO_2$ and maintained at 37 °C (pH 7.4) to achieve an optimal tension (TA 10 mN, RA and MA 3 mN). Each segment was allowed to equilibrate for 60 min. Curve recording was performed with LabChart™ software (AD-Instruments, Shanghai, China) by using a PowerLab Data Acquisition System™ for data acquisition. After equilibration, segments were pre-contracted with 60 mM KCl twice, and then contracted with phenylephrine (10 μM). Once a sustained tension was reached, acetylcholine (ACh, 0.01–10 μM) was added cumulatively to evoke endothelium-dependent relaxations. TAs with intact endothelia was incubated for 30 min with each of the following inhibitors: 100 μM L-NAME (an NOS inhibitor), 1 μM indomethacin (a non-selective COX inhibitor), 100 nM 1400 W (an iNOS inhibitor) and 3 μM ODQ before the contraction with phenylephrine. In organ culture experiments, aortic rings were incubated in DMEM/F12 supplemented with 10% FBS oxygenated with 95% $O_2$ and 5% $CO_2$ and maintained at 37 °C. After pre-incubation with 10 μM STA or vehicle for 12 h, aortic rings were mounted in Myograph system to measure the ACh-induced relaxations.

## Quantitative reverse transcriptase-PCR (qRT-PCR)

Total RNA was isolated using TRIzol (Invitrogen, Carlsbad, CA), reverse transcribed into cDNA by using iScript cDNA synthesis kit (Bio-rad, Hercules, CA). Real-time PCR was performed by using SYBR Green Supermixes (Bio-rad) and a 7500 Real-time PCR machine (Applied Biosystems, Foster City, CA). Fold changes of gene expression were calculated

using the $2^{-\Delta\Delta Ct}$ method. The qRT-PCR primers used were as follows: GTPCH1 forward primer: 5'-TTGGAAAGGTC CATATCGGT-3', reverse primer: 5'-ATTGTGCTCGTCA CGGTTCT-3'; DHFR forward primer: 5'-AAGAACGG AAACCTGCCCTG-3', reverse primer: 5'-GCCTCCCACT ATCCAAACCA-3'; Nrf2 forward primer: 5'-AGC AC ACCCAGTCAGAAACCAG-3'; reverse primer: 5'-TCTAC AAACGGGAATGTCG-3'; β-actin forward primer: 5'-CGAGCATTCCCAAAGTTCTACAGTG-3', reverse primer: 5'- CTACATACTTCCGAAAACCAGGGG-3'. β-actin was used as an internal control.

## Western blotting

Whole protein samples were extracted with lysis buffer (50 mM Tris-HCl, pH 7.5, 15 mM EGTA, 100 mM NaCl, 0.1% Triton X-100 and the protease inhibitors). Cytoplasmic protein samples were extracted with hypotonic lysis buffer (10 mM Tris-HCl, pH 7.5, 1.5 mM $MgCl_2$, 10 mM KCl, and 0.5% NP40). Nuclear protein samples were extracted with high-salt buffer (20 mM Tris-HCl, 1.5 mM $MgCl_2$, 420 mM NaCl, 10% glycerol, and 0.2 mM EGTA). And then separated on 10% SDS-PAGE and blotted onto PVDF membranes. The blots were incubated with primary antibodies and HRP-conjugated secondary antibodies, and then visualized by using the ECL chemoluminescence system. The intensity of the bands was quantified by using Image Pro Plus software. The eNOS dimerizations were assayed by using low-temperature SDS-PAGE (LT-PAGE) as described previously (Klatt et al., 1995). The protein lysates were mixed with loading buffer (without β-mercaptoethanol) and loaded on gels without boiling. Electrophoresis and gel transferring were kept at 4 °C during the whole procedure.

## Small interfering RNA and transfection

For small interfering RNA (siRNA)-mediated gene knockdown, the siRNA targeting the human Nrf2 gene was synthesized: sense: 5'-GCCCAUUGAUGUUUCUG AUTT-3', antisense: 5'-AUCAGAAACAUCAAUGGGC TT-3'. The siRNAs were transfected into cells using Lipofectamine2000 (Invitrogen). A scrambled siRNA was used as negative control (NC).

## Statistical analysis

Quantitative data are expressed as mean ± SEM, and data analyses were carried out independently by the third party without knowledge of treatments. Student's $t$ test or ANOVA was used to analyze the differences between two or among more groups, respectively. Relaxation curves were analyzed by using two-way ANOVA followed by Bonferroni post-tests. Bonferroni post hoc tests were run when F achieved $P < 0.05$ and there was no significant inhomogeneity. Non-quantitative results were representative of at least five independent experiments.

## Results
### STA improved Hcy-impaired vascular relaxation
In order to examine the effect of Hcy on vasorelaxation, rat TA, MA and RA rings were incubated with Hcy (500 µM) or control medium for 1 h before measuring the ACh-induced endothelium-dependent relaxation. The effects of STA were assessed by the pre-incubation of artery rings with STA (10 µM) for 12 h before the exposure to Hcy. As shown in Fig. 1, Hcy significantly impaired the vasorelaxations in response to ACh in all three types of arteries. Clearly, STA effectively restored the vascular relaxation to ACh. Figure 1b–f are representative traces of endothelium-dependent relaxations as in A, C and E. In uninjured rat TA, MA and RA, STA only slightly affected the vasorelaxation (Additional file 1: Figure S1A-C). Taken together, these results suggest that STA protected endothelial function impaired by Hcy.

In addition, we assessed the effects of STA on endothelial dysfunction induced by Ang II and PA, the two common injurious factors associated with metabolic disorders such as hypertension and obesity. in In rat thoracic aortas, exposure to either Ang II (1 µM, 1 h) or PA (200 µM, 1 h) significantly impaired vasorelaxations (Additional file 2: Figure S2A and B). However,

pretreatment with STA (10 µM, 12 h) effectively protected the vascular relaxation against Ang II and PA.

### STA-improved relaxation was dependent on endothelium-derived NO
To define the contribution of NO in the STA-improved relaxation, the artery rings were treated with different pharmacological inhibitors before the measurement of relaxation. As shown in Fig. 2, either L-NAME (an inhibitor of NOS) or ODQ (an inhibitor of the NO-sensitive soluble guanylyl cyclase, sGC) abolished the effect of STA on the relaxation of endothelium-intact rat thoracic arterial rings. In contrast, neither indomethacin (a non-selective COX inhibitor) nor 1400 W (an iNOS inhibitor) affect the STA effect (Fig. 2). These results indicated that protective effect of STA was dependent on NO signaling.

### STA increased NO, cGMP and BH4 production
Thus, we examined the effect of STA on NO production in ECs. In cultured BAECs, treatment with STA (0–20 µM for 24 h) had no significant effect on cell viability, as measured with the MTT assay (Fig. 3a). The production of NO was significantly reduced in BAECs after the exposure to Hcy (500 µM for 12 h). However, pretreatment with STA (10 µM, 12 h) effectively attenuated the detrimental effect of Hcy on NO production (Fig. 3b). The effect of STA on NO production was confirmed with laser confocal microscopy using a specific fluorescence dye

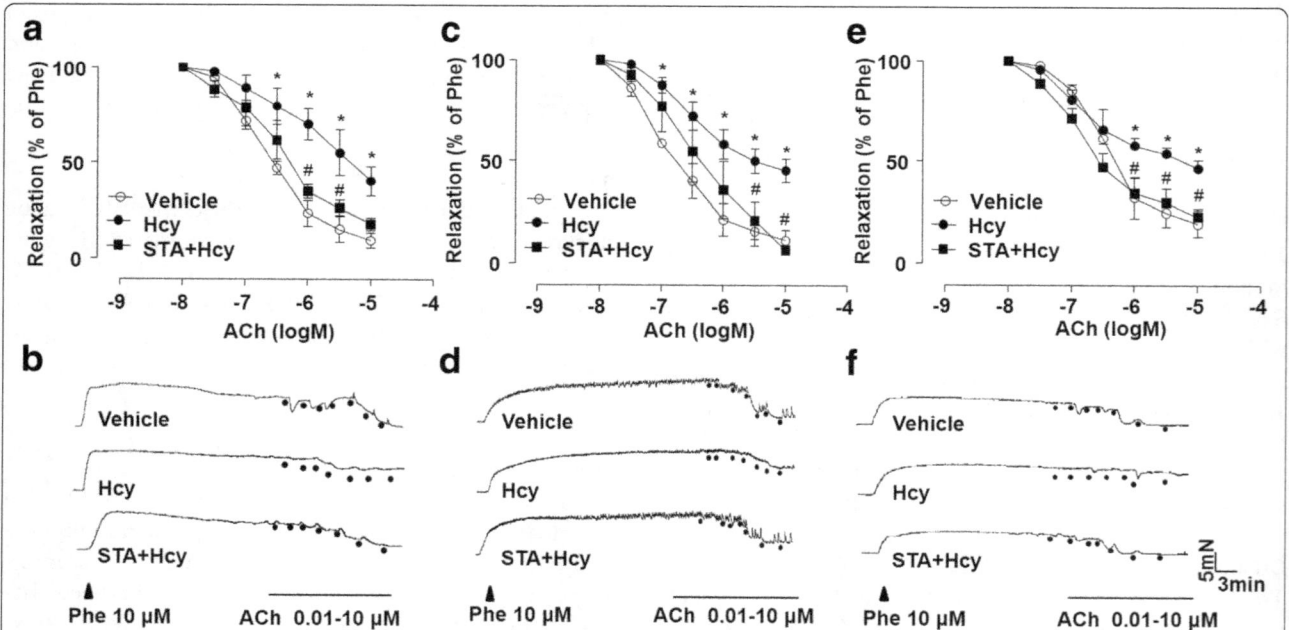

**Fig. 1** STA improved Hcy-impaired vascular relaxation. After pre-treatment of TA (**a**), MA (**c**) and RA (**e**) rings with STA (10 µM, 12 h), the arterial rings were exposed to Hcy (500 µM, 60 min). The cumulative concentration-response curves for ACh-induced relaxations of the phenylephrine-pre-contracted arterial rings were shown. **b**, **d** and **f** Representative traces of endothelium-dependent relaxations as in (**a**, **c** and **e**). Data were shown as mean ± SEM; $n = 5$ for each group, $^*P < 0.05$ vs. Vehicle; $^\#P < 0.05$ vs. Hcy

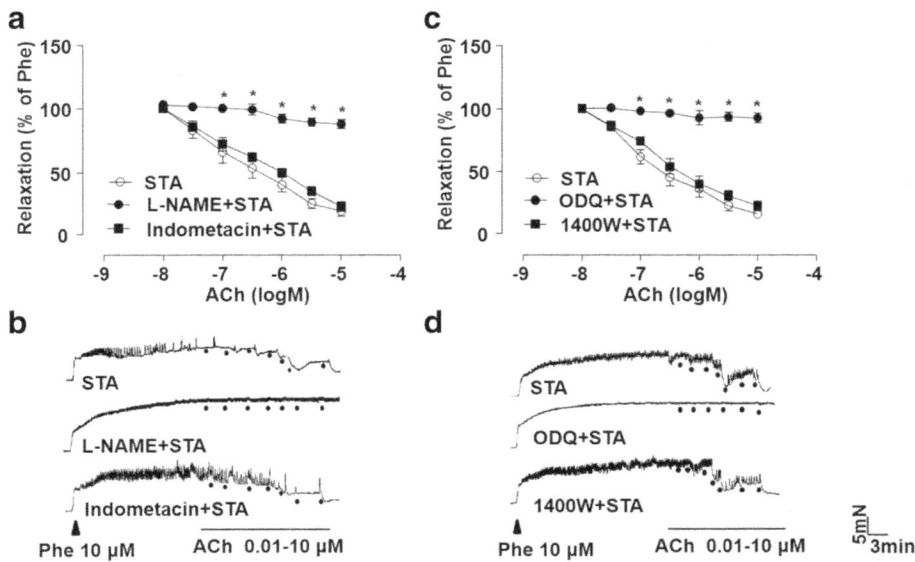

**Fig. 2** STA-improved relaxation was dependent on endothelium-derived NO. Rat thoracic artery rings were incubated with STA (10 µM) for 12 h and exposed to L-NAME (100 µM), indometacin (1 µM) (**a**), 1400 W (100 nM) or ODQ (3 µM) (**c**) for 30 min before the PE-contraction and ACh-induced relaxation. **b** and **d** Representative traces of endothelium-dependent relaxations as in (**a** and **c**). Data were shown as mean ± SEM; n = 5, *P < 0.05 vs. Vehicle

DAF-FM (Fig. 3c and d). Since endothelium-derived NO acts on arterial walls to promotes vasorelaxation by producing cGMP via the activation of sGC (Papapetropoulos et al., 2015), we further determined the cGMP levels in arterial rings treated with STA. As shown in Fig. 3e, The Hcy-decreased cGMP production was prevented by STA. BH4 is an essential cofactor for eNOS to completely

couple NADPH oxidation to NO production. As shown in Fig. 3f, treatment with Hcy (500 µM, 12 h) significantly reduced BH4 production compared with vehicle control. However, pretreatment with STA effectively restored the BH4 level in BAECs. These results suggest that increase of BH4 and the ensuing activation of NO pathway may contribute to the protective effect of STA.

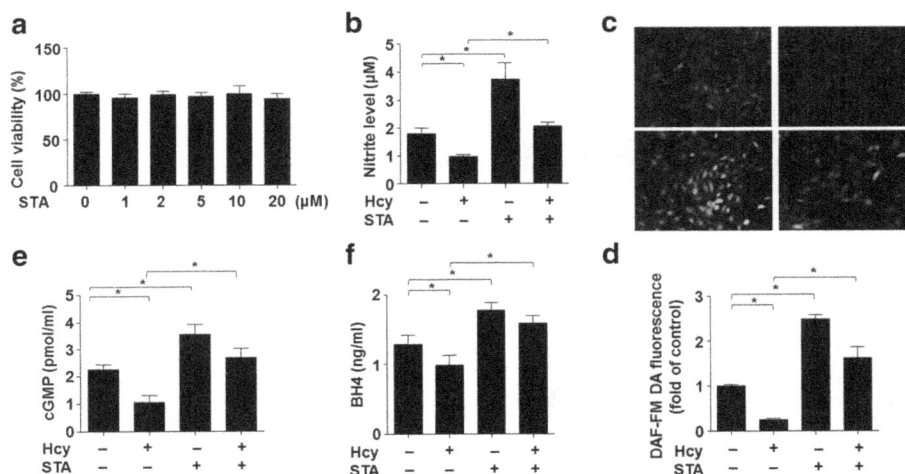

**Fig. 3** STA increased NO, cGMP and BH4 production. **a** BAECs were treated with indicated concentrations of STA for 24 h, and cell viability was measured by using MTT. **b** BAECs were pre-incubated with STA (10 µM) or vehicle for 12 h, and then exposed to Hcy (500 µM, 12 h). NO concentration in supernatants was measured by using the Griess reagent. **c** Intracellular NO was detected by using DAF-FM probe (40× objective). **d** The mean fluorescence intensity was evaluated as in (**c**). **e** Rat thoracic artery rings pre-incubated with STA or vehicle were exposed to Hcy. The cGMP production was measured by using an enzyme immunoassay kit. **f** Intracellular levels of BH4 were measured by using BH4 ELISA Kit. Data shown were mean ± SEM, n = 5, *P < 0.05

## STA ameliorated Hcy-induced eNOS uncoupling

It is established that BH4 plays an important role in facilitating eNOS dimerization, which is necessary for its normal catalytic function. Thus, we investigated the effects of STA on eNOS dimerization. As shown in Fig. 4a and b, the ratio of eNOS dimers to monomers, assayed by low-temperature SDS-PAGE, was significantly decreased in Hcy-treated ECs. However, pretreatment with STA ameliorated Hcy-decreased ratio of eNOS dimer to monomer. In fact, we observed that STA increased the dimer/monomer ratio in a dose-dependent manner (Fig. 4c and d). These results suggest that STA attenuated Hcy-induced eNOS uncoupling.

## STA increased the levels of GTPCH1 and DHFR

GTPCH1 and DHFR are the two key catalyzing the biosynthesis of BH4 and NO. Therefore, we further assessed the effect of STA on the expression of these two genes in ECs by using qRT-PCR and Western blotting. As shown in Fig. 5a-c, Hcy reduced the mRNA and protein levels of GTPCH1 and DHFR, which were significantly reversed by STA pretreatment. Furthermore, STA increased mRNA and protein levels of GTPCH1 and DHFR in dose- and time-dependent manners (Fig. 5d-h). These results suggested that induction of GTPCH1 and DHFR may contribute to the protection against the Hcy-impaired BH4 and NO production.

## STA increased the expressions of GTPCH1 and DHFR via activation of Nrf2

Nuclear factor erythroid 2–related factor 2 (Nrf2) transcriptionally controls the gene expression of many cytoprotective enzymes, such as heme oxygenase-1 (HO-1) (Swamy et al., 2016) and NAD(P)H:quinone reductase (NQO1) (Rohrer et al., 2014). Particularly, it was shown that Nrf2 regulated-GTPCH1/BH4 axis ameliorated skin injury (Xue et al., 2017). To test whether Nrf2 is involved in the effects of STA on the induction of expressions of GTPCH1 and DHFR, BAECs were treated with STA (10 µM) for different time periods and the Nrf2 levels were detected by using western blotting. As shown in Fig. 6a, STA increased the total Nrf2 protein level. Furthermore, STA treatment rapidly increased Nrf2 protein level in the nuclear portions (Fig. 6b and c), suggesting that Nrf2 is activated and likely translocated into the nuclear compartment in response to STA exposure. Furthermore, Nrf2 knockdown by siRNA abrogated STA-increased levels of GTPCH1 and DHFR (Fig. 6d and e). These results indicated that activation of Nrf2 might act as a transcriptional regulator to mediate the STA-induced gene expression of GTPCH1 and DHFR.

## Discussion

Endothelial dysfunction has been implicated in the pathogenesis of CVDs such as atherosclerosis, diabetes and hypertension (Martin-Timon et al., 2014). STA is belongs to naturally occurring alkaloids. Among their diverse pharmacological properties such as anti-microbial, anti-tumor, anti-diabetic and anti-inflammatory effects, many natural alkaloids have been reported to possess vascular protective activities (Kittakoop et al., 2014; Cushnie et al., 2014). However, the molecular mechanisms underlying such vascular benefit remain largely unknown. In the present study, we for the first time provided both in vitro and ex vivo evidence that STA protects against the Hcy-impaired endothelial dysfunction.

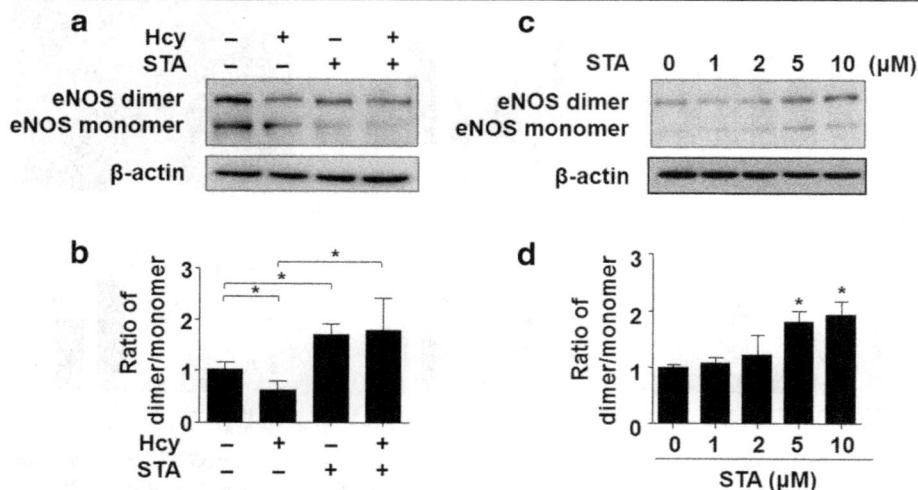

**Fig. 4** STA ameliorated Hcy-induced eNOS uncoupling. **a** BAECs were pre-incubated with STA (10 µM, 12 h) or vehicle and, then exposed to Hcy (500 µM, 12 h). Protein levels of eNOS dimers and monomers were detected by using low-temperature SDS-PAGE/western blotting. **c** BAECs were exposed to indicated concentrations of STA for 24 h, cell lysates were analyzed to determine eNOS dimers and monomers protein levels. **b** and **d** Quantification of eNOS dimer/monomer levels. Data were shown as mean ± SEM, $n = 5$. $^*P < 0.05$

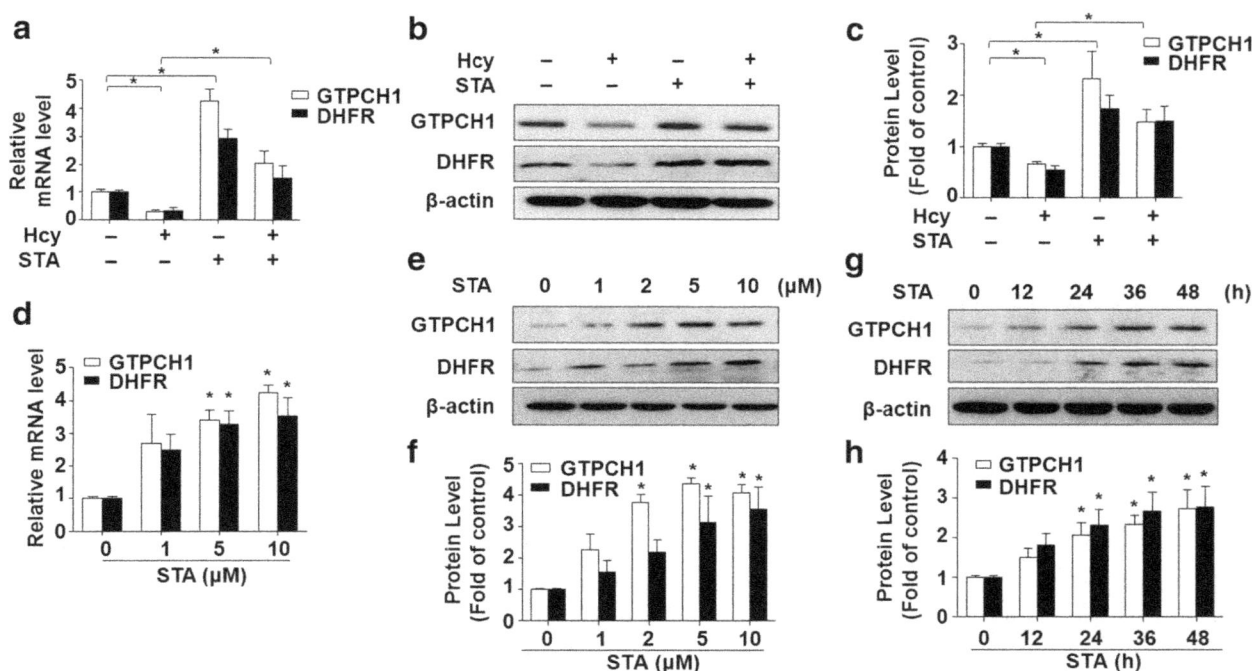

**Fig. 5** STA increased the levels of GTPCH1 and DHFR. **a** Relative mRNA levels of GTPCH1 and DHFR were assessed by using qRT-PCR. **b** Protein levels were assessed by using Western blotting. **c** Quantification of GTPCH1 and DHFR protein levels, which was normalized to the β-actin levels. **d** The mRNA levels of GTPCH1 and DHFR were assessed by using qRT-PCR. **e** GTPCH1 and DHFR protein levels were assessed by using Western blotting. **f** Quantification of GTPCH1 and DHFR protein levels as in (**e**). **g** BAECs were incubated with 10 μM STA for indicated time periods, GTPCH1 and DHFR protein levels were assessed by using Western blotting. **h** Quantification of GTPCH1 and DHFR protein levels as in (**g**). Data shown were mean ± SEM, n = 5. *P < 0.05

Most importantly, we defined the novel mechanisms by which STA enhances eNOS coupling and NO bioavailability via up-regulation of GTPCH1 and DHFR, the genes for two major enzymes responsible for the de novo biosynthesis and salvage pathways of BH4. Given the critical roles of NO signaling in the vascular homeostasis and diseases, these findings are of pathophysiological importance to our understanding of the pharmacological mechanisms, by which the naturally occurring compounds exert their vascular actions.

Hcy is an intermediate metabolite in the metabolic pathway of cysteine and methionine (Gurda et al., 2015). Elevated level of plasma Hcy is an independent risk factor of CVD and Hcy contributes to the development of CVD as it causing endothelial dysfunction (Ivanov et al., 2015). In our study, we found that STA prevented Hcy-induced impairment of endothelium-dependent relaxation (Fig. 1). L-NAME, a NOS inhibitor, suppressed the relaxation of STA, indicating that the vasorelaxant effect of STA was associated with NO release. This notion is corroborated with the result that ODQ, a NO-sensitive guanylyl cyclase inhibitor that blocks the signaling pathway of the endothelium-derived NO, also reduced STA-induced relaxation. By contrast, iNOS did not play any roles in the enhanced NO release, which was confirmed

using the iNOS inhibitor 1400 W (Fig. 2). These results clearly demonstrated that STA can elicit a NO-dependent vasodilation.

ECs produce a variety of vasoactive substances, such as NO, endothelium-derived hyperpolarizing factor (EDHF), prostacyclin, or endothelin-1 (ET-1), Ang II, thromboxane A2 and prostaglandin H2, to keep the delicate balance between vasodilation and vasoconstriction (Husain et al., 2015). Among these endothelial-derived vasodilators, NO is the most important one because of its key role in inhibiting platelet aggregation, inflammation, oxidative stress, vascular smooth muscle cell migration and proliferation, and leukocyte adhesion (Zhao et al., 2015). In our study, we showed that the impaired production of NO by Hcy was rescued by STA (Fig. 3). NO-induced relaxation is associated with increased levels of cGMP in vascular smooth muscle cells. An elevation in intracellular cyclic GMP levels leads to vasorelaxation. Our findings indicated that the effect of STA-induced relaxation via NO-dependent cGMP production. eNOS catalyzes the biosynthesis of NO in endothelial cells whereas BH4 is a critical determinant of eNOS activity. We demonstrated that STA prevented the Hcy-induced BH4 decrease and that STA increased BH4 production in ECs (Fig. 3). BH4 bioavailability in the vasculature appears to be regulated by both a de

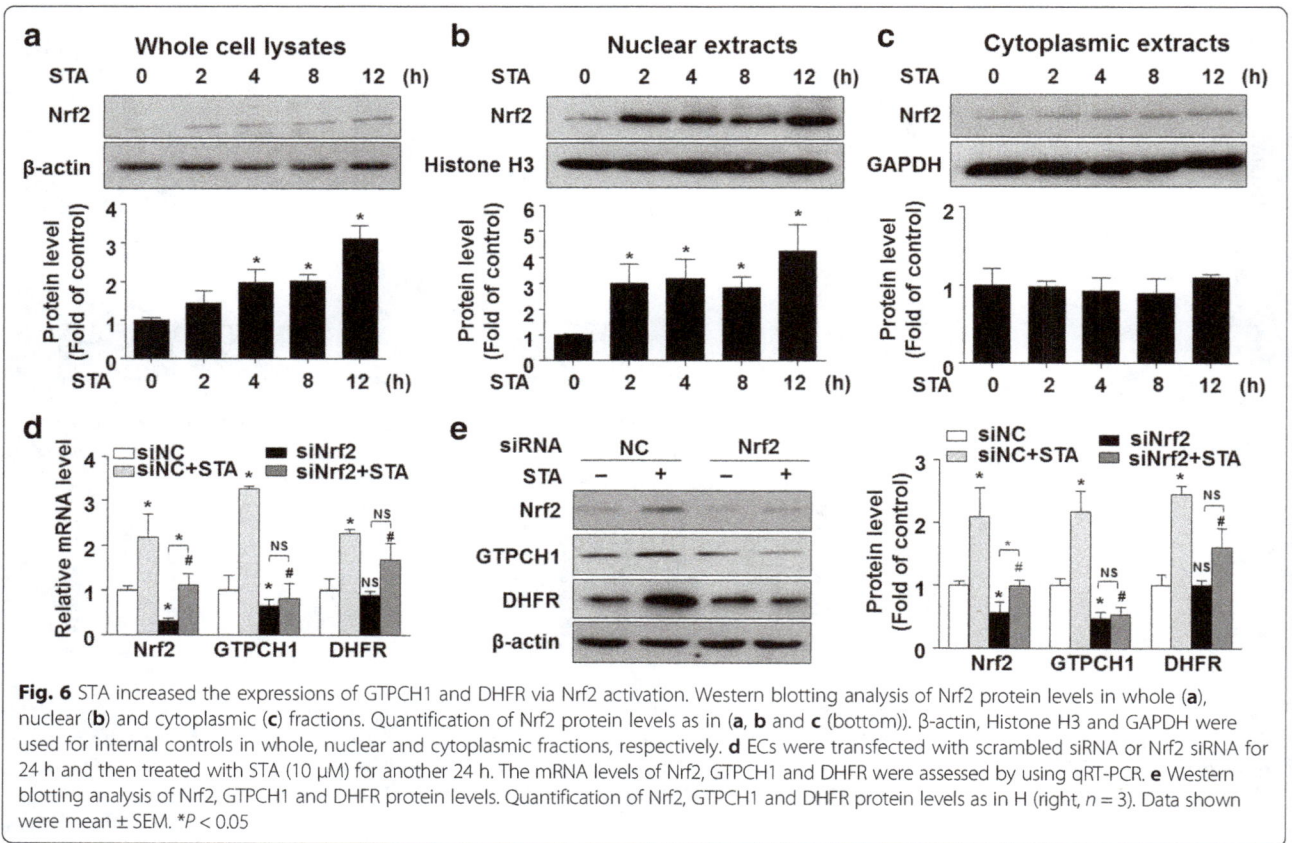

**Fig. 6** STA increased the expressions of GTPCH1 and DHFR via Nrf2 activation. Western blotting analysis of Nrf2 protein levels in whole (**a**), nuclear (**b**) and cytoplasmic (**c**) fractions. Quantification of Nrf2 protein levels as in (**a**, **b** and **c** (bottom)). β-actin, Histone H3 and GAPDH were used for internal controls in whole, nuclear and cytoplasmic fractions, respectively. **d** ECs were transfected with scrambled siRNA or Nrf2 siRNA for 24 h and then treated with STA (10 μM) for another 24 h. The mRNA levels of Nrf2, GTPCH1 and DHFR were assessed by using qRT-PCR. **e** Western blotting analysis of Nrf2, GTPCH1 and DHFR protein levels. Quantification of Nrf2, GTPCH1 and DHFR protein levels as in H (right, $n = 3$). Data shown were mean ± SEM. $*P < 0.05$

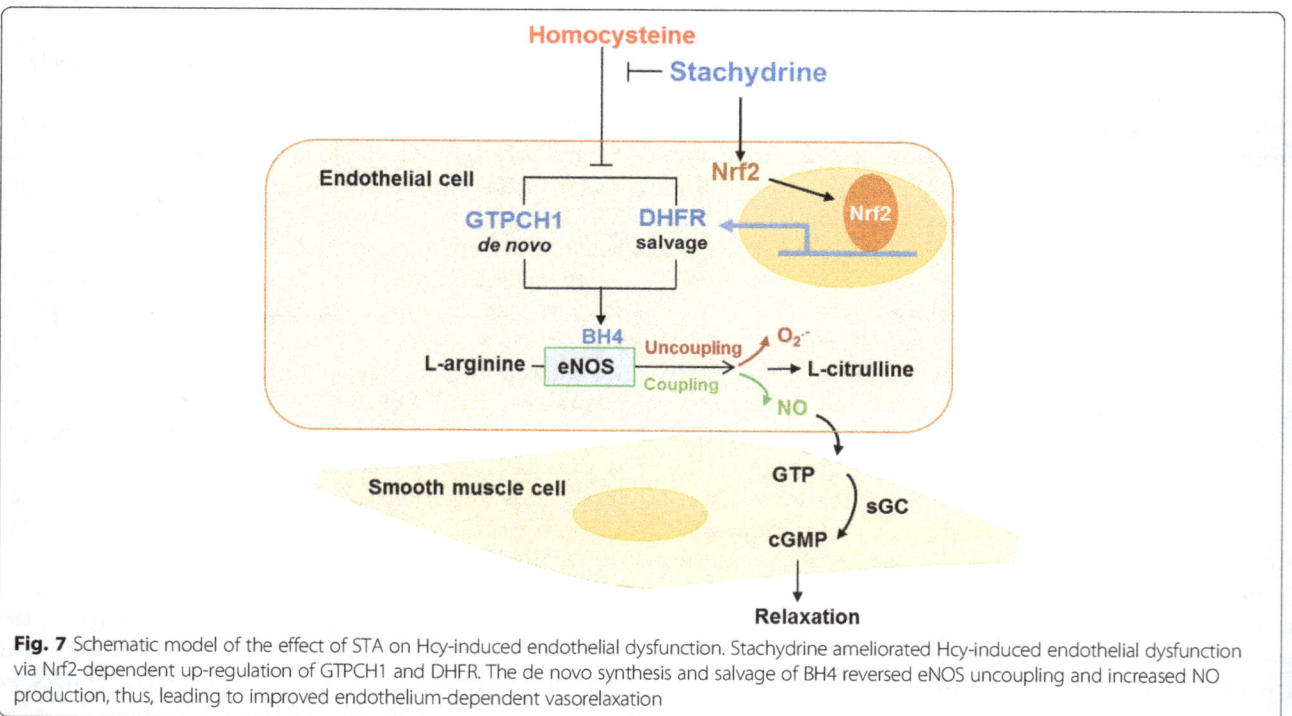

**Fig. 7** Schematic model of the effect of STA on Hcy-induced endothelial dysfunction. Stachydrine ameliorated Hcy-induced endothelial dysfunction via Nrf2-dependent up-regulation of GTPCH1 and DHFR. The de novo synthesis and salvage of BH4 reversed eNOS uncoupling and increased NO production, thus, leading to improved endothelium-dependent vasorelaxation

novo pathway using the rate-limiting enzyme GTP-cyclohydrolase I (GTPCH1) and a salvage pathway from the synthetic pterin, sepiapterin, which is metabolized to BH4 by sepiapterin reductase (SR) and endothelial dihydrofolate reductase (DHFR) (Bendall et al., 2014). It has been previously demonstrated that depletion of BH4 renders uncoupling eNOS uncoupled from L-arginine oxidation, resulting in generation of $O2^-$ rather than NO. Such an "eNOS uncoupling" status is thought to contribute to vascular oxidative stress and endothelial dysfunction (Hsieh et al., 2014). In fact, it was previously described that homocysteine exposure could lead to eNOS uncoupling in EC (Topal et al., 2004). The mechanisms underlying the suppressive effects of NO bioavailability and eNOS uncoupling are still incompletely understood. In light of the previous findings that Hcy significantly reduced intracellular BH4 level in ECs and that ascorbic acid, a BH4 regenerator, rescued the NO production in Hcy-exposed ECs (Topal et al., 2004), a decreased in BH4 level or, more importantly, the BH4:BH2 ratio (Crabtree et al., 2009), may account for the deleterious effect of homocysteine. Interestingly, we found STA markedly increased eNOS coupling, as suggested by the increased levels of NO production, dimerized eNOS, BH4:BH2 ratio, as well as GTPCH1 and DHFR expression in ECs (Figs. 4 and 5).

Nrf2 is sequestered in the cytoplasmic portion and bind to its repressor molecule, Keap1 (Soares et al., 2016). Under stressful conditions such as oxidative or ER stress, Nrf2 dissociates from the Nrf2-Keap1 complex. Subsequently, Nrf2 undergoes nuclear translocation to transcriptionally activate its target genes. In the present study, Nrf2 was rapidly increased by STA in ECs. Nrf2 was increased in the nuclear portion within 2 h after the STA treatment, indicating that Nrf2 activation is an early event in the STA signaling. A critical role of Nrf2 was further supported by the results that gene silencing of Nrf2 attenuated the STA induction of both GTPCH1 and DHFR (Fig. 6). Given that both GTPCH1 and DHFR genes harbor the cognate cis-elements within the 5′-flanking regions, we speculate that STA may activate Nrf2 to transcriptionally up-regulate the gene expression of GTPCH1 and DHFR, which are responsible for the de novo biosynthesis and salvage pathways of BH4; such a coordinated gene induction result in increased BH4 and NO bioavailability, thus protecting endothelial-dependent vascular function against such metabolic risk factor as homocysteinemia, saturated free fatty acids and Ang II (Fig. 7).

## Conclusion
Taken together, our results demonstrated that stachydrine ameliorated Hcy-induced endothelial dysfunction via Nrf2 dependent up-regulation of GTPCH1 and DHFR and increase in bioavailabilities of BH4 and NO. These results revealed a new mechanism by which the natural alkaloids STA protect endothelial function in response to such risk factors as increased concentration of homocysteine.

### Abbreviations
BH4: Tetrahydrobiopterin; CVDs: Cardiovascular diseases; DHFR: Dihydrofolate reductase; ECs: Endothelial cells; eNOS: Endothelial nitric oxide synthase; GTPCH1: Guanosine triphosphate cyclohydrolase-1; Hcy: Homocysteine; L-NAME: NG-nitro-L-arginine methylester; MA: Mesenteric arteries; NO: Nitric oxide; Nrf2: Nuclear factor erythroid 2–related factor 2; ODQ: 1H- [1, 2, 4] Oxadiazolo [4,3-a] quinoxalin-1-one; RA: Renal arteries; STA: Stachydrine; TA: Thoracic aortas

### Acknowledgements
We would like to thank Yahan Liu and Lei Qian for helpful discussion.

### Funding
This study was supported by grants from the National Science Foundation of China (31430045, 81770497, 81470373 and 81220108005).

### Authors' contributions
XX performed most of experiments, analyzed the data and wrote the draft of the manuscript. ZZ, XW and ZL performed a part of experiments. BL contributed new reagents or analytic tools. LX and NW designed the experiments, provided funding, and wrote the manuscript. All authors read and approved the final manuscript.

### Competing interests
The authors declare that they have no competing interests as defined by *Molecular Medicine* or other interests that might be perceived to influence the results and discussion reported in this paper.

### References
Almudever P, et al. Role of tetrahydrobiopterin in pulmonary vascular remodelling associated with pulmonary fibrosis. Thorax. 2013;68:938–48.

Baggott JE, Tamura T. Homocysteine, iron and cardiovascular disease: a hypothesis. Nutrients. 2015;7:1108–18.

Bendall JK, Douglas G, McNeill E, Channon KM, Crabtree MJ. Tetrahydrobiopterin in cardiovascular health and disease. Antioxid Redox Signal. 2014;20:3040–77.

Cheng Z, et al. Hyperhomocysteinemia and hyperglycemia induce and potentiate endothelial dysfunction via mu-calpain activation. Diabetes. 2015;64:947–59.

Crabtree MJ, et al. Quantitative regulation of intracellular endothelial nitric-oxide synthase (eNOS) coupling by both tetrahydrobiopterin-eNOS stoichiometry and biopterin redox status: insights from cells with tet-regulated GTP cyclohydrolase I expression. J Biol Chem. 2009;284:1136–44.

Cushnie TP, Cushnie B, Lamb AJ. Alkaloids: an overview of their antibacterial, antibiotic-enhancing and antivirulence activities. Int J Antimicrob Agents. 2014;44:377–86.

Gurda D, Handschuh L, Kotkowiak W, Jakubowski H. Homocysteine thiolactone and N-homocysteinylated protein induce pro-atherogenic changes in gene expression in human vascular endothelial cells. Amino Acids. 2015;47:1319–39.

Haruki H, Hovius R, Pedersen MG, Johnsson K. Tetrahydrobiopterin biosynthesis as a potential target of the kynurenine pathway metabolite Xanthurenic acid. J Biol Chem. 2016;291:652–7.

Hsieh HJ, Liu CA, Huang B, Tseng AH, Wang DL. Shear-induced endothelial mechanotransduction: the interplay between reactive oxygen species (ROS) and nitric oxide (NO) and the pathophysiological implications. J Biomed Sci. 2014;21:3.

Hu Y, He K, Zhu H. Chinese herbal medicinal ingredients affect secretion of NO, IL-10, ICAM-1 and IL-2 by endothelial cells. Immunopharmacol Immunotoxicol. 2015;37:324–8.

Hu YY, He KW, Guo RL. Six alkaloids inhibit secretion of IL-1alpha, TXB(2), ET-1 and E-selectin in LPS-induced endothelial cells. Immunol Investig. 2012;41:261–74.

Husain K, Hernandez W, Ansari RA, Ferder L. Inflammation, oxidative stress and renin angiotensin system in atherosclerosis. World J Biol Chem. 2015;6:209–17.

Hussein D, et al. Validating the GTP-cyclohydrolase 1-feedback regulatory complex as a therapeutic target using biophysical and in vivo approaches. Br J Pharmacol. 2015;172:4146–57.

Ivanov AN, Puchinyan DM, Norkin IA. Vascular endothelial barrier function. Usp Fiziol Nauk. 2015;46:72–96.

Karolczak K, Kamysz W, Karafova A, Drzewoski J, Watala C. Homocysteine is a novel risk factor for suboptimal response of blood platelets to acetylsalicylic acid in coronary artery disease: a randomized multicenter study. Pharmacol Res. 2013;74:7–22.

Kittakoop P, Mahidol C, Ruchirawat S. Alkaloids as important scaffolds in therapeutic drugs for the treatments of cancer, tuberculosis, and smoking cessation. Curr Top Med Chem. 2014;14:239–52.

Klatt P, Schmidt K, Lehner D, Glatter O, Bachinger HP, Mayer B. Structural analysis of porcine brain nitric oxide synthase reveals a role for tetrahydrobiopterin and L-arginine in the formation of an SDS-resistant dimer. EMBO J. 1995;14:3687–95.

Kuchta K, Volk RB, Rauwald HW. Stachydrine in Leonurus cardiaca, Leonurus japonicus, Leonotis leonurus: detection and quantification by instrumental HPTLC and 1H-qNMR analyses. Die Pharmazie. 2013;68:534.

Martin-Timon I, Sevillano-Collantes C, Segura-Galindo A, Del CF. Type 2 diabetes and cardiovascular disease: have all risk factors the same strength? World J Diabetes. 2014;5:444–70.

Papapetropoulos A, Hobbs AJ, Topouzis S. Extending the translational potential of targeting NO/cGMP-regulated pathways in the CVS. Br J Pharmacol. 2015; 172:1397–414.

Rohrer PR, Rudraiah S, Goedken MJ, Manautou JE. Is nuclear factor erythroid 2-related factor 2 responsible for sex differences in susceptibility to acetaminophen-induced hepatotoxicity in mice? Drug Metab Dispos. 2014;42:1663–74.

Servillo L, et al. Stachydrine ameliorates high-glucose induced endothelial cell senescence and SIRT1 downregulation. J Cell Biochem. 2013;114:2522–30.

Soares MA, et al. Restoration of Nrf2 signaling normalizes the regenerative niche. Diabetes. 2016;65:633–46.

Swamy SM, Rajasekaran NS, Thannickal VJ. Nuclear factor-Erythroid-2-related factor 2 in aging and lung fibrosis. Am J Pathol. 2016;186:1712–23.

Takimoto E, et al. Oxidant stress from nitric oxide synthase-3 uncoupling stimulates cardiac pathologic remodeling from chronic pressure load. J Clin Invest. 2005;115:1221–31.

Topal G, et al. Homocysteine induces oxidative stress by uncoupling of NO synthase activity through reduction of tetrahydrobiopterin. Free Radic Biol Med. 2004;36:1532–41.

Wejksza K, et al. Kynurenic acid production in cultured bovine aortic endothelial cells. Homocysteine is a potent inhibitor. Naunyn Schmiedeberg's Arch Pharmacol. 2004;369:300–4.

Xue J, et al. The Nrf2/GCH1/BH4 Axis ameliorates radiation-induced skin injury by modulating the ROS Cascade. J Invest Dermatol. 2017;137:2059–68.

Yin J, et al. Stachydrine, a major constituent of the Chinese herb leonurus heterophyllus sweet, ameliorates human umbilical vein endothelial cells injury induced by anoxia-reoxygenation. Am J Chin Med. 2010;38:157–71.

Zhao Y, Vanhoutte PM, Leung SW. Vascular nitric oxide: Beyond eNOS. J Pharmacol Sci. 2015;129:83–94.

# 17

# The effects of lncRNA MALAT1 on proliferation, invasion and migration in colorectal cancer through regulating *SOX9*

Yuanlin Xu[1], Xihong Zhang[2], Xiufeng Hu[3], Wenping Zhou[1], Peipei Zhang[1], Jiuyang Zhang[1], Shujun Yang[1] and Yanyan Liu[1*]

## Abstract

**Background:** For the study, we determine the potential biomarkers and uncover the regulatory mechanisms of lncRNA MALAT1 / miR-145 / *SOX9* axis on the abilities of cell growth and cell metastasis of colorectal cancer.

**Methods:** Previously published dataset GSE18105 from GEO database was used for microarray analysis to identify differential-expressed lncRNAs and mRNAs. The miRNA which had targeted relationships with both lncRNA and mRNA was predicted using miRCode and Targetscan. The association between lncRNA and miRNA, miRNA and mRNA was verified using dual-luciferase reporter assay.
Expression levels of lncRNA MALAT1, miR-145 and *SOX9* were examined by quantitative RT-PCR analysis. The cell viability of two cancer cell lines was compared by CCK-8 assay. Colony formation was hired to detected cell proliferation. The cell cycle distribution and apoptotic cell rate were conducted by flow cytometry assay. Wound healing as well as transwell assay were compare the cell migration and cell invasion respectively among groups. The effect of MALAT1 on colorectal cancer in vivo was constructed by xenograft model.

**Results:** Significantly dysregulated lncRNAs and mRNAs were identified by microarray analysis. By experimental verification, MALAT1 and *SOX9* were expressed in a high percentage of colorectal cancer tumors and cells, while miR-145 was in a low expression. We also identified miR-145 as a target of MALAT1 and *SOX9*. MALAT1 played a role in regulating cancer process by functioning as a competing endogenous RNA. Silencing MALAT1 could effectively decrease the expression level of *SOX9*, thus suppress cell viability and metastasis. Down-regulated MALAT1 could induce resistance of G1 phase in cell cycle, and facilitation of colorectal cancer cell apoptosis. Nude mice injected with cells transfected with si-MALAT1 had smaller tumor on size and weight.

**Conclusions:** The regulatory function of lncRNA MALAT1 / miR-145 / *SOX9* axis was revealed in colorectal cancer based on bioinformatics analysis. LncRNA MALAT1 could facilitate colorectal cancer cell proliferation, invasion and migration by down-regulating miR-145 and up-regulating *SOX9*. LncRNA MALAT1 could suppress cell cycle and apoptosis through MALAT1 / miR-145 / *SOX9* axis.

**Keywords:** lncRNA MALAT1, miR-145, *SOX9*, Colorectal cancer

* Correspondence: drsl954@163.com
[1]Department of Lymphatic Comprehensive Internal Medicine, Affiliated Cancer Hospital of Zhengzhou University, No.127 Dongming Road, Zhengzhou 450001, Henan, China
Full list of author information is available at the end of the article

## Background

Colorectal cancer is at the third place which leads to death worldwide (Siegel et al. 2014), with a high capacity for tumor invasion and migration. The development of colorectal cancer from normal epithelial cells to malignant carcinomas is considered to be a polystage process involving disruption of cell survival mechanisms, such as cell proliferation, differentiation and apoptosis (Rupnarain et al. 2004). Although metastasis has been recognized as the most deadly attributes of colorectal tumors (Rasool et al. 2013), the molecular underpinnings of colorectal cancer proliferation still remain incompletely understood. Accordingly, the identification of novel molecules which are differentially expressed in colorectal cancer may afford insights into the mechanisms involved.

Long non-coding RNAs (LncRNAs), greater than 200 nucleotides in length, are arbitrarily defined as RNA molecules that do not contain any apparent protein-coding potential determined largely via bioinformatics (Bergmann and Spector 2014). Although lncRNAs were previously regarded as spurious transcriptional noise on account of RNA polymerase II low specificity (Struhl 2007), they were recently elucidated to involve in the modulation of gene expression through dosage compensation, nuclear organization, transcriptional regulation and imprinting (Bonasio and Shiekhattar 2014). MALAT-1, metastasis associated lung adenocarcinoma transcript-1, named after its function that was initially discovered, is transcribed from the nuclear-enriched transcript 2 (NEAT2) for about 8.1 kb in length (Ji et al. 2003). MALAT-1 was later notarized as a transcript with abundant nuclear enrichment (Hutchinson et al. 2007) and expressed in the lungs, nerve system, pancreas and other human organs (Hutchinson et al. 2007). High expression of MALAT1 has been reported in multiple cancers. For instance, up-regulation of long non-coding RNA MALAT-1 conferred poor prognosis and influenced cell proliferation and apoptosis in acute monocytic leukemia (Huang et al. 2017). In addition, it indicated a poor prognosis and induced migration and carcinoma growth in non-small cell lung cancer (Schmidt et al. 2011). In lung adenocarcinoma cells, MALAT-1 was also reported enhancing cell motility by affecting the expression quantity of motility-related genes (Tano et al. 2010). Besides, over-expression of MALAT-1 was found in colorectal cancer, (Yang et al. 2015). With the enhancement of kinase (PRKA) anchor protein 9 (AKAP-9) expression, MALAT-1 could accelerate cell proliferation, migration and invasion in vitro (Yang et al. 2015), which implied that MALAT1 acted as a potential role in the progression of colorectal cancer.

*Sex-determining region Y (SRY)-box 9 (SOX9)*, a transcription factor, was critical for cancer progression and reported as oncogene (Qian et al. 2017). Recent studies presented that uncontrolled expression of *SOX9* was found in many kinds of cancers, such as glioma (Liu et al. 2016a), lung cancer (Li et al. 2017), colorectal cancer (Carrasco-Garcia et al. 2016) and so on. More importantly, *SOX9* with up-regulated expression was indicated poor prognosis in colorectal cancer, glioma and lung cancer (Liu et al. 2017; Bruun et al. 2014; Zhou et al. 2012). *SOX9* over-expressed in colorectal cancer was reported by (Javier et al. 2016; Montorsi et al. 2016 and Shi et al. 2015). However, the mechanisms underlying *SOX9* mediated tumorigenesis remain elusive.

MicroRNAs (miRNAs) were small endogenous non-coding RNA molecules which played a crucial role in regulating gene expression by interaction of specific transcripts (Yang et al. 2017). MiR-145 was verified to suppress tumor development and found decreased in colorectal cancer (Sheng et al. 2017). In the further studies, miR-145 has been demonstrated that it took part in the progression of colorectal cancer by controlling a series of related gene expressions participated in oncogenesis and metastasis (Wang et al. 2016; Li et al. 2016). As for upstream regulation, Arun et al. discovered that MALAT1 regulated miR-145 in gastric cancer as a competing endogenous RNA (ceRNA) (Arun et al. 2018). Nevertheless, molecular mechanisms of the ceRNA axis of MATAL1 and miR-145 modulating colorectal cancer process were rarely explored.

Taken together, to make an investigation on the critical function and mechanism of MALAT1/miR-145/*SOX9* in colorectal cancer, the expression and the correlation among MALAT1, miR-145 and *SOX9* were determined. Then we investigated the influence on cell proliferation, invasion, migration, cell cycle and apoptosis of colorectal cancer through MALAT1 / miR-145 / *SOX9*. Better understandings of the role of competing endogenous RNA MALAT1, miR-145 and *SOX9* will have translational potential for early diagnosis and may lead to the progress of novel treatment strategy against malignant colorectal tumor.

## Methods
### Human tissue samples
Forty pairs of freshly frozen colorectal tumors and corresponding normal mucous tissue (5 cm away from the cancer lesions) were collected from colorectal cancer patients who underwent colorectal resection at Affiliated Cancer Hospital of Zhengzhou University. Each AJCC classification (I-IV) had ten cases. Tissue samples were stored at a low-temperature environment until further use. Tumor samples contained more than 80% of tumor cells. Specimens are handled with very close attention to maintaining integrity and isolation. For this study tissues were held briefly at − 80 °C during frozen sectioning, using 100% ethanol to clean the blade between all samples. For each of the 40 subjects in our study, one tumor section and one matched adjacent tissue were analyzed,

totaling 80 samples. The pathological diagnosis of colorectal cancer specimens and confirmation of the adjacent normal intestinal mucosa specimens were performed by at least two pathologists. No pre-operative chemotherapy or radiotherapy treatments were taken on patients. The Clinical Research Ethics Committee of Affiliated Cancer Hospital of Zhengzhou University approved the research protocols. All patients were signed the informed consents.

## Bioinformatics analysis

GSE418105 dataset containing lncRNA and mRNA expression profiles were retrieved from the Gene Expression Omnibus (GEO) database (http://www.ncbi.nlm.nih.gov/geo/). LncRNAs and mRNAs differentially expressed in colorectal cancer tissues from normal tissues were obtained through microarray analysis. Microarray type used in the microarray analysis was HG-U133_Plus_2, obtained from GEO. A total of 85 samples were adopted. The target relationships between miRNA and the selected lncRNA and mRNA were found using miRCode and Targetscan (Whitehead Institute, Cambridge, MA, USA). GO analysis was performed to explore the relationship between differential genes and molecular function, and to show the gene enrichment in different biological processes like migration, apoptosis, cell cycle and so on.

## Cell culture

Human normal colorectal epithelial cell line NCM-460 and cell lines for colorectal cancer DLD-1, HT-29 (BNCC, Beijing, China) were cultured in RPMI-1640 medium (Haoranbio, Shanghai, China) supplemented with 10% fetal bovine serum (FBS; Hyclone, Logan, UT, USA; 100 mg/L). A humidified incubator containing 5% $CO_2$ was used to incubate cells at 37 °C.

## Vector construction

Small interference RNA (siRNA) and negative control (Invitrogen, Carlsbad, CA, USA) was hired to knockdown MALAT1, *SOX9* and controls. The following siRNAs were used to target human MALAT1: sense: 5′-CACAGGGAA AGCGAGTGGTTGGTAA-3′ and antisense: 5′-TTACCA ACCACTCGCTTTCCCTGTG-3′. The following siRNAs were used to target human *SOX9*: sense: 5′-GGGUCUCUU CUCGCUCUCGUU-3′ and antisense: 5′-AACGAGAGC GAGAAGAGACCC-3′. The sequence of the negative control was: 5′-TTCTCCGAACGTGTCACGT-3′. The full-length *SOX9* was inserted into the clone pcDNA3.1 (−) for further use. The restriction enzyme cutting sites were *Not*I and *EcoR*I. The clone pGCSIL-GFP slow virus expression vector (GeneChem, Shanghai, China) was inserted.

## Cell transfection

In logarithmic phase DLD-1 and HT-29 cells were obtained and resuspended in RPMI-1640 medium (Hyclone, South Logan, UT, USA) supplemented with 10% FBS (Hyclone, Logan, UT, USA). Cells with the destiny of $6 \times 10^5$/well were seeded in 24-well plates at for 24 h before transfection. Adherent cells were transfected with interference sequences and pGCSIL-GFP recombinant vector using Lipofectamine 2000 reagent (Invitrogen). 48 h later, transfection efficiency was tested.

## qRT-PCR

Total RNA, including the small RNA fraction, was extracted from collected tissues and each cell lines with TRIZOL reagent (Invitrogen). Next, reverse transcription reactions were carried out with PrimeScript RT Reagent kit (Takara, Dalian, China), and quantitative real-time PCR (qRT-PCR) was performed using SYBR Premix DimerEraser (Takara, Dalian, China) and the Step One Plus Real-time PCR system (Applied Biosystems, Foster City, CA, USA). Primers (Shanghai Generay Biotechnology Co., Ltd.) were listed in Table 1. Quantitative PCR was performed using TaqMan 2×universal master mix (Applied Biosystems, Foster City, CA, USA) and using the following cycle conditions: 95 °C for 30 s, 95 °C for 5 s and 40 cycles of 62 °C for 40 s. GAPDH was employed as the endogenous control. The $2^{-\Delta\Delta C_t}$ method was used to calculate the relative expression.

## Western blot

NCM-460, DLD-1 and HT-29 cells together with the corresponding transfection cells in logarithmic phase were obtained. Proteins from tissue samples and colorectal cancer cell lines were extracted with lysis buffer. The BCA Protein Assay kit (both from Beyotime Institute of Biotechnology, Haimen, Jiangsu, China) was utilized to determine the protein concentration. Protein lysate was separated on 12% SDS-PAGE gels, and then transferred onto PVDF membranes (Millipore, Billerica, MA, USA). After that, 5% non-fat dried milk was made use of blocking the membrane. Next, membranes were incubated with rabbit anti *SOX9* monoclonal antibody (ab6721; Abcam, Cambridge, MA, USA) or GAPDH (ProteinTech, Chicago,

**Table 1** The sequences of primers

| cDNA | Sequences (5′-3′) |
| --- | --- |
| MALAT1 (forward) | 5′-TGCGAGTTGTTCTCCGTCTA-3′ |
| MALAT1 (reverse) | 5′-TATCTGCGGTTTCCTCAAGC-3′ |
| SOX9 (forward) | 5′-TGCAGGAGGAGAAGAGAAGG-3′ |
| SOX9 (reverse) | 5′-GTGGCCAGTTCACAGCTGC-3′ |
| GAPDH (forward) | 5′-CTGGGCTACACTGAGCACC-3′ |
| GAPDH (reverse) | 5′-AAGTGGTCGTTGAGGGCAATG-3′ |

IL, USA) overnight, then washed with Tris-buffered saline with Tween (TBST) four times, and cultured with horse radish peroxidase (HRP) labeled goat anti-rabbit secondary antibody for 2 h. Enhanced chemiluminescence (ECL) reagent (Pierce, Rockford, IL, USA) was taken to reveal protein bands.

## Dual-luciferase reporter assay

Wild type MALAT1 and wild type *SOX9* were connected to pmiR-RB-REPORORT™ Vector (Ribobio, Guangzhou, China). MUT-MALAT1 and MUT-*SOX9* were used as the control. The mutation vectors of MALAT1 3'UTR and *SOX9* 3'UTR were constructed and the recombinant plasmid sequences were identified. The restriction enzyme cutting sites were *Xho*I and *Not*I. Mutation was performed using QuikChange II XL Site-Directed Mutagenesis Kit (Strategene, La Jolla, CA, USA). For the luciferase assay, NCM-460 cells were grown in DMEM medium (Invitrogen) and collected after digestion. Several 96-well plates were employed to seed cells. Plasmid DNA (0.2 μg) and Fugene HD (0.3 μl) were added into miR mimics after mixing. Each group had three compound holes. 0.15 μg sensor reporter genes and 0.9 μl FugeneHD were diluted by 30 μl Opti-MEM medium. Groups included NC-MUT-MALAT1, NC-WT-MALAT1, miR-mimics-MUT-MALAT1, miR-mimics-WT-MALAT1, NC-MUT-*SOX9*, NC-WT-*SOX9*, miR-mimics-MUT-*SOX9* and miR-mimics-WT- *SOX9*. After cells being transfected for 48 h, lysis buffer was diluted by double distilled water and the medium was abandoned. 80 μl lysis buffer was added into each hole and centrifuged for 1 h. Sediment was collected and added into non-transparent 96-well plates with firefly luciferase and sea cucumber luciferin substrate. Luciferase activities were gauged by a Dual-Luciferase Reporter Assay Kit (Promega, Madison, WI, USA).

## Scratch wound healing assay

Scratch wound healing assay was performed for analysis of cell migration in vitro. Briefly, DLD-1 and HT-29 cells transfected with si-MALAT1, miR-145 inhibitor, si-MALAT1 + miR-145 inhibitor, si-*SOX9*, pcDNA3.1-*SOX9*, si-*SOX9* + miR-145 inhibitor and negative control miRNA or mRNA. In order to further understand the effect of MALAT1 / miR-145 / *SOX9* axis on cell migration, wound healing assays were also conducted in the presence of the cell proliferation inhibitor mitomycin C (MMC, Sigma-Aldrich, St. Louis, MO). The DLD-1 and HT-29 cells were cultured in 6-well plates ($5 \times 10^5$/well) and incubated overnight. Culture inserts were removed after appropriate cell attachment and washed twice using PBS. Afterwards, cells were added in the DMEM medium with 10% FBS. At 0 and 24 h after scratch would formation, images were obtained using an inverted microscope (Nikon, Tokyo, Japan) at a magnification of

200× and measured by Image-Pro Plus software (Media Cybernetics, Inc., Rockville, MD, USA).

## Colony formation assay

DLD-1 and HT-29 cells transfected with si-MALAT1, miR-145 inhibitor, si-MALAT1 + miR-145 inhibitor, si-*SOX9*, pcDNA3.1-*SOX9*, si-*SOX9* + miR-145 inhibitor were obtained. Cells were digested by trypsin solution and then added into RPMI1640 (Hyclone, South Logan, UT, USA) medium. The cell suspension was seeded into a petri dish with appropriate concentration. Petri dishes were gently vibrated to let the cells spread evenly and placed at a constant temperature to cultivate cells for 14–21 days at a routine culture environment. The culture was terminated when visible cells were observed. PBS was used to wash cells and 10% methanol and 10% acetic acid were utilized to fix cells. Then 0.4% crystal violet was used to stain cells. Then the staining was removed. The colony numbers were counted using ColCounte colony counter (Oxford Optronix Ltd., Abingdon, UK). Sensitivity was set to cell number > 50. The efficiency of plating (PE) was calculated by the following formula: PE = the number of colonies/number of plated cells. PE was standardized to the blank group. The following formula was taken to calculate survival rate (SF): SF = the number of colonies/the number of plated cells × PE.

## Cell invasion assay by transwell

For the invasion assay, DLD-1 and HT-29 cells were put into the upper chamber of each well of a 24-well transwell polycarbonate membrane (8-mm pore size; Costar, Cambridge, MA, USA) coated with Matrigel (BD Biosciences, San Jose, CA, USA). Medium containing 10% FBS, served as a chemoattractant, was put into the lower chambers. After wells were incubated for 16 h at 37 °C, the surface of cells on the upper membrane were removed. Cells were then fixed and stained with 0.2% crystal violet solution for 30 min. An inverted microscope (IX71; Olympus, Japan, Toyoko) was applied to count (five high-power fields per chamber) the invading cells attached the adaxial surface of the filter were counted.

## Cell proliferation assay by CCK-8

Cell Counting Kit-8 (CCK-8) was performed to test cell viability. Cells were put into 96-well plates at $1 \times 10^4$/well in complete medium and cultured for 24 h. The medium was then replaced with medium containing 10% FBS, with or without treatment. After incubation, 10 μL of CCK-8 reagent was inserted to each well, and the plates were further incubated for 4 h. Proliferation rates were determined every 12 h after transfection. The spectrophotometric absorbance at 450 nm was measured for each sample. All the experiments were performed at least three times and the mean was calculated.

## Cell cycle and apoptosis assays by flow cytometry

For cycle analysis, the test was performed using the cell cycle kit (#A10798; Invitrogen, Carlsbad, CA, USA). Cells were cultured in 6-well plates at the destiny of approximate $5 \times 10^4$ cells/well. Cells with 72 h transfection were digested with pancreatin and centrifuged for about 5 min at 1200 rpm. After mediums were abandoned, the cells were washed and centrifuged for 5 min at 1000 rpm and then collected. After being fixed in the refrigerator with 1 ml pre-cooled 70% alcohol at 4 °C overnight, cells were washed twice with PBS and incubated with 100 μl of RnaseA in the dark at 37 °C for 30 min. The flow cytometry was conducted after cells were treated with 50 μl PI for 1 h in darkness.

For apoptosis analysis, cells were put in 6-well plates at the destiny of approximate $5 \times 10^4$/well. Cells transfected for 48 h were collected, washed twice with cold PBS and re-suspended in binding buffer with a density of $1 \times 10^6$/mL. Cells were next stained with FITC (BioVision, San Francisco, CA, USA) and PE (Beyotime). The signal was acquired by a FACS Calibur flow cytometer (BD Biosciences) and was analyzed with FACS Diva software (BD Biosciences). Experiments were conducted in triplicate.

## Xenograft model

DLD-1 and HT-29 cells were transfected with si-NC and si-MALAT1. $2 \times 10^5$ cells were injected into female BALB/c-nu nude mice (weighing 15–20 g, Department of Laboratory Animal, Fudan University). Each group had 5 mice. Tumor size of the mice was measured and calculated at the interval of 7 days. After 28 days, the mice were decapitated and the tumors were excised. The growth of tumors in vivo was visualized and imagined using GFP imaging system (Lighttools, Encinitas, Canada), and the tumor volume was measured with vernier caliper. Animal experiments were approved by the Institutional Animal Care and Use Committee of Affiliated Cancer Hospital of Zhengzhou University and performed following the Institutional Guidelines and Protocols.

## Statistical analysis

Statistical analysis was using SPSS 20.0 and GraphPad Prism 6.0 (GraphPad Software, San Diego, CA). Data were presented in the form of the "mean ± standard". Student's t-test was used to assess differences between two groups. One-way analysis of variance (ANOVA) was used to compare differences among three groups or more. Rank-sum test was used to evaluate heterogeneity of variance. All experiments were with 3 repetitions for each group. $P < 0.05$ was considered statistically significant.

## Results

### MALAT1 and SOX9 were high expressed in colorectal cancer tissues

According to the volcano plot, 111 lncRNAs and 3465 mRNAs were found to be up-regulated in colorectal cancer tissues by microarray analysis (Fig. 1a and c). 16 lncRNAs and 18 mRNAs with the largest differences were exhibited in the heat map (Fig. 1b and d). Among them, the expression of lncRNA MALAT1 in cancerous tissues was increased to 2.16 folds compared with that

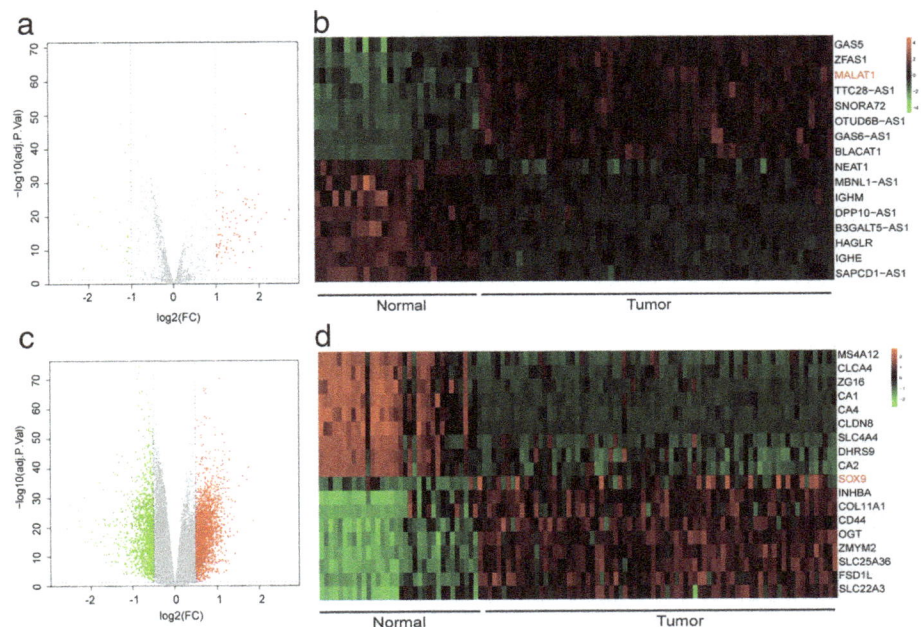

Fig. 1 Microarray analysis and verification a Volcano plot of lncRNAs. b Heat map of lncRNAs. c Volcano plot of mRNAs. d Heat map of mRNAs

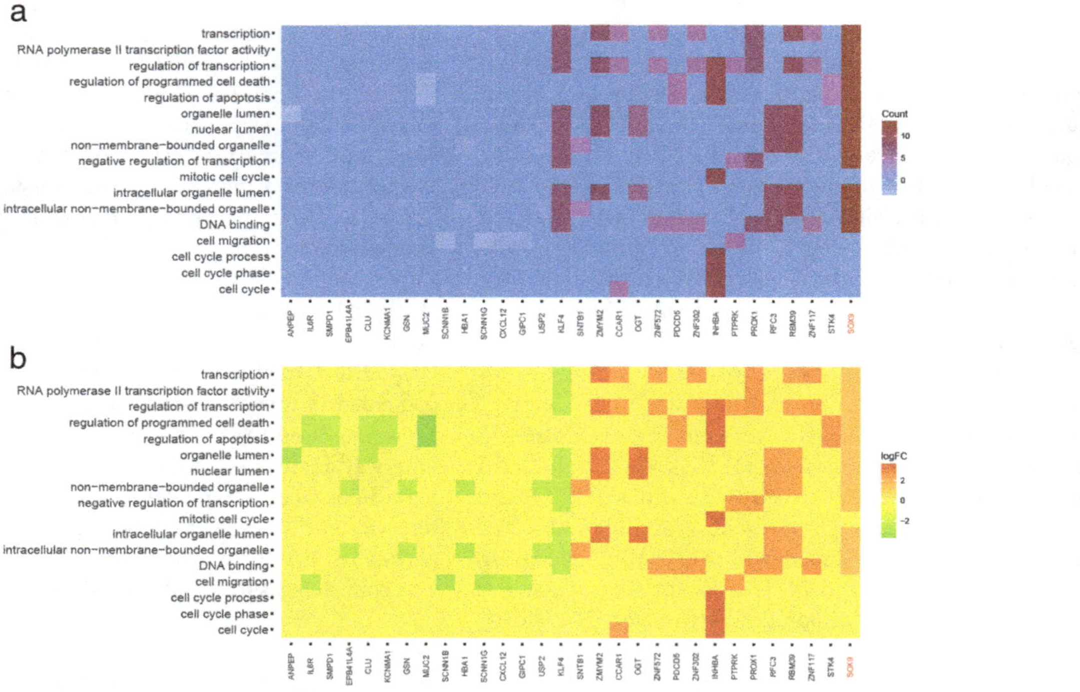

**Fig. 2** GO analysis and gene enrichment **a** Heat map of GO analysis arranged by count value. **b** Heat map of GO analysis arranged by logFC value

of paracancerous tissues, and the expression of *SOX9* was 1.86 folds greater than that of paracancerous tissues (Fig. 1b and d). Heat map of GO analysis showed the result of gene enrichment in different GO terms. *SOX9* was participated in biological processes like transcription, cell death, apoptosis, migration and so on (Fig. 2a-b). After microarray analysis, a series of differential lncRNAs and genes including MALAT1/SOX9

had been screened out. Then, bioinformatics prediction was performed and we discovered miR-145 was the target of both MALAT1 and SOX9. Among the differential lncRNAs and genes which could establish lncRNA-miRNA-mRNA regulatory axis, MALAT1 and SOX9 were found to be close to colorectal cancer progress through references. Therefore, MALAT1 and *SOX9* were selected as our subsequent study objects.

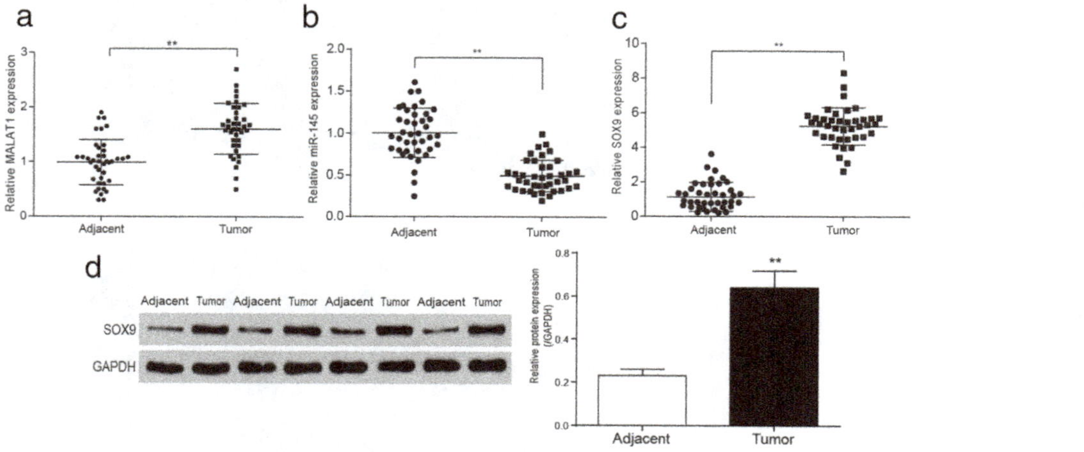

**Fig. 3** MALAT1 and *SOX9* were highly expressed in colorectal cancer tissues while miR-145 was low expressed **a** The relative MALAT1 expression in colorectal cancer tissues and adjacent tissues. **b** the expression of miR-145 in colorectal cancer tissues and adjacent tissues. **c** qRT-PCR detected the expression of *SOX9* in colorectal cancer tissues and adjacent tissues. **d** western blot detected the expression of *SOX9* in colorectal cancer tissues and adjacent tissues. $^{**}P < 0.01$, compared with "Adjacent" group

**Table 2** Correlation between MALAT1/SOX9 expression and clinicopathologic characteristics in 40 cases of colorectal cancer tissues

| Characteristics total cases | N of cases 40 | MALAT1 expression | | $P$ value[a] | SOX9 expression | | $P$ value[a] |
|---|---|---|---|---|---|---|---|
| | | Low | High | | Low | High | |
| Age (years) | | | | 0.5092 | | | 0.7471 |
| ≤ 60 | 24 | 9 | 15 | | 11 | 13 | |
| > 60 | 16 | 8 | 8 | | 6 | 10 | |
| Gender | | | | 0.5306 | | | 0.1074 |
| Male | 15 | 5 | 10 | | 9 | 6 | |
| Female | 25 | 12 | 13 | | 8 | 17 | |
| AJCC stage | | | | 0.012[*] | | | 0.0038[**] |
| I | 10 | 8 | 2 | | 8 | 2 | |
| II | 10 | 5 | 5 | | 4 | 6 | |
| III | 10 | 3 | 7 | | 5 | 5 | |
| IV | 10 | 1 | 9 | | 0 | 10 | |
| Tumor size | | | | 0.7471 | | | 0.1043 |
| ≤ 3 cm | 24 | 11 | 13 | | 13 | 11 | |
| > 3 cm | 16 | 6 | 10 | | 4 | 12 | |
| Vascular invasion | | | | 0.0172[*] | | | 0.0921 |
| Yes | 14 | 2 | 12 | | 3 | 11 | |
| No | 26 | 15 | 11 | | 14 | 12 | |
| Distant metastasis | | | | 0.0786 | | | 0.0008[***] |
| $M_0$ | 29 | 15 | 14 | | 17 | 12 | |
| $M_1$ | 11 | 2 | 9 | | 0 | 11 | |

*AJCC* American joint committee on cancer
[*]$P < 0.05$, [**]$P < 0.01$, [***]$P < 0.001$
[a]Chi-square test

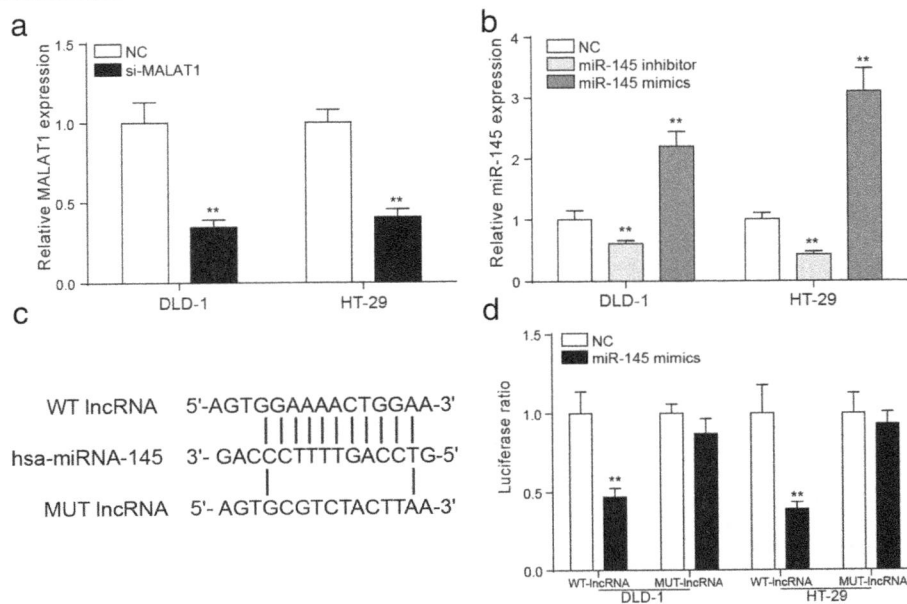

**Fig. 4** MiR-145 was the target of MALAT1 **a** the relative expression level of MALAT1 after the transfection of si-MALAT1. **b** the relative expression level of miR-145 after the transfection of miR-145 inhibitor or miR-145 mimics. **c** the binding sites of lncRNA and miRNA. **d** it was verified by the dual luciferase reporter that miR-145 was the target gene of MALAT1. [**]$P < 0.01$, compared with NC group

## Expressions of MALAT1, *SOX9* increased while miR-145 decreased in colorectal cancer tissues

MiR-145, which had targeted relationships with MALAT1 and *SOX9*, was found by miRCode and Targetscan. According to Fig. 3a, the expression of MALAT1 in cancerous tissues significantly increased compared with that of adjacent tissues in the 40 cases of colorectal cancerous tissues, and the difference was statistical ($P < 0.01$). The results of qRT-PCR displayed that miR-145 was low expressed in colorectal cancerous compared with that of adjacent tissues (Fig. 3b, $P < 0.01$). *SOX9* was in a high expression in colorectal cancer compared with that of adjacent tissues (Fig. 3c, $P < 0.01$). Expressions of *SOX9* in colorectal cancerous tissues and

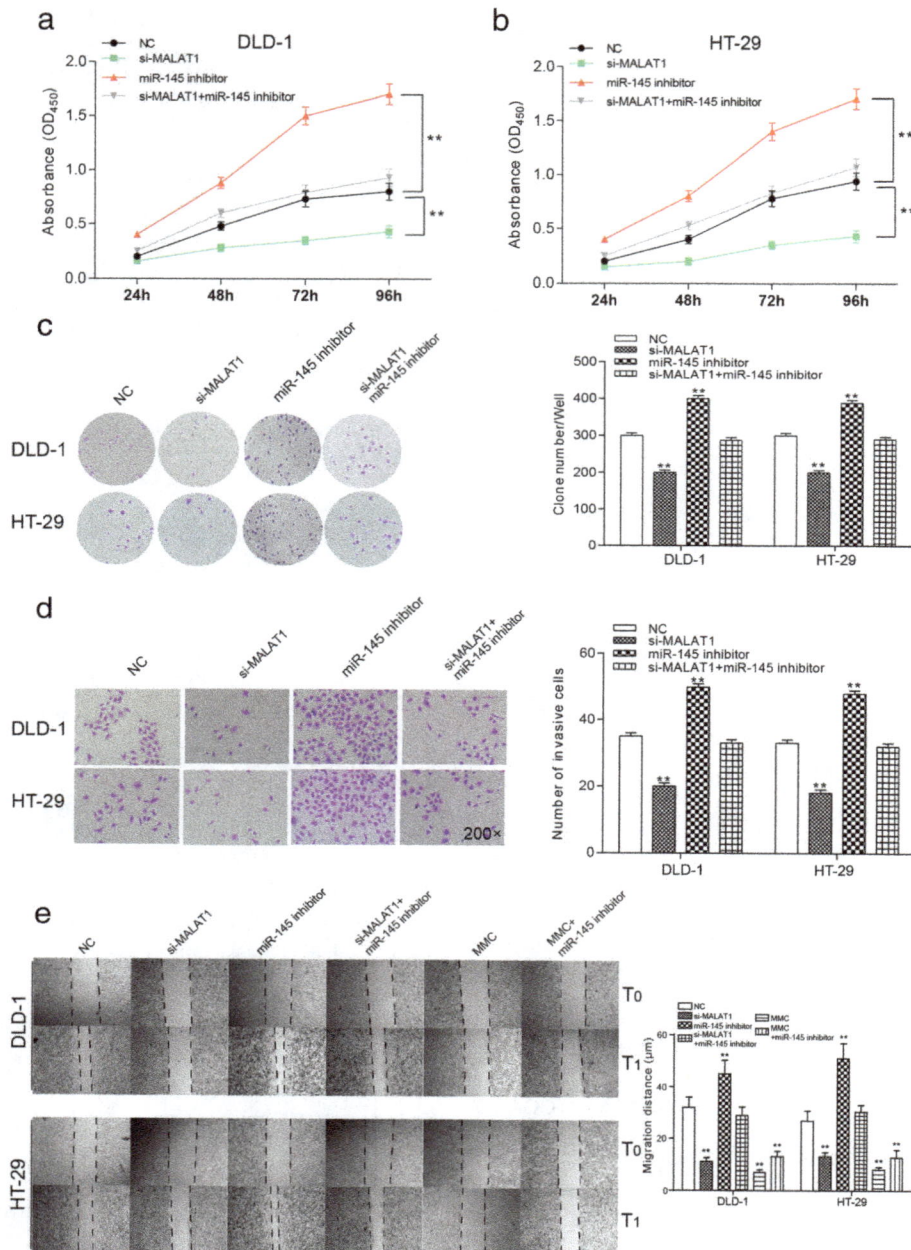

**Fig. 5** The effects of MALAT1 on proliferation, invasion and migration of colorectal cancer cells through regulating miR-145 **a** and **b** cell proliferation of DLD-1 and HT-29, cell proliferation of si-MALAT1 group was the lowest, NC group and si-MALAT1 + miR-145 inhibitor group was comparative and miR-145 inhibitor group was the highest. **c** colony formation of DLD-1 and HT-29 cells, the number of clone cells was the least in si-MALAT1 group. The miR-145 inhibitor group had the most clone cells. The number of clone cells was comparative in si-MALAT1 + miR-145 inhibitor group and NC group. **d** invasion assay of DLD-1 and HT-29 cells. **e** wound healing assay of DLD-1 and HT-29 cells. $^{**}P < 0.01$, compared with NC group

paracarcinoma tissues were detected by western blot, the results suggested that the expression of *SOX9* in colorectal cancer tissues was significantly increased than that of adjacent tissues (Fig. 3d, $P < 0.01$). The correlation between MALAT1 / *SOX9* and clinicopathologic characteristic of patients was showed in Table 2. Chi-square test demonstrated that MALAT1 / *SOX9* had a close relation with disease progress like cell invasion and metastasis.

**MiR-145 was the target of MALAT1**

QRT-PCR was applied to detect the transfection efficiencies of si-MALAT1, miR-145 inhibitor and miR-145 mimics. The results of qRT-PCR showed that MALAT1 was significantly down regulated in DLD-1 and HT-29 cells after the transfection of si-MALAT1 (Fig. 4a, $P < 0.01$). The expression of miR-145 in DLD-1 and HT-29 cells changed conspicuously after the addition of miR-145 inhibitor of miR-145 mimics (Fig. 4b, $P < 0.01$). The bioinformatics

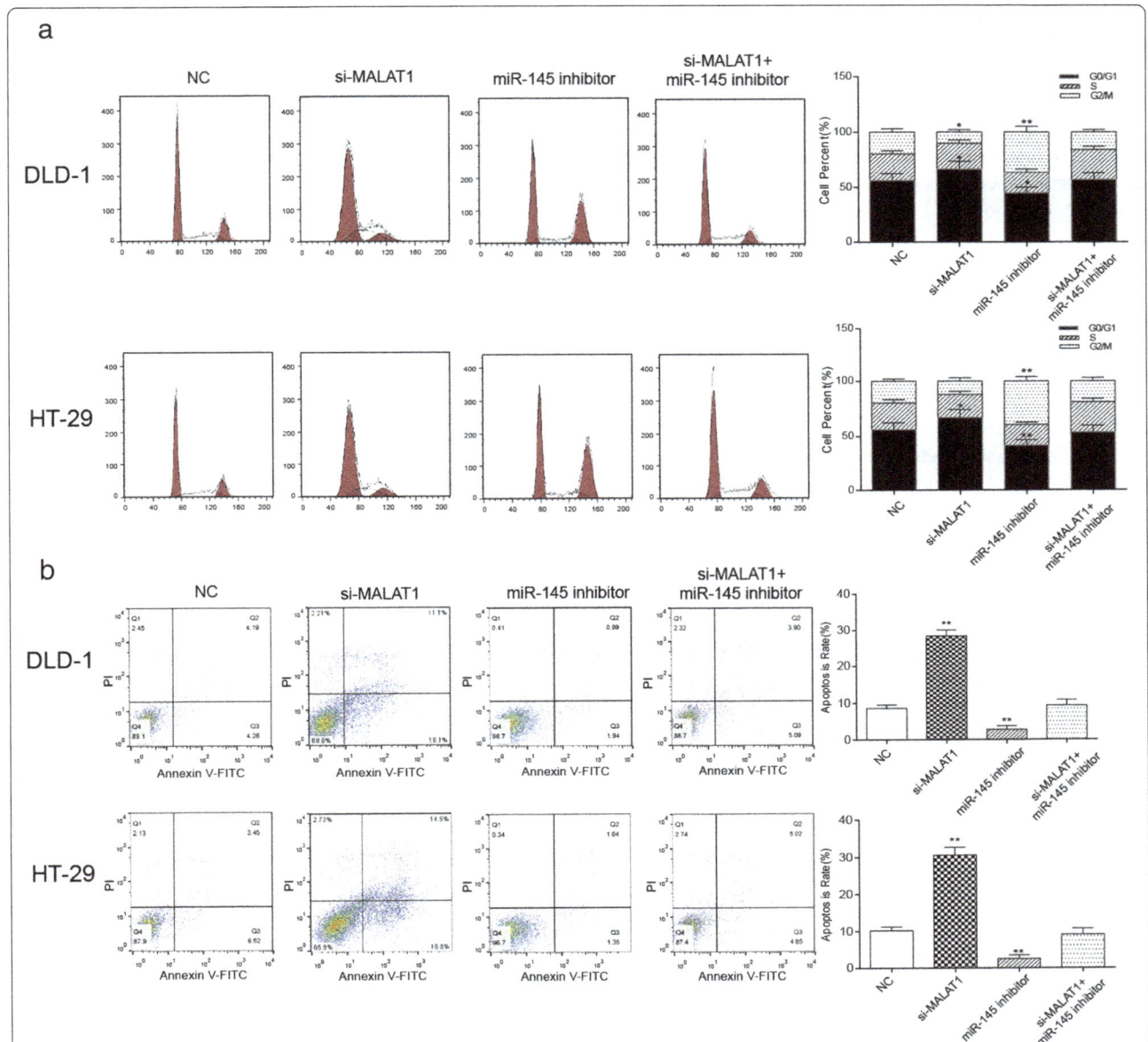

**Fig. 6** The effects of MALAT1 on cell cycle and apoptosis of cancer cells through regulating miR-145 **a** the experimental results of cell cycle of the two types of cells under different interference conditions, si-MALAT1 group had the most cells in G1 phase and the least cells in G2 phase. The number of cells in G2 phase was the most in miR-145 inhibitor group **b** experimental results of apoptosis of two types of cells under different interference conditions, the apoptosis ratio of si-MALAT1 group was the highest, and the miR-145 inhibitor group was the lowest, the si-MALAT1 + miR-145 inhibitor group and the NC group was comparative. *$P < 0.05$, **$P < 0.01$, compared with NC group

method was used to predict that miR-145 might be the target gene of MALAT1 and the binding site was shown (Fig. 4c). In consideration of structure and cytoplasmic distribution of MALAT1 in colorectal cancer cell, we hypothesized that MALAT1 may function as a competing endogenous RNA to miR-145. Dual-luciferase reporter assay was conducted to detect the targeted relationship between miR-145 and MALAT1. In the mutant group, the fluorescence signal intensity of the NC group and miR-145mimics group was comparative. In the wild-type group, the fluorescence signal intensity of miR-145 mimics group was strikingly lower than that in the NC group (Fig. 4d, $P < 0.01$), indicating that miR-145 was the target of MALAT1.

## MALAT1 accelerated the cell growth, invasion and migration of colorectal cancer cells through down-regulating miR-145

The OD value of si-MALAT1 cells was the least in the two types of cell lines. The OD value of cells transfected with miR-145 inhibitor was the largest. The proliferation ability of si-MALAT1 + miR-145 inhibitor group and NC group was comparative (Fig. 5a-b, $P < 0.01$). The number of clone cells was the fewest in si-MALAT1 group. The miR-145 inhibitor group had the most clone cells. The number of clone cells was comparative in si-MALAT1 + miR-145 inhibitor group and the NC group (Fig. 5c, $P < 0.01$). The invasive cells were the least in si-MALAT1 group, si-MALAT1 + miR-145 inhibitor group and NC group took the second place. MiR-145 inhibitor group had the most invasive cells (Fig. 5d, $P < 0.01$). According to Fig. 5e, the migration distance was the shortest in si-MALAT1 group while the longest in miR-145 inhibitor group ($P < 0.01$). Cell migration was significantly suppressed in MCC group and the condition was not changed conspicuously with the addition of miR-145 inhibitor. But there was a big difference between miR-145 inhibitor group and MMC group. No notable difference was revealed between si-MALAT1 + miR-145 inhibitor group and the NC group. These results manifested that low-expression of MALAT1 inhibited proliferation, invasion and migration of colorectal cancer cells.

## Knockdown of MALAT1 induced cell cycle arrest at G1 phase and apoptosis of colorectal cancer cells through up-regulating miR-145

In DLD-1 and HT-29, the number of cancer cells in the G1 phase increased in the si-MALAT1 group while decreased in miR-145 inhibitor group in contrast to the NC group. The cell number of in the G1 phase in the NC group and the si-MALAT1 + miR-145 inhibitor group was comparable. In addition, cancer cells in the G2 phase increased in miR-145 inhibitor group and decreased in the si-MALAT1 group compared with the NC group (Fig. 6a, $P < 0.05$). These results indicated that down-regulation of MALAT1 induced the G1 phase arrest of colorectal cancer cells. As shown in Fig. 6b, compared with the NC group, the apoptosis ratio was significantly rose in the si-MALAT1 group but obviously reduced in miR-145 inhibitor group ($P < 0.01$). The apoptosis rate of the si-MALAT1 + miR-145 inhibitor group had no significant difference from that of the NC group. These indicated that the knockdown of MALAT1 could promote apoptosis of cells, while the down-regulation of miR-145 inhibited cell apoptosis.

## SOX9 was the target gene of miR-145

The bioinformatics method was used to predict that miR-145 might be the target gene of MALAT1 and the binding site was shown in Fig. 7a. According to Fig. 7b, in the mutant group, the luciferase ratio of miR-145 mimics group was comparative to that of NC group ($P < 0.01$). But in wild-type group, it was lower in miR-145 mimics group than in the NC group. It uncovered that miR-145 had a targeted relationship with *SOX9*. The qRT-PCR analysis showed that *SOX9* expression changed conspicuously after the transfection of si-*SOX9* or pcDNA3.1-*SOX9* (Fig. 7c, $P < 0.01$).

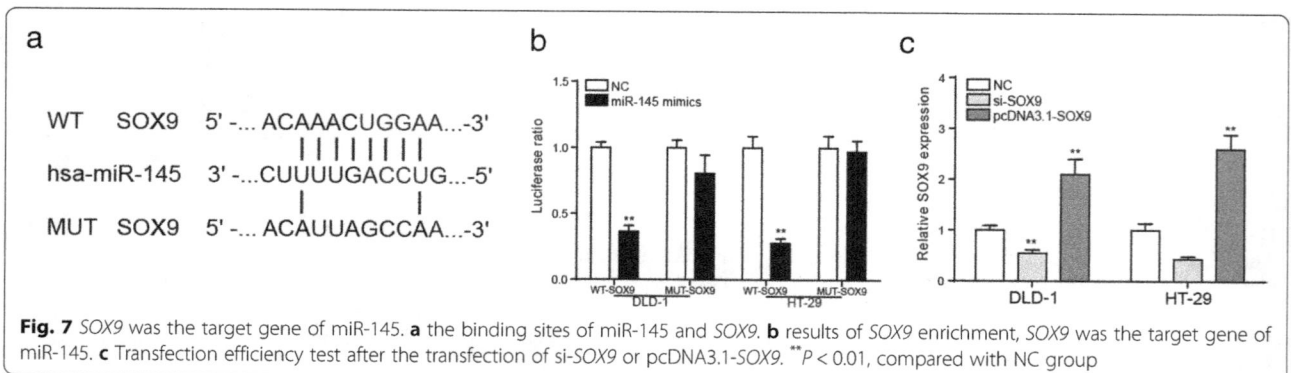

**Fig. 7** *SOX9* was the target gene of miR-145. **a** the binding sites of miR-145 and *SOX9*. **b** results of *SOX9* enrichment, *SOX9* was the target gene of miR-145. **c** Transfection efficiency test after the transfection of si-*SOX9* or pcDNA3.1-*SOX9*. $^{**}P < 0.01$, compared with NC group

### SOX9 could promote proliferation, invasion and migration of colorectal cancer cells

After 96 h, OD value was the lowest in si-*SOX9* group, and highest in pcDNA3.1-*SOX9* group. The OD value of si-*SOX9* + miR-145 inhibitor group showed no significant change compared with the NC group, suggesting that the down-regulation of *SOX9* inhibited the proliferation of colorectal cancer cells (Fig. 8a-b, $P < 0.01$).

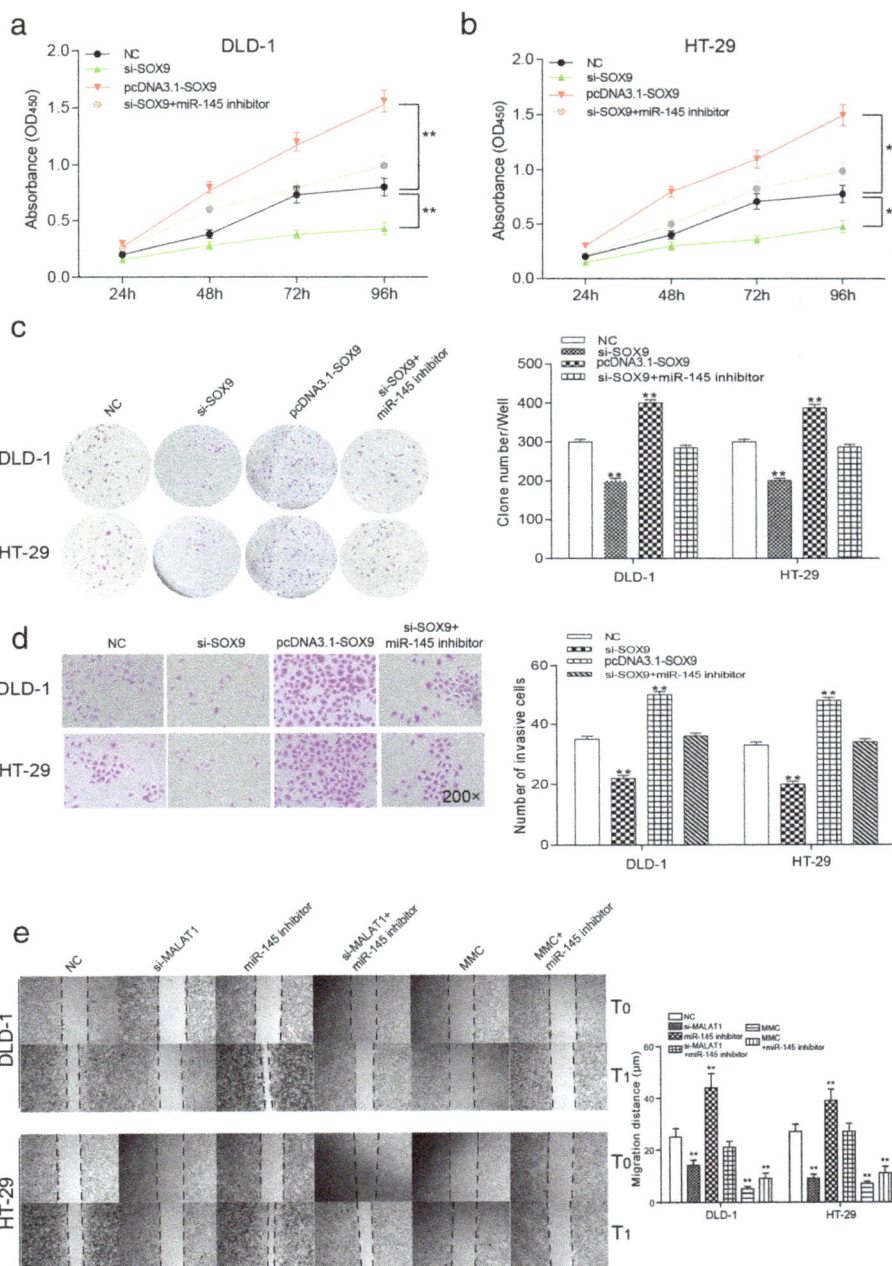

**Fig. 8** Effects of *SOX9* on proliferation, invasion and migration of colorectal cancer cells **a** and **b** the cell proliferation of colorectal cancer cell lines DLD-1 and HT-29 transfected with different interference sequences, cell proliferation was the weakest in si-*SOX9* group, and pcDNA3.1-*SOX9* group had the strongest cell proliferation ability compared with NC group. The cell proliferation of si-*SOX9* + miR-145 inhibitor group and NC group was comparative. **c** cell colony formation of colorectal cancer, the formation rate of colorectal cancer cells in the si-*SOX9* group was remarkably slower than that of the NC group. The cell formation rate was significantly higher in pcDNA3.1-*SOX9* group than that of NC group, and the cell formation in si-*SOX9* + miR-145 inhibitor group and NC group had no significant difference. **d** invasion assays of two kinds of cancer cells under different interference conditions. **e** the scratch wound healing assays of two kinds of cancer cells under different interference conditions. **$P < 0.01$, compared with NC group

Similarly, in the two groups of cell lines in the colony formation assay, the clone number of colorectal cancer cells with the knockdown of *SOX9* was significantly smaller than that of the NC group. After the over-expression of *SOX9*, the clone number was significantly improved. The clone number in si-*SOX9* + miR-145 inhibitor group and NC group had no significant difference (Fig. 8c, *P* < 0.01). Twenty-four hours after transfection, the number of invasive cells and migration

distance significantly decreased in si-*SOX9* group but increased in pcDNA3.1-*SOX9* group compared with that of the NC group. Migration distance and number of invasion cells were undifferentiated in si-*SOX9* + miR-145 inhibitor group and the NC group (Fig. 8d-e, *P* < 0.01). There was a big difference between miR-145 inhibitor group and MMC group. These results suggested that down-regulation of *SOX9* could effectively suppress proliferation, invasion and migration of colorectal cancer cells.

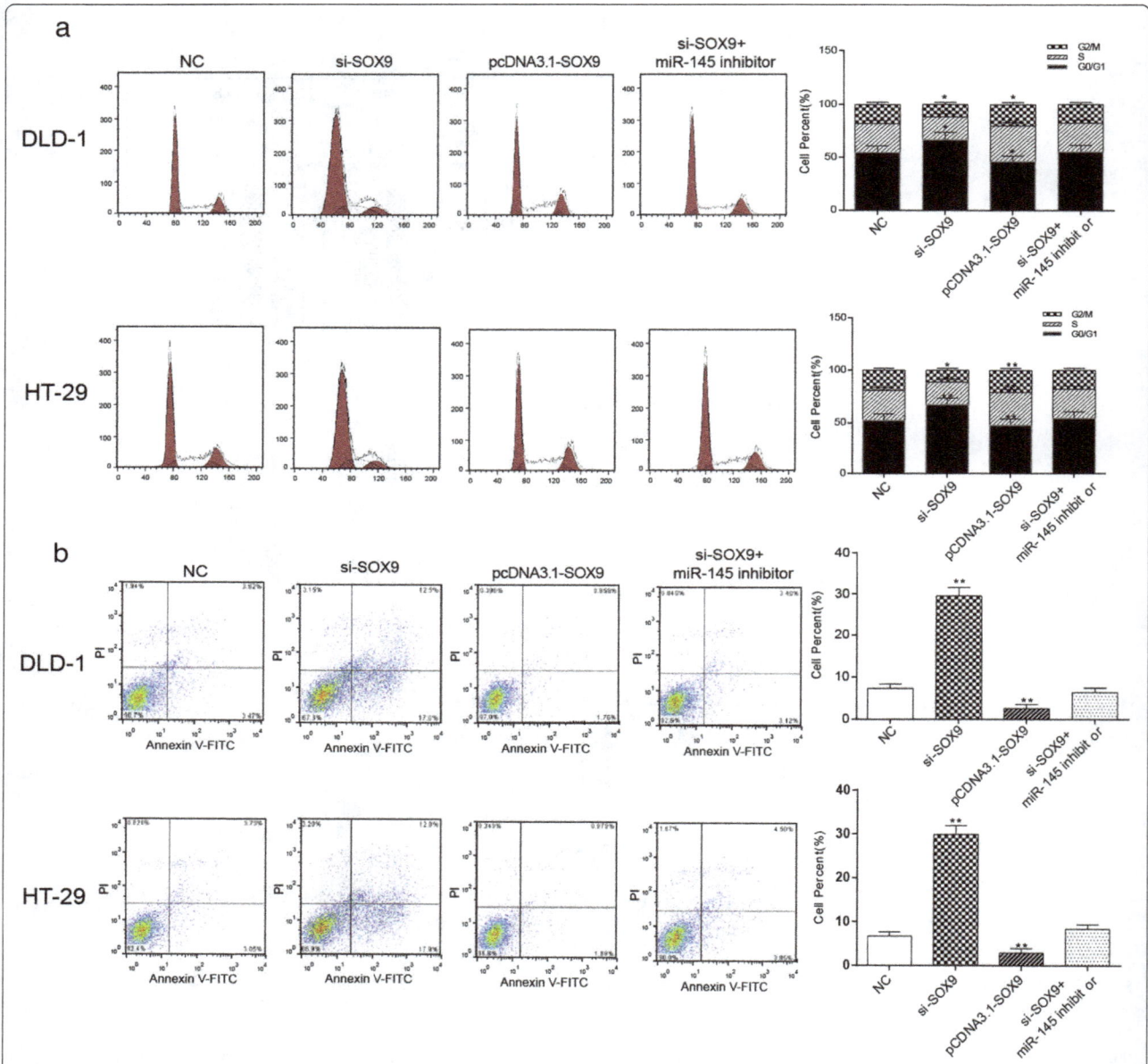

**Fig. 9** Effects of *SOX9* on cycle and apoptosis of colorectal cancer cells **a** the cell cycle was assessed by flow cytometry, the number of cells in G1 phase was the most in the si-*SOX9* group and was the least in pcDNA3.1-*SOX9* group, the si-*SOX9* + miR-145 inhibitor group was comparative to the NC group. **b** The apoptosis rate which measured by flow cytometry of pcDNA3.1-*SOX9* group was the highest, si-*SOX9* + miR-145 inhibitor group and NC group took the second place, and si-*SOX9* group had the lowest apoptosis rate. *P* < 0.05, **P* < 0.01, compared with NC group

## Knockdown of *SOX9* could induce cell cycle arrest at G1 phase and apoptosis of colorectal cancer cells

As Fig. 9a revealed, the number of cells in G1 phase was obviously increased in the si-*SOX9* group, remarkably decreased in pcDNA3.1-*SOX9* group and didn't change much in si-*SOX9* + miR-145 inhibitor group compared with the NC group ($P < 0.05$). The apoptosis rate of pcDNA3.1-*SOX9* group was significantly higher than that of the NC group, si-*SOX9* + miR-145 inhibitor group and NC group took the second place, and si-*SOX9* group had the lowest apoptosis rate (Fig. 9b, $P < 0.01$). We might draw the conclusion that down-regulation of *SOX9* promoted cell apoptosis and induced G1 cell cycle arrest of colorectal cancer.

## Down-regulating MALAT1 could prevent cell proliferation of colorectal cancer by up-regulating miR-145 in vivo

The nude mice were subcutaneously injected with DLD-1 and HT-29 cells that transfected with si-NC and si-MALAT1. The tumor size was smaller in si-MALAT1 group. And in this group, the tumor volume were lower than that in the NC group (Fig. 10a and b, $P < 0.01$). The weight of the tumor had the similar trend of the NC group (Fig. 10a and c, $P < 0.01$). We could see that in si-MALAT1 group, the expression of miR-145 was higher and *SOX9* was lower than NC group, further verifying the knockdown of MALAT1 inhibited the growth of colorectal cancer in vivo by up-regulating miR-145 and down-regulating *SOX9* (Fig. 10d-f, $P < 0.01$).

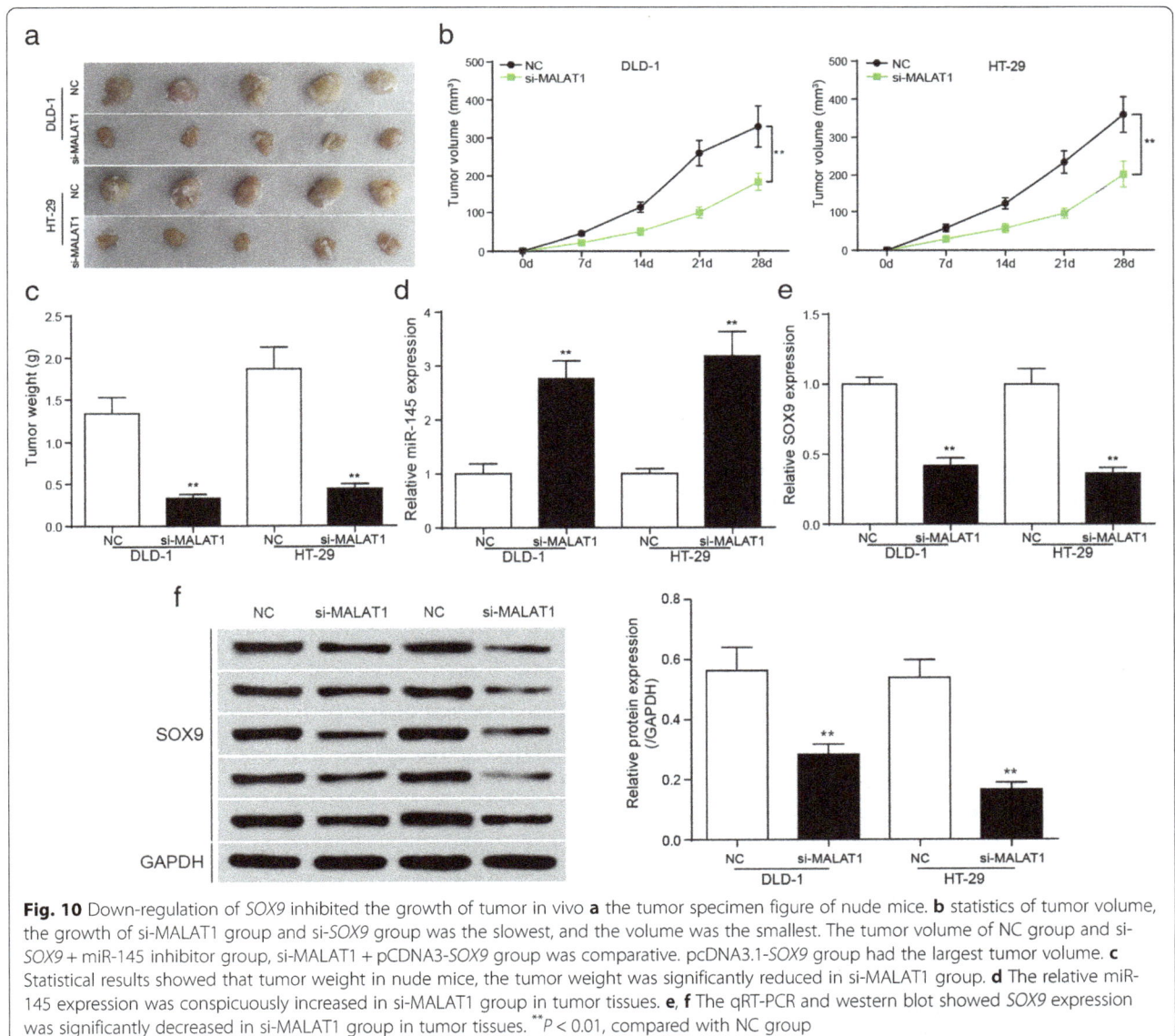

**Fig. 10** Down-regulation of *SOX9* inhibited the growth of tumor in vivo **a** the tumor specimen figure of nude mice. **b** statistics of tumor volume, the growth of si-MALAT1 group and si-*SOX9* group was the slowest, and the volume was the smallest. The tumor volume of NC group and si-*SOX9* + miR-145 inhibitor group, si-MALAT1 + pCDNA3-*SOX9* group was comparative. pcDNA3.1-*SOX9* group had the largest tumor volume. **c** Statistical results showed that tumor weight in nude mice, the tumor weight was significantly reduced in si-MALAT1 group. **d** The relative miR-145 expression was conspicuously increased in si-MALAT1 group in tumor tissues. **e**, **f** The qRT-PCR and western blot showed *SOX9* expression was significantly decreased in si-MALAT1 group in tumor tissues. $^{**}P < 0.01$, compared with NC group

---

## Discussion

In this present study, we noted that significantly up-regulated MALAT1 expression was observed in colorectal cancer tissues and cells. Moreover, over-expression of MALAT1 enhanced the cell growth of colorectal cancer cells, whereas miR-145 showed the opposite effect through repressing SOX9 expression. The down-regulation of miR-145 by competing endogenous RNA MALAT1 led to up-regulation of SOX9. Our results showed that MALAT1 might play an essential role via the miR-145-SOX9-mediated pathway in the development of colorectal cancer.

MALAT1, which is also known as PRO2853, HCN, NCRNA00047, and NEAT2, is one of the first lncRNAs described to play a significant role in cancer metastasis (Ji et al. 2003). We found that MALAT1 up-regulated in colorectal cancerous cells and tissues, which were coincident with previously reports. MALAT-1 has been demonstrated to be up-regulated in many types of cancer, such as prostate cancer (Ren et al. 2013), breast cancer (Jadaliha et al. 2016) and monocytic leukemia (Huang et al. 2017). In this study, endogenous competition function of MALAT1 was verified through down-stream miR-145 expression. Silencing MALAT1 significantly inhibited cell growth, migration and invasion. Consistent with results of our experiments, previous studies also suggested that higher expression of MALAT1 significantly correlated with metastasis in patients with cancers through the transcriptional and post-transcriptional modulation. For instance, MALAT1 RNA promoted migration and tumor growth of non-small cell lung cancer (Schmidt et al. 2011). Additionally, MALAT1 has been demonstrated to enhance cell motility of lung adenocarcinoma cells (Tano et al. 2010) and promote the migration and invasion of gastric cancer cells via EMT (Chen et al. 2017). MALAT1 also played an important role in cell cycle and cell apoptosis (Gutschner et al. 2013). It was illustrated that down-regulation of MALAT1 significantly increased G1 phase and decreased S phase in cervical cancer, and resulted in cell apoptosis increased obviously (Guo et al. 2010). Similar to these findings, our study also identified that knockdown of MALAT1 promoted cell cycle arrest and cell apoptosis.

Up to now, studies on tumor metastasis have reported that miRNAs play a role in regulating oncogenes and tumor suppressors (Dalmay and Edwards 2006; Lim et al. 2005). There have been several studies examining the expression patterns of miRNAs and its role in the progression of cancers (Asangani et al. 2008). In the present study, miR-145 expression was significantly decreased in colorectal cancer tissues. This study further demonstrated that down-regulation of miR-145 promoted the development of colorectal cancer, indicating a potential role for miR-145 in tumor invasion and metastasis. Consistent with our results, reports showed that in colorectal cancer,

miR-145 inhibited tumor growth and metastasis via regulating fascin-1 (Feng et al. 2014). Besides, miR-145 was identified in clinical colorectal cancer samples, which showed that miR-145 weakened the migrating and invading ability of cancer cells by targeting an ETS-related gene (Li et al. 2016). Hence, the specific biological function of miR-145 in the process of colorectal cancer metastasis remained to be importantly and necessarily studied. All these above can provide a powerful reference for clinical treatment.

SOX9, one target of miR-145, has been reported up-regulated in many carcinomas and has been regarded to be an important oncogene which promotes migration (Liu et al. 2017; Xiong et al. 2017) found that SOX9 functioned as a tumor promotion in hepatocellular carcinoma partially induced by miR-138 (Liu et al. 2016b). Contrary to these reports, in our study, miR-145 led to down-regulation of SOX9, which resulted in the suppression of colorectal cancerous cell growth, migration and invasion. We speculate that this inconsistency may result from the insufficient number of cases or that SOX9 may have a special role in colorectal cancer.

## Conclusions

To sum up, our study tested and verified that MALAT1 was highly expressed in colorectal cancer tissues and cells. MALAT1 regulated miR-145 expression as a competing endogenous RNA and down-regulation of MALAT1 suppressed proliferation and invasion, promoted cell cycle G1 phase and apoptosis of cancerous cells by increasing the expression of miR-145 and decreasing SOX9 expression. Therefore, MALAT1, miR-145 and SOX9 are indicated to be novel promising candidates for developing effective therapeutic strategies for colorectal cancer.

**Abbreviations**
ANOVA: Analysis of variance; ECL: Enhanced chemiluminescence; GEO: Gene Expression Omnibus; miRNAs: MicroRNAs; PE: The efficiency of plating; SF: Survival rate; TBST: Tris-buffered saline with Tween

**Authors' contributions**
Contributing to the conception and design: YLX, XH Z, WP Z, SJ Y; Analyzing and interpreting data: XF H, PP Z, JY Z; Drafting the article: YL X; Revising it critically for important intellectual content: YY L; Approving the final version to be published: All authors.

**Competing interests**
The authors declare that they have no competing interests.

**Author details**
[1]Department of Lymphatic Comprehensive Internal Medicine, Affiliated Cancer Hospital of Zhengzhou University, No.127 Dongming Road,

Zhengzhou 450001, Henan, China. ²Department of Gynaecology and Obstetric, Pepole's Hospital of Henan University of Chinese Medicine (Pepole's Hospital of Zhengzhou), Zhengzhou 450003, Henan, China. ³Department of Respiratory, Affiliated Cancer Hospital of Zhengzhou University, Zhengzhou 450001, Henan, China.

## References

Arun K, et al. Comprehensive analysis of aberrantly expressed lncRNAs and construction of ceRNA network in gastric cancer. Oncotarget. 2018;9: 18386–99.

Asangani IA, et al. MicroRNA-21 (miR-21) post-transcriptionally downregulates tumor suppressor Pdcd4 and stimulates invasion, intravasation and metastasis in colorectal cancer. Oncogene. 2008;27:2128–36.

Bergmann JH, Spector DL. Long non-coding RNAs: modulators of nuclear structure and function. Curr Opin Cell Biol. 2014;26:10–8.

Bonasio R, Shiekhattar R. Regulation of transcription by long noncoding RNAs. Annu Rev Genet. 2014;48:433–55.

Bruun J, et al. Prognostic significance of beta-catenin, E-cadherin, and SOX9 in colorectal Cancer: results from a large population-representative series. Front Oncol. 2014;4:118.

Carrasco-Garcia E, et al. SOX9-regulated cell plasticity in colorectal metastasis is attenuated by rapamycin. Sci Rep. 2016;6:32350.

Chen D, et al. The role of MALAT-1 in the invasion and metastasis of gastric cancer. Scand J Gastroenterol. 2017;52:790–6.

Dalmay T, Edwards DR. MicroRNAs and the hallmarks of cancer. Oncogene. 2006;25:6170–5.

Feng Y, et al. MicroRNA-145 inhibits tumour growth and metastasis in colorectal cancer by targeting fascin-1. Br J Cancer. 2014;110:2300–9.

Guo F, et al. Inhibition of metastasis-associated lung adenocarcinoma transcript 1 in CaSki human cervical cancer cells suppresses cell proliferation and invasion. Acta Biochim Biophys Sin. 2010;42:224–9.

Gutschner T, Hammerle M, Diederichs S. MALAT1 -- a paradigm for long noncoding RNA function in cancer. J Mol Med. 2013;91:791–801.

Huang JL, et al. Upregulation of long non-coding RNA MALAT-1 confers poor prognosis and influences cell proliferation and apoptosis in acute monocytic leukemia. Oncol Rep. 2017;38:1353–62.

Hutchinson JN, et al. A screen for nuclear transcripts identifies two linked noncoding RNAs associated with SC35 splicing domains. BMC Genomics. 2007;8:39.

Jadaliha M, et al. Functional and prognostic significance of long non-coding RNA MALAT1 as a metastasis driver in ER negative lymph node negative breast cancer. Oncotarget. 2016;7:40418–36.

Javier BM, et al. Recurrent, truncating SOX9 mutations are associated with SOX9 overexpression, KRAS mutation, and TP53 wild type status in colorectal carcinoma. Oncotarget. 2016;7:50875–82.

Ji P, et al. MALAT-1, a novel noncoding RNA, and thymosin beta4 predict metastasis and survival in early-stage non-small cell lung cancer. Oncogene. 2003;22:8031–41.

Li S, et al. miR-145 suppresses colorectal cancer cell migration and invasion by targeting an ETS-related gene. Oncol Rep. 2016;36:1917–26.

Li Z, Li B, Niu L, Ge L. miR-592 functions as a tumor suppressor in human non-small cell lung cancer by targeting SOX9. Oncol Rep. 2017;37:297–304.

Lim LP, et al. Microarray analysis shows that some microRNAs downregulate large numbers of target mRNAs. Nature. 2005;433:769–73.

Liu N, et al. MicroRNA-101 inhibits proliferation, migration and invasion of human glioblastoma by targeting SOX9. Oncotarget. 2017;8:19244–54.

Liu X, et al. MicroRNA-105 targets SOX9 and inhibits human glioma cell progression. FEBS Lett. 2016a;590:4329–42.

Liu Y, et al. miR-138 suppresses cell proliferation and invasion by inhibiting SOX9 in hepatocellular carcinoma. Am J Transl Res. 2016b;8:2159–68.

Montorsi L, et al. Loss of ZFP36 expression in colorectal cancer correlates to wnt/ ss-catenin activity and enhances epithelial-to-mesenchymal transition through upregulation of ZEB1, SOX9 and MACC1. Oncotarget. 2016;7:59144–57.

Qian Y, Xia S, Feng Z. Sox9 mediated transcriptional activation of FOXK2 is critical for colorectal cancer cells proliferation. Biochem Biophys Res Commun. 2017; 483:475–81.

Rasool S, Kadla SA, Rasool V, Ganai BA. A comparative overview of general risk factors associated with the incidence of colorectal cancer. Tumour Biol. 2013;34:2469–76.

Ren S, et al. Long noncoding RNA MALAT-1 is a new potential therapeutic target for castration resistant prostate cancer. J Urol. 2013;190:2278–87.

Rupnarain C, Dlamini Z, Naicker S, Bhoola K. Colon cancer: genomics and apoptotic events. Biol Chem. 2004;385:449–64.

Schmidt LH, et al. The long noncoding MALAT-1 RNA indicates a poor prognosis in non-small cell lung cancer and induces migration and tumor growth. J Thorac Oncol. 2011;6:1984–92.

Sheng N, et al. MiR-145 inhibits human colorectal cancer cell migration and invasion via PAK4-dependent pathway. Cancer Med. 2017;6:1331–40.

Shi Z, et al. Context-specific role of SOX9 in NF-Y mediated gene regulation in colorectal cancer cells. Nucleic Acids Res. 2015;43:6257–69.

Siegel R, Desantis C, Jemal A. Colorectal cancer statistics, 2014. CA Cancer J Clin. 2014;64:104–17.

Struhl K. Transcriptional noise and the fidelity of initiation by RNA polymerase II. Nat Struct Mol Biol. 2007;14:103–5.

Tano K, et al. MALAT-1 enhances cell motility of lung adenocarcinoma cells by influencing the expression of motility-related genes. FEBS Lett. 2010;584:4575–80.

Wang W, et al. Epigenetically regulated miR-145 suppresses colon cancer invasion and metastasis by targeting LASP1. Oncotarget. 2016;7:68674–87.

Xiong Y, et al. microRNA-130a promotes human keratinocyte viability and migration and inhibits apoptosis through direct regulation of STK40-mediated NF-kappaB pathway and indirect regulation of SOX9-mediated JNK/MAPK pathway: a potential role in psoriasis. DNA Cell Biol. 2017;36:219–26.

Yang J, et al. Expression analysis of microRNA as prognostic biomarkers in colorectal cancer. Oncotarget. 2017;8:52403–12.

Yang MH, et al. MALAT1 promotes colorectal cancer cell proliferation/migration/invasion via PRKA kinase anchor protein 9. Biochim Biophys Acta. 2015;1852:166–74.

Zhou CH, et al. Clinical significance of SOX9 in human non-small cell lung cancer progression and overall patient survival. J Exp Clin Cancer Res. 2012;31:18.

# 18

# Differential effect of surgical manipulation on gene expression in normal breast tissue and breast tumor tissue

Inge Søkilde Pedersen[1,5,6*†] (iD), Mads Thomassen[2†], Qihua Tan[2], Torben Kruse[2], Ole Thorlacius-Ussing[3,5,6], Jens Peter Garne[4] and Henrik Bygum Krarup[1,5]

## Abstract

**Background:** Gene expression profiles of normal and tumor tissue reflect both differences in biological processes taking place in vivo and differences in response to stress during surgery and sample handling. The effect of cold (room temperature) ischemia in the time interval between surgical removal of the specimen and freezing is described in a few studies. However, not much is known about the effect of warm (body temperature) ischemia during surgery.

**Methods:** Three women with primary operable breast cancer underwent in situ biopsies from normal breast and tumor tissue prior to radical mastectomy. Ex vivo biopsies from normal and tumor tissue were collected immediately after surgical excision. The putative effects on gene expression of malignancy (tumor versus normal), surgical manipulation (post- versus pre-surgical) and interaction between the two (differences in effect of surgical manipulation on tumor and normal samples) were investigated simultaneously by Generalized Estimating Equation (GEE) analysis in this self-matched study.

**Results:** Gene set enrichment analysis (GSEA) demonstrates a marked difference in effect of surgical manipulation on tumor compared to normal tissue. Interestingly, a large proportion of pathways affected by ischemia especially in tumor tissue are pathways considered to be specifically up regulated in tumor tissue compared to normal.

**Conclusion:** The results of this study suggest that a large contribution to this differential expression originates from altered response to stress in tumor cells rather than merely representing in vivo differences. It is important to bear this in mind when using gene-expression analysis to deduce biological function, and when collecting material for gene expression profiling.

**Keywords:** Specimen handling, Ischemia, Gene expression, Cell cycle, Cancer

## Introduction

Several multigene classifiers are currently commercially available for breast cancer, among them MammaPrint (Agendia, The Netherlands), Oncotype DX (Genomic Health, USA) and PAM50 (Nano String, USA). However, caution should be taken interpreting gene signatures, when sampling conditions are suboptimal (i.e. prolonged delay of sample preservation after surgery), since sample handling and preservation methods affect gene expression. This has been shown previously by snap freezing aliquots of breast tumor tissue at different time points after surgical removal in a few studies. De Cecco et al. (2009) investigated breast tumor tissue from 11 patients. For each patient 4 aliquots were analyzed, 1 was frozen immediately and the remaining left at room temperature for 2, 6 and 24 h respectively. No major effect on RNA integrity was observed. However, expression levels of 461 genes were significantly altered. Borgan et al. (2011) observed significantly altered expression of 1788 mRNAs and 56 miRNAs in a study with delayed freezing of 0.5,

* Correspondence: isp@rn.dk
†Inge Søkilde Pedersen and Mads Thomassen contributed equally to this work.
[1]Molecular Diagnostics, Clinical Biochemistry, Aalborg University, Aalborg, Denmark
[5]Clinical Cancer Research Center, Aalborg University Hospital, Aalborg, Denmark
Full list of author information is available at the end of the article

1, 2, 3 and 6 h when compared to the breast tumor tissue frozen immediately post surgery. Aktas et al. (2014) investigated the difference between preservation of breast tumor tissue in RNAlater and freezing on dry ice in prechilled vials, they found expression of 481 transcripts to be significantly altered. In addition, they observed an effect of delayed preservation on 41 transcripts. In a previous study on the same samples, comparing preservation methods, it was concluded that RNAlater improves RNA yield and quality (Hatzis et al., 2010). Recently the sparse literature on the effect of cold ischemia has been reviewed (Grizzle et al., 2016).

As pointed out by Grizzle et al., warm ischemia may be the more important variable, however this is not easily controlled and data on the effect of warm ischemia is rarely available (Grizzle et al., 2016) . To our knowledge no study has investigated the effect of surgical manipulation on gene expression profiles in breast tissue. In animal studies a difference between effect of ischemic stress at room temperature and body temperature has been shown (Almeida et al., 2004). In addition, a study investigating gene expression in histologically benign prostate tissue before and after surgery demonstrated substantial gene expression changes as a result of surgical manipulation with a median warm ischemia time of 28 min during surgery (Lin et al., 2006). Albeit, the effect is likely to be at least partly contributable to ischemia, other factors may also affect gene expression. The best studied example being anesthesia (Lucchinetti et al., 2007). Since environmental changes cause the cell to adjust its regulatory mechanisms which in turn alters the way it reacts to external input, tumor and normal cells are not only different per se, they could also be expected to react differently when exposed to stress such as surgical manipulation. The current study has been designed to investigate the effect of surgical manipulation in both normal breast tissue and breast tumor tissue by comparing gene expression profiles before and after surgery using a self-matched study design for increased statistical power.

## Materials and methods
### Patient material
Participants were 3 women with primary operable breast cancer. None of the participants had received anti-cancer treatment prior to surgery. Time between biopsy was approximately 1 h in the 3 cases. Clinical and pathological characteristics of the patients are summarized in Table 1. The study protocol was approved by the Research Ethics Committee of the North Denmark Region (N-20090029). All participants gave written informed consent.

### Tissue collection
Biopsies from normal and tumor tissue were taken in situ immediately after induction of anesthesia (by *intra-venous*

injection of fentanyl and propofol) prior to radical mastectomy. All tumors in this study were well defined and easily palpable. Biopsies from normal tissue were taken as far from the tumor as possible. After surgical excision 4 biopsies were taken ex vivo, 3 from normal (to test for variation among replicate samples) and 1 from tumor tissue. Origin (tumor or normal) of the biopsies was confirmed by macroscopic inspection. All biopsies were snap frozen in liquid nitrogen and subsequently kept at $-80$ °C until RNA extraction.

### RNA isolation and expression profiling
Total RNA was extracted using RNeasy Micro kit (Qiagen, Hilden, Germany) according to manufacturer's instructions. RNA concentration and purity was determined by UV spectrometry on a NanoDrop 2000 (Thermo Scientific, Waltham, Massachusetts, USA). Amplified RNA was synthesized from 300 ng total RNA using the MessageAmpTM III RNA amplification kit and fragmented according to manufacturer's instructions (Ambion, Austin, TX, USA). Fragmented amplified RNA was hybridized to Human Genome U133 Plus 2.0 GeneChip® (Affymetrix, Santa Clara, California, USA), washed and scanned as recommended by the manufacturer. Data are available from Gene Expression Omnibus (http://www.ncbi.nlm.nih.gov/geo; accession no. GSE71053).

### Data analysis and statistics
The affy package (www.bioconductor.org), implemented in the statistical programming language R version 3.1.1 was applied for initial data analysis. Robust multi-array average expression measure (rma) (Irizarry et al., 2003) was applied to perform background correction, quantile normalization, and expression index calculation of all microarrays. Only perfect match probes were used for data analysis.

Hierarchical clustering of genes was carried out using MultiExperiment Viewer (MeV; http://www.tm4.org) with Pearson correlation as distance metric and average linkage.

The experimental design is factorial with 3 putative effects on gene expression investigated simultaneously by GEE analysis. GEE was chosen because it allows analysis of interaction. The following analyses were performed. 1) Effect of ischemia during surgery on tumor tissue compared to normal (interaction). 2) Effect of surgical manipulation irrespective of tissue type/malignancy state (time). 3) Effect of malignancy state comparing tumor to normal tissue irrespective of whether samples had been collected pre or post surgery (tissue). A false discovery rate (FDR) of 0.01 was used for cut-off to identify differentially expressed genes. Subsequently, GSEA analysis was carried out to identify pathways differentially expressed in the same 3 comparisons using the GEE

**Table 1** Patient cilincal ad pathological charcteristics and details of sample collection

| Patient ID | Age at diagnosis, years | Histology at diagnosis | ER status | HER2 status | Pathological lymph node status | Tumor size, mm | Histological grade |
|---|---|---|---|---|---|---|---|
| 1 | 61 | IDC | N | P | N | 31 | 3 |
| 2 | 60 | IDC | P | N | P | 29 | 2 |
| 3 | 48 | IDC | P | P | N | 30 | 1 |

*IDC* Invasive Ductal Carcinoma, *N* negative, *P* positive

ranked data and the preranking option in GSEA. The GSEA method takes the entire rank of genes into account allowing identification of pathways not only represented among most differentially regulated genes, but also pathways supported by a larger number of moderately differentially expressed genes. The Reactome pathway collection from MSigDB was used for all GSEA analyses. For the ease of presentation of data a more stringent FDR cut-off of 0.005 was emploid for the GSEA analyses. Out of 674 gene sets, 486 passed a criterion of at least 15 genes represented in the data set.

In order to compare our results with a previous publication investigating the effect of cold ischemia on gene expression in tumor tissue, GSEA analysis was used to compare tumor tissue before and after surgical manipulation. Genes were in this analysis ranked according to differentially expression in tumor post-surgery compared to pre-surgery, using the statistical parameter $d$, derived from Significance Analysis of Microarray (SAM). Pathways with a FDR value below 0.0005 were considered significant.

## Results

Hierarchical clustering of pre surgery samples using all genes (Fig 1a) shows a combined effect of individual and tissue type, with no distinct clustering of tumor and normal. Post surgery there is a more pronounced effect of tissue origin with tumor samples clustering separately from normal samples (Fig 1b). The 3 biopsies taken from normal tissue post surgery cluster together for each patient, as expected for tissue of the same tissue type handled identically. In order to analyze the interaction of ischemia (pre/post-surgery) and tissue (tumor/normal) GEE was applied. This analysis of the interaction identified 3179 differentially expressed genes. Top 50 up- and down-regulated genes are listed in additional material (Additional file 1 and Additional file 2). Pathway analysis of interaction, including all genes ranked by GEE and performed with GSEA, revealed significant up-regulation of 29 pathways and down-regulation of 1 pathway (Fig 2). Among the pathways specifically upregulated in tumor as a consequence of surgical manipulation were several cell cycle related pathways. Enrichment plots and information on pathways significantly affected by interaction are provided as additional material (Additional file 3 and Additional file 4).

The analysis of ischemia, i.e. surgical manipulation, on tissue regardless of malignancy state identified 667 differentially expressed genes Top 50 up- and down-regulated genes are listed in additional material (Additional file 5 and Additional file 6). GSEA demonstrated 6 pathways upregulated after ischemia, including pathways involved in adipocyte differentiation, lipid mobilization, cell interactions and immune system pathways (Fig 3). Enrichment plots and information on pathways significantly affected by surgical manipulation are provided as additional material (Additional file 7 and Additional file 8).

The comparison of tumor tissue (pre- and post-surgery) and normal tissue (pre- and post-surgery) identified a total of 6166 differentially expressed genes. Top 50 up- and down-regulated genes are listed in additional material (Additional file 9 and Additional file 10). Pathway analysis demonstrated 22 pathways that were upregulated in tumor tissue compared to normal tissue (Fig 4). Among these pathways are pathways characteristic for invasive tumors such as extracellular matrix degradation, PDGF signaling and immune system pathways. Enrichment plots and information on pathways significantly affected by tissue type are provided as additional material (Additional file 11 and Additional file 12).

We next wanted to perform validation of our findings in external data sets. Since no data of warm ischemia are available, we used the data set from Aktas et al.'s study of cold eschemia in tumor tissue (Aktas et al., 2014). This provided a strong validation of observed effect in tumor tissue (Fig 5) with 30 of 36 pathways being affected in the same direction, and 1 of these pathways (REGULATION_OF_MITOTIC_CELL_CYCLE) had a nominal $p$-value of less than 0.05.

## Discussion

Our study reveals a remarkable effect of surgical manipulation, such as warm ischemia and anesthesia. It is not possible from the current study to deduce the specific contribution of these variables. In our hierarchical clustering analysis it is only for the post-surgery samples that tumor samples cluster separately from normal samples, indicating a differential effect of surgical manipulation on gene expression profiles in normal and tumor tissue. Indeed GSEA analysis identifies several pathways which are differentially affected by warm ischemia between tumor and normal tissue. This is in keeping with

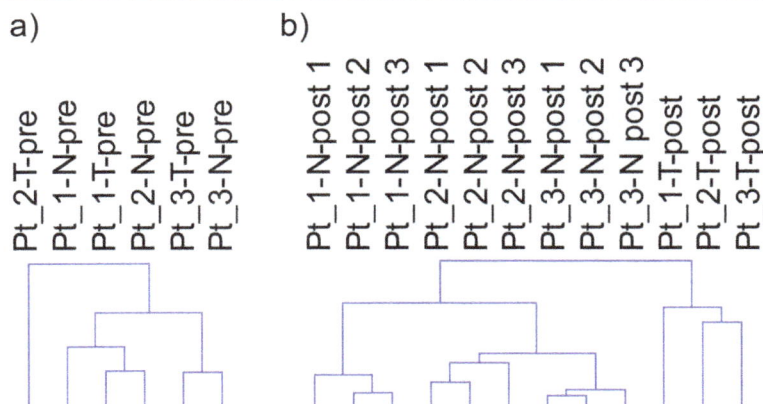

**Fig. 1** Hierarchical clustering dendrograms. Dendrograms based on hierarchical clustering of all genes on pre (**a**) and post (**b**) surgery samples. Patient samples are numbered Pt_1, Pt_2 and Pt_3, N for normal, T for tumor and pre/post for pre surgery and post-surgery respectively

observations of cell type specific response to environmental stress such as hypoxia (Chi et al., 2006) and a likely consequence of different pre-conditioning as a result of the different milieu of tumor cells compared to normal. Interestingly, immune system pathways are up-regulated both as a result of surgical manipulation and when comparing tumor and normal tissue. This is in agreement with what has already been documented in the literature. (Grigoryev et al., 2006; Bottai et al., 2017; Liu et al., 2017). However, immune system pathways are not significantly affected in the interaction analysis, indicating activation of a similar immune response in

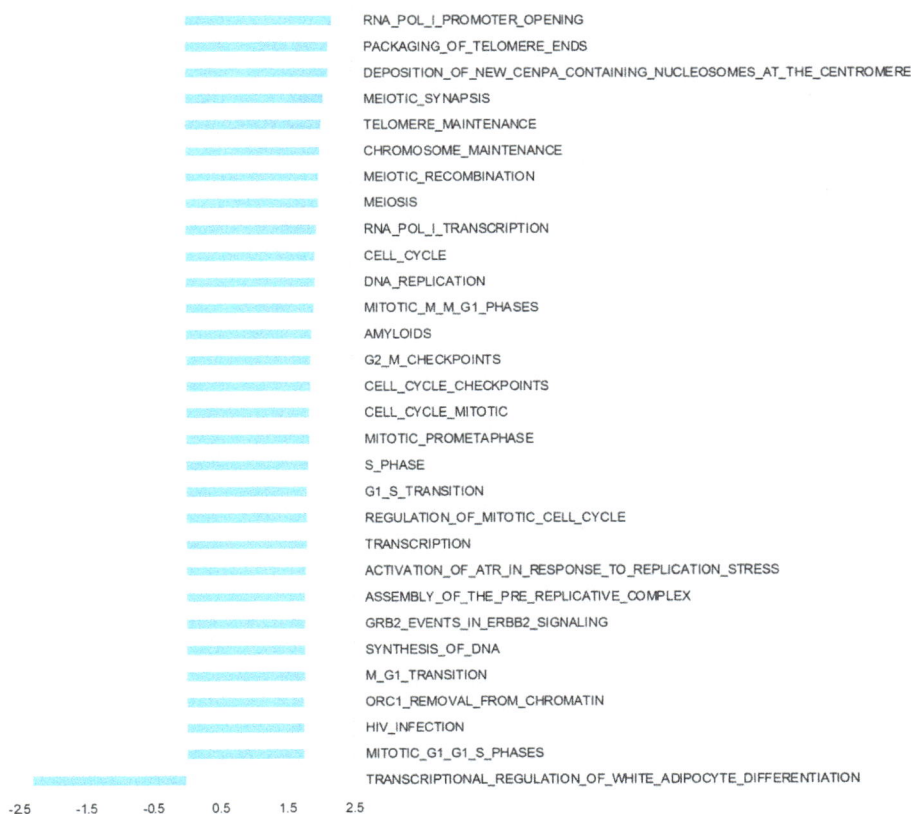

**Fig. 2** Pathway analysis of interaction. Pathway analysis was performed with GSEA using ranking of genes according to the interaction term from GEE. The Normalized Enrichment Scores (NES) is depicted for all Reactome pathways significantly altered in tumor tissue as a result of surgical manipulation compared to surgical manipulation of normal tissue

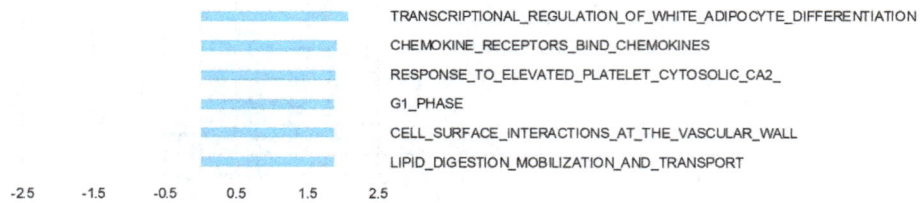

TRANSCRIPTIONAL_REGULATION_OF_WHITE_ADIPOCYTE_DIFFERENTIATION

CHEMOKINE_RECEPTORS_BIND_CHEMOKINES

RESPONSE_TO_ELEVATED_PLATELET_CYTOSOLIC_CA2_

G1_PHASE

CELL_SURFACE_INTERACTIONS_AT_THE_VASCULAR_WALL

LIPID_DIGESTION_MOBILIZATION_AND_TRANSPORT

-2.5    -1.5    -0.5    0.5    1.5    2.5

**Fig. 3** Pathway analysis of the effect of surgical manipulation (warm ischemia). Pathway analysis was performed with GSEA using ranking of genes according to the time term from GEE. NES depicted for all Reactome pathways significantly altered in samples collected post-surgery compared to samples collected pre-surgery irrespective of whether it was normal or tumor tissue

tumor and normal tissue as a consequence of surgical manipulation.

Pathways preferentially enriched in tumor compared to normal tissue as a result of surgical manipulation are pathways involved in cell cycling. Despite it being well documented for neurons to re-enter cell cycling in response to ischemia (Love, 2003), this is a somewhat counterintuitive response for actively replicating cells. However, when restricting analysis to the effect of surgical manipulation on tumor tissue, 1 of the cell-cycle related pathways up regulated in tumor tissue as a result of surgery was found to be significantly up regulated as a result of 40 min cold ischemia of breast tumor tissue post surgery in a previous study by Aktas et al. (Aktas et al., 2014). Furthermore, there is a significant correlation between direction of the effect of warm and cold ischemia, with 30 out of 36 pathways affected in the same direction in both studies, providing strong validation of the observed effect on cell cycle pathways of ischemia on tumor tissue. Differences between this study and

previous studies could be explained both by a differential effect of cold and warm ischemia and differences in baseline, since up regulation of different genes have been shown to peak at different time points after tissue resection (Spruessel et al., 2004). In previous studies baseline has been within minutes of surgery, effectively the endpoint of the current study. For the purpose of the current study it was of utmost importance to ensure immediate preservation of baseline samples. In other studies samples were pathologically evaluated before mincing into smaller fragments and dividing into aliquots for freezing at different time points (Aktas et al., 2014; Hatzis et al., 2010). This procedure minimizes intra-tumoral variation. However, it introduces a median delay prior to stabilization of 40 min, and hence would not be suitable in our set up. On the other hand, lack of control over tissue composition adds some degree of uncertainty to our results. It is also important to keep in mind that the three tumors in this study represent three different histopathological entities (Table 1). This could

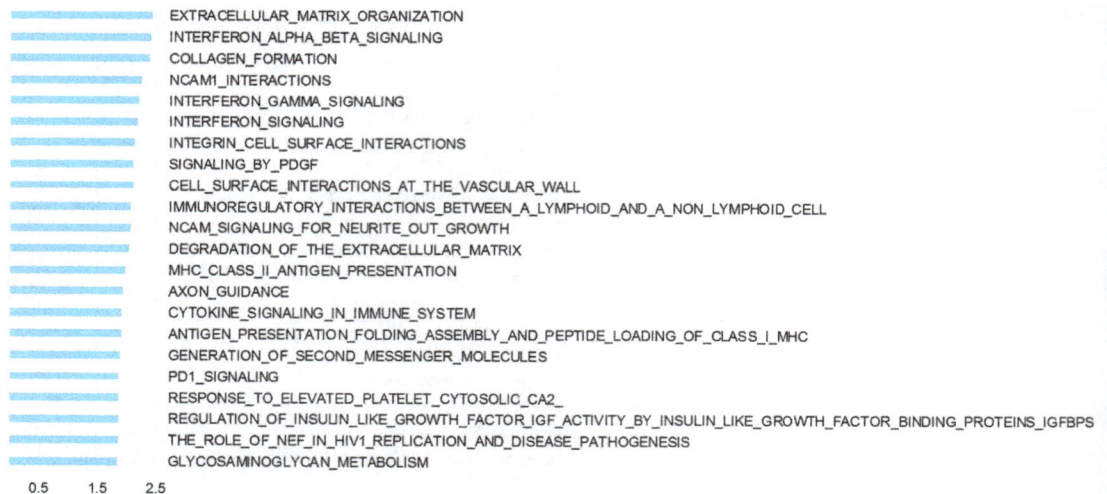

EXTRACELLULAR_MATRIX_ORGANIZATION
INTERFERON_ALPHA_BETA_SIGNALING
COLLAGEN_FORMATION
NCAM1_INTERACTIONS
INTERFERON_GAMMA_SIGNALING
INTERFERON_SIGNALING
INTEGRIN_CELL_SURFACE_INTERACTIONS
SIGNALING_BY_PDGF
CELL_SURFACE_INTERACTIONS_AT_THE_VASCULAR_WALL
IMMUNOREGULATORY_INTERACTIONS_BETWEEN_A_LYMPHOID_AND_A_NON_LYMPHOID_CELL
NCAM_SIGNALING_FOR_NEURITE_OUT_GROWTH
DEGRADATION_OF_THE_EXTRACELLULAR_MATRIX
MHC_CLASS_II_ANTIGEN_PRESENTATION
AXON_GUIDANCE
CYTOKINE_SIGNALING_IN_IMMUNE_SYSTEM
ANTIGEN_PRESENTATION_FOLDING_ASSEMBLY_AND_PEPTIDE_LOADING_OF_CLASS_I_MHC
GENERATION_OF_SECOND_MESSENGER_MOLECULES
PD1_SIGNALING
RESPONSE_TO_ELEVATED_PLATELET_CYTOSOLIC_CA2_
REGULATION_OF_INSULIN_LIKE_GROWTH_FACTOR_IGF_ACTIVITY_BY_INSULIN_LIKE_GROWTH_FACTOR_BINDING_PROTEINS_IGFBPS
THE_ROLE_OF_NEF_IN_HIV1_REPLICATION_AND_DISEASE_PATHOGENESIS
GLYCOSAMINOGLYCAN_METABOLISM

-2.5    -1.5    -0.5    0.5    1.5    2.5

**Fig. 4** Pathway analysis of the effect of tissue type. Pathway analysis was performed with GSEA using ranking of genes according to the tissue term from GEE. NES depicted for all Reactome pathways significantly altered in tumor samples compared to normal samples irrespective of whether samples were collected pre- or post-surgery

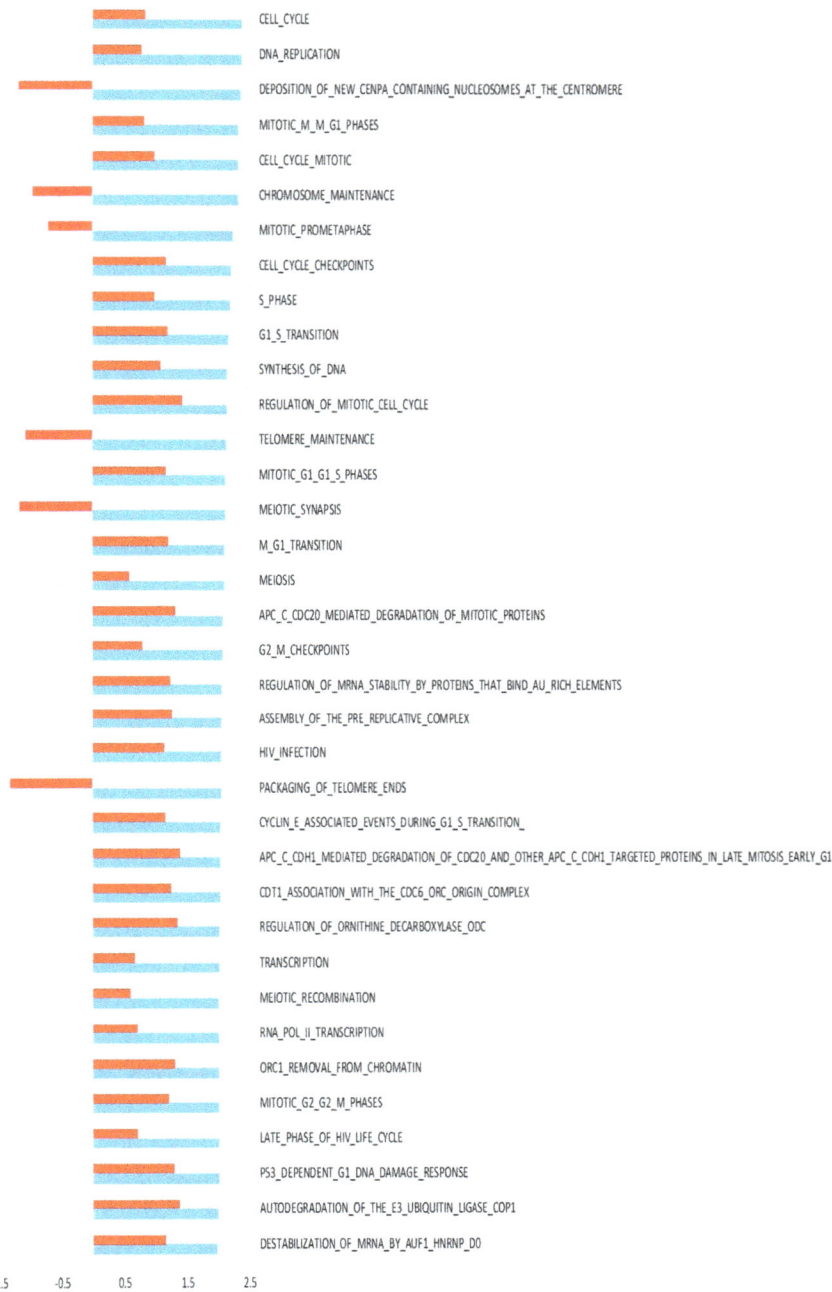

**Fig. 5** Comparison of GSEA on effect of warm and cold ischemia on tumor tissue. NES depicted in blue for all Reactome pathways significantly altered in tumor tissue collected post-surgery compared to pre-surgery (warm ischemia). To illustrate concordance with previously published data by Aktas et al. (2014) NES from tumor tissue subjected to 40 min cold ischemia post surgery are represented by red bars. One pathway had a nominal *p*-value < 0.05 in the dataset from Aktas: REGULATION_OF_MITOTIC_CELL_CYCLE

potentially affect the analysis and may explain the lack of clustering of tumor samples pre-surgery. Interestingly, our results suggest a distinct response of this heterogeneous group to surgical manipulation.

In order to elucidate differences in gene expression between tumor and normal tissue in addition to what is evident from hierarchical clustering, GSEA was carried out and 22 pathways displayed differential representation. This shows a difference between normal and tumor samples when it comes to pathways involved in organization and degradation of extracellular matrix and interferon signaling.

Speculatively, it may not be surprising that the differences between normal and tumor tissue in vivo are less pronounced than the differences after being subjected to ischemic stress. After all, the cells have to carry out more or less the same functions in order to survive. Pronounced difference in reaction to changes in external environment could putatively be what constitutes the main difference between normal cells and tumor cells. Activation of cell cycling genes during stress could be an acquired response of a cancer cell no longer reacting as expected to environmental signals. Similar to what is seen in cell cultures where normal cells stop growing when reaching confluence whereas tumor cells keep dividing.

Reported differential expression of pathways between tumor and normal tissue almost exclusively refers to post surgery samples. This has been proven to work well for several multigene classifiers. Our results open the possibility that differences observed in post-surgical specimens not necessarily mirrors differences present in vivo, and whereas difference in response to stress may be an equally good measurement for classifying tumors into subgroups, it requires standardized control over sampling conditions and information about surgical procedures. Furthermore, when it comes to investigating biological differences of tumor and normal cells and considering possible therapeutical targets, caution should be taken deducing in vivo differences based on gene expression profiles from tissue sampled after surgery.

## Conclusions

The current study is to our knowledge the first study to simultaneously investigate the effect of surgical manipulation, malignancy state and the interaction of these two parameters on gene expression profiling in breast tissue. The self-matched design gives added statistical power compared to a case-control design, and even with a limited number of samples we are able demonstrate an effect on a large number of pathways and a differential response between tumor and normal tissue. The majority of pathways affected primarily in tumor tissue are pathways that have previously been implicated in oncogenesis. It is of great interest that the well documented up regulation of gene sets involved in cell cycling may in fact primarily reflect altered reaction to surgical manipulation/ischemic stress of tumor cells compared to normal cells rather than reflecting the state of cells in the body.

## Additional files

**Additional file 1:** Top 50 up-regulated genes (interaction). The top 50 genes up-regulated in the GEE interaction analysis. (PDF 30 kb)

**Additional file 2:** Top 50 down-regulated genes (interaction). The top 50 genes down-regulated in the GEE interaction analysis. (PDF 31 kb)

**Additional file 3:** GSEA enrichment plots – interaction. GSEA enrichment plots of pathways significantly affected by interaction. (TIF 3730 kb)

**Additional file 4:** Significantly affected pathways – interaction. Information on rank and enrichment scores of significantly affected pathways in the GSEA analysis on interaction. (PDF 27 kb)

**Additional file 5:** Top 50 up-regulated genes (surgical manipulation). The top 50 genes up-regulated in the GEE surgical manipulation analysis. (PDF 31 kb)

**Additional file 6:** Top 50 down-regulated genes (surgical manipulation). The top 50 genes down-regulated in the GEE surgical manipulation analysis. (PDF 30 kb)

**Additional file 7:** GSEA enrichment plots – surgical manipulation. GSEA enrichment plots of pathways significantly affected by surgical manipulation. (TIF 1173 kb)

**Additional file 8:** Significantly affected pathways - surgical manipulation. Information on rank and enrichment scores of significantly affected pathways in the GSEA analysis on surgical manipulation. (PDF 9 kb)

**Additional file 9:** Top 50 up-regulated genes (tissue type). The top 50 genes up-regulated in the GEE tissue type analysis. (PDF 35 kb)

**Additional file 10:** Top 50 down-regulated genes (tissue type). The top 50 genes down-regulated in the GEE tissue type analysis. (PDF 35 kb)

**Additional file 11:** GSEA enrichment plots – tissue type. GSEA enrichment plots of pathways significantly affected by tissue type. (TIF 3588 kb)

**Additional file 12:** Significantly affected pathways - tissue type. Information on rank and enrichment scores of significantly affected pathways in the GSEA analysis on tissue type. (PDF 21 kb)

## Abbreviations
FDR: False Discovery Rate; GEE: Generalized Estimating Equation; GSEA: Gene Set Enrichment Analysis; MeV: MultiExperiment Viewer; rma: Robust multi-array average expression measure; SAM: Significance Analysis of Microarray

## Acknowledgements
We thank technician Anne Bentzen-Petersen for her assistance in collecting the samples and Bettina Andersen for help with the figures.

## Funding
This work was supported by "Det Obelske Familiefond" [grant number 29190941].

## Authors' contributions
ISP and HBK conceived of the study, designed and coordinated it. ISP drafted the manuscript. MT and QT carried out data analysis and contributed in drafting of the manuscript. TK were involved in data interpretation and revised the manuscript. OTU and JPG were involved in study design and revised the manuscript. JPG collected samples. All authors read and approved the manuscript.

## Competing interests
The authors declare they have no competing interests as defined by Molecular Medicine or other interests that may be perceived to influence the results and discussion reported in this paper.

## Author details
[1]Molecular Diagnostics, Clinical Biochemistry, Aalborg University, Aalborg, Denmark. [2]Department of Clinical Genetics, Odense University Hospital, Odense, Denmark. [3]Department of Gastrointestinal Surgery, Aalborg University Hospital, Aalborg, Denmark. [4]Department of Breast Surgery,

Aalborg University Hospital, Aalborg, Denmark. [5]Clinical Cancer Research
Center, Aalborg University Hospital, Aalborg, Denmark. [6]Department of Clinical
Medicine, Aalborg University, Aalborg, Denmark.

## References

Aktas B, et al. Global gene expression changes induced by prolonged cold
  ischemic stress and preservation method of breast cancer tissue. Mol Oncol.
  2014;8(3):717–27.

Almeida A, Paul Thiery J, Magdelénat H, Radvanyi F. Gene expression analysis by
  real-time reverse transcription polymerase chain reaction: influence of tissue
  handling. Anal Biochem. 2004;328(2):101–8.

Borgan E, et al. Ischemia caused by time to freezing induces systematic microRNA
  and mRNA responses in cancer tissue. Mol Oncol. 2011;5(6):564–76.

Bottai G, et al. Integrated MicroRNA–mRNA profiling identifies Oncostatin M as a
  marker of mesenchymal-like ER-negative/HER2-negative breast Cancer. Int J
  Mol Sci. 2017;18(1):194.

Chi J-T, et al. Gene expression programs in response to hypoxia: cell type
  specificity and prognostic significance in human cancers. PLoS Med. 2006;
  3(3):e47.

De Cecco L, et al. Impact of biospecimens handling on biomarker research in
  breast cancer. BMC Cancer. 2009;9:409.

Grigoryev DN, Liu M, Cheadle C, Barnes KC, Rabb H. Genomic profiling of kidney
  ischemia-reperfusion reveals expression of specific Alloimmunity-associated
  genes: linking "immune" and "nonimmune" injury events. Transplant Proc.
  2006;38(10):3333–6.

Grizzle WE, Otali D, Sexton KC, Atherton DS. Effects of cold ischemia on gene
  expression: a review and commentary. Biopreserv Biobank. 2016;14(6):548–58.

Hatzis C, et al. Effects of tissue handling on rna integrity and microarray
  measurements from resected breast cancers. J Natl Cancer Inst. 2010;103(24):
  1871–83.

Irizarry RA, et al. Exploration, normalization, and summaries of high density
  oligonucleotide array probe level data. Biostatistics. 2003;4(2):249–64.

Lin DW, et al. Influence of surgical manipulation on prostate gene expression:
  implications for molecular correlates of treatment effects and disease
  prognosis. J Clin Oncol. 2006;24(23):3763–70.

Liu JC, Zacksenhouse M, Eisen A, Nofech-Mozes S, Zacksenhaus E. Identification
  of cell proliferation, immune response and cell migration as critical pathways
  in a prognostic signature for HER2+;ERα- breast cancer. PLoS One. 2017;12(6):
  e0179223.

Love S. Apoptosis and brain ischaemia. Prog Neuro-Psychopharmacol Biol
  Psychiatry. 2003;27(2):267–82.

Lucchinetti E, et al. Gene regulatory control of myocardial energy metabolism
  predicts postoperative cardiac function in patients undergoing off-pump
  coronary artery bypass graft surgery: inhalational versus intravenous
  anesthetics. Anesthesiology. 2007;106(3):444–57.

Spruessel A, et al. Tissue ischemia time affects gene and protein expression
  patterns within minutes following surgical tumor excision. Biotechniques.
  2004;36(6):1030–7.

# 19

# Protective role of down-regulated microRNA-31 on intestinal barrier dysfunction through inhibition of NF-κB/HIF-1α pathway by binding to HMOX1 in rats with sepsis

Cheng-Ye Zhan, Di Chen[*], Jin-Long Luo, Ying-Hua Shi and You-Ping Zhang

## Abstract

**Background:** Intestinal barrier dysfunction is a significant clinical problem, commonly developing in a variety of acute or chronic pathological conditions. Herein, we evaluate the effect of microRNA-31 (miR-31) on intestinal barrier dysfunction through NF-κB/HIF-1α pathway by targeting HMOX1 in rats with sepsis.

**Methods:** Male Sprague-Dawley rats were collected and divided into the sham group, and the cecum ligation and perforation group which was subdivided after CACO-2 cell transfection of different mimic, inhibitor, or siRNA. Levels of serum D-lactic acid, diamine oxidase and fluorescence isothiocyanate dextran, FITC-DX concentration, and bacterial translocation were detected. Superoxidedismutase (SOD) activity and malondialdehyde (MDA) content were evaluated using the colorimetric method and an automatic microplate reader, respectively. Additionally, the levels of tumor necrosis factor, interleukin (IL)-6, and IL-10 were tested using enzyme-linked immunosorbent assay. The expression of miR-31, HMOX1, NF-κB, HIF-1α, IκB, ZO-1 and Occludin were assessed by reverse transcription quantitative polymerase chain reaction and Western blot analysis.

**Results:** Inhibition of miR-31 decreased intestinal mucosal permeability and intestinal barrier function. The increased levels of miR-31 could cause oxidative damage and affect the expression of inflammatory factors in intestinal tissue of rats. HMOX1 was confirmed as a target gene of miR-31. MiR-31 affected intestinal mucosal permeability and intestinal barrier function, as well as oxidative damage and inflammation level by regulating HMOX1. Down-regulation of miR-31 inhibited NF-κB/HIF-1α pathway related genes by regulating HMOX1 expression. Furthermore, inhibition of miR-31 increased survival rates of rats.

**Conclusion:** Overall, the current study found that inhibition of miR-31 protects against intestinal barrier dysfunction through suppression of the NF-κB/HIF-1α pathway by targeting HMOX1 in rats with sepsis.

**Keywords:** microRNA-31, Sepsis, HMOX1, NF-κB/HIF-1α pathway, Intestinal barrier dysfunction

* Correspondence: cdchendi2018@126.com
Intensive Care Unit, Tongji Hospital Affiliated to Tongji Medical College of Huazhong University of Science and Technology, No. 1095, Jiefang Road, Qiaokou District, Wuhan 430030, Hubei Province, People's Republic of China

## Background

Sepsis, a life-threatening clinical syndrome, is characterized by the presence of both infection and a systemic inflammatory response (Tiruvoipati et al. 2010). The common clinical manifestations of sepsis are correlated with systemic inflammatory response syndrome and organ dysfunction, including hemodynamic instability, hypoxemia, and intestinal barrier dysfunction (Melvan et al. 2010). In addition, the intestine contains endogenous and exogenous microorganisms which have been reported to be the potential pathogens of sepsis, and it can also be susceptible to ischaemia-reperfusion injuries because of sepsis (Jiang et al. 2013). Moreover, intestinal barrier dysfunction can result in secondary bacterial translocation and various clinical syndromes of multiple organ dysfunctions in sepsis (Fredenburgh et al. 2011). Previous studies have demonstrated that anti-inflammatory genes targeting intestinal barrier dysfunction and relevant pathogenic factors can decrease bacterial translocation and unfavourable inflammatory responses, which thereby can increase survival rate in sepsis (Jiang et al. 2013). Importantly, microRNA (miRNA) dysregulation was reported to be correlated with clinical manifestations and inflammation, which thereby could serve as a potential therapeutic target against sepsis (Zhou et al. 2015).

MiRNAs are small noncoding RNAs, post-transcriptionally inhibiting target gene expression by base paring to their 3'untranslated region (3'UTR) (Bartel 2009). They are involved in gene regulatory networks managing almost all cellular functions, and are essential in some diseases like inflammation as well as cancer (Montano 2011; O'Connell et al. 2012; Schetter et al. 2010). Recently, miR-31 was confirmed to be a regulator of hypoxia-inducible factor (HIF)-1$\alpha$ and nuclear factor-kappa B (NF-$\kappa$B) which was closely correlated key transcription factor families (Creighton et al. 2010; Valastyan et al. 2009). MiR-31 stimulates the HIF pathway by targeting factor-inhibiting HIF-1$\alpha$ (FIH) in human head and neck carcinoma (Liu et al. 2010), and inhibits the noncanonical NF-$\kappa$B pathway in adult T cell leukemia by suppressing NF-$\kappa$B–inducing kinase (NIK) (Yamagishi et al. 2012). Heme oxygenase (HMOX) 1 is essential in the defense of the body against oxidant-induced injury during inflammatory processes, in which elevated plasma concentrations of HMOX1 have been observed in septic patients and experimental models of sepsis syndrome (Takaki et al. 2010). As a cytoprotective enzyme, HMOX1 has anti-inflammatory, antioxidant, anti-apoptotic, and antiproliferative effects (Hou et al. 2010). HMOX1 can be induced by oxidative stress-promoting agents such as heme, hyperoxia, hypoxia, heat shock, endotoxins, hydrogen peroxide, heavy metals, and nitric oxide (Vazquez-Armenta et al., 2013). A recent study has shown that lower expression of miR-31 in CD4+ T Cells contributed to immunosuppression in human sepsis by promoting TH2 skewing (van der Heide et al. 2016). From all above, it can be hypothesized that the miR-31, HMOX1, and the HIF-1$\alpha$/NF-$\kappa$B pathway exert certain effects on sepsis. Thereby, the current study aims to investigate the effect of miR-31 on intestinal barrier dysfunction through the NF-$\kappa$B/HIF-1$\alpha$ pathway by targeting HMOX1 in sepsis.

## Methods

### Ethical statement

All experimental procedures and the use of animals were approved by the Ethics committee on animal experiments of Tongji Hospital Affiliated to Tongji Medical College of Huazhong University of Science and Technology. All efforts were made to minimize the suffering of the included animals.

### Cell culture

CACO-2 cells (Shanghai Suer Biotechnology Co. Ltd., Shanghai, China) were incubated in Dulbecco's modified eagle medium (DMEM) high sugar medium (Life Technologies Corporation, California, USA) (containing 10% fetal bovine serum, 1% non-essential amino acids (NEAA), 2.5 mg/mL plasmocin), and cultured in a humidified incubator at 37 °C with 5% $CO_2$ in air. The medium was replaced every two days. When cell confluency reached 80%, the cells were treated with 0.25% trypsin (Gibco Company, Gaitherburg, MD, USA) and were further subcultured for three generations.

### Dual-luciferase reporter assay

The biology prediction website, *microRNA.org* was used to predict the possible target gene of miR-31 and to obtain the sequence fragments containing the site of action. The DNA content was extracted from human colorectal adenocarcinoma cells (CACO-2 cells) according to the instructions of the PureLink® Genomic DNA Mini Kit (Item No. K182001, Thermo Fisher Scientific, Massachusetts, USA), and the HMOX1 3'UTR wild-type sequence (HMOX1–3'-UTR-wt), and the mutant sequence of HMOX1–3'-UTR (HMOX1–3'-UTR-mut) with a deleted miR-31 binding site were designed. Next, a luciferase reporter plasmid vector was constructed, and the miR-31 mimic was transfected into CACO-2 cells (Shanghai Suer Biotechnology Co., Ltd., Shanghai, China). The sample luciferase activity was detected using a dual-luciferase reporter gene assay reagent. After transfection for 48 h, the medium was removed, and the sample was rinsed twice with phosphate buffer saline (PBS). The cells were treated with passive lysis buffer (PLB) (100 μL/well), shaken slightly for 15 min at room temperature, and then the cell lysate was collected. The program was pre-read for 2 s and the value was read for 10 s. The luciferase assay reagent II (LARII) and Stop & Glo® Reagent (Promega Corporation, Madison, WI, USA) (100 μL/sample intake) were prepared, and added to the luminous tube or plate of the cell lysate

(20 μL/sample), and then tested using a bioluminescent detector (Modulus™, Sunnyvale, CA, USA).

## Cell transfection

The 3rd generation of CACO-2 cells were transfected with the miR-31 mimic, the miR-31 inhibitor and the negative control (50 nM of final concentration) in accordance with the instructions of lipofectamine 2000 (Shanghai Heng Fei Biotechnology Co., Ltd., Shanghai, China). After being cultured for 24 ~ 48 h, the expression of HMOX1 gene was detected using reverse transcription quantitative polymerase chain reaction (RT-qPCR) and Western blot analysis. The transfection sequences were synthesized by Shanghai GenePharma Co., Ltd. (Shanghai, China). Primer sequences are shown in Table 1.

## Experiment animals and cecum ligation and perforation (CLP) model establishment

Male Sprague-Dawley (SD) rats (weight: 250 ~ 350 g) were provided by the Department of Laboratory Animal Science of Tongji Hospital Affiliated to Tongji Medical College of Huazhong University of Science and Technology. The laboratory animals were fed for more than 3 days for acclimatization, and fasted for 6 h prior to the experiment with free access to water. The CLP model of sepsis was established as follows. A median incision (2 cm) was made in the middle of the abdomen to open the abdominal cavity. The No. 1 silk thread was used for cecal ligation 0.5 cm under the ileocecal valve in the cecum and proximal colon, and then the No.8 syringe needle was perforated through the edge of the mesenterium in the cecum. No. 1 silk thread was left for preventing pinhole from closing. The sham group was underwent dissociation, without ligation and perforation. After concluding the surgery, Ringer's solution (50 mL/kg) was subcutaneously injected to supplement the loss of intraoperative fluid. Rats in each group were gave free access to food. Positive intestinal microflora was detected in blood about 6 h after the CLP surgery and clinical signs of the sepsis emerged, which suggested modeling success (Rittirsch et al. 2009).

## Animal grouping

The rats were divided into the following 7 groups ($n = 25$): sham group (sham group, 1 ml normal saline was injected intravenously 24 h before the surgery), sepsis group (CLP model rats, 1 ml normal saline was injected intravenously 24 h before the surgery), negative control (NC) group (CLP model rats, 10 μg NC sequence was injected intravenously 24 h before the surgery), miR-31 mimic group (CLP model rats, 10 μg miR-31 mimic was injected intravenously 24 h before the surgery), miR-31 inhibitor group (CLP model rats, 10 μg miR-31 inhibitor was injected intravenously 24 h before the surgery), siRNA-HMOX1 group (CLP model rats, 10 μg siRNA-HOMX1 was injected intravenously 24 h before the surgery), and miR-31 inhibitor + siRNA-HMOX1 group (CLP model rats, 10 μg miR-31 mimic and 10 μg sRNA-HOMX1 were injected intravenously 24 h before the surgery). All siRNA, mimic, and inhibitor were processed by the in vivo RNA reagent (Engreen, 18,668–11-2, Engreen Biosystem Co. Ltd., Beijing, China). The operation was carried out in accordance with the instructions. A total of 15 rats in each group were randomly selected in order to observe the physiological activities and the survival rate at 72 h, and the remaining rats in each group (10 rats for each group) were used for other experiments (Zhao et al. 2016).

## Specimen collection

Twenty-four hours after the surgery, 5 rats were randomly selected from each group, and were anesthetized with 1% pentobarbital injections (0.2 mL/100 g) into the abdominal cavity. The abdominal cavity was incised opened and the abdominal aorta was separated. After separation, blood samples were collected using blood collection needles. The blood was centrifuged at 1812×g for 15 min, and the supernatant was collected to detect

**Table 1** RT-qPCR primer sequences

| mRNA | Forward primers (5'-3') | Reverse primers (5'-3') |
|---|---|---|
| miR-31 | CAGCTATGCCAGCATCTTGCCT | ATATGGAACGCTTCACGAATT |
| NF-κB | GGGCATGGGAATTTCCAACTC | GCAGAAGTAACTTTCCGAGAGG |
| IκB | TTGCTGAGGCACTTCTGAAAG | TCTGCGTCAAGACTGCTACAC |
| HIF-1α | GTCGGACAGCCTCACCAAACAG | TAGGTAGTGAGCCACCAGTGTCC |
| HMOX-1 | CTCAAACCTCCAAAAGCC | TCAAAAACCACCCCAACCC |
| ZO-1 | CCATTCTTTGGACCGATTGCTG | TAATGCCCGAGCTCCGATG |
| Occludin | ACGGTGCCATAGAATGAGATGTTG | CAGCTAGTTGTTCATTTCTGCACCA |
| GADPH | TTCACCACCATGGAGAAGGC | GGCATGGACTGTGGTCATGA |
| U6 | CTCGCTTCGGCAGCACA | AACGCTTCACGAATTTGCGT |

Note: *RT-qPCR* Reverse transcription quantitative polymerase chain reaction, *miR-31* microRNA-31, *NF-κB* nuclear factor-kappa B, *IκB* inhibitor of NF-κB, *HIF-1α* hypoxia inducible factor-1α, *HMOX-1* heme oxygenase 1, *ZO-1* zonula occludens-1, *GADPH* glyceraldehyde-3-phosphate dehydrogenase

serum indexes. Next, the intestinal tissues were incised under aseptic conditions to detect the levels of inflammatory factors and to observe the histological changes. The liver, spleen, mesenteric lymph nodes and ileal tissue of the rats were removed quickly under aseptic condition. Western blot analysis and RT-qPCR were employed in order to test the expression of related genes and proteins.

### Detection of intestinal mucosal permeability function

The serum D-lactic acid levels of rats were tested by coupled liquid chromatography and UV-visible spectrophotometry. The D-lactic acid was oxidized specifically using D-Lactate dehydrogenase, and then the colored oxidation product was produced, which was detected by automatic microplate reader at excitation wavelength of 450 nm. All specific experimental steps were carried out in accordance with the instructions. The absorbance was measured at 450 nm using a microplate reader (Bio-Rad 550, Hercules, CA, USA). A standard curve was plotted, and the levels of D-lactic acid were evaluated. The experiment was conducted three times to obtain the mean values.

The levels of Diamine oxidase (DAO) were tested using enzyme-linked immunosorbent assay (ELISA). All specific experimental steps were conducted according to the instructions. The absorbance was measured at excitation wavelength of 450 nm using a microplate reader (Bio-Rad 550, Hercules, CA, USA). A standard curve was plotted, and the levels of DAO were evaluated. The experiment was conducted three times to obtain the mean value.

Rats from each group were treated with gavage administration of 750 mg/kg FD-40 18 h after the surgery. After gavage administration for 6 h, venous blood samples were collected from the mesentery of rats with the serum separated. The absorbance was measured by a fluorescence spectrophotometer (Beckman, Palo Alto, CA, USA) at excitation wavelength of 490 nm and emission wavelength of 520 nm. A standard curve was plotted, and the levels of FD-40 of the venous blood in mesentery were evaluated. The experiment was conducted three times to obtain the mean value.

### Detection of intestinal barrier function

A total of 5 rats were randomly selected in each group 20 h after modeling, and were treated with gavage administration of 0.6 mg/g FITC-DX (Item No. DX500-BNFC-1, DMD BioMed Ltd., Suzhou, Jiangsu, China) under conditions void of light. Four hours later, the rats were anesthetized and 1 mL blood samples were collected by heart puncture. The obtained blood was centrifuged at 201×g for 10 min at 4 °C, and the supernatant was collected and tested using a fluorescence spectrophotometer (F-7000, Yi De science instrument Co., Ltd., Guangdong, Guangzhou, China) at an excitation wavelength of 490 nm and emission

wavelength of 520 nm. A standard curve was plotted, and the levels of FITC-DX were evaluated. The experiment was conducted three times to obtain the mean value.

The liver, spleen, mesenteric lymph nodes of the rats were placed in a sterile homogenizer, and sterile 0.85% sodium chloride solution was added at a 1: 10 ratio to make tissue homogenates. The tissue homogenates (0.1 mL) were collected, and 15 mL blood agar medium at 55 °C were added into a sterile plate, all of which were incubated at 37 °C for 24 h. Then, the organs with bacteria cultured were counted as the positive organs. Next, the rates of bacterial translocation (number of positive organs/total number of cultured organs) were counted. The experiment was conducted three times to obtain the mean value.

### Malondiadehyde (MDA) content and superoxide dismutase (SOD) activity

Intestinal tissues obtained from the sham group or 24 h after CLP were added with 1 mol/L HCI solutions, ground into tissue homogenates, and centrifuged at 1812×g for 10 min to collect the supernatant. In accordance with the instructions of the employed SOD test kit (HL70042, Shanghai haling biotechnology Co., Ltd., Shanghai, China) and MDA test kit (HLTO1013, Shanghai haling biotechnology Co., Ltd., Shanghai, China), the SOD activity and MDA content were evaluated using the colorimetric method by an automatic microplate reader (Beckman Coulter, Fullerton, CA, USA). The cells in each group were collected, and centrifuged after ultrasonic cell disruption. The supernatant (100 μL) was obtained to test the optical density (OD) value using an automatic microplate reader in accordance with the instructions of the SOD and MDA test kit, and the vitalities were calculated. The experiment was conducted three times to obtain the mean value.

### Detection of inflammatory factors

The intestinal tissues obtained from the sham group or 24 h after CLP were treated with a homogenizer. The supernatant was separated after centrifugation at 20128×g for 15 min at 4 °C. The levels of tumor necrosis factor (TNF-α), interleukin (IL)-6, and IL-10 were tested using an ELISA test kit (TWp022566, TWp028583, TWp028605, Shanghai Tong Wei Biological Technology Co., Ltd., Shanghai, China). The operations were carried out in strict accordance with the kit instructions. The test kit was maintained at room temperature for 20 min, and the detergents were prepared. A total of 10 standard wells (including 2 blank control wells, no samples and enzyme labeling reagents) were set on the enzyme-labeled plate, and the standard curve was plotted after standard dilution. The samples were diluted, and then placed into the sample wells of the enzyme-labeled plate. The plates were shaken gently after the addition of samples, and then sealed for incubation for 30 min at 37 °C. The liquid in the wells were removed, detergents were added and removed after 30 s. The process was repeated 5 times, and then the samples were dried. The enzyme labeling reagents (50 μL) was added and incubated for 30 min at 37 °C. Then the liquid in the wells were removed, the detergents were added and removed after 30 s. The process was repeated for 5 times and then the sample was dried. Next, Chromogenic agent A (50 μL) was added to each well, then Chromogenic agent B (50 μL). After gentle mixing, the samples were incubated at 37 °C for 15 min, and 50 μL stop buffer was added. The OD value per well was measured respectively at an excitation wavelength of 450 nm using a microplate reader (Bio-Rad, Hercules, CA, USA) within 10 min with the blank well serving as the control. The concentration standard curve was plotted, and the sample concentration was recorded according to the standard curve. The experiment was conducted three times to obtain the mean value.

## Hematoxylin and eosin (HE) staining

The middle parts of intestinal tissues of rats from each group were fixed with 4% formaldehyde for 6 h, and embedded in paraffin wax. The paraffin-embedded tissues were sliced into 3 μm sections. After being baked at 60 °C, the sections were dewaxed in xylene I and xylene II, for 20 min each time. After that, the sections were placed in 100%, 95%, 80%, 70% ethanol respectively for 5 min and then rinsed with distilled water for 3 min. Next, the samples were stained with hematoxylin for 10 min, washed under tap water for about 15 min, and then stained with eosin for 30 s. The double distilled water was used for washing until red coloration was all washed away. Then the sections were dehydrated in alcohol, cleaned with xylene and sealed with neutral gum. A light microscope was employed for histopathological examination and photographing, and them the tissue coloration and the staining intensity were observed. The pathological damage of rats was scored according to the standard of Chiu's intestinal injury (Chiu et al. 1970). The experiment was repeated three times to obtain the mean value.

## RT-qPCR

Rats in each group were sacrificed by cervical dislocation, and a section of the ileal tissues was extracted. After analyzing the quality, the RNA content of the sample was extracted using Trizol in accordance with the Trizol instructions (Item: 15596–018, Invitrogen, Carlsbad, CA, USA). The RNA content was dissolved in ultra-pure water treated with diethylpyrocarbonate (DEPC) (A100174–0005, Shanghai Sangon Biotech Co., Ltd., Shanghai, China), and absorbance at 260 nm and 280 nm were measured using an ND-1000 UV/Vis spectrophotometer (Thermo Scientific, Massachusetts, CA, USA) in order to evaluate the quality of the total RNA. Reverse transcription of the extracted RNA

was completed with a two-step method according to the kit instructions (Thermo Scientific, Massachusetts, CA, USA). The reaction conditions were as follows: 10 min at 70 °C, 2 min in ice bath and then 60 min at 42 °C, and finally 10 min at 70 °C. The cDNA obtained from the reverse transcription was temporarily stored in a refrigerator at − 80 °C. The TaqMan probe method was used in RT-qPCR, and the reaction system was operated according to the kit instructions (MBI Fermentas, Vilnius, Lithuania). The primer sequences are shown in Table 1, and the reaction conditions were as follows: pre-denaturation at 95 °C for 30 s, denaturation at 95 °C for 10 s, annealing at 60 °C for 20 s and extension at 70 °C for 10 s, for a total of 40 cycles. The reaction system was as follows: 12.5 μL Premix Ex Taq or SYBR Green Mix, 1 μL Forward Primer, 1 μL Reverse Primer, 1– 4 μL DNA template, and added with $ddH_2O$ for a total of 25 μL reaction system. A real-time fluorescence quantitative PCR (Bio-Rad, Model Bio-Rad iQ5, Hercules, CA, USA) instrument was for testing. Glyceraldehyde-3-phosphate dehydrogenase (GAPDH) was regarded as the internal reference for the genes. The $2^{-\Delta\Delta Ct}$ method represents the ratio of the expression of the target gene in the experiment group and the control group. The formula was as follows: $\Delta\Delta CT = \Delta Ct_{\text{experiment group}} - \Delta Ct_{\text{control group}}$, $\Delta Ct = Ct_{\text{target gene}} - Ct_{\text{GADPH}}$. The experiment was repeated three times to obtain the mean value.

## Western blot analysis

Rats in each group were sacrificed by cervical dislocation, and a section of the ileal tissues were selected and weighed, and then added with 200 μL pre-cooled radio-immunoprecipitation assay (RIPA) lysate (R0020, Beijing Solarbio Life Sciences Co., Ltd., Beijing, China) (containing 1 mmol/L phenylmethylsulfonyl fluoride) The samples were gently shaken to make the cell lysate and the cells in full contact, with the transfer liquid gun treated a few times, and then cracked on ice for 30 min. The protein lysate was placed into a new centrifuge tube, and centrifuged at 289845×g for 5 min at 4 °C with the upper protein extracted. The protein concentration was tested using a bicinchoninic acid (BCA) protein assay kit (AR0146, Boster Biological Technology Co., Ltd., Wuhan, Hubei, China). The protein extracted from the ileal tissue was added to the loading buffer, 30 μg per well, and then boiled at 95 °C for 10 min. The 10% polyacrylamide gel (mc0001, Shanghai McKinang Biotechnology Co., Ltd., Shanghai, China) electrophoresis was used to separate the proteins. After electrophoresis, the protein was transferred to poly (vinylidene fluoride) (PVDF) membrane (P2438, Sigma, St Louis, MO, USA) using the semi-dry electrotransfer method, and the membrane was sealed with 5% bovine serum albumin (BSA) at room temperature for 1 h. Then, the PVDF membrane was incubated with the addition of the following antibodies anti-rabbit monoclonal antibody NF-κB (1: 1000;

ab32360), rabbit polyclonal antibody IκB (1: 500; ab64813), rabbit monoclonal antibody HIF-1α (1: 500; ab51608), rabbit polyclonal antibody ZO-1 (1: 100; ab59720), rabbit monoclonal antibody Occludin (1: 50000; ab167161), and the rabbit monoclonal antibody HMOX1 (1: 2000; ab52947) at 4 °C overnight. All the above mentioned antibodies were purchased from Abcam Inc. (Cambridge, MA, USA). The next day, the membrane was washed 3 times with Tris-buffered saline with Tween 20 (TBST) (5 min/time), and the goat anti-rabbit second antibody was added to the membrane for incubation at room temperature for 1 h. And then, the membrane was rinsed 3 times (5 min/time), and developed using a chemiluminescent reagent (Research Biology Co., Ltd., Shanghai, China) with GADPH serving as the internal reference. The Bio-rad Gel Dol EZ Imager (GEL DOC EZ IMAGER, Bio-Rad, Hercules, CA, USA) was employed to analyze the obtained images. The gray scale of the target protein band was analyzed using Image J (National Institutes of Health), and the ratio of the gray value of the target protein band to the gray value of the internal reference protein was used as the levels of the target protein. The experiment was repeated three times to obtain the mean value.

### Statistical analysis

Statistical analyses were processed using SPSS 21.0 software (IBM Corp., Armonk, NY, USA). Measurement data were expressed as mean ± standard deviation. The $t$-test was applied for comparisons between two groups, and one-way analysis of variance (ANOVA) for comparisons among groups. Count data was expressed as a percentage or rate, and the $x^2$ test was used for comparison. ANOVA was used for comparisons between multiple groups, and homogeneity test of variances was used. When the ANOVA presented with significant differences, the q test was used for further comparisons, otherwise, the nonparametric rank sum was used, and the significance level $\alpha = 0.05$. $p < 0.05$ was considered to be statistically significant.

### Results

#### miR-31 affects intestinal mucosal permeability and intestinal barrier function

Rats were subjected to CPL and administration of during sepsis in order to detect the role of miR-31 in intestinal mucosal permeability. Next, serum samples were obtained 24 h after injection in order to determine the levels of D-lactic acid, DAO and FD-40. The results are shown in Fig. 1. The levels of D-lactic acid, DAO and FD-40 in serum in the other groups were found to be significantly higher than in the sham group ($p < 0.05$). The levels of D-lactic acid, DAO and FD-40 were evidently increased in the miR-31 mimic group ($p < 0.05$), while significantly decreased in the miR-31 inhibitor group in comparison to the sepsis group ($p < 0.05$).

After administration of miR-31 mimic or inhibitor, FITC-DX content and bacterial translocation rate were detected in order to determine the effect of miR-31 on intestinal barrier function (Table 2). The FITC-DX content and the bacterial translocation rate were found to be significantly higher in other groups than those in the sham group (all $p < 0.05$). In addition, the levels of FITC-DX and the bacterial translocation rate were found to be markedly higher in the miR-31 mimic group while obviously lower in the miR-31 inhibitor group when compared with those in the sepsis group. The above results showed that intestinal mucosal permeability and intestinal barrier function could be negatively affected by the level of miR-31.

### Levels of miR-31 can cause oxidative damage and affect the expression of inflammatory factors in intestinal tissue of rats

Additionally, the MDA content and SOD activity were measured in order to detect the effect of miR-31 on oxidative damage of intestinal tissue of rats. To further study the oxidative damage caused by miR-31 in rat small intestine tissue, MDA was regarded as an indicator to indirectly reflect the damage of oxygen free radicals to cells, and SOD to reflect the antioxidant capacity of the cells. The results showed that the MDA content in the intestine tissues in other groups was found to be significantly higher while the SOD activity significantly was lower than that in the sham group (all $p < 0.05$). Compared with the sepsis group, the MDA content in the intestine tissues was evidently increased and the SOD activity was significantly decreased in the miR-31 mimic group (all $p < 0.05$), while the miR-31 inhibitor group exhibited opposite trends (all $p < 0.05$) (Fig. 2a and b).

Furthermore, the contents of TNF-α, IL-6 and IL-10 were detected in order to study the inflammation induced by miR-31 on the small intestine of rats. The levels of TNF-α, IL-6 and IL-10 in the intestine tissues in each group are shown in Fig. 2c-e. The levels of TNF-α and IL-6 and IL-10 in the intestine tissues in the other groups were found to be significantly higher than those in the sham group (all $p < 0.05$). The levels of TNF-α, IL-6 and IL-10 were significantly higher in the miR-31 mimic group (all $p < 0.05$) while significantly lower levels were observed in the miR-31 inhibitor group when compared with the sepsis group (all $p < 0.05$). The above results showed that oxidative damage of intestinal tissue of rats could be caused by treatment with miR-31, and the expression of inflammatory factors in intestinal tissue of rats was also regulated by miR-31.

### Confirmation of HMOX1 as a target gene of miR-31

HMOX1 was confirmed as a target gene of miR-31 by the biology predicted website, *microRNA.org* (Fig. 3a).

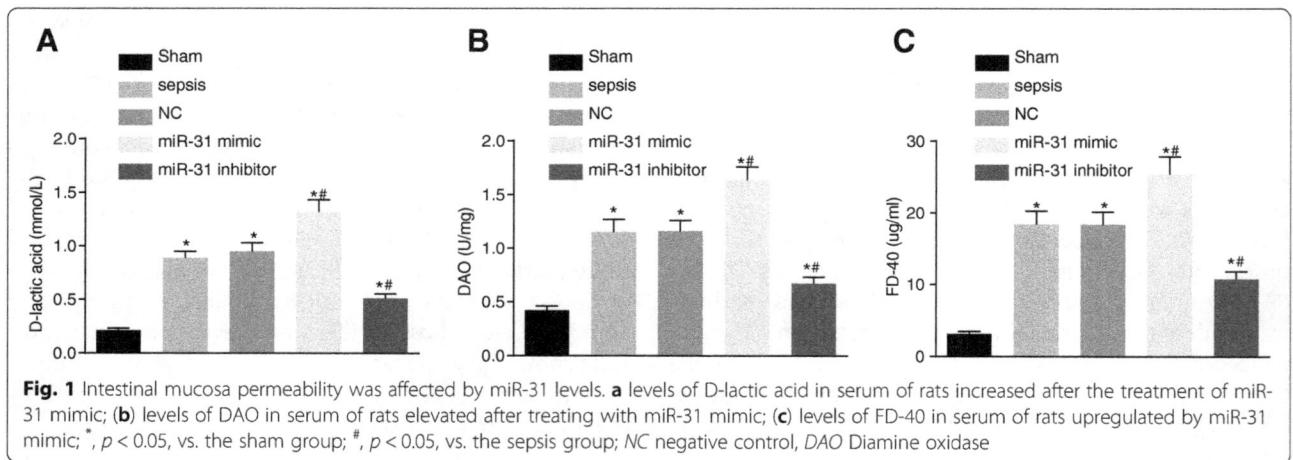

**Fig. 1** Intestinal mucosa permeability was affected by miR-31 levels. **a** levels of D-lactic acid in serum of rats increased after the treatment of miR-31 mimic; (**b**) levels of DAO in serum of rats elevated after treating with miR-31 mimic; (**c**) levels of FD-40 in serum of rats upregulated by miR-31 mimic; *, $p < 0.05$, vs. the sham group; #, $p < 0.05$, vs. the sepsis group; NC negative control, DAO Diamine oxidase

The results of dual-luciferase reporter gene assay (Fig. 3b) showed that the fluorescence signal of the miR-31 mimic + pHMOX1-Wt group was decreased by approximately 50% (all $p < 0.05$) when compared with the other three groups, and the miR-31 mimic + pHMOX1-Mut presented with no significant differences in the luciferase signal compared with the miR-31 mimic NC + pHMOX1-Mut group and the miR-31 mimic NC + pHMOX1-Wt group (all $p > 0.05$). In addition, western blot analysis was applied in order to detect the expression of HMOX1 in CACO-2 cells. It was found that (Fig. 3c, d) compared with the NC group, the expression of HMOX1 in the miR-31 mimic group was significantly down-regulated ($p < 0.05$), while obviously up-regulated in the miR-31 inhibitor group ($p < 0.05$). These findings suggested that miR-31 could target HMOX1.

### MiR-31 affects intestinal mucosal permeability and intestinal barrier function by regulating HMOX1

In order to further study the effect of miR-31 on intestinal mucosal permeability and intestinal barrier function in rats by regulating HMOX1, we interfered with HMOX1 with siRNA. The detection results of intestinal mucosal permeability function are shown in Fig. 4. Compared with the NC group, the contents of D-lactic acid, DAO and FD-40 in serum were found to be significantly increased in the siRNA-HMOX1 group (all $p < 0.05$). There were no significant differences in the contents of D-lactic acid, DAO and

FD-40 between the miR-31 inhibitor + siRNA-HMOX1 group and the NC group ($p > 0.05$).

The results of intestinal barrier function in each group are shown in Table 3. Compared with the NC group, the siRNA-HMOX1 group presented with elevated FITC-DX content and increased bacterial translocation rate in each organ. There were no obvious differences in FITC-DX content and bacterial translocation rate between the miR-31 inhibitor + siRNA-HMOX1 group and the NC group (all $p > 0.05$). These results suggested that intestinal mucosal permeability and intestinal barrier function could be influenced by miR-31 through the regulation of HMOX1.

### MiR-31 affects oxidative damage and inflammation level in rat small intestine tissues through HMOX1

The content of MDA and SOD activity in the small intestine of rats was measured in order to detect oxidative damage. The results are shown in Fig. 5a and b. In comparison to the NC group, the content of MDA was found to be remarkably increased while SOD activity was obviously reduced in the siRNA-HMOX1 group (all $p < 0.05$). There were no significant differences in the content of MDA and SOD activity between the miR-31 inhibitor + siRNA-HMOX1 group and the NC group ($p > 0.05$). These findings showed that miR-31 can affect MDA content and SOD activity in rat small intestine through HMOX-1.

**Table 2** Intestinal barrier function of the rats is affected by miR-31

| Group | FITC-DX (µg/mL) | Numbers | Visceral organ | | | Bacterial translocation rate (%) |
| --- | --- | --- | --- | --- | --- | --- |
| | | | Liver | Spleen | Mesenteric lymph node | |
| Sham | 0.27 ± 0.01 | 5 | 0 | 0 | 1 | 6.67% |
| Sepsis | 1.93 ± 0.13* | 5 | 3 | 3 | 4 | 66.67%* |
| NC | 1.99 ± 0.14* | 5 | 5 | 3 | 3 | 73.33%* |
| miR-31 mimic | 2.71 ± 0.19*# | 5 | 4 | 5 | 5 | 93.33%* |
| miR-31 inhibitor | 0.78 ± 0.06*# | 5 | 5 | 2 | 2 | 40.00%* |

Notes: *, $p < 0.05$, vs. the sham group; #, $p < 0.05$, vs. the sepsis group; NC negative control

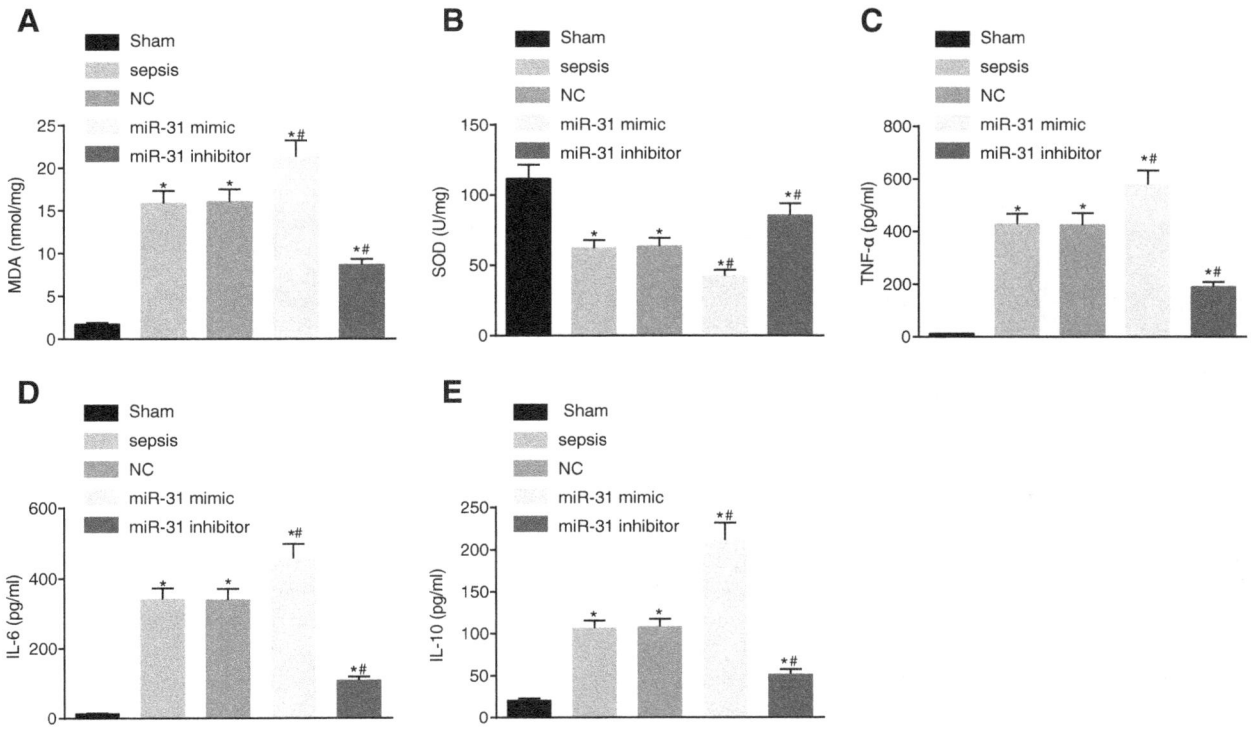

**Fig. 2** MiR-31 caused oxidative damage and affected the levels of inflammatory factors in intestinal tissue of rats. **a** content of MDA increased after treating with miR-31 mimic; (**b**) SOD activity was inhibited by miR-31 mimic; (**c**) elevated levels of TNF-α after the treatment of miR-31 mimic; (**d**) increased levels of IL-6 following the treatment of miR-31 mimic; (**e**), increased levels of IL-10 by miR-31 mimic; *, $p < 0.05$, vs. the sham group; #, $p < 0.05$, vs. the sepsis group; *MDA* malondiadehyde, *SOD* superoxidedismutase, *NC* negative control, *TNF* tumor necrosis factor, *IL* interleukin

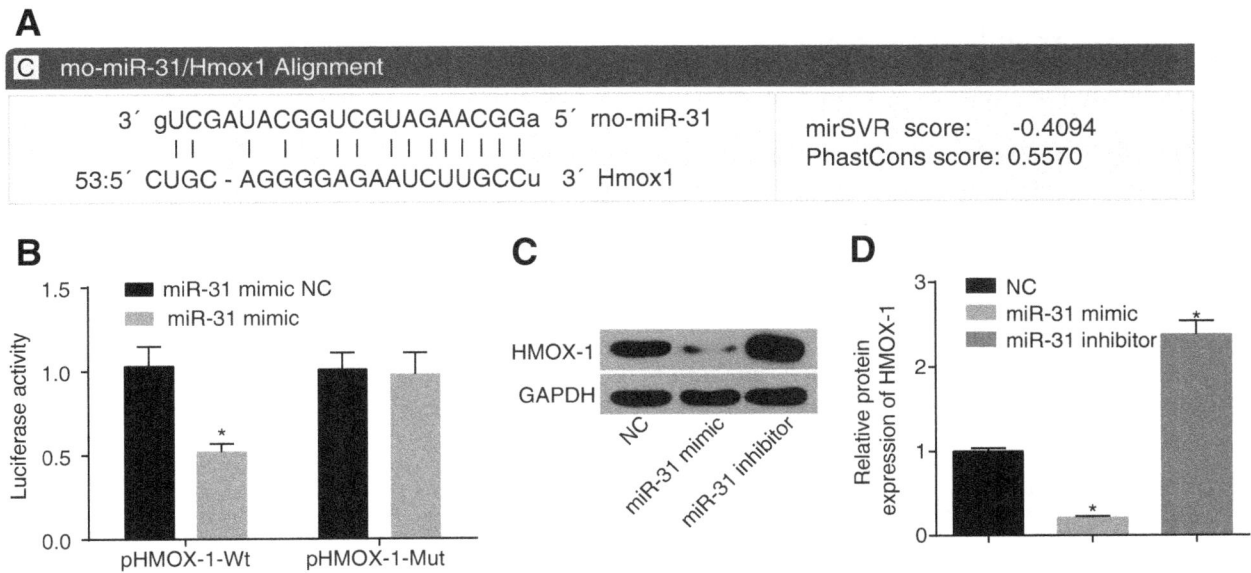

**Fig. 3** HMOX1 was the target gene of miR-31. **a** HMOX1 was confirmed as a target gene of miR-31 by the biology predicted website microRNA.org; (**b**) dual-luciferase reporter assay showed HMOX1 was a target gene of miR-31; (**c**) Western blot analysis detected that protein levels of HMOX1 were significantly increased after treating miR-31 inhibitor; (**d**) inhibition of miR-31 could increase protein levels of HMOX1; *, $p < 0.05$, vs. the corresponding control group

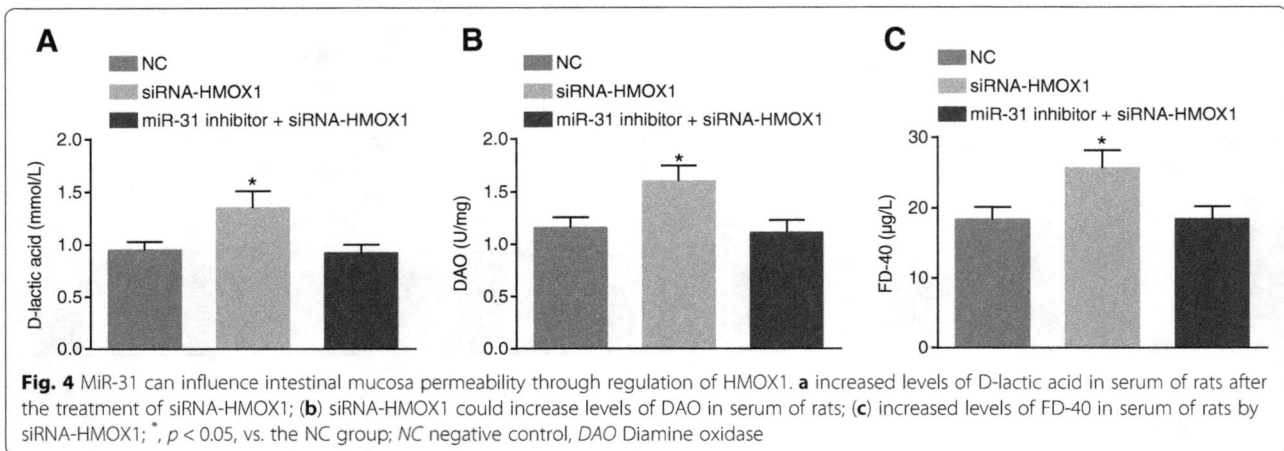

**Fig. 4** MiR-31 can influence intestinal mucosa permeability through regulation of HMOX1. **a** increased levels of D-lactic acid in serum of rats after the treatment of siRNA-HMOX1; (**b**) siRNA-HMOX1 could increase levels of DAO in serum of rats; (**c**) increased levels of FD-40 in serum of rats by siRNA-HMOX1; *, $p < 0.05$, vs. the NC group; *NC* negative control, *DAO* Diamine oxidase

In addition, the content of TNF-α, IL-6 and IL-10 in rats was detected in order to study the inflammation induced by miR-31 on the small intestine of rats through HMOX1. The results are shown in Fig. 5c-e. In comparison to the NC group, the siRNA-HMOX1 group presented with significantly increased TNF-α, IL-6 and IL-10 content in rats (all $p < 0.05$). There were no significant differences in the contents of TNF-α, IL-6 and IL-10 between the miR-31 inhibitor + siRNA-HMOX1 group and the NC group ($p > 0.05$). These findings showed that miR-31 can induce oxidative damage in rat small intestine, and furthermore affect the expression of inflammatory factors through HMOX-1.

### Relatively mild histopathological changes in intestine tissues after transfection with miR-31 inhibitor

HE staining was employed in order to detect histopathological changes of the intestine tissues in rats. The results of HE staining in the intestine tissues in each group are shown in Fig. 6. The rats in the sham group exhibited normally structured intestines under light microscope observation, without tissue edema, and presented with normal villus structure and clear edge of microvilli, with a pathological injury score of $0.90 \pm 0.32$. In the sepsis group, the intestinal wall was noted to be thinner, the mucosa was atrophied, in addition to intestinal mucosal necrosis, shedding and occurrence of villous rupture in some areas, as well as a pathological injury score of $4.20 \pm 0.42$, which was significantly different compared with the sham group

($p < 0.05$). The histopathological changes of the rats in the NC group and the miR-31 inhibitor + siRNA-HMOX1 group were consistent with the sepsis group, with pathological injury scores of $4.60 \pm 0.52$ and $4.10 \pm 0.32$, respectively. The intestinal wall and mucosal atrophy of rats in the miR-31 mimic group and the siRNA-HMOX1 group were more obvious, with more intestinal mucosal necrosis, shedding and occurrence of villous rupture in more areas, the pathological injury scores of $6.20 \pm 0.42$ and $6.40 \pm 0.70$, respectively. There were statistically significant differences compared with the sham and sepsis groups ($p < 0.05$). The rats in the miR-31 inhibitor group exhibited partial intestinal mucosal necrosis and shedding, but the intestinal mucosal lesions were relatively mild, with a pathological injury score of $2.20 \pm 0.42$. The above results suggested that miR-31 could cause the above mentioned histopathological changes of the intestine tissues.

### Inhibition of HMOX1 expression by miR-31 affects the expression of NF-κB/HIF-1α pathway related genes

RT-qPCR and western blot analysis were employed in order to determine the mRNA and protein levels of the NF-κB/HIF-1α pathway related. The levels of miR-31 and mRNA levels of NF-κB, HIF-1α, and HMOX1 in ileal tissues of each group are shown in Fig. 7. The levels of miR-31 in the ileal tissues in the other groups were found to be significantly increased compared to that in the sham group (all $p < 0.05$). The levels of miR-31 were significantly higher in the miR-31 mimic group than in

**Table 3** MiR-31 influences intestinal barrier function of the rats by regulating HMOX1

| Group | FITC-DX (μg/mL) | Numbers | Visceral organ | | | Bacterial translocation rate (%) |
| --- | --- | --- | --- | --- | --- | --- |
| | | | Liver | Spleen | Mesenteric lymph node | |
| NC | 1.99 ± 0.14 | 5 | 5 | 3 | 3 | 73.33% |
| siRNA-HMOX1 | 2.83 ± 0.21* | 5 | 5 | 5 | 5 | 100%* |
| miR-31 inhibitor + siRNA-HMOX1 | 1.96 ± 0.11 | 5 | 5 | 2 | 3 | 66.67% |

Note: *, $p < 0.05$, vs. the NC group; *NC* negative control, *HMOX1* heme oxygenase 1

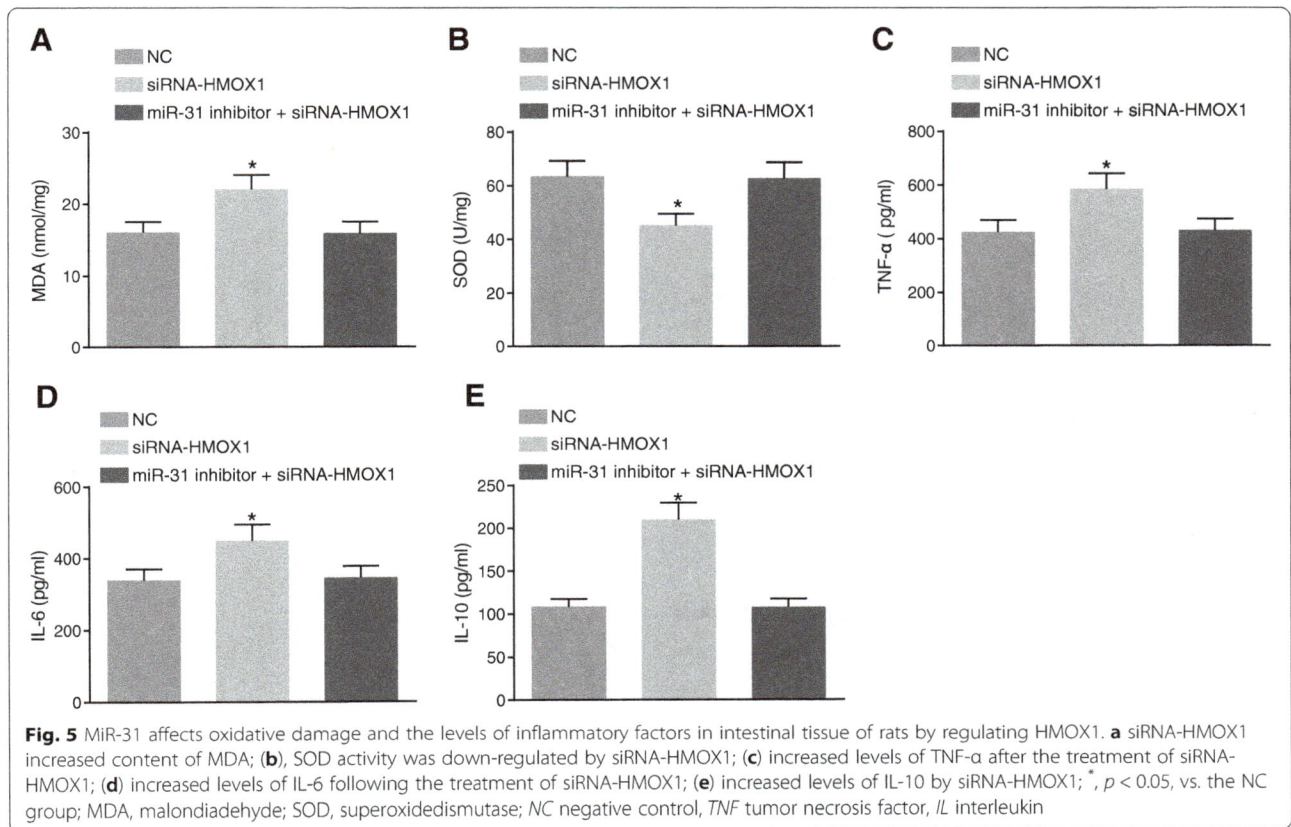

**Fig. 5** MiR-31 affects oxidative damage and the levels of inflammatory factors in intestinal tissue of rats by regulating HMOX1. **a** siRNA-HMOX1 increased content of MDA; (**b**), SOD activity was down-regulated by siRNA-HMOX1; (**c**) increased levels of TNF-α after the treatment of siRNA-HMOX1; (**d**) increased levels of IL-6 following the treatment of siRNA-HMOX1; (**e**) increased levels of IL-10 by siRNA-HMOX1; *, $p < 0.05$, vs. the NC group; MDA, malondiadehyde; SOD, superoxidedismutase; *NC* negative control, *TNF* tumor necrosis factor, *IL* interleukin

the sepsis group, and significantly decreased in the miR-31 inhibitor and miR-31 inhibitor + siRNA-HMOX1 groups (all $p < 0.05$). Compared with the sham group, the expression of NF-κB and HIF-1α mRNA and protein in ileal tissues were significantly higher in the other groups (all $p < 0.05$), in addition to significantly decreased mRNA and protein levels of IκB, ZO-1 and Occludin (all $p < 0.05$). Compared with the sepsis group, the expression of

NF-κB and HIF-1α mRNA and protein in ileal tissues were found to be significantly increased, while IκB, ZO-1 and Occludin mRNA and protein were significantly decreased in the miR-31 mimic group and the siRNA-HMOX1 group (all $p < 0.05$). The expression of NF-κB and HIF-1α mRNA and protein in ileal tissues were found to be remarkably decreased, and IκB, ZO-1 and Occludin mRNA and protein were significantly increased in the

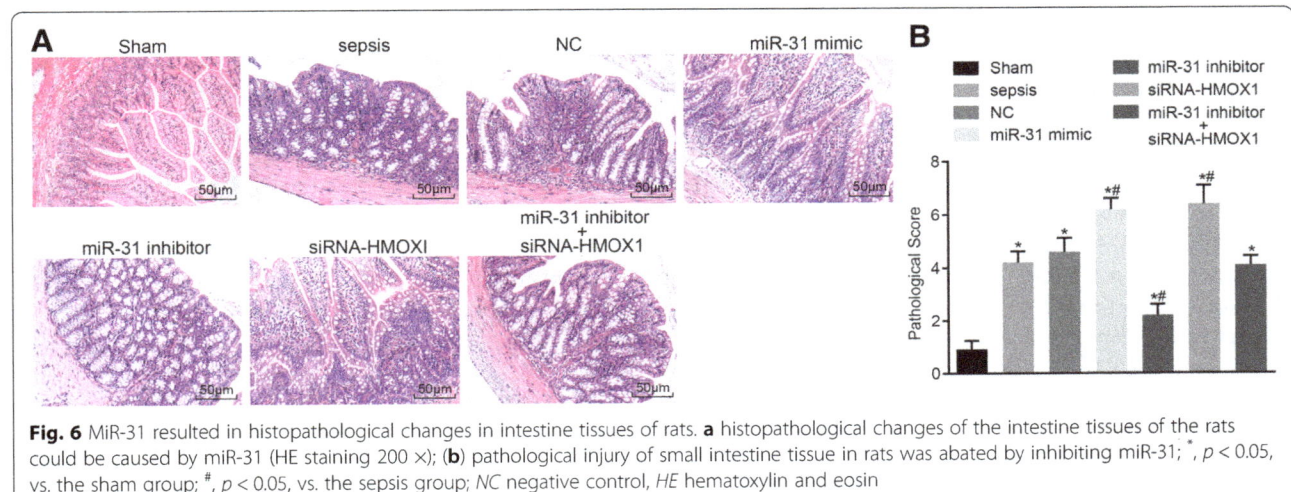

**Fig. 6** MiR-31 resulted in histopathological changes in intestine tissues of rats. **a** histopathological changes of the intestine tissues of the rats could be caused by miR-31 (HE staining 200 ×); (**b**) pathological injury of small intestine tissue in rats was abated by inhibiting miR-31; *, $p < 0.05$, vs. the sham group; #, $p < 0.05$, vs. the sepsis group; *NC* negative control, *HE* hematoxylin and eosin

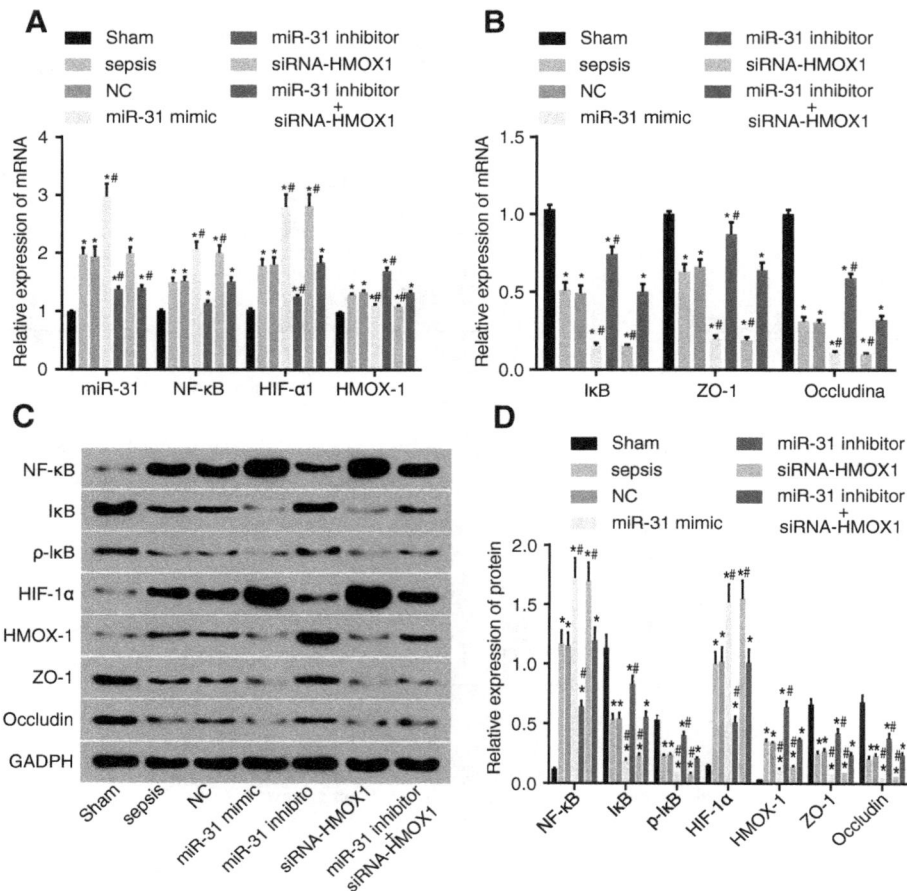

**Fig. 7** MiR-31 regulated expression of the NF-κB/HIF-1α pathway related genes by inhibiting HMOX1. **a-b** RT-qPCR detected that the mRNA levels of NF-κB, HIF-1α, HMOX1, IκB, ZO-1, and Occludin in the ileal tissue of the rats were affected by miR-31 through HMOX1; (**c-d**), Western blot analysis detected that protein levels of IκB, p-IκB, ZO-1, HMOX1, HIF-1α, NF-κB, and Occludin in the ileal tissue of the rats were regulated by miR-31 via HMOX1; *, $p < 0.05$, vs. the sham group; #, $p < 0.05$, vs. the sepsis group; NC negative control

miR-31 inhibitor group (all $p < 0.05$). Compared with the sham group, the mRNA and protein levels of HMOX1 in the ileal tissues in other groups were evidently elevated (all $p < 0.05$). In comparison to the sepsis group, the expression of HMOX1 mRNA and protein in the ileal tissues in the miR-31 mimic and siRNA-HMOX1 groups were significantly lower (all $p < 0.05$), whereas significantly higher levels were observed in the miR-31 inhibitor group. The mRNA and protein levels of relative genes in the ileal tissues in the sepsis, NC, and miR-31 inhibitor + siRNA-HMOX1 groups exhibited no significant differences (all $p > 0.05$). The mRNA and protein levels of NF-κB, HIF-1α, HMOX1, IκB, ZO-1, and Occludin (except miR-31) in the ileal tissues in the miR-31 mimic group and siRNA-HMOX1 group presented with no significant differences (all $p > 0.05$). The above results showed that the levels of the NF-κB/HIF-1α pathway related genes could be affected by miR-31 through inhibition of HMOX1.

### Inhibition of miR-31 can increase survival rates of rats

The rats in the sham group were awoken after anesthetization and fed with a normal diet, and the rats presented with normal stool and body temperature, smooth and shiny hair, and quick response. When the sepsis rats were awoken after anesthetization, the rats were observed to be dull, slow, and presenting with shortness of breath and bloating. Then, the rats died and accompanied by different symptoms during the process. The survival curves of rats at 0–72 h in each group are shown in Fig. 8. The non-parametric estimation of survival rates was based on the Kaplan-Meier method. The median survival time and the 95% confidence interval (CI) of each group were as follows: the sham group, no death; the sepsis group, 95% CI (44.458–64.342); the NC group, 95% CI (43.909–64.624); the miR-31 mimic group, 95% CI (28.571–51.429); the miR-31 inhibitor group, 95% CI (61.860–72.540); the siRNA-HMOX group, 95% CI (31.088–52.112); the miR-31 inhibitor + siRNA-HMOX1 group, 95% CI (45.338–65.062).

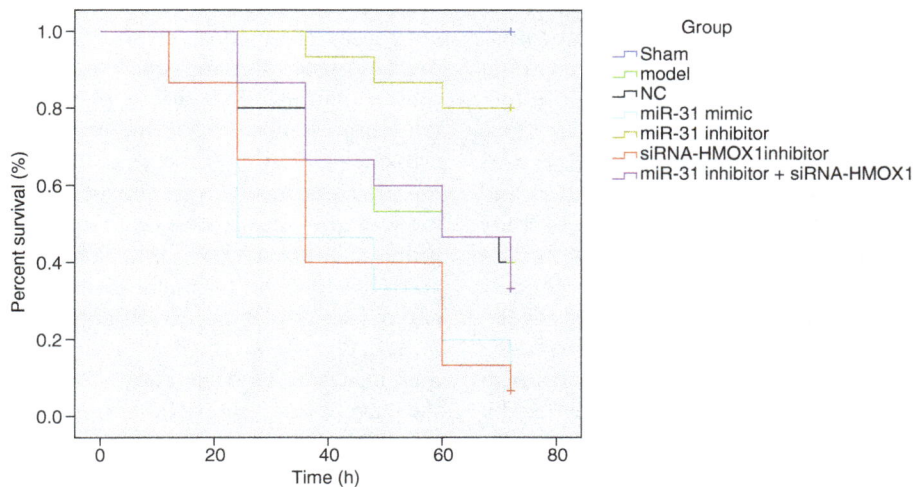

**Fig. 8** MiR-31 reduced the survival rates of rats. $n = 15$

The survival curves of the different groups were compared using the Log-rank test. The survival analysis showed that the survival curves in the seven groups were different. There were no deaths in the sham group. Compared with the sham group, the survival rates of rats in other groups were found to be reduced significantly. There were rat deaths at the 12 h time interval in the miR-31 mimic and siRNA-HMOX1 groups, and the number of deaths increased and survival rate decreased with time. In the miR-31 inhibitor group, rat deaths were observed at the 36 h time interval. In the sepsis, NC and miR-31 inhibitor + siRNA-HMOX1 groups, the rats died at the 24 h time interval. These findings suggested that inhibition of miR-31 reduced survival rates of rats.

## Discussion

Sepsis, a life-threatening condition, is arisen when the body's response to infection results in injury to its own tissues and organs, causing multiple organ dysfunctions like intestinal barrier dysfunction (Ma et al. 2013; Singer et al. 2016). Previously, miRNAs have been regarded to be essential for the regulation of numerous cellular processes, including inflammation and immunity (Ma et al. 2013). The current study aimed to investigate whether miR-31 has effects on intestinal barrier dysfunction by targeting HMOX1 through the NF-κB/HIF-1α pathway in sepsis. The results of our study demonstrated that intestinal barrier dysfunction can be improved through suppressing the expression of miR-31 by targeting HMOX1 through inhibition of the NF-κB/HIF-1α pathway.

Firstly, the current study found that sepsis rats exhibited increased expressions of D-lactic acid, DAO, bacterial translocation, MDA, TNF-α, IL-6, and IL-10, in addition to decreased SOD activity. D-lactic acid is a metabolic product of intestinal flora, and a recent study has shown that

patients suffering from chronic fatigue syndrome presented with increased D-lactic acid intestinal bacteria (Sheedy et al. 2009). Serum DAO, acting as a marker for mammalian intestinal mucosa, was found to be significantly higher in rats with irritable bowel syndrome as noted by increased DAO activity (Liu et al. 2012). The intestines are a primary source for endogenous bacteria, and recent evidences have shown that elevated bacterial translocation rates are found in intestinal barrier dysfunction (Gomez-Hurtado et al. 2011). Similarly, decreased SOD activity with increased MDA levels were observed for intestinal barrier function damage in pancreatitis rats (Mirmalek et al. 2016). Interestingly, a previous study suggested that intestinal epithelial barrier dysfunction is triggered by a mechanism that involves mast cell dependent TNF-α and protease release and disruption of paracellular tight junctions, owing to findings of increased TNF-α in intestinal epithelial barrier function (Overman et al. 2012). In addition, data indicated that for obvious pathological damages in the intestine, the levels of TNF-α, IL-6, and IL-10 were elevated (Zhongkai et al. 2012).

Additionally, the current study showed that the miR-31 inhibitor group exhibited decreased expressions of D-lactic acid, DAO, FITC-DX, TNF-α, IL-6, and IL-10, in addition to increased expressions of SOD. A recent study showed that damage to the intestinal mucosa barrier may result in intestinal bacterial and endotoxin translocation, leading to local and systemic inflammation, and furthermore, FITC-DX and D-lactic acid were respectively the markers for changes in intestinal permeability and intestinal barriers (Bao et al. 2014). Similarly, the expression of inflammatory cytokines like TNF-α, DAO and D-lactic acid, and IL-1 were found to be significantly lower in normal conditions in intestinal mucosa compared to intestinal mucosal injury (Shu et al. 2016) and inflammatory cytokines also included

IL-6, IL-8, IL-10, and TNF-α (Piantadosi et al. 2011; Terasaka et al. 2010). It was also reported that inhibition of endogenous miR-31 in psoriasis (a common chronic inflammatory skin disease) inhibits the production of inflammatory mediators (Xu et al. 2013). Thus, in the current study, it was assumed that miR-31 was related to intestinal mucosal permeability function and intestinal barrier function. Moreover, another study found that HO-1 and CORM-2 exerted a protective role in intestinal epithelial barrier function by reducing cell apoptosis and intestinal inflammation through regulation of NF-κB (Zhang et al. 2017). Furthermore, increasing evidences have shown that the activity of DAO was high in intestinal villous cells, and reduced activity was noted if injury to intestinal epithelial cells had ensued, so changes of intestinal mucosa integrity, permeability and the barrier function can be shown by DAO activity (Han et al. 2016). Another study also indicated that the expression of SOD in the cytosol was down-regulated by miR-398 during growth on low copper (Higashi et al. 2013).

Furthermore, the current study showed that the rats with sepsis exhibited higher expressions of miR-31, HMOX1, NF-κB, and HIF-1α in addition to decreased expressions of IκB, ZO-1, and Occludin. Whereas, the rats transfected with miR-31 inhibitor presented with higher expressions of IκB, ZO-1, Occludin, and HMOX1 and lower expressions of miR-31, NF-κB, and HIF-1α. Previously, it has been found that miR-31 is expressed widely in different cell types, and has been studied in different diseases (Peng et al. 2012). It was also demonstrated that miR-31 expression is up-regulated in human cervical, colorectal, liver, and head-and-neck squamous cell carcinomas, indicating the role of miR-31 in various cancers (Guo et al. 2016). Additionally, miR-31 was found to be up-regulated in colorectal cancer (Slaby et al. 2007). Indicating correlations, miR-31 was found to negatively regulate the noncanonical NF-κB pathway, and higher expression of Polycomb proteins resulted in lower expression of miR-31 in an epigenetic fashion, causing activation of NF-κB and apoptosis resistance (Yamagishi et al. 2012). miR-31 contributes to colorectal cancer development by targeting factor inhibiting HIF-1α (Chen et al. 2014). In addition, the expression of IκB was found to be decreased in cardiac dysfunction in mice with chronic kidney disease, and lung inflammation and systemic inflammatory response resulted from lipopolysaccharide administration (Chen et al. 2017). As previously reported, it was found an impaired tight junction and decreased expression of occludin and ZO-1 in the intestinal epithelial cells (Yu et al. 2016). Moreover, inhibition of miR-122a increased intestinal occludin expression and protected mice from alcoholic liver disease (Zhao et al. 2015). From the previous studies, induction of HMOX1 by inflammation like in sepsis, is related both to

an anti-inflammatory response and to mitochondrial biogenesis (Piantadosi et al. 2011), and HMOX1 can promote pro-inflammatory cytokine secretion and suppress inflammation-induced phenotypic maturation in the immune effector cells and enhance anti-inflammatory cytokine production (Ozen et al. 2015). Another study also reported that over-expression of HO-1 promoted sepsis induced immunosuppression at the late stages of sepsis by promoting polarization of anti-inflammatory gene Th2 and Treg function to inhibit excessive immune responses and maintain tolerance to self-antigens (Yoon et al. 2017). HMOX1 was confirmed as a target gene of miR-31 by dual-luciferase reporter assay. Therefore, the findings of the current study showed that suppression of miR-31 alleviates intestinal barrier dysfunction by targeting HMOX1.

## Conclusion

In conclusion, the current study demonstrated that inhibition of miR-31 exerted positive effects on intestinal barrier dysfunction in sepsis, and HMOX1 was the target gene of miR-31. It should be noted that the specific mechanism of targeted correlation required further exploration. However, it can be expected to be a new target gene for treating intestinal barrier dysfunction in sepsis in order to raise the quality of life of patients suffering from this disease.

### Acknowledgements

We acknowledge and appreciate our colleagues for their valuable efforts and comments on this paper.

### Funding

This work was supported by Natural Science Foundation of Hubei Province (2014CFB970).

### Authors' contributions

CZ, DC, JL and YS designed the study. CZ and DC designed and developed the database, carried out data analyses and produced the initial draft of the manuscript. JL, YS and YZ collated the data and contributed to drafting the manuscript. All authors have read and approved the final submitted manuscript.

### Competing interest

The authors declare that they have no competing interests.

### References

Bao J, Tan S, Yu W, Lin Z, Dong Y, Chen Q, et al. The effect of peritoneal air exposure on intestinal mucosal barrier. Gastroenterol Res Pract. 2014;2014:674875.

Bartel DP. MicroRNAs: target recognition and regulatory functions. Cell. 2009;136: 215–33.

Chen J, Kieswich JE, Chiazza F, Moyes AJ, Gobbetti T, Purvis GS, et al. IkappaB kinase inhibitor attenuates Sepsis-induced cardiac dysfunction in CKD. J Am Soc Nephrol. 2017;28:94–105.

Chen T, Yao LQ, Shi Q, Ren Z, Ye LC, Xu JM, et al. MicroRNA-31 contributes to colorectal cancer development by targeting factor inhibiting HIF-1alpha (FIH-1). Cancer Biol Ther. 2014;15:516–23.

Chiu CJ, McArdle AH, Brown R, Scott HJ, Gurd FN. Intestinal mucosal lesion in low-flow states. I. a morphological, hemodynamic, and metabolic reappraisal. Arch Surg. 1970;101:478–83.

Creighton CJ, Fountain MD, Yu Z, Nagaraja AK, Zhu H, Khan M, et al. Molecular profiling uncovers a p53-associated role for microRNA-31 in inhibiting the proliferation of serous ovarian carcinomas and other cancers. Cancer Res. 2010;70:1906–15.

Fredenburgh LE, Velandia MM, Ma J, Olszak T, Cernadas M, Englert JA, et al. Cyclooxygenase-2 deficiency leads to intestinal barrier dysfunction and increased mortality during polymicrobial sepsis. J Immunol. 2011;187:5255–67.

Gomez-Hurtado I, Santacruz A, Peiro G, Zapater P, Gutierrez A, Perez-Mateo M, et al. Gut microbiota dysbiosis is associated with inflammation and bacterial translocation in mice with CCl4-induced fibrosis. PLoS One. 2011;6:e23037.

Guo H, Qi RQ, Lv YN, Wang HX, Hong YX, Zheng S, et al. miR-31 is distinctively overexpressed in primary male extramammary Paget's disease. Oncotarget. 2016;7:24559–63.

Han J, Xu Y, Yang D, Yu N, Bai Z, Bian L. Effect of polysaccharides from Acanthopanax senticosus on intestinal mucosal barrier of Escherichia coli lipopolysaccharide challenged mice. Asian-Australas J Anim Sci. 2016;29:134–41.

Higashi Y, Takechi K, Takano H, Takio S. Involvement of microRNA in copper deficiency-induced repression of chloroplastic CuZn-superoxide dismutase genes in the moss Physcomitrella patens. Plant Cell Physiol. 2013;54:1345–55.

Hou W, Tian Q, Zheng J, Bonkovsky HL. MicroRNA-196 represses Bach1 protein and hepatitis C virus gene expression in human hepatoma cells expressing hepatitis C viral proteins. Hepatology. 2010;51:1494–504.

Jiang L, Yang L, Zhang M, Fang X, Huang Z, Yang Z, et al. Beneficial effects of ulinastatin on gut barrier function in sepsis. Indian J Med Res. 2013;138:904–11.

Liu CJ, Tsai MM, Hung PS, Kao SY, Liu TY, Wu KJ, et al. miR-31 ablates expression of the HIF regulatory factor FIH to activate the HIF pathway in head and neck carcinoma. Cancer Res. 2010;70:1635–44.

Liu Y, Xu W, Liu L, Guo L, Deng Y, Liu J. N-acetyl glucosamine improves intestinal mucosal barrier function in rat. Bangladesh Journal of Pharmacology. 2012;7: 281–4.

Ma Y, Vilanova D, Atalar K, Delfour O, Edgeworth J, Ostermann M, et al. Genome-wide sequencing of cellular microRNAs identifies a combinatorial expression signature diagnostic of sepsis. PLoS One. 2013;8:e75918.

Melvan JN, Bagby GJ, Welsh DA, Nelson S, Zhang P. Neonatal sepsis and neutrophil insufficiencies. Int Rev Immunol. 2010;29:315–48.

Mirmalek SA, Gholamrezaei Boushehrinejad A, Yavari H, Kardeh B, Parsa Y, Salimi-Tabatabaee SA, et al. Antioxidant and anti-inflammatory effects of coenzyme Q10 on L-arginine-induced acute pancreatitis in rat. Oxidative Med Cell Longev. 2016;2016:5818479.

Montano M. MicroRNAs: miRRORS of health and disease. Transl Res. 2011;157:157–62.

O'Connell RM, Rao DS, Baltimore D. microRNA regulation of inflammatory responses. Annu Rev Immunol. 2012;30:295–312.

Overman EL, Rivier JE, Moeser AJ. CRF induces intestinal epithelial barrier injury via the release of mast cell proteases and TNF-alpha. PLoS One. 2012;7:e39935.

Ozen M, Zhao H, Lewis DB, Wong RJ, Stevenson DK. Heme oxygenase and the immune system in normal and pathological pregnancies. Front Pharmacol. 2015;6:84.

Peng H, Hamanaka RB, Katsnelson J, Hao LL, Yang W, Chandel NS, et al. MicroRNA-31 targets FIH-1 to positively regulate corneal epithelial glycogen metabolism. FASEB J. 2012;26:3140–7.

Piantadosi CA, Withers CM, Bartz RR, MacGarvey NC, Fu P, Sweeney TE, et al. Heme oxygenase-1 couples activation of mitochondrial biogenesis to anti-inflammatory cytokine expression. J Biol Chem. 2011;286:16374–85.

Rittirsch D, Huber-Lang MS, Flierl MA, Ward PA. Immunodesign of experimental sepsis by cecal ligation and puncture. Nat Protoc. 2009;4:31–6.

Schetter AJ, Heegaard NH, Harris CC. Inflammation and cancer: interweaving microRNA, free radical, cytokine and p53 pathways. Carcinogenesis. 2010;31: 37–49.

Sheedy JR, Wettenhall RE, Scanlon D, Gooley PR, Lewis DP, McGregor N, et al. Increased d-lactic acid intestinal bacteria in patients with chronic fatigue syndrome. In Vivo. 2009;23:621–8.

Shu X, Zhang J, Wang Q, Xu Z, Yu T. Glutamine decreases intestinal mucosal injury in a rat model of intestinal ischemia-reperfusion by downregulating HMGB1 and inflammatory cytokine expression. Exp Ther Med. 2016;12:1367–72.

Singer M, Deutschman CS, Seymour CW, Shankar-Hari M, Annane D, Bauer M, et al. The third international consensus definitions for Sepsis and septic shock (Sepsis-3). JAMA. 2016;315:801–10.

Slaby O, Svoboda M, Fabian P, Smerdova T, Knoflickova D, Bednarikova M, et al. Altered expression of miR-21, miR-31, miR-143 and miR-145 is related to clinicopathologic features of colorectal cancer. Oncology. 2007;72:397–402.

Takaki S, Takeyama N, Kajita Y, Yabuki T, Noguchi H, Miki Y, et al. Beneficial effects of the heme oxygenase-1/carbon monoxide system in patients with severe sepsis/septic shock. Intensive Care Med. 2010;36:42–8.

Terasaka Y, Miyazaki D, Yakura K, Haruki T, Inoue Y. Induction of IL-6 in transcriptional networks in corneal epithelial cells after herpes simplex virus type 1 infection. Invest Ophthalmol Vis Sci. 2010;51:2441–9.

Tiruvoipati R, Ong K, Gangopadhyay H, Arora S, Carney I, Botha J. Hypothermia predicts mortality in critically ill elderly patients with sepsis. BMC Geriatr. 2010;10:70.

Valastyan S, Reinhardt F, Benaich N, Calogrias D, Szasz AM, Wang ZC, et al. A pleiotropically acting microRNA, miR-31, inhibits breast cancer metastasis. Cell. 2009;137:1032–46.

van der Heide V, Mohnle P, Rink J, Briegel J, Kreth S. Down-regulation of MicroRNA-31 in CD4+ T cells contributes to immunosuppression in human Sepsis by promoting TH2 skewing. Anesthesiology. 2016;124:908–22.

Vazquez-Armenta G, Gonzalez-Leal N, J Vázquez-de la Torre M, Munoz-Valle JF, Ramos-Marquez ME, Hernandez-Canaveral I, et al. Short (GT)n microsatellite repeats in the heme oxygenase-1 gene promoter are associated with antioxidant and anti-inflammatory status in Mexican pediatric patients with sepsis. Tohoku J Exp Med. 2013;231:201–9.

Xu N, Meisgen F, Butler LM, Han G, Wang XJ, Soderberg-Naucler C, et al. MicroRNA-31 is overexpressed in psoriasis and modulates inflammatory cytokine and chemokine production in keratinocytes via targeting serine/threonine kinase 40. J Immunol. 2013;190:678–88.

Yamagishi M, Nakano K, Miyake A, Yamochi T, Kagami Y, Tsutsumi A, et al. Polycomb-mediated loss of miR-31 activates NIK-dependent NF-kappaB pathway in adult T cell leukemia and other cancers. Cancer Cell. 2012;21:121–35.

Yoon SJ, Kim SJ, Lee SM. Overexpression of HO-1 contributes to Sepsis-induced immunosuppression by modulating the Th1/Th2 balance and regulatory T-cell function. J Infect Dis. 2017;215:1608–18.

Yu T, Lu XJ, Li JY, Shan TD, Huang CZ, Ouyang H, et al. Overexpression of miR-429 impairs intestinal barrier function in diabetic mice by down-regulating occludin expression. Cell Tissue Res. 2016;366:341–52.

Zhang L, Zhang Z, Liu B, Jin Y, Tian Y, Xin Y, et al. The protective effect of Heme Oxygenase-1 against intestinal barrier dysfunction in Cholestatic liver injury is associated with NF-kappaB inhibition. Mol Med. 2017;23:215–24.

Zhao H, Zhao C, Dong Y, Zhang M, Wang Y, Li F, et al. Inhibition of miR122a by lactobacillus rhamnosus GG culture supernatant increases intestinal occludin expression and protects mice from alcoholic liver disease. Toxicol Lett. 2015; 234:194–200.

Zhao H, Zhao M, Wang Y, Li F, Zhang Z. Glycyrrhizic acid prevents Sepsis-induced acute lung injury and mortality in rats. J Histochem Cytochem. 2016;64:125–37.

Zhongkai L, Jianxin Y, Weichang C. Vasoactive intestinal peptide promotes gut barrier function against severe acute pancreatitis. Mol Biol Rep. 2012;39:3557–63.

Zhou J, Chaudhry H, Zhong Y, Ali MM, Perkins LA, Owens WB, et al. Dysregulation in microRNA expression in peripheral blood mononuclear cells of sepsis patients is associated with immunopathology. Cytokine. 2015;71:89–100.

# Permissions

All chapters in this book were first published in MM, by BioMed Central; hereby published with permission under the Creative Commons Attribution License or equivalent. Every chapter published in this book has been scrutinized by our experts. Their significance has been extensively debated. The topics covered herein carry significant findings which will fuel the growth of the discipline. They may even be implemented as practical applications or may be referred to as a beginning point for another development.

The contributors of this book come from diverse backgrounds, making this book a truly international effort. This book will bring forth new frontiers with its revolutionizing research information and detailed analysis of the nascent developments around the world.

We would like to thank all the contributing authors for lending their expertise to make the book truly unique. They have played a crucial role in the development of this book. Without their invaluable contributions this book wouldn't have been possible. They have made vital efforts to compile up to date information on the varied aspects of this subject to make this book a valuable addition to the collection of many professionals and students.

This book was conceptualized with the vision of imparting up-to-date information and advanced data in this field. To ensure the same, a matchless editorial board was set up. Every individual on the board went through rigorous rounds of assessment to prove their worth. After which they invested a large part of their time researching and compiling the most relevant data for our readers.

The editorial board has been involved in producing this book since its inception. They have spent rigorous hours researching and exploring the diverse topics which have resulted in the successful publishing of this book. They have passed on their knowledge of decades through this book. To expedite this challenging task, the publisher supported the team at every step. A small team of assistant editors was also appointed to further simplify the editing procedure and attain best results for the readers.

Apart from the editorial board, the designing team has also invested a significant amount of their time in understanding the subject and creating the most relevant covers. They scrutinized every image to scout for the most suitable representation of the subject and create an appropriate cover for the book.

The publishing team has been an ardent support to the editorial, designing and production team. Their endless efforts to recruit the best for this project, has resulted in the accomplishment of this book. They are a veteran in the field of academics and their pool of knowledge is as vast as their experience in printing. Their expertise and guidance has proved useful at every step. Their uncompromising quality standards have made this book an exceptional effort. Their encouragement from time to time has been an inspiration for everyone.

The publisher and the editorial board hope that this book will prove to be a valuable piece of knowledge for researchers, students, practitioners and scholars across the globe.

# List of Contributors

A. Armakolas, A. Dimakakos, C. Loukogiannaki, E. Papageorgiou, M. Stathaki, D. Spinos and M. Koutsilieris
Physiology Laboratory, Medical School, National & Kapodistrian University of Athens, 115 27 Goudi-Athens, Greece

N. Armakolas and A. Antonopoulos
Third orthopaedic clinic, KAT General Hospital, 145 61 Kifisia, Attiki, Greece

C. Florou and D. Pektasides
Oncology Section, Second Department of Internal Medicine, Hippokration Hospital, 115 27 Athens, Greece

P. Tsioli, T. P. Alexandrou and E. Patsouris
Department of Pathology, University of Athens, Medical School, 115 27 Athens, Greece

Fuhua Wang, Haiyi Yu, Bo Zuo, Zhu Song, Ning Wang and Guisong Wang
Department of Cardiology, Peking University Third Hospital, Key Laboratory of Cardiovascular Molecular Biology and Regulatory Peptides, Ministry of Health, Key Laboratory of Molecular Cardiovascular Sciences, Ministry of Education. Beijing Key Laboratory of Cardiovascular Receptors Research, 9, Hua Yuan Bei Road, Hai Dian District, Beijing 100191, People's Republic of China

Huan Wang, Xuejing Liu and Wei Huang
Institute of Cardiovascular Sciences and Key Laboratory of Molecular Cardiovascular Sciences, Ministry of Education, Peking University Health Science Center, 38, XueYuan Road, HaiDian District, Beijing 100191, People's Republic of China

Jyotsna Bhattacharya, Cynthia Aranow, Meggan Mackay and Betty Diamond
The Feinstein Institute for Medical Research, Center for Autoimmune, Musculoskeletal and Hematopoietic Diseases, 350 Community Dr, Manhasset, NY 11030, USA

Karalyn Pappas
Department of Statistical Science, Cornell University, Ithaca, NY, USA

Bahtiyar Toz
Department of Internal Medicine, Istanbul University, Istanbul, Turkey

Peter K. Gregersen
The Feinstein Institute for Medical Research, Center for Genomics and Human Genetics, Manhasset, NY, USA

Ogobara Doumbo
Malaria Research and Training Center, Bamako, Mali

Abdel Kader Traore
Deputy of the Department of Internal Medicine, University Hospital, Bamako, Mali

Martin L. Lesser
The Feinstein Institute for Medical Research, Center of Biostatistics Unit Manhasset, Manhasset, NY, USA

Maureen McMahon
UCLA David Geffen School of Medicine, Los Angeles, CA 90095, USA

Tammy Utset
University of Chicago Medical Center, Chicago, IL, USA

Earl Silverman and Deborah Levy
Hospital for Sick Children, University of Toronto, Toronto, ON M5G 1X8, Canada

William J. McCune
University of Michigan, Ann Arbor, MI 48109, USA

Meenakshi Jolly
Rush University Medical Center, Chicago, IL 60612, USA

Daniel Wallace and Michael Weisman
Cedars Sinai Medical Center, Los Angeles, CA 90048, USA

Juanita Romero-Diaz
Instituto Nacional de Ciencias Medicas y Nutrician Salvador Zubiran, Mexico City, Mexico

**Lamia Heikal, Pietro Ghezzi and Manuela Mengozzi**
Brighton and Sussex Medical School Department of Clinical and experimental investigation, University of Sussex, Falmer East Sussex, Brighton BN1 9PS, UK

**Gordon Ferns**
Brighton and Sussex Medical School Department of Clinical and experimental investigation, University of Sussex, Falmer East Sussex, Brighton BN1 9PS, UK
Brighton and Sussex Medical School Department of Medical Education, Mayfield House, Falmer East Sussex, Brighton BN1 9PH, UK

**Jiaqin Yan, Xudong Zhang, Xin Li, Ling Li, Zhaoming Li, Lei Zhang, Jingjing Wu, Xinhua Wang, Zhenchang Sun, Xiaorui Fu, Yu Chang, Feifei Nan, Hui Yu, Xiaolong Wu, Xiaoyan Feng and Mingzhi Zhang**
Department of Oncology, The First Affiliated Hospital, Zhengzhou University, No. 1 Jianshe East Road, Zhengzhou, Henan 450052, People's Republic of China

**Junhui Zhang**
Department of Otorhinolaryngology, The Third Affiliated Hospital of Zhengzhou University, Zhengzhou, Henan 450052, People's Republic of China

**Renyin Chen and Wencai Li**
Department of pathology, The First Affiliated Hospital, Zhengzhou University, Zhengzhou, Henan 450052, People's Republic of China

**Sujun Li, Fang Liang and Youzhou Tang**
Department of Hematology and Key Laboratory of non-resolving inflammation and cancer of Human Province, The 3rd Xiangya Hospital, Central South University, Changsha, Hunan province 410000, People's Republic of China

**Kevin Kwan, Jianhua Li, Huan Yang, Sangeeta S. Chavan and Kevin J. Tracey**
Laboratory of Biomedical Science, Feinstein Institute for Medical Research, 350 Community Drive, Manhasset, NY 11030, USA

**Yiting Tang**
Department of Physiology, School of Basic medical research, Central South University, Changsha, Hunan province, People's Republic of China

Key Laboratory of Medical Genetics, School of Biological Science and Technology, Central South University, Changsha, Hunan province 410000, People's Republic of China

**Xiangyu Wang and Ben Lu**
Department of Hematology and Key Laboratory of non-resolving inflammation and cancer of Human Province, The 3rd Xiangya Hospital, Central South University, Changsha, Hunan province 410000, People's Republic of China
Key Laboratory of Medical Genetics, School of Biological Science and Technology, Central South University, Changsha, Hunan province 410000, People's Republic of China

**Haichao Wang**
Department of Emergency Medicine, North Shore University Hospital, Manhasset, NY 11030, USA

**Ulf Andersson**
Department of Women's and Children's Health, Karolinska Institute, 171 76 Stockholm, Sweden

**Valentina Maria Sofia, Cecilia Surace, Anna Cristina Tomaiuolo, Antonio Novelli and Adriano Angioni**
Laboratory of Medical Genetics Unit, "Bambino Gesù" Children's Hospital, IRCCS, Viale di San Paolo 15, 00146 Rome, Italy

**Vito Terlizzi and Cesare Braggion**
Department of Pediatrics, Tuscany Regional Centre for Cystic Fibrosis, Anna Meyer Children's Hospital, Florence, Italy

**Letizia Da Sacco**
Multifactorial Diseases and Complex Phenotypes Research Area, "Bambino Gesù" Children's Hospital, IRCCS, Rome, Italy

**Federico Alghisi and Vincenzina Lucidi**
Cystic Fibrosis Unit, "Bambino Gesù" Children's Hospital, IRCCS, Rome, Italy

**Antonella Angiolillo**
Department of Medicine and Health Sciences "Vincenzo Tiberio", University of Molise, Campobasso, Italy

**Natalia Cirilli**
Regional Cystic Fibrosis Centre, United Hospitals, Mother – Child Department, Ancona, Italy

**Carla Colombo**
Cystic Fibrosis Regional Centre (Lombardia), IRCCS Ca' Granda Foundation, University of Milan, Milan, Italy

**Antonella Di Lullo**
CEINGE-Biotecnologie Avanzate, Naples, Italy
Department of Neuroscience, ORL Section, University of Naples Federico II, Naples, Italy

**Rita Padoan**
Cystic Fibrosis Support Centre, Pediatric Department, Children's Hospital, ASST Spedali Civili, Brescia, Italy

**Serena Quattrucci**
Cystic Fibrosis Regional Centre (Lazio), Sapienza University and Policlinico Umberto I, Rome, Italy

**Valeria Raia**
Cystic Fibrosis Regional Centre (Campania), Department of Medical Transalational Sciences, Section of Pediatrics, University of Naples Federico II, Naples, Italy

**Giuseppe Tuccio**
Cystic Fibrosis Regional Centre, Soverato Hospital, Catanzaro, Italy

**Federica Zarrilli**
Department of Biosciences and Territory, University of Molise, Isernia, Italy

**Marco Lucarelli**
Department of Cellular Biotechnologies and Hematology, Sapienza University of Rome, Rome, Italy
Pasteur Institute, Cenci Bolognetti Foundation, Sapienza University of Rome, Rome, Italy

**Giuseppe Castaldo**
CEINGE-Biotecnologie Avanzate, Naples, Italy
Department of Molecular Medicine and Biotechnologies, University of Naples Federico II, Naples, Italy

**Hauke Thomsen and Miguel Inacio da Silva Filho**
Division of Molecular Genetic Epidemiology, German Cancer Research Center (DKFZ), Im Neuenheimer Feld 580, 69120 Heidelberg, Germany

**Subhayan Chattopadhyay**
Division of Molecular Genetic Epidemiology, German Cancer Research Center (DKFZ), Im Neuenheimer Feld 580, 69120 Heidelberg, Germany
Faculty of Medicine, University of Heidelberg, Heidelberg, Germany

**Niels Weinhold**
Department of Internal Medicine V, University of Heidelberg, Heidelberg, Germany
Myeloma Institute, University of Arkansas for Medical Sciences, Little Rock, AR, USA

**Per Hoffmann**
Institute of Human Genetics, University of Bonn, Bonn, Germany
Department of Biomedicine, University of Basel, Basel, Switzerland

**Markus M. Nöthen**
Institute of Human Genetics, University of Bonn, Bonn, Germany
Department of Genomics, Life & Brain Research Center, University of Bonn, Bonn, Germany

**Arendt Marina, Karl-Heinz Jöckel, Börge Schmidt and Sonali Pechlivanis**
Institute for Medical Informatics, Biometry and Epidemiology, University Hospital Essen, University of Duisburg-Essen, Essen, Germany

**Christian Langer**
Department of Internal Medicine III, University of Ulm, Ulm, Germany

**Hartmut Goldschmidt**
Department of Internal Medicine V, University of Heidelberg, Heidelberg, Germany
National Centre of Tumor Diseases, Heidelberg, Germany

**Kari Hemminki and Asta Försti**
Division of Molecular Genetic Epidemiology, German Cancer Research Center (DKFZ), Im Neuenheimer Feld 580, 69120 Heidelberg, Germany
Center for Primary Health Care Research, Lund University, Malmö, Sweden

**Rui Zhang, Xiaojun Zhou and Chunmei Xu**
Department of Endocrinology, Shandong Provincial Qianfoshan Hospital, Shandong University, Jinan, Shandong, China

**Zhiwei Zou**
Department of Endocrinology, Qilu Hospital of Shandong University, Jinan, Shandong, China

**Xue Shen and Tianyue Xie**
Division of Endocrinology, Department of Internal Medicine, Shandong University of Traditional Chinese Medicine, Jinan, Shandong, China

**Jianjun Dong**
Department of Endocrinology, Qilu Hospital of Shandong University, Jinan, Shandong, China
Department of Internal Medicine, Division of Endocrinology, Qilu Hospital of Shandong University, No. 107, Wenhuaxi Road, Jinan, Shandong, China

**Lin Liao**
Department of Endocrinology, Shandong Provincial Qianfoshan Hospital, Shandong University, Jinan, Shandong, China
Department of Internal Medicine, Division of Endocrinology, Shandong Provincial Qianfoshan Hospital, Shandong University, No. 16766, Jingshi Road, Jinan, Shandong, China

**Xin-Rui Han, Xin Wen, Yong-Jian Wang, Shan Wang, Min Shen, Zi-Feng Zhang, Shao-Hua Fan, Qun Shan, Liang Wang, Meng-Qiu Li, Bin Hu, Chun-Hui Sun, Dong-Mei Wu, Jun Lu and Yuan-Lin Zheng**
Key Laboratory for Biotechnology on Medicinal Plants of Jiangsu Province, School of Life Science, Jiangsu Normal University, No. 101, Shanghai Road, Tongshan District, Xuzhou 221116, Jiangsu Province, People's Republic of China
College of Health Sciences, Jiangsu Normal University, No. 101, Shanghai Road, Tongshan District, Xuzhou 221116, Jiangsu Province, People's Republic of China

**Natasha Fillmore, Jody L. Levasseur, Arata Fukushima, Cory S. Wagg, Wei Wang, Jason R. B. Dyck and Gary D. Lopaschuk**
Cardiovascular Research Centre, Mazankowski Alberta Heart Institute University of Alberta, Edmonton, Canada

**Heng Jiang, Tao Lin, Wei Shao, Yichen Meng, Jun Ma, Ce Wang, Rui Gao and Xuhui Zhou**
Department of Orthopedics, Changzheng Hospital, Second Military Medical University, No.415 Fengyang Road, Shanghai, People's Republic of China

**Fu Yang**
Department of Medical Genetics, Second Military Medical University, Shanghai, People's Republic of China
Shanghai Key Laboratory of Cell Engineering (14DZ2272300), Shanghai, People's Republic of China

**Mingzhu He, Tom R. Coleman and Yousef Al-Abed**
Center for Molecular Innovation, The Feinstein Institute for Medical Research, 350 Community Drive, Manhasset, New York 11030, USA

**Marco E. Bianchi**
Chromatin Dynamics Unit, Division of Genetics and Cell Biology, San Raffaele University and San Raffaele Scientific Institute IRCCS, Via Olgettina 58, 20132 Milan, Italy

**Kevin J. Tracey**
Center for Biomedical Science, and Center for Bioelectronic Medicine, The Feinstein Institute for Medical Research, 350 Community Drive, Manhasset, New York 11030, USA

**Armin Zlomuzica, Friederike Preusser, Marcella L. Woud and Jürgen Margraf**
Mental Health Research and Treatment Center, Ruhr-Universität Bochum, 150, 44780 Bochum, Germany

**Susanna Roberts and Thalia C. Eley**
Institute of Psychiatry, Psychology and Neuroscience, MRC Social, Genetic and Developmental Psychiatry Centre, King's College London, London, UK

**Kathryn J. Lester**
Institute of Psychiatry, Psychology and Neuroscience, MRC Social, Genetic and Developmental Psychiatry Centre, King's College London, London, UK
School of Psychology, University of Sussex, Brighton, UK

**Ekrem Dere**
Teaching and Research Unit. Life Sciences (UFR927), University Pierre and Marie Curie, Paris, France
Clinical Neuroscience, Max Planck Institute of Experimental Medicine, Göttingen, Germany

**Rong Zhou, Shuya Zhang, Xuejiao Gu, Yuanyuan Ge, Dingjuan Zhong, Yuling Zhou, Lingyun Tang, Xiao-Ling Liu and Jiang-Fan Chen**
Institute of Molecular Medicine, School of Optometry and Ophthalmology and Eye Hospital, Wenzhou Medical University, 270 Xueyuan Road, Wenzhou 325027, Zhejiang, China
State Key Laboratory Cultivation Base and Key Laboratory of Vision Science, Ministry of Health, China and Zhejiang Provincial Key Laboratory of Ophthalmology and Optometry, Wenzhou Zhejiang, China

**Xinya Xie, Zihui Zhang, Xinfeng Wang, Zhenyu Luo, Baochang Lai and Lei Xiao**
Cardiovascular Research Center, School of Basic Medical Sciences, Xi'an Jiaotong University, Xi'an 710061, China

**Nanping Wang**
The Advanced Institute for Medical Sciences, Dalian Medical University, Dalian 116044, China

**Yuanlin Xu, Wenping Zhou, Peipei Zhang, Jiuyang Zhang, Shujun Yang and Yanyan Liu**
Department of Lymphatic Comprehensive Internal Medicine, Affiliated Cancer Hospital of Zhengzhou University, No.127 Dongming Road, Zhengzhou 450001, Henan, China

**Xihong Zhang**
Department of Gynaecology and Obstetric, Pepole's Hospital of Henan University of Chinese Medicine (Pepole's Hospital of Zhengzhou), Zhengzhou 450003, Henan, China

**Xiufeng Hu**
Department of Respiratory, Affiliated Cancer Hospital of Zhengzhou University, Zhengzhou 450001, Henan, China

**Inge Søkilde Pedersen**
Molecular Diagnostics, Clinical Biochemistry, Aalborg University, Aalborg, Denmark
Clinical Cancer Research Center, Aalborg University Hospital, Aalborg, Denmark
Department of Clinical Medicine, Aalborg University, Aalborg, Denmark

**Mads Thomassen, Qihua Tan and Torben Kruse**
Department of Clinical Genetics, Odense University Hospital, Odense, Denmark

**Ole Thorlacius-Ussing**
Department of Gastrointestinal Surgery, Aalborg University Hospital, Aalborg, Denmark
Clinical Cancer Research Center, Aalborg University Hospital, Aalborg, Denmark
Department of Clinical Medicine, Aalborg University, Aalborg, Denmark

**Jens Peter Garne**
Department of Breast Surgery, Aalborg University Hospital, Aalborg, Denmark

**Henrik Bygum Krarup**
Molecular Diagnostics, Clinical Biochemistry, Aalborg University, Aalborg, Denmark
Clinical Cancer Research Center, Aalborg University Hospital, Aalborg, Denmark

**Cheng-Ye Zhan, Di Chen, Jin-Long Luo, Ying-Hua Shi and You-Ping Zhang**
Intensive Care Unit, Tongji Hospital Affiliated to Tongji Medical College of Huazhong University of Science and Technology, No. 1095, Jiefang Road, Qiaokou District, Wuhan 430030, Hubei Province, People's Republic of China

# Index

www.ingramcontent.com/pod-product-compliance
Lightning Source LLC
Chambersburg PA
CBHW082040190326
41458CB00010B/3416